# Sports Injuries

## Examination, Imaging and Management

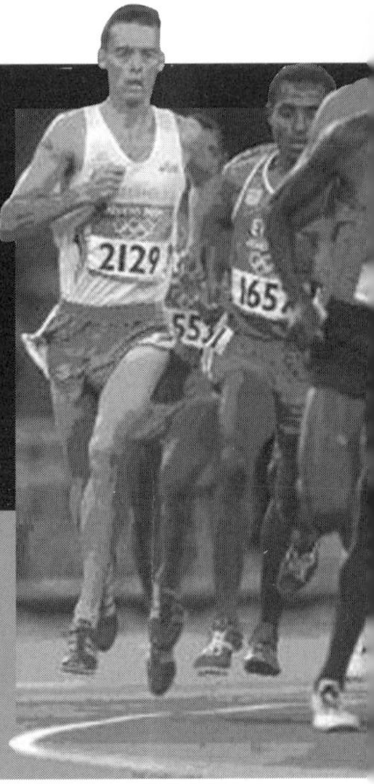

To Nicola, Sarah, Emma, Jack and Nick Eustace for tolerating hours at the computer over again, love and thanks to all.

To Fiona, Ciara, Sorca, Aisling and Fergal O'Byrne … for more patience than could have been expected! Love to all.

To the Johnston Family up North, thank you for your love and support.

To Eilish for enduring support, all my love.

To Caroline, James and Amelia Eustace, all my love.

*For Elsevier:*

*Senior Commissioning Editor:* Sarena Wolfaard
*Development Editor:* Dinah Thom
*Project Manager:* Morven Dean
*Designer:* Sarah Russell
*Illustration Manager:* Bruce Hogarth

# Sports Injuries

## Examination, Imaging and Management

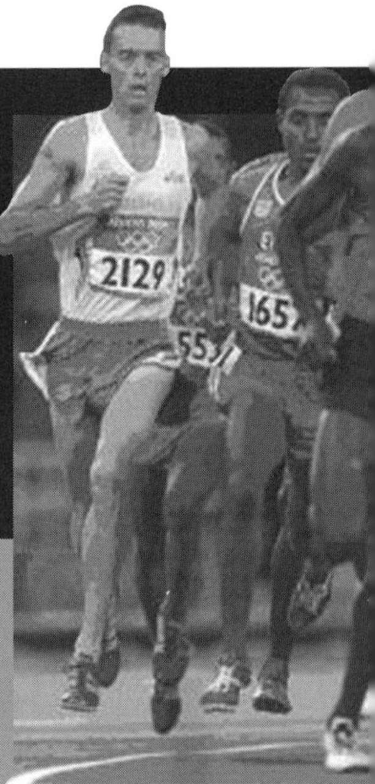


**Stephen Eustace**
MB, MSC(Hons), MRCPI, FFR(RCSI), FRCR, FFSEM(RCSI)
Professor of Musculoskeletal Radiology, Cappagh National Orthopaedic and Mater Misericordiae Hospitals, and University College Dublin, Ireland

**Ciaran Johnston** MSC(Rad Sci), MRCPI, FRCR
Musculoskeletal Radiologist, Cappagh National Orthopaedic Hospital, Dublin, Ireland

**Pat O'Neill** MSC(sports Med), FFSEM, RCPI, RCSI
Consultant Sports Medicine Physician, Mater Private Hospital, Dublin, Ireland

**John O'Byrne** MCH, FRCSI, FFSEM, RCPI, RCSI
Professor of Orthopaedic Surgery, Cappagh National Orthopaedic Hospital and Royal College of Surgeons in Ireland, Dublin, Ireland

*With contributions from*

**Nicholas Eustace** MMed Sci, FCARCSI, DIBICM
Consultant Anaesthetist, Cappagh National Orthopaedic & Temple Street Children's Hospitals, Dublin, Ireland

**Deirdre Duke** MRCPI, FFR, RCSI
Musculoskeletal Radiologist, Cappagh National Orthopaedic and Mater Misericordiae Hospitals, Dublin, Ireland

**Peter MacMahon** MRCPI
Registrar, Cappagh National Orthopaedic and Mater Misericordiae Hospitals, and University College Dublin, Ireland

**Conor Shortt** MRCPI FFR RCSI
Musculoskeletal Radiologist, Cappagh National Orthopaedic and Mater Misericordiae Hospitals, Dublin, Ireland

*Foreword by*

**Conor McCarthy** MD FRCPI FFSEM
Consultant Rheumatologist, Mater Misericordiae Hospital, Dublin, Ireland and Medical Director of the Irish Rugby Football Union

CHURCHILL LIVINGSTONE
ELSEVIER

Edinburgh London New York Oxford Philadelphia St Louis Sydney Toronto 2007

CHURCHILL
LIVINGSTONE
ELSEVIER

An imprint of Elsevier Limited



First published 2007

ISBN-10 0-443-10203-1
ISBN-13 978-0-443-10203-5

**British Library Cataloguing in Publication Data**
A catalogue record for this book is available from the British Library

**Library of Congress Cataloging in Publication Data**
A catalog record for this book is available from the Library of Congress

**Notice**
Knowledge and best practice in this field are constantly changing. As new research and experience broaden our knowledge, changes in practice, treatment and drug therapy may become necessary or appropriate. Readers are advised to check the most current information provided (i) on procedures featured or (ii) by the manufacturer of each product to be administered, to verify the recommended dose or formula, the method and duration of administration, and contraindications. It is the responsibility of the practitioner, relying on their own experience and knowledge of the patient, to make diagnoses, to determine dosages and the best treatment for each individual patient, and to take all appropriate safety precautions. To the fullest extent of the law, neither the publisher nor authors assume any liability for any injury and/or damage to persons or property arising out or related to any use of the material contained in this book.

***The Publisher***



The publisher's policy is to use **paper manufactured from sustainable forests**

Printed in the UK

# Contents

# Foreword

It is an honour to be asked to write the foreword to *Sports Injuries* by my long-term friend and colleague, Professor Stephen Eustace. We have known each other for more than 20 years and have worked closely together, at the same institution, over the last 7 years. His academic achievements are many and I believe there are few who can match his publication and research record. His specific expertise is in musculoskeletal radiology, particularly in the use of magnetic resonance imaging (MRI) in the evaluation of bone, joint and muscle disease. His clinical opinion has been invaluable to me on many occasions; he is always willing to make the difficult calls on diagnostic dilemmas but never forgets that the patient is central to the process. Above all, his enthusiasm for radiology is a constant source of encouragement to his colleagues, trainees and medical students alike. This enthusiasm for radiology is only matched by his enthusiasm for sport!

Professor Eustace's latest publication on sports injuries with co-authors Johnston, O'Neill and O'Byrne is an excellent reference book for the sports medicine physician. The most common types of sports injuries are presented by anatomic location in summary tables that facilitate easy access. Differential diagnoses and the appropriate treatments for various injuries and clinical scenarios are clearly laid out. Each chapter has an excellent set of accompanying images. The MRI images, in particular, demonstrate clearly the typical radiological findings for many different types of sports injuries. The chapter on groin injuries gives clarity to this difficult clinical condition and provides information that is essential to anyone involved in treating athletes with this type of injury.

The timing of this publication is fortuitous given the significant developments that have occurred in sports medicine in Ireland over the last few years. These developments include the formation of a Faculty of Sports and Exercise Medicine. The Faculty is an important focus for the development of training programs and the provision of ongoing education to physicians involved in sports medicine. The Faculty is now the recognized body for the accreditation of training programs in sports and exercise medicine in Ireland. Both their Professor Eustace and Dr Pat O'Neill were members of the inaugural board of this Faculty and there input proved invaluable. This textbook will be on the reading list for the Faculty and should be included in all good medical libraries and sporting organizations.

Sport and exercise is becoming increasingly popular in our society. Opportunities for sports participation have improved. Sports facilities have increased in number. This increase in sports participation and facilities will add to the demands for expertise in sports medicine. In addition, improvements in sports science and the development of 'High Performance Units' and 'Sports Institutes' are pushing athletes to a level where maximum performance can only be achieved by the assistance and integration of a number of experts; the sports physician should be central to this process, particularly when it is necessary to advise the athlete and coaches on the safe return to full participation following a sports injury.

Inevitably, the increasing popularity in sport and exercise leads to an increase in injuries that require skilled management. The clinical demands of the injured athlete, in particular, continue to increase as athletes endeavour to maximize their performance in sport. Improvements in sports science and the development of 'High Performance Units' and 'Sports Institutes' will result in a greater role for the sports physician at the top end of the sports spectrum. The sports medicine physician is central in the coordination of investigations and rehabilitation programs to allow the athlete to return to their pre-injury state and safely return to full participation. Furthermore, the role of the sports medicine physician has evolved from the provision of medical care to the elite athlete into the broader remit of exercise as a prescription: the promotion of a healthy lifestyle and disease prevention.

Sports medicine physicians will find this textbook accessible and invaluable in the management of those injured through sport or exercise. Professor Eustace and his co-authors Johnston, O'Neill and O'Byrne have produced an impressive textbook on the diagnosis and management of sports injuries. Reading this textbook has enhanced my knowledge of sports injuries and I would have no hesitation in recommending it to anyone who has an interest in the treatment and management of sports injuries. Sports medicine physicians will find it accessible and invaluable in the management of those injured through sport or exercise.

Conor McCarthy
*Medical Director*
*Irish Rugby Football Union*
*Dublin, Ireland*

# Preface

With the formation of the Faculty of Sport and Exercise Medicine in Dublin in 2003, closely followed by specialty recognition, it seemed timely to produce a concise but up-to-date review of sports injuries, embracing clinical examination, methods of diagnosis, and current approaches to injury management. As specialists in physical medicine, imaging and sports orthopedics have developed more sophisticated practice, the gaps between each professional group have grown. The purpose of this book is to bridge those gaps in one publication integrating clinical examination and approaches to imaging, and to review current approaches to management as defined by findings at both examination and imaging.

In merging the ideas of a dedicated sports medicine physician, Dr Pat O'Neill, the Professor of Orthopedics in the Royal College of Surgeons, Professor John O'Byrne, and of two radiologists with special interests in sports, Dr Ciaran Johnston and Professor Stephen Eustace, we have attempted to produce a balanced text in a form suited to both practical and didactic use.

Dr Pat O'Neill is the public relations officer of the medical division of the Gaelic Athletic Association, and is both a former player and manager of the Dublin County Football Team. Professor John O'Byrne is the orthopedic surgeon to the Football Association of Ireland, and is the medical director of the Irish Para-Olympic Team. Professor Stephen Eustace is the musculoskeletal radiologist to the Football Association of Ireland, provides support for the Irish Rugby Football Union and is a member of the Gaelic Athletic Medical Society.

Stephen Eustace
Dublin 2006

# Acknowledgment

Throughout this book there are several sporting figures within the text. These are reproduced with permission of Sportsfile.

# 1

# Mechanism of Injury and Tissue Healing



## BONE

### Histology

The skeletal system protects soft visceral organs and is the framework for movement. It is not an inert scaffolding system but a dynamic system that is very active at a cellular and molecular level. Bone alters its physical shape and biomechanical properties in response to changes in demand. Age, exercise, injury and disease also influence bone geometry and metabolism.

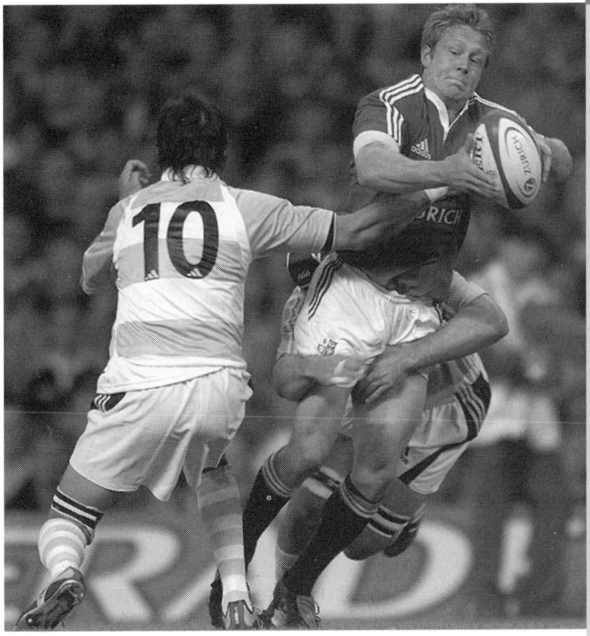


**Fig. 1.1** Sportsfile.

Bone is organized into **cancellous bone**, which is trabecular, and metabolically active and **cortical bone**, which is dense and has greater biomechanical resistance to bending, torsion and compression forces. Microscopically bone is divided into woven, immature bone, which is cellular with a random cellular arrangement, and lamellar bone, which is more mature and organized. The unit of bone in the haversian system is the osteon, which consists of a branching cylinder with a neurovascular central canal surrounded by layers of bone matrix with cells. Non-articular bone is covered by a layer of connective tissue called periosteum.

The three cell types are osteoblasts, osteocytes and osteoclasts:

1. Osteoblasts form bone, line the surface and communicate with the osteocytes deep in the matrix by cellular processes in the canaliculi in the haversion system. Osteoblasts produce type I collagen, osteocalcin, osteopontin, osteonectin and other regulatory factors, and they secrete osteoid.
2. Osteocytes are mature osteoblasts encased in a mineralized matrix, arranged around the central lumen of the osteon. The cytoplasmic processes of osteocytes extend to the blood vessels through the canaliculi. The osteocytes are important in calcium and phosphate metabolism.
3. Osteoclasts are multinucleate cells. They resorb bone and lie in resorbed cavities called Howship's lacunae. When active, they attach to the bone and form a space where bone resorption occurs. The pH drops and the crystals dissolve and the organic components of bone are resorbed.

Bone cells have differential receptors to parathyroid hormone, 1,25-dihydroxycholecalciferol (1,25-dihydroxyvitamin $D_3$) and glucocorticoids. Bone cells orchestrate the bone metabolism but the matrix also controls some of the processes. The matrix consists of 65% inorganic material (predominantly hydroxyapatite), water (5–10%) and an organic matrix, which is mainly collagen.

## Formation and growth

Long bones grow in length by endochondral ossification and in width by intramembraneous ossification. Bone is constantly remodeling. The osteoclast resorbs by cutting cones through the bone. Behind this are osteoblasts and a capillary loop that forms osteoid and new osteons. Formation and resorption are carefully coupled.

The dominant blood supply to bone is via the nutrient artery, which enters the midshaft and gives ascending and descending branches. Blood supply is also from a plexus of vessels around the metaphysis or periarticular area. The third and lesser source is from direct periosteal attachments. The clinical relevance of this is highlighted by fractures around the metaphysis, which usually heal well compared to open fractures around the diaphysis with soft-tissue stripping and the disruption of nutrient vessels, which frequently lead to delayed union or non-union.

## Injury and healing

Bone injury is caused by energy absorption. It is important to realize that energy is also absorbed by adjacent soft tissues which can also be damaged. Low-velocity injuries generally lead to simple fracture patterns with little soft tissue envelope destruction while high-velocity injuries are associated with comminution and frequent significant soft-tissue disruption. The bone is broken and soft tissue attachments and blood supply to the fragments are severed. Different parts of different bones can absorb different amounts of energy without breaking (Fig. 1.2). Depending on the type of force applied to the bone, a different fracture pattern may emerge. Some fracture patterns have more intrinsic stability than others and may require less elaborate fixation (Fig. 1.3).

Damage to internal trabeculae and to their associated neurovascular bundles without damage to the overlying cortex is termed a bone bruise. Impaction trauma leads to concertina compression of multiple trabeculae and extensive hemorrhage leading to a globular poorly marginated bone bruise. In contrast, applied distraction forces exceeding the elastic modulus of trabeculae lead to disruption at a single point in multiple trabeculae to produce local hemorrhage and bruising linearly perpendicular to the axis of stress. Shear forces produce obliquely oriented bruises (Figs 1.4–1.6).

The general principles of fracture treatment are to:

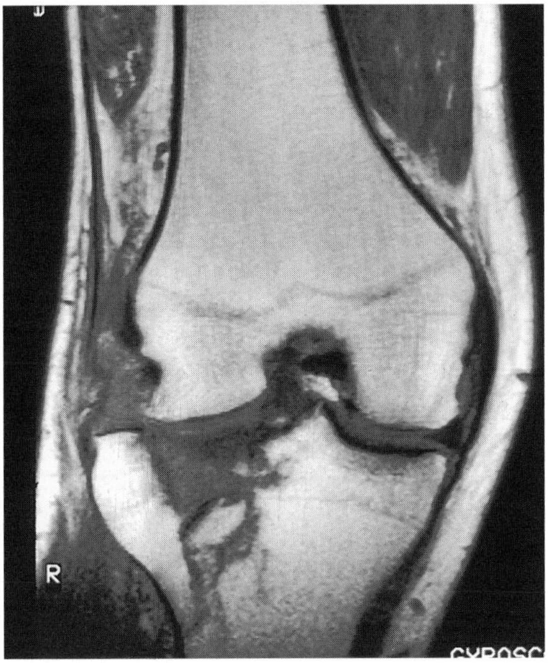


**Fig. 1.2** Coronal $T_1$-weighted MRI showing a lateral tibial plateau fracture complicating an acute valgus impaction injury in a footballer (soccer player). Lateral fracture has decompressed the valgus forces and protected the medial collateral ligament.

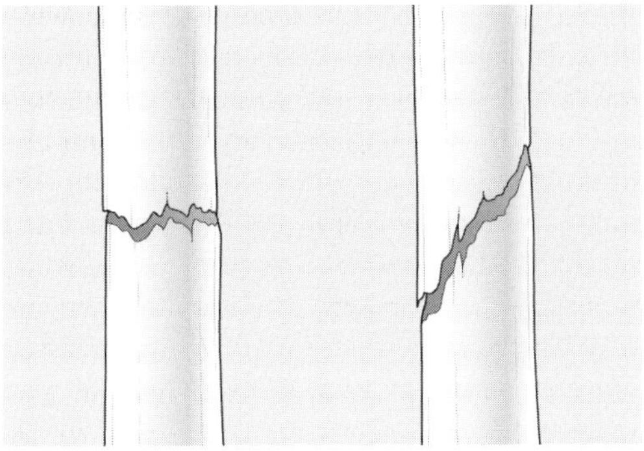

(a) (b)

**Fig. 1.3** (**a**) Transverse fracture pattern: more axial stability and smaller fracture interface. (**b**) Long oblique fracture pattern: poor axial stability and large fracture interface.

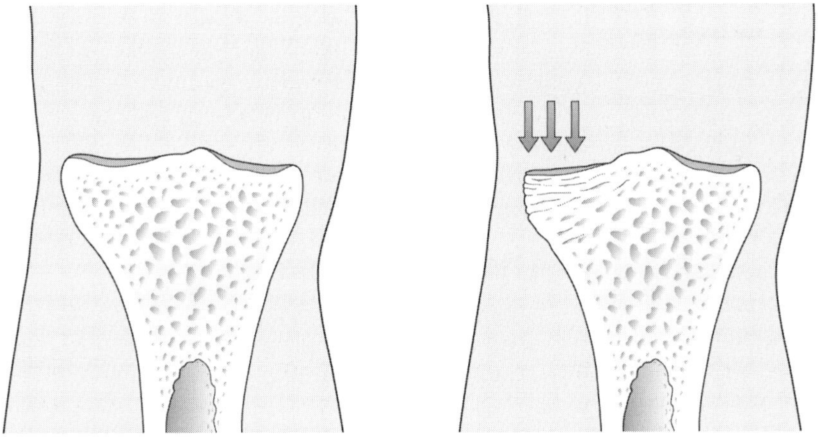

**Fig. 1.4** Impaction forces produce a concertina compression of multiple trabeculae resulting in an associated disruption of capillaries, hemorrhage and edema, producing a globular bone bruise.

- achieve satisfactory reduction
- maintain reduction
- mobilize and rehabilitate.

## Biology of fracture repair

Bleeding into the fracture brings fibrin, platelets, polymorphonuclear neutrophils and macrophages followed by fibroblasts and osteoprogenitor cells. There is vascular ingrowth which dominates, and collagen is formed. In the chondroid phase, cartilage is formed and type II collagen appears. Calcified bars then appear in the chondroid–osteoid step. In the osteogenic phase, more mature bone is formed. By the third week mineralization of the fracture callus begins. Growth factors, including transforming growth

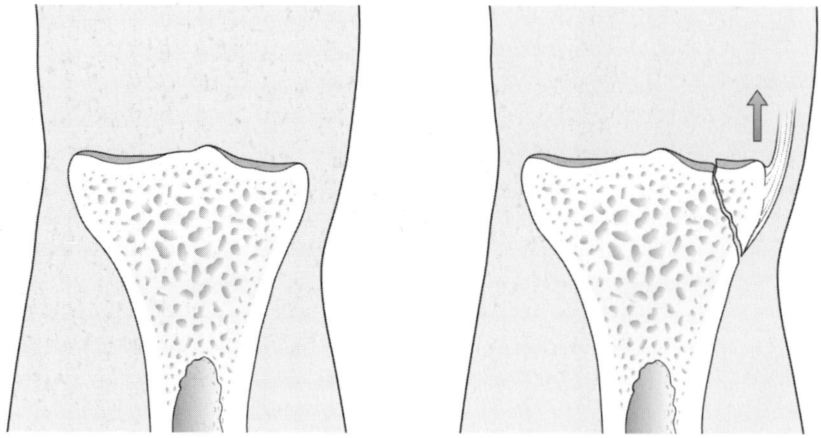

**Fig. 1.5** Distraction forces result in disruption of trabeculae at a single point with local hemorrhage and edema with an orientation perpendicular to the axis of distraction, producing a linear distraction bone bruise.

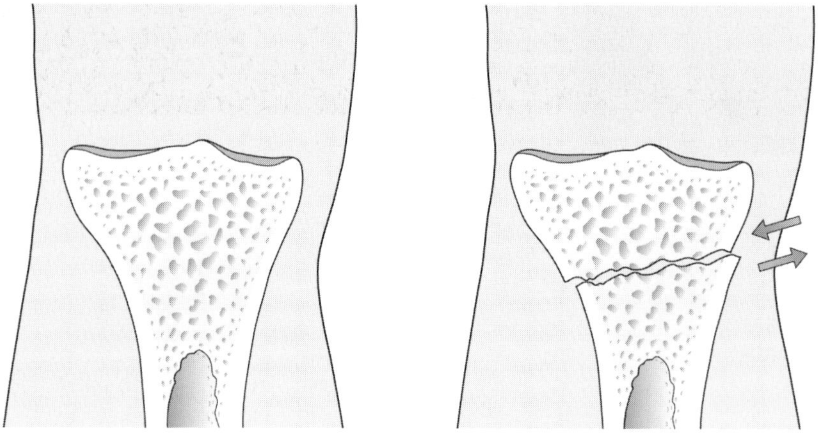

**Fig. 1.6** Shear forces lead to disruption of trabeculae with a linear axis and a similar bone bruise with an oblique orientation along the axis of stress.



factor (TGF), are found in the fracture hematoma and influence cartilage and bone formation. Multiple systemic influences can disrupt bone healing, e.g. cigarettes, diabetes, steroids and malnutrition (Fig. 1.7).

Bone morphogenic protein is an osteoinductive factor which encourages mesenchymal cells to become active osteoblasts. The magnitude of cellular response and callus formation is proportional to the degree of stability at the fracture site. This explains the large amount of callus around a comminuted midshaft clavicle fracture compared to the minimal callus formation seen around a fractured lateral malleolus that has healed following open reduction and internal fixation. In the clavicle fracture, copious amounts of cartilaginous callus must form and then convert to bone by endochondral ossification. When the bone ends are in direct contact, very little cartilage will form and a small amount of hard callus is seen (endosteal healing) (Fig. 1.8).

## The growth plate

Bone formation at the growth plate is described as endochondral. The growth plate lies between the epiphysis and the metaphysis and has three zones:

1. Reserve zone – this is adjacent to the epiphysis and has cells with copious endoplasmic reticulum but little cellular proliferation.
2. Proliferative zone – this zone produces cells in a columnar fashion and produces proteoglycans; longitudinal growth occurs here.
3. Hypertrophic zone – these cells are ten times the size of those in the proliferative zone and are very active metabolically; this zone prepares for and contributes to matrix calcification.

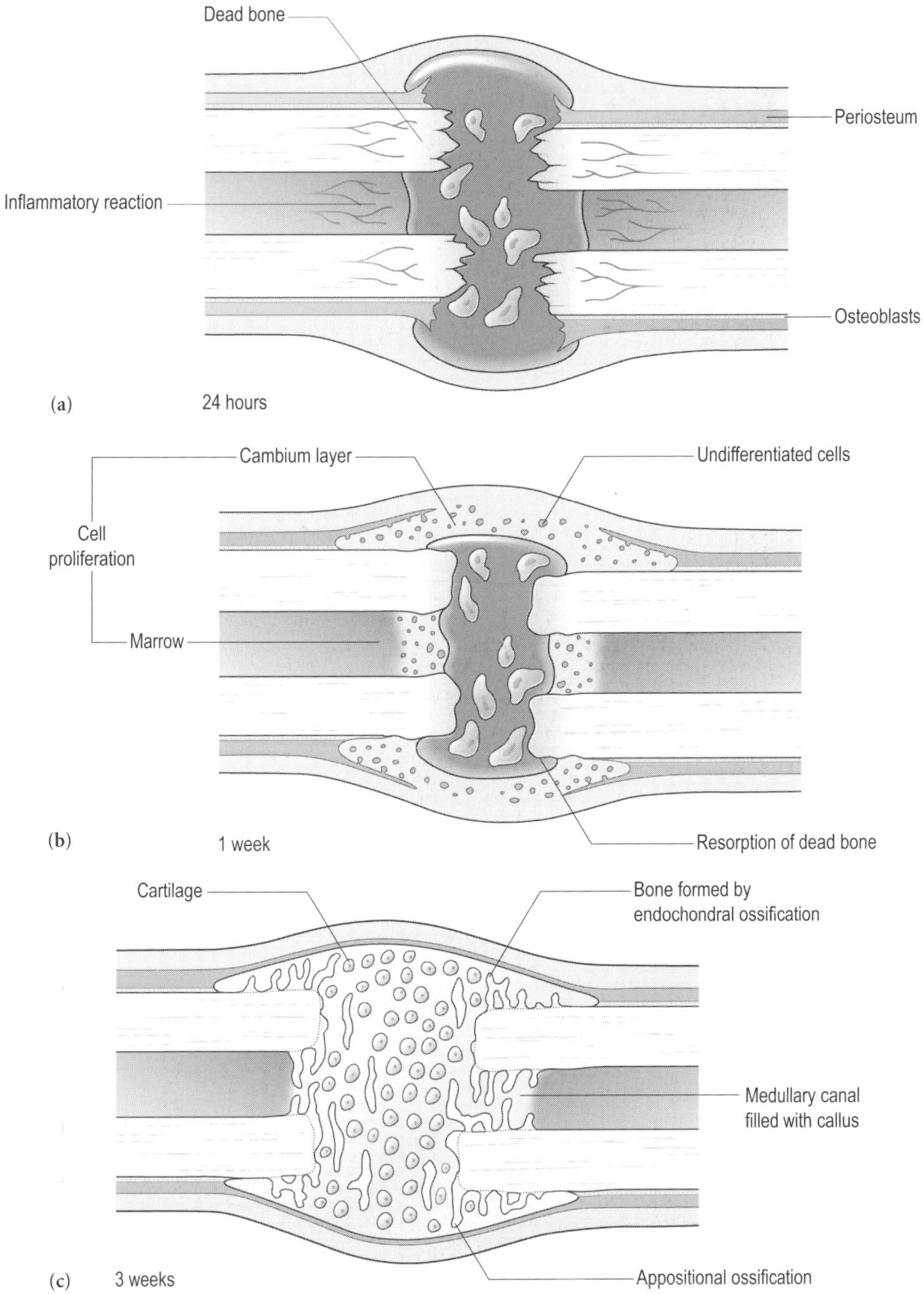


**Fig. 1.7** **(a–c)** These show immediate local hemorrhage at the site of fracture, followed by early callus formation at 1 week and endochondral bone formation at 3 weeks.

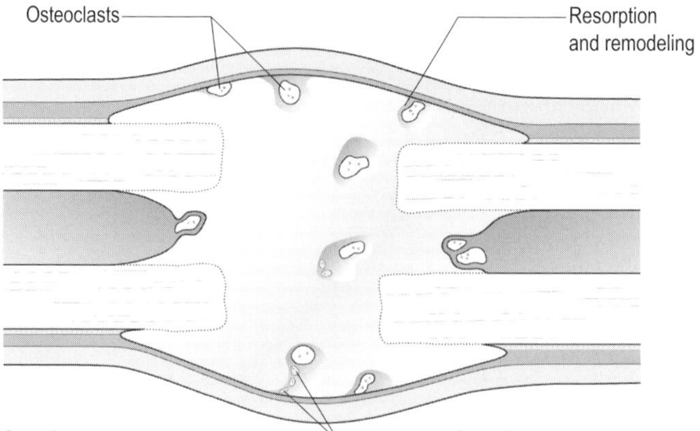


(d) 6 weeks

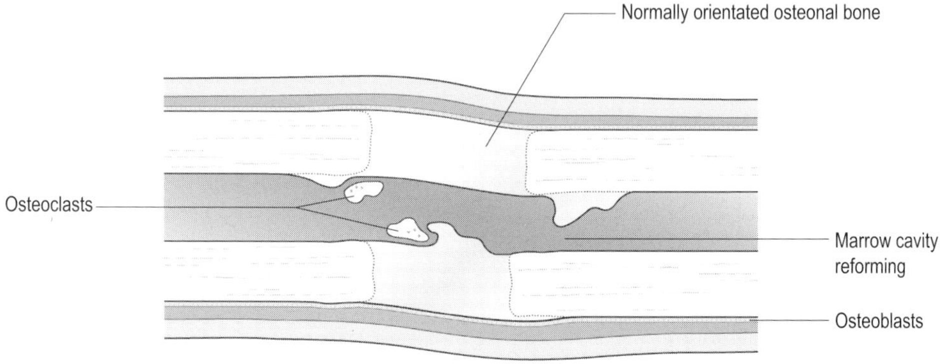


(e) 1 year



**Fig. 1.7 (d, e)** These show early bone formation at 6 weeks, which progressively remodels over the following months with restoration of anatomic alignment.

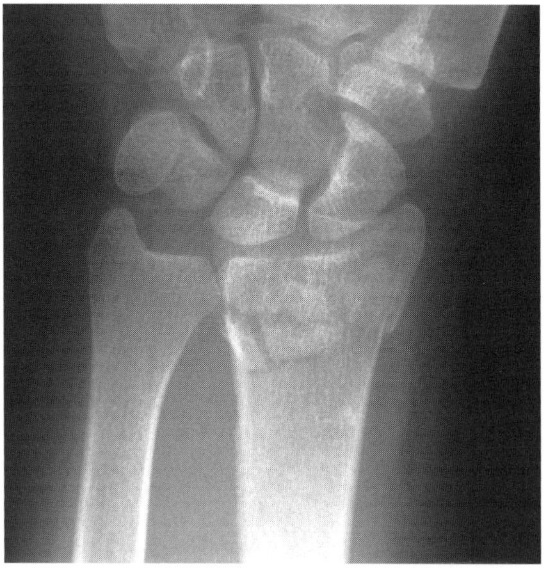

**Fig. 1.8** Radiograph showing an impaction fracture of the distal radius in an adult following a skiing injury with a fall on the outstretched hand.

## Growth plate injuries

The Salter–Harris classification identifies growth plate injuries:

1. Type I – there is no associated bony injury (Fig. 1.9). The fracture line is in the lower hypertrophic zone therefore the growth plate is unlikely to be permanently damaged.
2. Type II – the fracture line runs along the hypertrophic zone and then into the metaphyseal bone (Fig. 1.10). Anatomical reduction is essential and, if achieved, the prognosis is good.

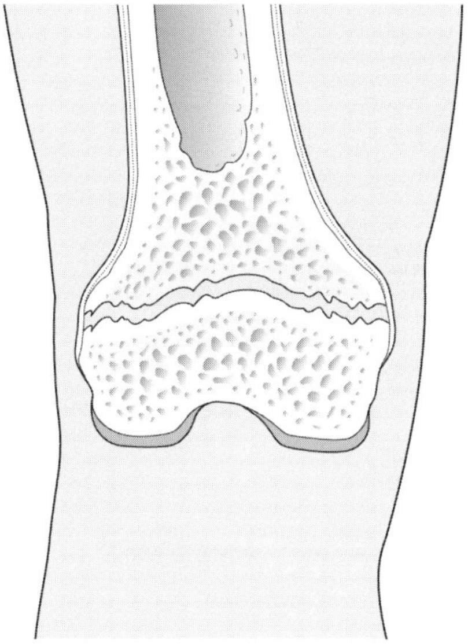

**Fig. 1.9** Type I Salter fracture.

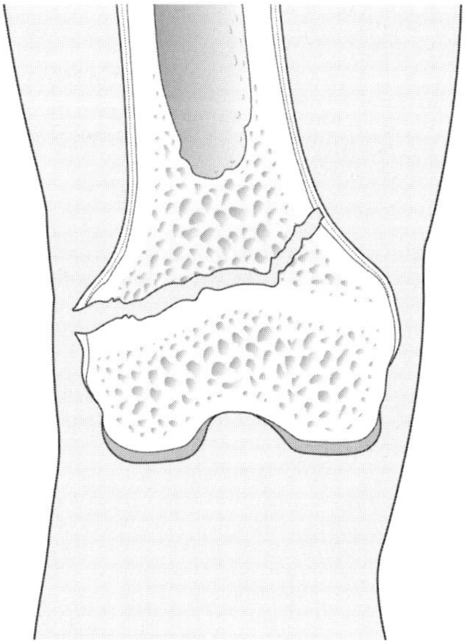

**Fig. 1.10** Type II Salter fracture.

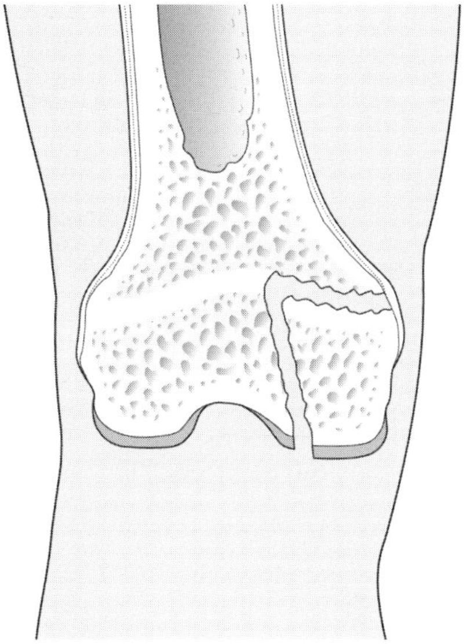

**Fig. 1.11** Type III Salter fracture.

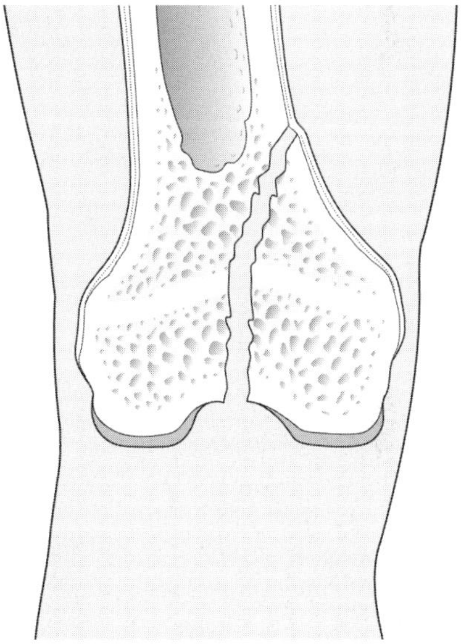

**Fig.1.12** Type IV Salter fracture.

3. Type III – the lower hypertrophic zone is cleared (Fig. 1.11) and the fracture extends to the joint. Prognosis is good.
4. Type IV – this fracture interface is predominately bony but crosses the growth plate (Figs 1.12 and 1.13). Excellent reduction usually leads to a good outcome.
5. Type V – this fracture crushes the cells of the reserve zone with a corresponding poor prognosis (Fig. 1.14).

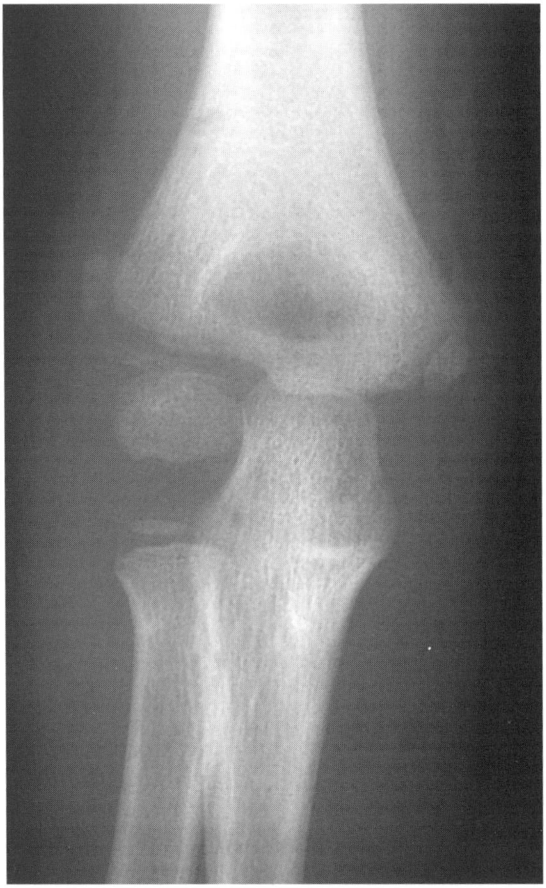

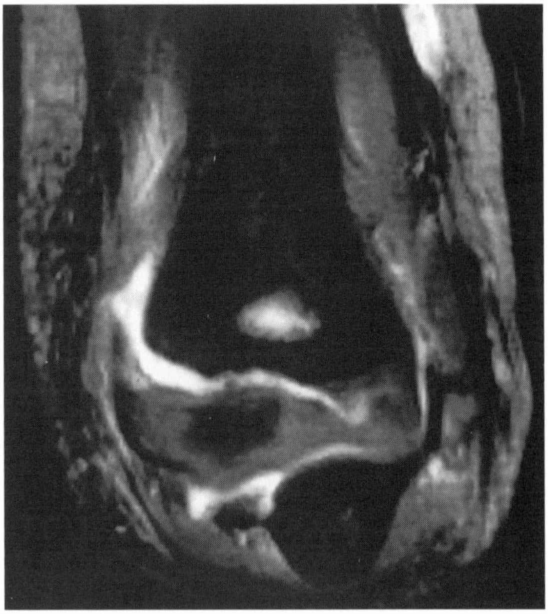

**Fig. 1.13** Radiograph (left) and $T_2$-weighted MRI showing a type IV Salter fracture of the elbow extending to the unossified cartilage of the trochlea.

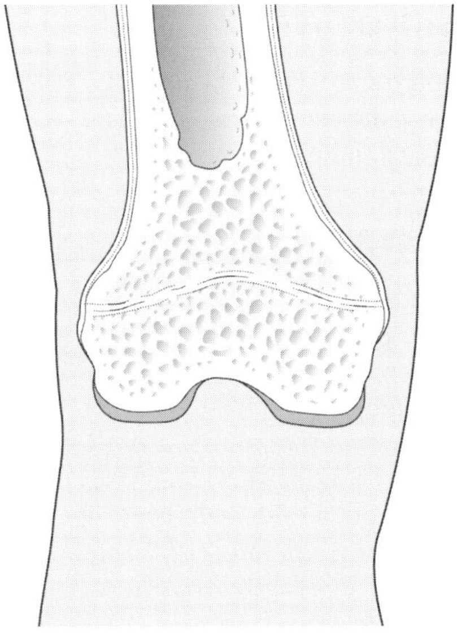

**Fig. 1.14** Type V Salter fracture.

## ARTICULAR CARTILAGE

Articular cartilage is more than just weight-bearing material. It also has lubrication and low-friction features that allow movement between adjacent bone ends. However, it has poor reparative capacity and when damaged (usually by trauma or degenerative disease) can progress to requiring surgical replacement.

### Structure

The extracellular matrix consists of water (65–80%) with proteoglycans and collagen. Chondrocytes are scattered through the matrix and secrete matrix components. In cross-section, the hyaline cartilage is divided into four zones (Fig. 1.15):

1. Superficial zone – the collagen fibrils are parallel to the surface with elongated chondrocytes.
2. Middle zone – the chondrocytes are more rounded with more randomly aligned thicker collagen fibrils.
3. Deep zone – the collagen fibers are perpendicular to the joint surface and chondrocytes form columns.

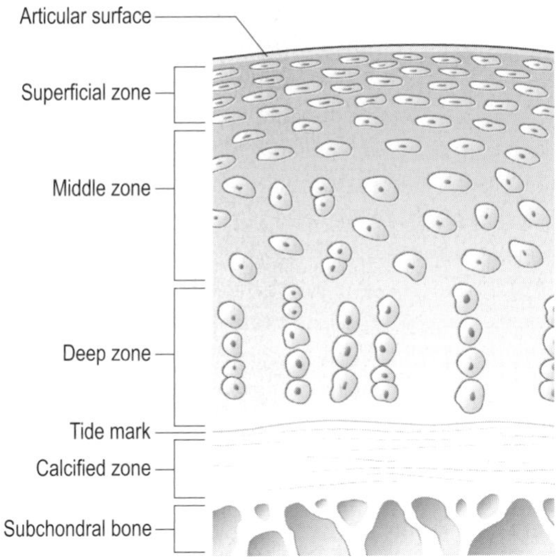


**Fig. 1.15** The basic structure of cartilage.

4. Calcified zone – the 'tidemark' separates the deep and calcified zones. In the calcified zone, the matrix is calcified and rich in opacities.

## Chondrocytes

Chondrocytes are mesenchymal cells whose activity levels vary during growth and as a response to mechanical or humeral stimuli. They are anaerobic.

## Function

The water content in the extracellular matrix is higher near the surface of the cartilage with very low permeability. This leads to high load-bearing features. Compression leads to some exudation of water and nutrients onto the surface leading to very low friction characteristics. Many types of collagen have been identified although type II is the dominant one. This gives tensile properties and interacts with proteoglycan. (Collagen molecular structure is described in 'Tendons' below.)

Proteoglycans are a protein core with polysaccharide chains attached. It mostly consists of a protein core with chondroitin sulfate, hyaluronate and glycosaminoglycan chains attached. Many protein cores can be attached to one long hyaluronate chain forming very large proteoglycans; proteoglycans are mostly concentrated in the transitional zone. Chondrocytes manufacture and secrete the matrix components. They respond to mechanical stimuli as well as soluble mediators such as growth factors and interleukins. Pathological behavior of the chondrocyte will lead to cartilage breakdown, possibly via altered production or production remodeling of the proteoglycans. Chondrocytes also produce proteinases that break down cartilage. Other factors that influence cartilage include growth factors (platelet-derived growth factor, fibroblast growth factor, insulin-like growth factor and TGF).

## Biomechanics

To understand the biomechanical features of articular cartilage, it should be regarded as having a fluid and a solid phase, i.e. biphasic. It has been shown that very high pressures are required to displace water through cartilage. The main resistance to compression is from fluid and this acts to protect the solid matrix. The flow of interstitial fluid as a response to compression is one of the mechanics responsible for the viscoelastic property of hyaline cartilage. The second mechanism reflects alteration in the collagen–proteoglycan interaction. The viscoelastic characteristic describes a time-dependent response to constant load. As load continues, the fluid phase gives way entirely to the solid phase provided by the collagen–proteoglycan matrix. Experimentally, this takes hours and physiologically almost never arises; fluid pressurization is the principle load-support mechanism. Damaged cartilage shows a diminished fluid pressurization response.

The random alignment of collagen fibers in the deep and middle zones reflects the mechanism for resisting shear forces on the cartilage. When compression is applied to the surface of the cartilage, these fibers absorb the spreading forces. If these fibers are overcome, the cartilage may shear off the bone (Fig. 1.16).

## Nutrition

The tidemark and calcified zone effectively prevent diffusion in the adult from the underlying bone. The superficial zone is poorly permeable; however, large molecules and growth factors easily perfuse through it. Large degradation molecules can also easily leave. The synovial fluid is therefore crucial for articular cartilage nutrition.

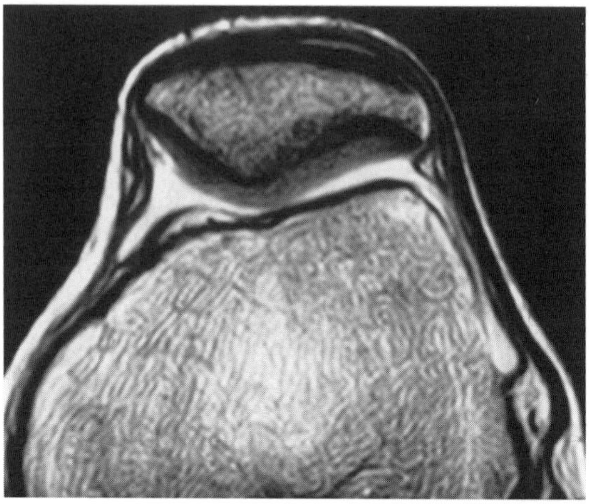

**Fig. 1.16** $T_2$-weighted MRI of the patellofemoral joint showing thick hyaline cartilage overlying the articular surfaces.

Small amounts of synovial fluid are present in normal joints and this fluid takes nutrients from the synovium to the articular surface, which it coats with a 10–20 mm thick layer. Clearly joint compression and movement circulates the synovial fluid and helps cartilage maintenance. If a joint is rigidly immobilized, the contact areas of cartilage undergo chondrocyte death. The adjacent non-contact areas show fibrillation and altered proteoglycan formation with increased water content. Rehabilitation reverses these changes. Excessive joint loading can also decrease the proteoglycan content and aggregate size. Any factor that leads to abnormal biomechanical forces, e.g. cruciate ligament injury, can lead to histological and biomechanical changes.



## Injury

This may be the result of acute injuries to the cartilage or fracture of the underlying bone with extension into the articular cartilage. A blunt or shear type of injury may delaminate or separate the articular cartilage from the underlying bone.

Chondromalacia refers to a softening of the cartilage with superficial fissuring and is most commonly seen on the patella.

## Repair

There are two major obstacles to regeneration of articular cartilage. First, there are no blood vessels that can mobilize an inflammatory response and, second, there are no undifferentiated mesenchymal cells that can synthesize a new matrix. The chondrocyte is very specialized, unable to replicate and not sufficiently active to reform new matrix. Experimental work has identified that lacerations to the layers superficial to the tidemark do not heal. There is no inflammatory response and the chondrocytes do not migrate into the lesion: the injury remains intact. If, however, the injury extends to the bone, the vessels from the bone bring fibrin to clot, and inflammatory mediators and cells. Multiple growth factors and undifferentiated mesenchymal cells flow into the injured zone. These cells differentiate into chondrocytes, which produce collagen and proteoglycans. The chondral defect fills in with hyaline and fibrous cartilage, and the bony injury heals with bone. This reparative process is the basis for the drilling or 'picking' of osteochondral lesions. This is a marrow-stimulating technique. Alternative surgical techniques for osteochondral defects include harvesting small dowels of articular cartilage and bone from less high-pressure areas and inserting them into the defect (mosaicplasty). Prepared cartilage is not as resilient as normal cartilage and does not show the normal collagen–proteoglycan features. Blunt injuries to the cartilage lead to chondrocyte death and occasionally separation from the underlying bone. Autologous chondrocyte implantation refers to the harvesting, culturing and subsequent reimplantation of chondrocytes into a chondral defect.

# TENDONS

Tendons are composed of densely packed type I collagen fibers with strong tensile strength but also elastic properties. Tendons are large and strong to resist mechanical forces, e.g. tendo Achillis, or lubricated by a tendon sheath to allow significant excursion, e.g. finger flexors. The tendon's fibers are embedded in a matrix of proteoglycans with a few fibroblasts, which lie in the spaces between the parallel collagen bundles. Type I collagen makes up 86% of the dry weight of collagen. Collagen consists of amino acids including glycine, proline and hydroxyproline. The chain of amino acids forms a left-handed helix, which is the secondary structure. Three of these helical chains coil together in a right-

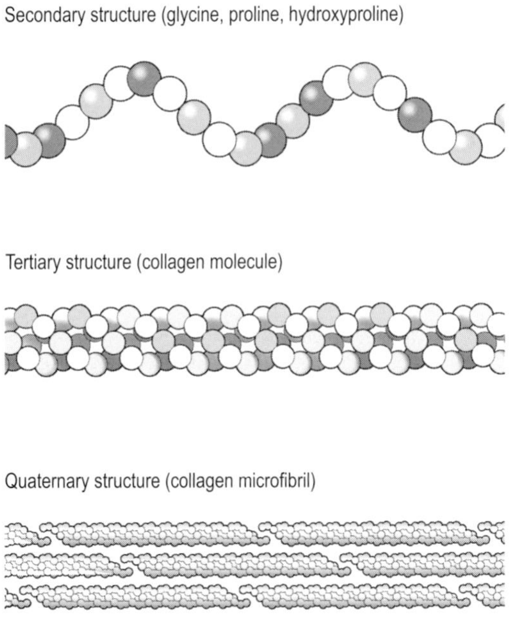


**Fig. 1.17** The structure of a tendon. (**a**) Secondary structure (glycine, proline, hydroxyproline). (**b**) Tertiary structure (collagen molecule). (**c**) Quaternary structure (collagen microfibril).

handed triple helix, which is held together by hydrogen and covalent bonds (tertiary structure) to form the collagen molecules. The molecules are staggered and attached by oppositely charged amino acids in very strong bonds. This staggered arrangement makes up the microfibril (quaternary structure) (Fig. 1.17).

The microfibrils are combined with proteoglycan and water and are grouped into subfibrils and then fibrils along the axis of force. As tendons age, there is less collagen synthesis, less dense collagen fibrils and less water leading to a stiffer tendon.

Tendons can be enclosed in tendon sheaths and sliding occurs in synovial fluid, e.g. finger flexors. Tendons that are not in sheaths are surrounded by loose connective tissue called paratenon. The blood supply to the tendon is from the attachment to muscle at one end and periosteum at the other end. The surrounding tissue can also provide a blood supply in paratenon-covered tendons. In the tendon sheath, synovial diffusion contributes to tendon nutrition. At the attachment of tendon to bone, the tendon merges into fibrocartilage, mineralized fibrocartilage and then bone.

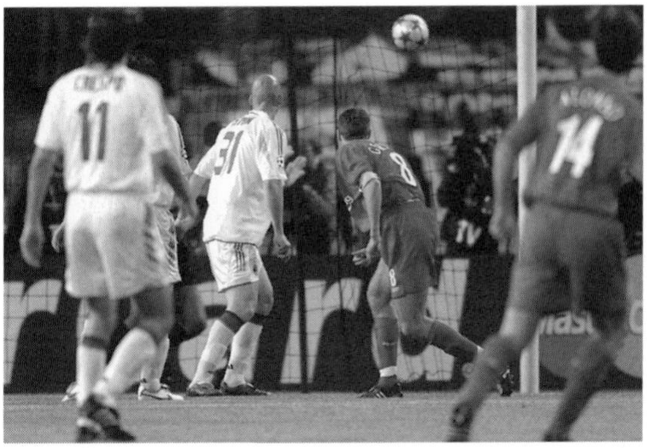

**Fig. 1.18** Sportsfile.

## Mechanical properties

Tensile strength is a key property in many tendons, e.g. the patellar tendon. Viscoelastic properties including stress relaxation and 'creep' can be identified. In isometric muscle contractions, the tendon can actually elongate (creep) decreasing the rate of muscle fatigue and enhancing muscle performance in isometric contraction. Mechanical properties are affected by the anatomic location of the tendon, exercise and age.

## Injury

Tendon injuries are usually overload injuries and usually occur at either end of the tendon. Midsubstance tendon ruptures are less common than avulsion bony injuries and rupture of the musculotendinous junction. Midsubstance injury frequently indicates a pre-existing pathology, e.g. tendo Achillis rupture or rotator cuff tear. Tendinopathy refers to a clinical scenario of pain, swelling and reduced function. Tendinosis refers to degeneration without inflammation and tendinitis refers to inflammation within a tendon. In chronic tendon injuries, contributing factors include pre-existing tendon abnormalities, age, weight and medications including steroids. Excessive or inappropriate training and incorrect equipment are also important contributors. Microscopically, there may be damage to the paratenon, which becomes thickened with fibroblasts and adhesions, and damage to the tendon itself. The relationship between paratenon pathology and tendon damage is still unclear (Fig. 1.19).

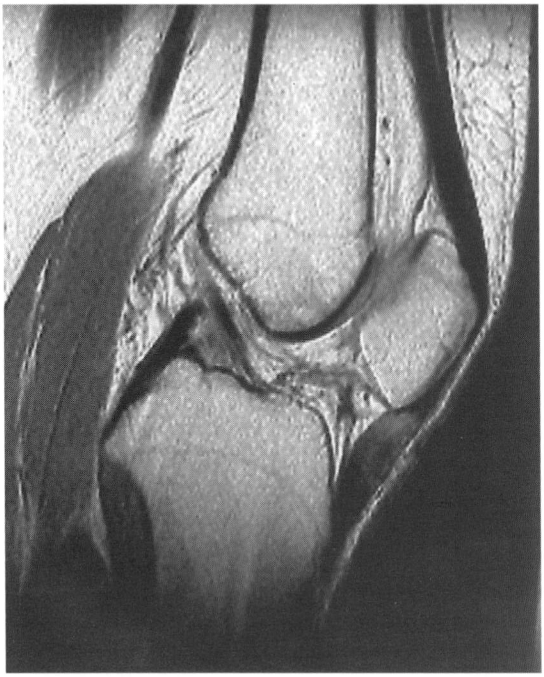

Fig. 1.19 Sagittal MRI showing a signal abnormality and thickening of the patellar tendon in a basketball player with a 'jumper's knee'.

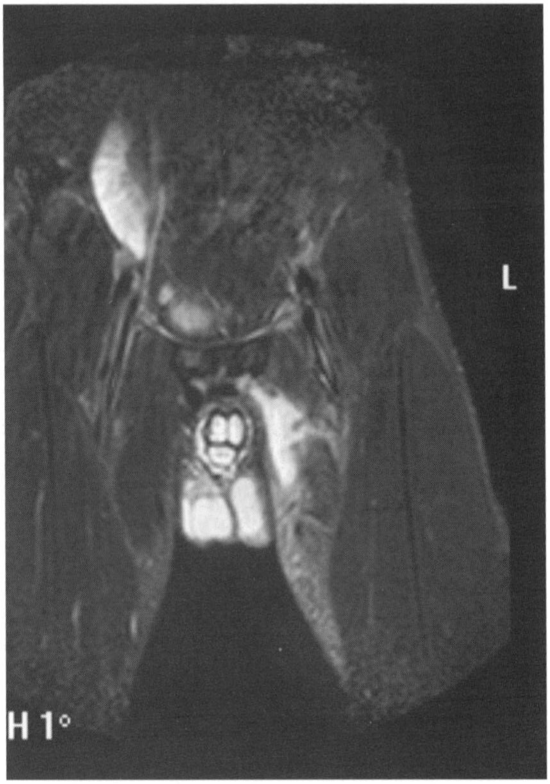


Fig. 1.20 Local hemorrhage and edema at the site of a grade 3 tear of the left adductor longus at the musculotendinous junction in a professional rugby player.



## Healing

Different patterns of healing occur in tendons enclosed in a synovial sheath as compared to those surrounded by paratenon (Fig. 1.20).

In paratenon-covered tendons (vascular), fibroblasts and capillaries invade the gap and collagen precursors are formed. A bridge of scar tissue is formed by two weeks and marked fibroblasts and vascular activity is seen. As healing continues, and particularly as stress is applied to the tendon, the fibroblasts and collagen fibers align along the mechanical axis and tensile strength increases.

In sheath-covered tendons (avascular) there is an intrinsic healing response from the epitenon which can heal these tendons in repaired tendons with passive motion post-operatively. If immobilized, healing has been shown to occur from the adjacent digital sheath and endotenon. Most of these tendon ruptures are treated by primary repair. Early mobilization following a strong repair with a smooth repaired surface is associated with a good functional outcome (Fig. 1.21).

# LIGAMENTS

Ligaments are bands of dense fibrous connective tissue similar to tendons. Microscopically they consist of fibroblasts surrounded by parallel bundles of predominantly type I collagen fibers. Elastin is present in varying amounts in different ligaments depending on the required mechanical properties of the ligament. For example, in the spinous ligaments more flexibility is required and the elastin content is higher.

Ligaments are made up of fascicles, which are bundles of subfasciculi. The subfascicle is surrounded by endotenon and is formed by collagen fibrils 150–250 nm across, which are grouped into fibers up to 20 μm in diameter.

The insertion of the ligament into the bone is frequently a source of injury; the ligament is attached to the bone either directly or indirectly. In the direct

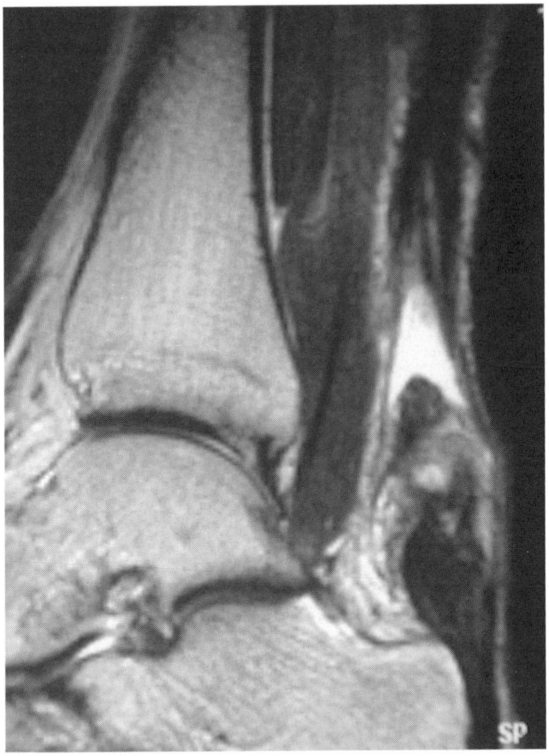


**Fig. 1.21** Sagittal $T_2$-weighted MRI showing a complete rupture of the Achilles tendon at the musculotendinous junction with retraction and interposed hemorrhage and clot at the site of tear occurring in a poorly conditioned middle-aged man following recreational indoor football (soccer).

attachment the superficial fibers merge with the periosteum and the deep fibers merge through a fibrocartilage zone, which becomes mineralized and attaches to the bone. Indirect ligament attachment involves a layer of ligaments attaching to the periosteum. The insertion of the ligament is also frequently the origin of the vascular supply to the ligament. There is a developed vascular system throughout the ligament, which maintains and repairs the matrix. There is also a well-developed innervation to ligaments including proprioception, nociception and pain fibers.

Ligaments, during inactivity, become more fluid filled but this fluid is extruded during activity. This means that the viscoelastic properties of ligaments following inactivity are different while the fluid is being extruded than after the fluid has been extruded. Following initial activity the fluid is extruded and the viscoelastic properties become predictable, i.e. preconditioning. The mechanical properties therefore alter with degree of activity as well as age.

Ligaments contribute stability to joints, and in different positions of the joint different ligaments can act as primary or secondary stabilizers.

The immobilization of ligaments can damage the normal parallel sliding pattern of the ligament fibers. It has been shown experimentally that immobilization affects tensile and elastic properties of ligaments. The insertion of the ligament to the bone is also weakened by immobilization. Exercise can subsequently revert the changes in the mechanical properties of the ligament relatively quickly. However, the damage to the insertion complex is slower to recover.

## Injury

1. Grade I – these are clinically regarded as mild sprains with no increase in translation of the affected joint. These injuries represent stretching of the ligaments and histologically demonstrate small hemorrhagic areas.
2. Grade II – histologically there is more tearing and hemorrhaging seen. Mild-to-moderate increased translation can be seen.
3. Grade III – there is complete disruption of the ligament, with clearly increased translation.



## Healing

Following damage and bleeding there is an initial inflammatory response. Necrotic tissue is removed and fibroblasts proliferate and lay down proteoglycan and collagen. Initially type III collagen is predominantly formed. The damaged zone is subsequently filled with more fibroblasts and capillary ingrowth. Type I collagen begins to predominate and organize itself along the mechanical axis of the ligament. With activity the tensile properties improve with increased collagen cross-linking and organization, which occurs over many months following the injury.

## MUSCLE

An understanding of the cellular structure of muscle and how it works helps care for the athlete in muscle preparation for optimum performance and in the treatment of muscle injuries. The muscle fiber is a fusion of muscle cells to give a large long fiber with multiple nuclei full of contractile proteins, principally actin and myosin, troponin and tropomysin. The fibers are parallel to the long axis of the muscle but can also run obliquely where high forces and less shortening is required.

Type I muscle fibers are slow-twitch oxidative endurance fibers and type II fibers are fast-twitch oxidative fibers. Each muscle fiber is surrounded by connective tissue called endomysium. The membrane that surrounds the fiber is sarcolemma. Satellite cells lie on the surface and become muscle cells following damage to the muscle fibers. Inside the fibers there are myofibrils made up of sacromeres. There are thick filaments of myosin and thin filaments of actin; troponin and tropomysin are attached to the actin molecules. The cell membrane has channels called sarcoplasmic reticulum, which reach into the cells.

The nerve contacts the muscle at the motor end-plate. When the nerve is fired, a chemical (acetylcholine) is released across the gap and binds to a receptor on the muscle membrane. This causes an electrical change on the surface membrane which spreads through the sarcoplasmic reticulum and which releases calcium. This release of calcium works through troponin to change the shape of tropomysin and alter the cross-linking between actin and myosin. Essentially, the overlap between the thick and thin filaments is altered. If the overlap is increased, the fiber shortens. An important point to understand is that the overlap can decrease while there is muscle contraction with subsequent lengthening of the fiber (eccentric contraction), e.g. the contraction of the quadriceps while descending stairs. This alteration in cross-linking is fuelled by adenosine triphosphate.

As the muscle fibers converge, the membranes 'infold'. As the actin filaments are attached by proteins to the membrane they fuse to form the musculotendinous junction. Muscle is viscoelastic tissue and can behave differently under different conditions. High resistance training leads to increased strength as each fiber hypertrophies and contains more contractile proteins. Repetitive training may increase the neuromuscular efficiency. Muscle fibers are adaptable and can respond differently to different training regimes. Endurance training can lead to cellular changes of increased mitochondria and changes to prolong energy supply. High-resistance training or short-term high-output training will lead to different cellular adaptive changes.

## Injury

The muscle can be injured directly, e.g. by a blunt or penetrating trauma, or more commonly indirectly during sports. The latter is usually related to excessive stretching. Following injury, neutrophils fill the injured area. Macrophages start to phagocytose injured tissue. The satellite cells on the membrane of the muscle cells become new muscle cells and myoblasts are formed. Connective tissue is then formed but if this occurs to excess it can interfere with full recovery. The motor end-plates must also regenerate (Fig. 1.22).

Muscle contusions result in bleeding into the muscle with hematoma formation. The hematoma can fill with connective tissue, which can lead to contraction, or, if severe, can occasionally result in bone formation (myositis ossificans). A short period of immobilization should be followed by mobilization for these injuries.

## Muscle strain

This is the most common injury and can indicate delayed muscle soreness, partial muscle tear or complete muscle tear. These injuries are commonly felt to be more common in fatigued muscles, which are not efficiently able to contract eccentrically, i.e. they are not able to lengthen in a controlled fashion. Incomplete tears are more common and associated with muscles that cross two joints (hamstring, gastrocnemius and rectus) and have predominantly type II fibers.

## Delayed muscle soreness

This is muscle pain 24–72 hours after intense physical activity. The intensity varies with the preexisting muscle condition and the exercise intensity. It usually occurs in eccentrically acting muscles and resolves in five days. Cell membrane destruction with calcium influx and inflammatory mediators and edema have been identified as a source of pain in this condition.

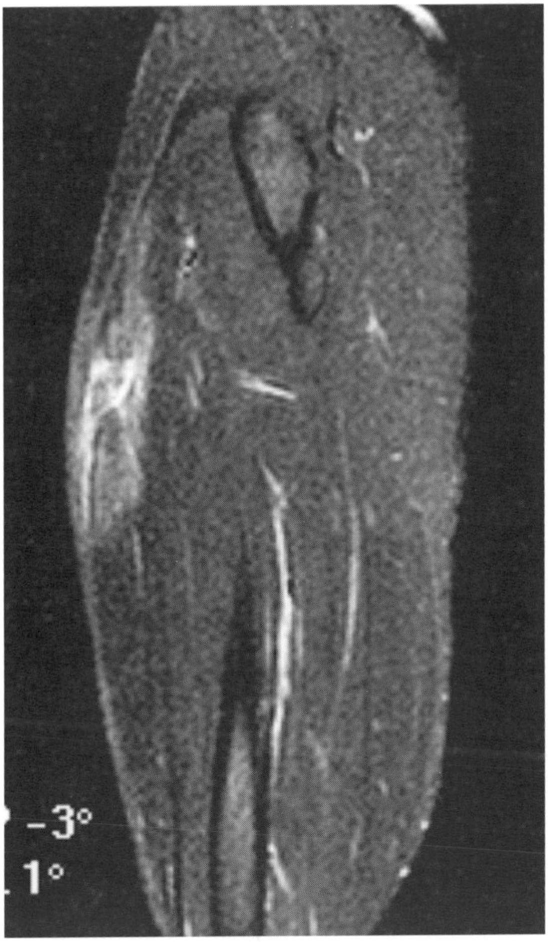


(a)

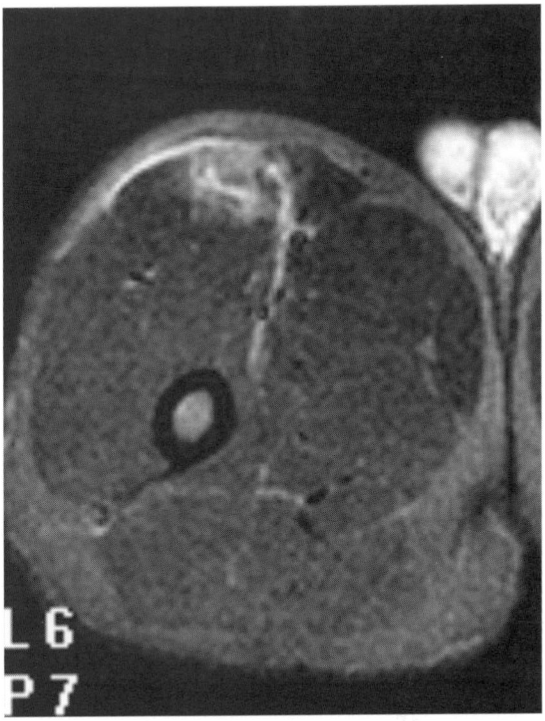


(b)

**Fig. 1.22** Grade 2 tear of the superficial belly of the proximal rectus femoris muscle in a professional rugby player. (**a**) Sagittal; (**b**) axial.



## Muscle cramps

This usually affects the gastrocnemius and is treated by stretching the muscle. This usually occurs with dehydration and altered electrolyte balance; the initiating abnormality may in fact be from the nerve.

## Immobilization

Immobilization of a muscle alters its girth, function and metabolism. The fibers atrophy and protein synthesis decreases. The muscle shows a lower load to failure. These changes are maximum if the muscle is immobilized under no tension.

## Further reading


Alms M. Fracture mechanics. J Bone Joint Surg 1961; 43B: 162–166.

De Lee JC, Drez, Jr D, Miller MD. Orthopaedic sports medicine, 2nd edn. Philadelphia, WB Saunders, 2003.

Eustace S. MRI of orthopaedic trauma. Philadelphia, Lippincott Williams & Wilkins, 1999.

Finnegan MA, Uhtoff HK. Healing of trabecular bone. In: Lang JM ed. Fracture healing, Churchill Livingstone, 1987; 33–38.

Fitzgerald RH, Kaufer H, Malkani AL. Orthopaedics. Oxford, Mosby/Elsevier, 2001.

Frankel VH, Burstein AH. Orthopedic biomechanics. Philadelphia, Lea & Febiger, 1970.

Hulth A. Current concepts of fracture healing. Clin Orthop 1989; 249: 265–284.

McKibbin B. The biology of fracture healing in long bones. J Bone Joint Surg 1978; 60B: 150–162.

Mink JH, Deutsch AL. Occult cartilage and bone injuries of the knee. Detection, classification and assessment with MR imaging. Radiology 1989; 170: 823–829.

Ogden JA. Injury to the growth mechanisms of the immature skeleton. Skeletal Radiol 1981; 6: 187–192.

Perkins G. Fractures and dislocations. London, Athlone Press, 1958.

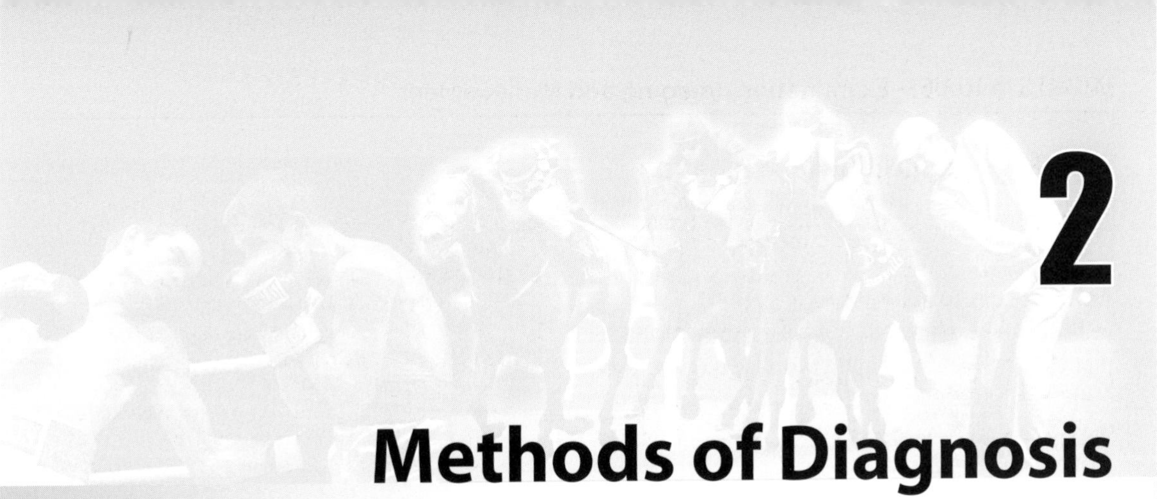

# 2

# Methods of Diagnosis



## CLINICAL INVESTIGATIONS

Despite extraordinary advances in imaging and related diagnostic investigations, history and clinical examination remain the foundation of patient assessment and management.

### History

A detailed record of symptoms, pattern of onset, duration, site and points of radiation, methods of relieving symptoms, a record of aggravating factors and of potential relief by medication should all be recorded.

### Examination

There are three phases in musculoskeletal clinical examination: observation; active motion; and passive motion. Observation requires an assessment of gait and posture. Passive examination involves passive movement of the joints. Active examination involves movement of joints by the clinician. At active examination an attempt should be made to elicit the presence or absence of swelling or excoriation, and it should determine the site of maximal discomfort, whether symptoms are aggravated by local palpation or only become apparent on deep manipulation, and whether symptoms are present on passive or resisted examination. Specific tests should be employed in the assessment of defined injuries reviewed under anatomic sites later in this book.

Examination in all cases should also include an assessment of the lungs, heart, central and peripheral nervous systems, abdomen, pelvis and groin.

## Specific tests at clinical examination

Expanded details are reviewed in the regional evaluation of injuries.

### Achilles rupture (Thompson's test)

Induced contraction of the calf muscles due to manual compression should produce plantar flexion of the forefoot if the Achilles tendon is intact.

### Anterior cruciate ligament tear (Lachman's test)

Anterior translation of the tibia relative to the femur may be induced in patients with an ACL tear. In health, the intact ligament prevents such an effect and attempted anterior translation is resisted by a firm endpoint.

### Patellar apprehension test

Lateral pressure applied to the patella with the knee in 5° of flexion. Induced pain suggests patellofemoral subluxation and chondromalacia.

### Superior labral tear of the hip

Pain induced by knee flexion and adduction with posterior hip loading.



### Trendelenburg's test

On weight bearing, the non-weight-bearing hip rises in normality. Secondary to gluteal weakness, or a short femur, the non-weight-bearing side of the pelvis tilts downwards.

### Osteitis pubis (squeeze test)

Groin pain induced by resisted adduction in flexion and to a lesser extent in extension. In simple terms, pain may be induced by compressing a clenched fist held between the knees.

Also, tenderness elicited on palpation at the teno-osseous attachment of the adductor and gracilis.

### Shoulder impingement (Hawkin's test)

Pain induced by 90° shoulder abduction and subsequent internal rotation of the arm.

### Shoulder impingement (Neer's test)

Pain induced by internal rotation with cross chest adduction.

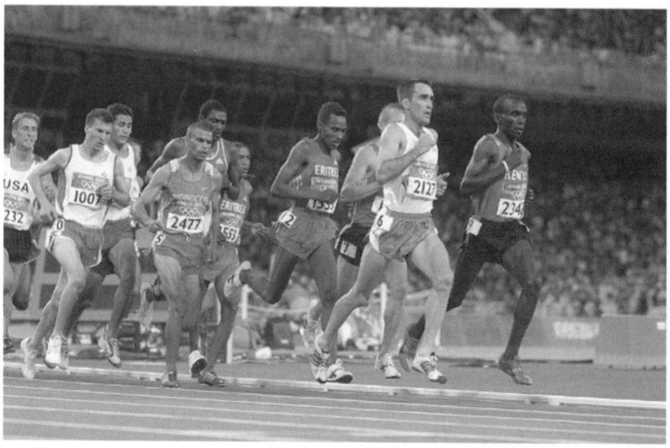


**Fig. 2.1** Sports file.

### Bicipitolabral complex (O'Brien's test)

Pain induced by arm adduction with internal rotation and resisted arm elevation and abduction.

### Lateral epicondylitis

Pain induced at the lateral epicondyle by resisted palmar extension or resisted extension of the long digit.

# CLINICAL IMAGING

## Radiographs

### Basic physics

Professor Wilhelm Konrad Roentgen is credited with the discovery of X-rays in 1895 at Würzburg University, Germany. He described the generation of penetrating electromagnetic waves by an interaction between an accelerated electron (generated by heat conduction through a tungsten filament and applied voltage between the filament and target) with a target material (tungsten) housed within an X-ray tube. When directed at materials of differing density, a beam of X-ray becomes attenuated according to tissue density. Differential attenuation of the beam is detected by the interaction between residual X-rays and silver halide crystals (in conventional X-ray film), a phosphor fluorescent plate (in computed radiography) or with digital cells (in direct digital radiography).

## Advantages
Widely available, excellent contrast between tissues of differing densities (such as bone and soft tissue) and excellent bone detail.

## Disadvantage
X-ray exposure produces mitogenesis and hence induces cancer. The relative risk of cancer induction reflects its cumulative exposure. Established dose limits protect the patient and physician.

## Clinical use in sports medicine
Despite the development of a range of sophisticated imaging techniques, radiographs still represent the most widely employed imaging technique, particularly when bone injury is suspected following clinical examination. When employed, the maximum diagnostic benefit is yielded by employing specific dedicated views tailored to improve visualization of particular pathologies.

The routine radiographic projections are listed in Table 2.1.

**Table 2.1** Routine radiographic projections

| Projection | Orientation |
|---|---|
| Digits | AP, Lat |
| Hand | AP, Lat (Obl in arthritis and occult trauma) |
| Wrist | AP, Lat (Obl in arthritis and occult trauma) |
| Forearm | AP, Lat |
| Elbow | AP, Lat (Obl in radial head trauma) |
| Shoulder | AP, Obl, Lat: axial; skyline; scapula Y; transthoracic |
| Acromioclavicular joint | AP 20° cephalad tilt; AP with/without weights |
| Sternoclavicular joint | AP, Lat, Obl |
| Cervical spine | AP, Lat, Odontoid peg view; (Obl if radicular pain) |
| Thoracic spine | AP, Lat |
| Lumbar spine | AP, Lat; Obl requested if spondylolysis suspected |
| Pelvis | AP (straight) |
| Hip | AP, Obl (supplemental views, Judet's and false profile) |
| Femur | AP, Lat |
| Knee | AP (weight bearing), Lat (supplemental views below) |
| Calf/Tibia and fibula | AP, Lat |
| Ankle | AP, Obl (mortice view), Lat |
| Subtalar joint | Lat, Axial (Harris–Beath view) |
| Midfoot | AP, Obl, Lat |
| Toes | AP, Lat |
| Facial bones | PA 30° tilt; occipitomental view |
| Skull | PA (occipitofrontal) 20° tilt, AP 30° tilt (Towne's view), Lat |

AP, anteroposterior; Lat, lateral; Obl, oblique.

## Sacroiliitis
Sacroiliac joints are best evaluated with views acquired perpendicular to the sacrum; in effect the view must be angled 25° caudally if acquired in the preferential posteroanterior (PA) plane or cephalad if acquired in the anteroposterior (AP) plane. Straight PA or AP films must be supplemented by oblique views to allow assessment of the joint space. Oblique views must be acquired of both sides (Fig. 2.2).

## Scaphoid fracture
The scaphoid is tilted volarly and appears foreshortened if the acquired film is in a straight PA or AP plain, the distal pole being projected over the scaphoid waist. It is critical that a specific view of the scaphoid is acquired angled perpendicular to the scaphoid with the wrist held in ulnar deviation (20° tilt) (Fig. 2.3).

## Spondylolysis and facet joint pain
This is best identified on images oblique to the posterior elements in the lumbar spine. Spondylolysis, if suspected following review of conventional radiographs, is best detected on axial computed tomography (CT) cuts angled to the posterior elements (reverse gantry) or on images reformatted from a multislice volumetric acquisition (multislice CT) (Fig. 2.4).

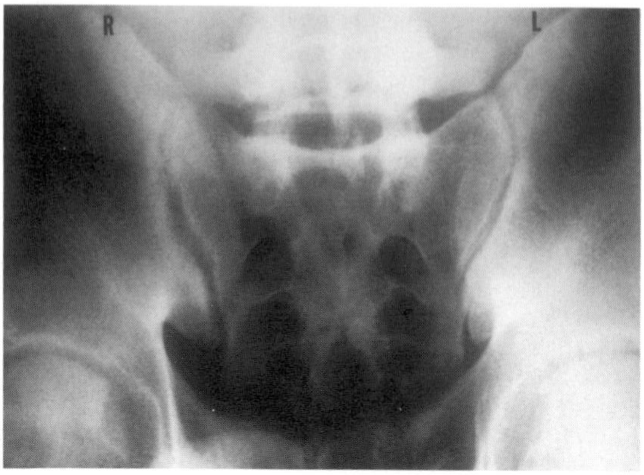


**Fig. 2.2** Posteroanterior angled view of the sacroiliac joints shows articular surface erosion on the right secondary to unilateral sacroiliitis.

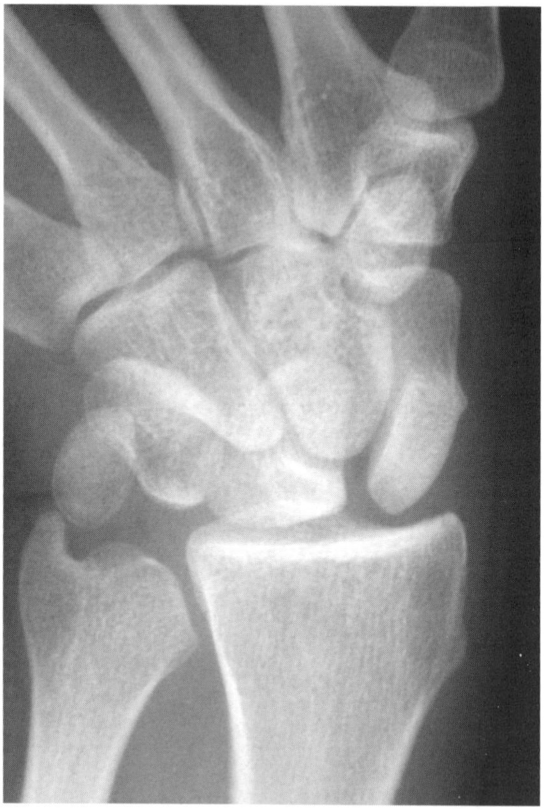

**Fig. 2.3** Posteroanterior view acquired with the wrist held in ulnar deviation and 20° of tube tilt, which produces an elongated view of the scaphoid.

## Cervical exit foramina

These are identified on oblique views. They should be obtained and assessed in patients with upper extremity radiculopathy.

## Acromioclavicular joint subluxation

Angled AP views (tilted or angled upwards 20°) of the symptomatic and asymptomatic sides may be supplemented by weight-bearing views. An imposed weight-bearing stress produces a widening of the joint space.

## Radial head fracture

When a radial head fracture is suspected, but not identified following identification of a post-traumatic elbow joint effusion, dedicated radial head views should be acquired in the oblique plain to throw the radial head off the adjacent osseous structures.

## Patellofemoral disease

Although patellar shape and crude alignment may be assessed with a skyline view, this is not a physiologic weight-bearing position. Improved assessment of the patellofemoral joint and associated tracking may be yielded by Merchant's views. These allow the assessment of patellofemoral alignment at varying degrees of flexion in weight-bearing positions through the use of a cassette holder placed immediately anterior to the mid tibia.

## Knee loose body or osteochondritis

Loose bodies within the knee may be identified on standard AP and lateral projections. Loose fragments within the intercondylar notch are often obscured on these projections and are best identified on a dedicated tunnel view.

## Acetabular injury

Although acetabular injury may be suspected on a standard AP radiograph, oblique views (Judet's views) allow improved assessment of the anterior and posterior acetabular columns and hence allow improved evaluation of suspected traumatic injury (Fig. 2.5).

## Hip joint space

Anteroposterior radiographs of the hip allow assessment of the superior and medial joint spaces. Joint space narrowing in osteoarthritis most frequently involves the anterosuperior joint space and can only be assessed on a false profile view (a true AP) of the hip, which allows assessment of the posterior, superior and anterior joint spaces.

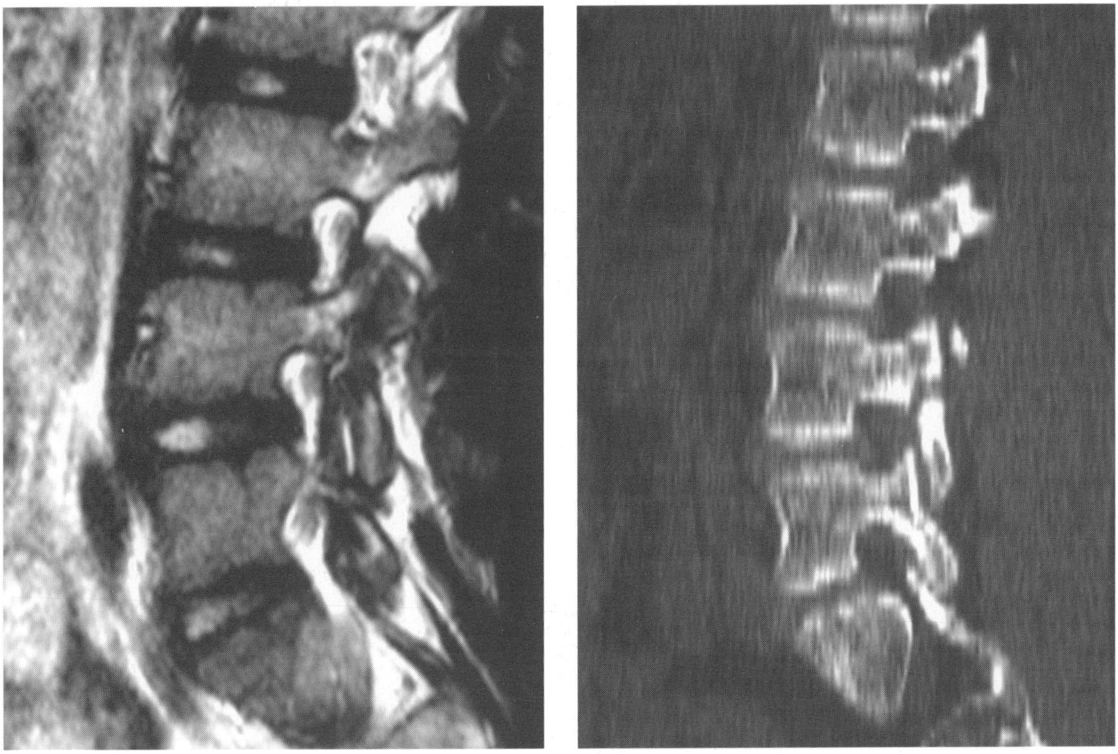

Fig. 2.4 Sagittal $T_2$-weighted MR image showing vertical lysis through the pars interarticularis of the L4 vertebral body (left) and sagittal reformatted image from a multislice CT acquisition showing oblique lysis through the pars interarticularis of L4 (right).



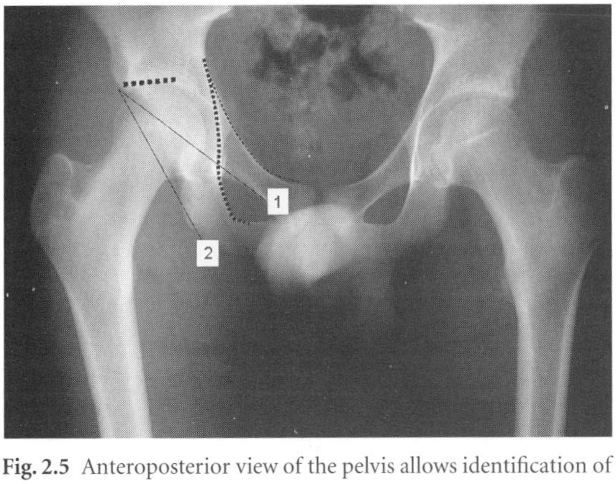


Fig. 2.5 Anteroposterior view of the pelvis allows identification of six acetabular lines. Line 1: the continuation of the inferior margin of the superior pubic ramus to the rim of the acetabulum demarcates the anterior wall of the acetabulum. Line 2: the continuation of the inferior margin of the inferior pubic ramus demarcates the posterior wall of the acetabulum.

## Knee joint space

Non-weight-bearing views are misleading. A true assessment of cartilage loss can only be achieved by review of weight-bearing AP and semiflexed lateral views.

## Shoulder dislocation

When dislocation is suspected, the loss of glenohumeral alignment is best appreciated on either an axial or scapula y view. Following dislocation patient positioning may be limited by pain and glenohumeral alignment in this setting is best appreciated by a transthoracic y view.

## C7 injury

Assessment of the lowest cervical vertebral body is often limited on standard lateral views by overlying shoulders. Visualization is best achieved in this setting by the swimmer's view.

## Odontoid peg

The odontoid peg is best visualized by the open mouth view although a clear assessment of the peg in this view may be limited by dentition. A clear

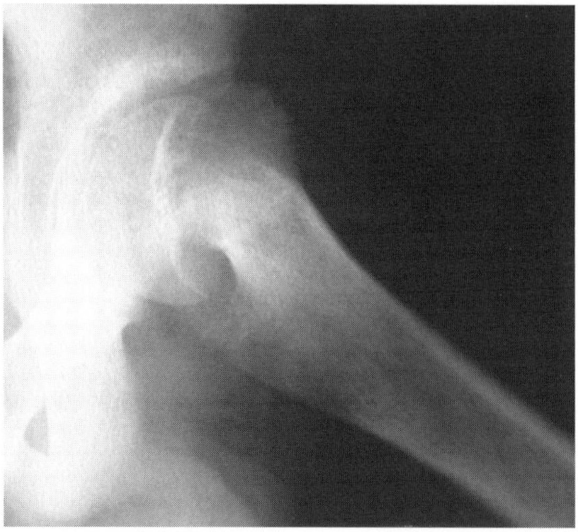

**Fig. 2.6** Oblique radiograph showing anteroinferior migration of the epiphysis in a patient with grade 1 slipped capital femoral epiphysis.

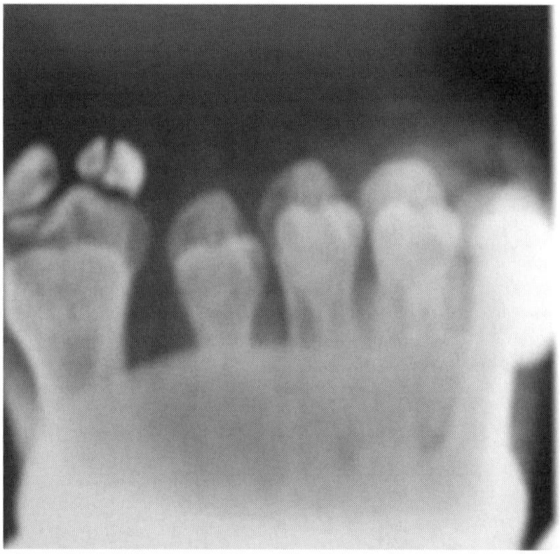

**Fig. 2.7** Sesamoid view showing a vertical fracture through the fibula sesamoid.

visualization of the odontoid peg may be achieved by an angled peg view (Fuchs' view) or by 'autotomography' in which an image of the peg is acquired with a prolonged exposure time during which the mandible is opened and closed.



### Slipped capital femoral epiphysis (SCFE)

An assessment of injury to the proximal femoral growth plate in patients with suspected SCFE is best achieved by the frog lateral projection. In this plane a line drawn along the lateral cortex should intersect the lateral third of the femoral epiphysis (Fig. 2.6).

### Ankle joint space

When injury to the talar dome is suspected it should be assessed by both a straight AP view and an oblique mortice view. The AP projection allows assessment of the superior tibiotalar joint space but limits evaluation of the medial and lateral joint spaces. An oblique mortice view opens out the medial and lateral tibiotalar joint spaces.

### Posterior subtalar joint (talocalcaneal coalition)

Evaluation of the posterior subtalar joint is achieved by a combined assessment of a direct lateral view and an axial view (Harris–Beath axial view), which permits the clear visualization of the posterior and middle subtalar joints.

### Sesamoid fracture (sesamoid views)

The tibial and fibula sesamoids at the base of the first metatarsophalangeal articulation represent the fulcrum for the long flexors during the toe-off phase of the gait cycle. Detection of fracture or infarction of the sesamoids is best yielded by lateral views or sesamoid views (Fig. 2.7).

## Scintigraphy

In contrast to radiographs derived by differential attenuation of an X-ray beam, 'scintiscans' are derived by recording the distribution of a gamma ray emitter (most frequently technetium 99m) following intravenous (i.v.) injection. The distribution of technetium may be predicted by binding it to a carrying agent such as methylene diphosphonate (MDP), which, when injected, becomes chemisorbed to apatite-coating active osteoblasts. In effect, MDP bound to technetium is the agent employed to provide an image of osteoblast activity, the isotope bone scan. Technetium bound to diethylenetriamine penta-acetic acid is preferentially excreted by the kidneys (rather than interacting with specific tissue

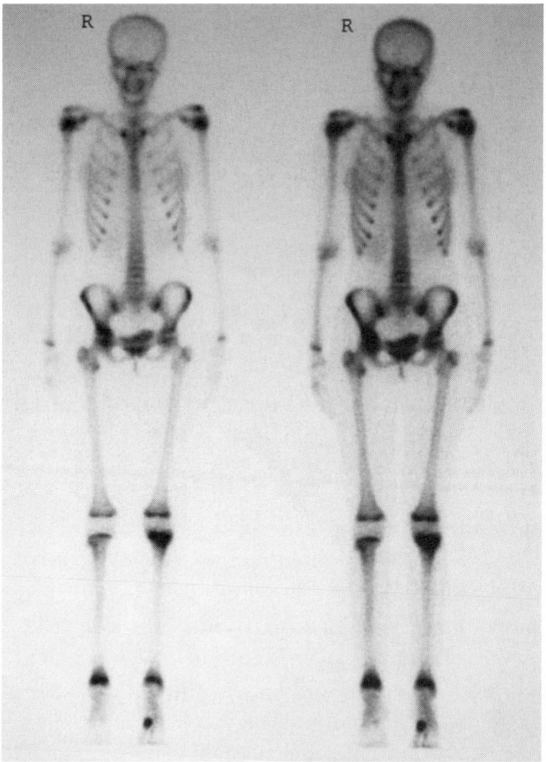


Fig. 2.8 Whole-body bone scan mapping skeletal osteoblastic activity. Increased activity is identified in the epiphysis of the right ankle, left knee and right hip due to multifocal epiphysiolysis in an adolescent schoolgirl playing sport 5 days a week.

components) and hence provides an agent for renal scans.

## Advantage

Isotope bone scanning is achieved by the widely available technetium 99m MDP tracer. It is cheap, provides a valuable map of osteoblast activity and is relatively low dose (as technetium has a short half-life of 6 hours). It provides a whole body image.

## Disadvantage

The uptake of technetium MDP indicates osteoblast activity. Since many pathologies can produce up-regulated osteoblast activity, trauma, tumors and inflammation, its uptake is somewhat non-specific. Although a low-dose technique (due to technetium's short half-life) and although it is rapidly excreted, repeated bone scans result in a cumulative dose with associated mitogenesis.

## Applications in sports medicine

Isotope bone scanning provides a whole body image of osteoblastic activity. It may therefore allow the detection of bone tumors, bone metastases, sites of bone infection or inflammation, and sites of traumatic injury. The most common applications of a bone scan are in the search for skeletal metastases, and in sports medicine in the detection of radiographically occult fractures. Although MRI now allows the detection of similar pathologies (and is favored), an isotope bone scan is still employed to detect abnormal osteoblastic activity in patients with shin splints (medial tibial stress syndrome), osteitis pubis, osteomyelitis and occult fractures of the extremities and spine. The detection of stress fractures of the spinal posterior element – spondylolysis – is best achieved by additional imaging in tomographic planes using single photon emission computed tomography (SPECT). (SPECT scans are acquired by rotation of a gamma detector around the patient allowing the reformatting of images by back projection in tomographic planes.) (Fig. 2.9).

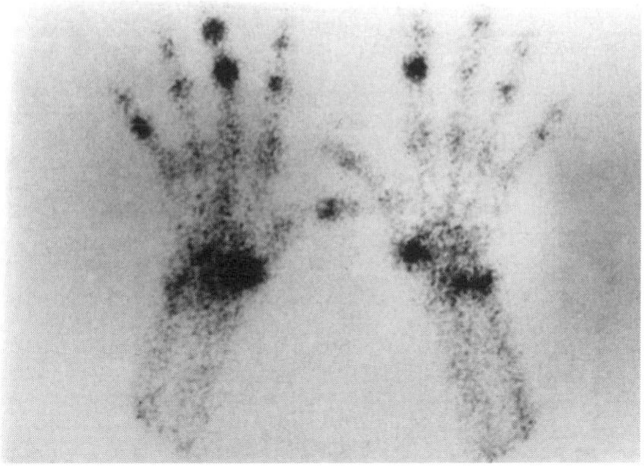

Fig 2.9 Bone scan showing radiotracer accumulation in the small joints of the hands in secondary to osteoarthritis.

**Box 2.1 Indications for isotope bone scan**

- Occult fracture detection
- Spondylolysis
- Osteitis pubis
- Medial tibial stress syndrome

# Ultrasound

Ultrasound employs sound waves in the megahertz frequency (3–20 Mhz) generated by the passage of a current through a piezoelectric crystal. Emitted sound passes freely through water but becomes reflected at soft-tissue interfaces, particularly by fat. Reflected echoes are received and recorded to generate a map of echoes and hence a diagnostic image. Ultrasound allows the useful evaluation of soft tissues, particularly those in the near field and hence is widely employed to assess tendon attachments and muscle tears. Being in real time, ultrasound allows the dynamic assessment of muscle contraction and of tendon–bone relationships during movement.

High-frequency probes offer exceptional near-field resolution at the expense of depth penetration and therefore are routinely used when ultrasound is employed as an imaging modality in sports medicine. The presence of Doppler ultrasound allows the assessment of vascular flow and therefore of soft-tissue vascularity or relative hyperemia (Fig. 2.10).

## Advantages

Ultrasound is cheap, non-ionizing and widely available. Allows the dynamic assessment of musculoskeletal structures.



## Disadvantage

The assessment of deep structures is limited when employing high-frequency probes, e.g. the assessment of bone is limited to the surface cortex. A coexistent injury to bone accompanying a muscle tear is often not appreciated with ultrasound.

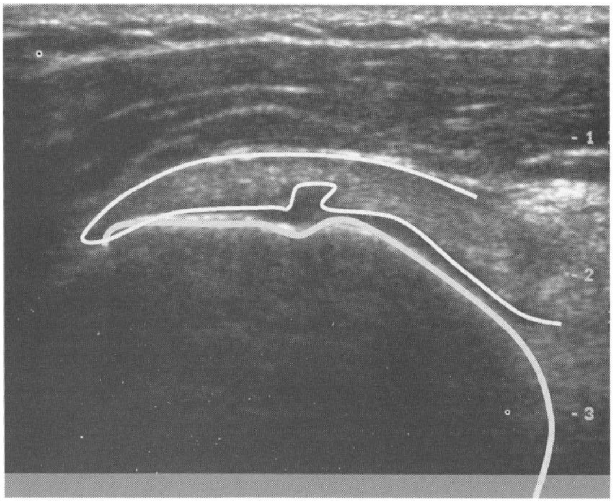


**Fig. 2.10** High-frequency ultrasound (14 MHz probe) showing a subtle undersurface tear in the distal supraspinatus tendon.

## Applications in sports medicine

- Rotator cuff assessment
- Lower limb knee extensor mechanism assessment
- Achilles tendon assessment
- Ankle tendon assessment
- Assessment of the unossified growth plate in children
- Guidance for tendon sheath injections
- Guidance for interventional biopsies or drainage.

# Computed tomography

Sir Godfrey Hounsfield (1919–2004) first described and developed computed tomography (CT) in 1973 in Northwick Park, London. He described the generation of images acquired in axial slices, yielded by the rotation of an X-ray tube held within a gantry around a patient. Relative attenuation of the beam at any place in the rotational arc can be mathematically calculated by back projection allowing an image to be created as a map of relative attenuation of the

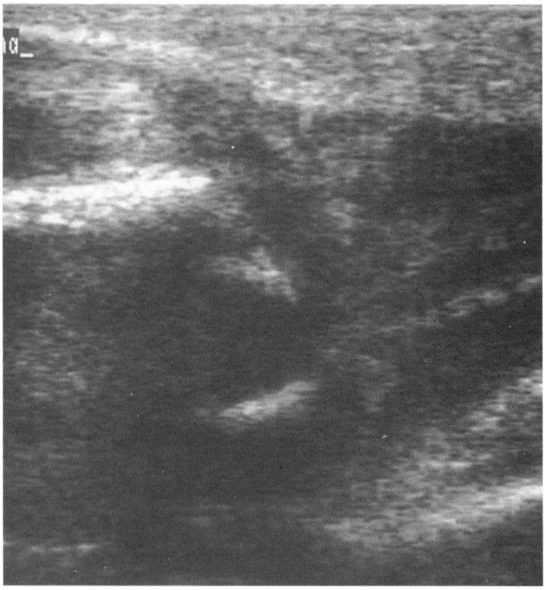

**Fig. 2.11** Ultrasound showing a transphyseal fracture of the distal humerus in a 2-year-old child. The cortex is demarcated by an echogenic reflective line; unossified cartilage of the epiphysis is hypoechoic. There is disruption of the anterior humeral line.

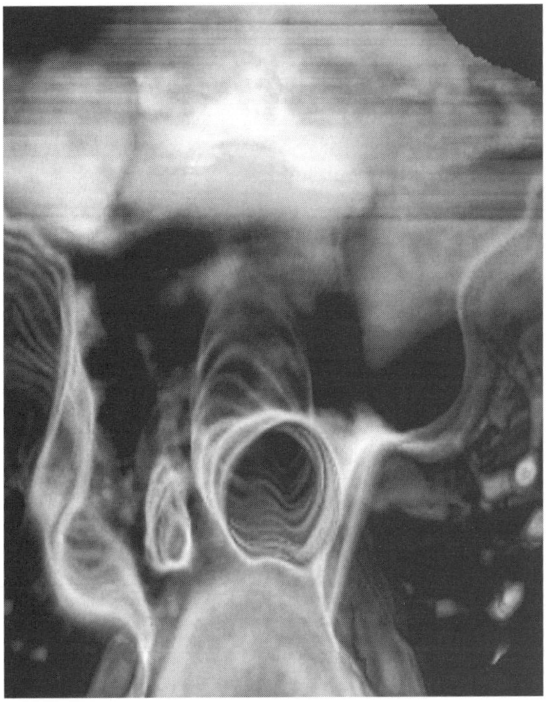

Fig. 2.12 Reformatted image from a CT acquisition in a basketball player following a posterior sternoclavicular dislocation showing encroachment of the cartilaginous rings of the trachea accounting for the presentation with dysphonia.

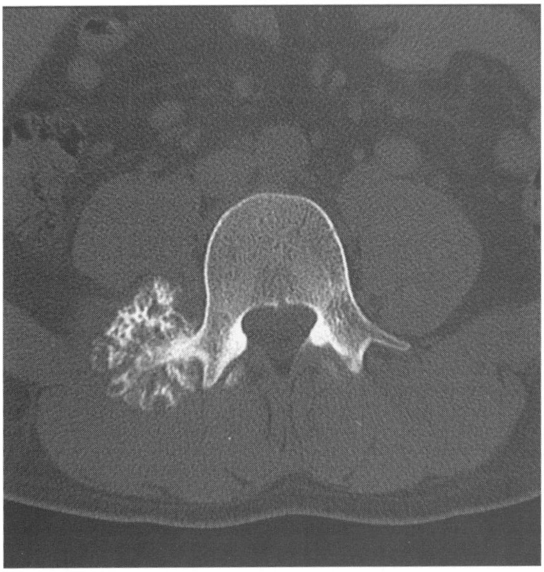

Fig. 2.14 Axial CT showing an incidental osteochondroma arising out of the right transverse process of the L3 vertebral body.

X-ray beam at each site in the slice. Digital units are applied to the attenuation map and these are subsequently coded by applied gray scales to generate a diagnostic image (Figs 2.12 and 2.13).

Initial CT scanners acquired images in individual single slices. A modification of conventional CT termed spiral CT allowed the acquisition of a volume of information, allowing more rapid image acquisition without omitting data in between conventionally acquired single slices. Spiral CT, by presenting a volume of data, allowed image reconstruction in off-axial planes and in the 3D mode, was favored for the assessment of bones and joints. Unfortunately data acquired in the spiral mode are acquired in anisotropic data sets, which limit fine detail in reconstructed images. This limitation has been overcome by the more recent development of multislice CT in which volumetric information data sets are acquired in an isotropic form. Isotropic data can be reformatted in any plane without loss of resolution or a noticeable impact or deterioration in image quality (Fig. 2.14).

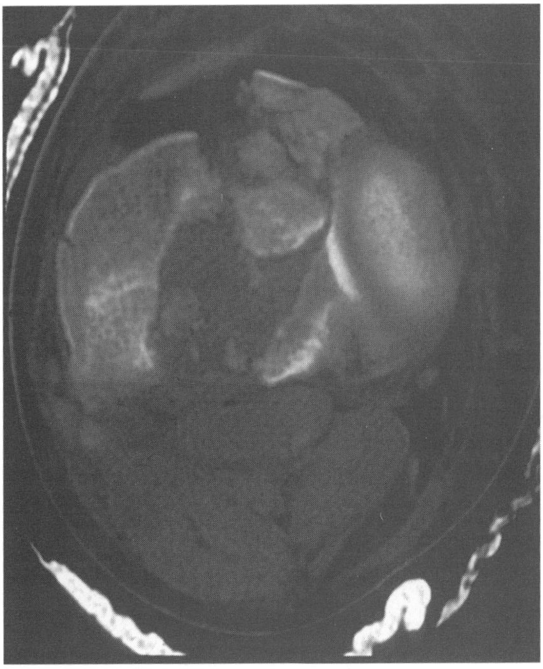

Fig. 2.13 Axial CT image showing a comminuted fracture of the tibial plateau.

Computed tomography images are essentially maps plotting the relative attenuation of an X-ray beam. The attenuation at a point in space allows the mathematical calculation of a decimal unit representation of attenuation, termed the Hounsfield unit (H). Image H values range from −1000 (in air) through to +60 (in soft tissue) through to +1000 (in compact bone). A gray-scale unit is applied to each H. In effect air is represented as black and soft tissue as gray, while bone is represented as white. Although a different gray-scale shade can be applied corresponding to each of the 2000 H, the eye can only differentiate between 16 shades. The range of H values over which the gray scales are spread is termed the window width. If the window width is wide, the 16 shades of gray perceived by the human eye will be spread over a wide range of H values densities. In this way, a perceived change in gray scale in an image will represent a large change in H values and fine-contrast resolution is limited. If fine-contrast resolution is required the window width is narrowed and the 16 gray-scale units are spread over a narrow range of H values or densities. The H value at the center of this window width is termed the window level. If, for example, an assessment of fine bone detail is required, the window level is set at the H value density of bone and the window is narrowly expanded around this level.



The technique of setting the window width and window level at CT allows one to review images with what are called bone windows, lung windows and soft-tissue windows.

### Advantages

Computed tomography image acquisition is rapid and robust. Derived data at multislice CT are isotropic and allow the postprocessing of images in off-axial planes and in the 3D format.

### Disadvantages

The ionizing dose. A potentially pregnant woman is prevented from harmful exposure by applying the 10-day rule.

### Applications in sports medicine

- Axial images of the spine and intervertebral disk
- Reverse gantry axial images are acquired to detect spondylolysis (now appreciated on lateral images generated from isotropic multislice CT data)
- Axial images of sternoclavicular joints
- Detailed assessment of fractures and of associated articular surface integrity
- Guidance for radiologic procedures and biopsies.

## Magnetic resonance imaging

Felix Bloch and Edward Purcell are credited with the initial description of the principles of magnetic resonance. They received Nobel prizes for their work in 1948 and 1952, respectively. During the following two decades magnetic resonance via spectroscopy was used to study the nature of chemical compounds. It was not until 1973, when three-dimensional magnetic resonance was described by Paul Lauterbur at Harvard, that the medium was first used to create a diagnostic image. The first clinical image was published in 1977 – an axial image of the wrist – by investigators at the University of Nottingham.

### Basic physics

When two poles of a magnet are apposed, they repel and are displaced (Fig. 2.15). In a similar way, protons magnetized within the bore of a magnetized large-bore coil are deflected by the brief application of an electromagnetic field in the form of a radiofrequency pulse. Deflected protons realign with the parent field following the cessation or removal of the applied magnetic field. This movement of protons, behaving like small magnets within the parent coil, generates current or an electromagnetic signal from which the diagnostic image is derived. In sequence, the generated electromagnetic signal is localized in space by rapidly switching three orthogonal magnetic gradients, it is converted from the frequency to the digital domain by using a Fourier transform, and it is finally converted to a diagnostic image by applying varying shades of gray according to the signal intensity recorded at points in space (Fig. 2.16).

Three physical components directly affect the quality of the derived image. The derived image is affected by the strength of the *parent magnetic field*, the strength, duration, frequency and pattern (pulse sequence) of the applied *excitatory electromagnetic pulse*, and the size, shape, configuration and location of the *receiver coil* used to sample the generated signal.

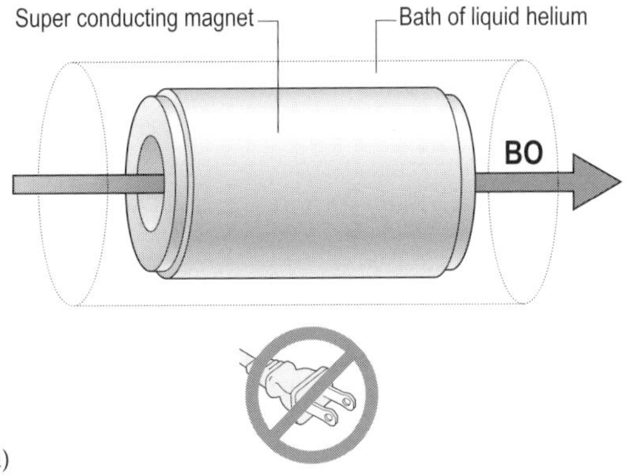


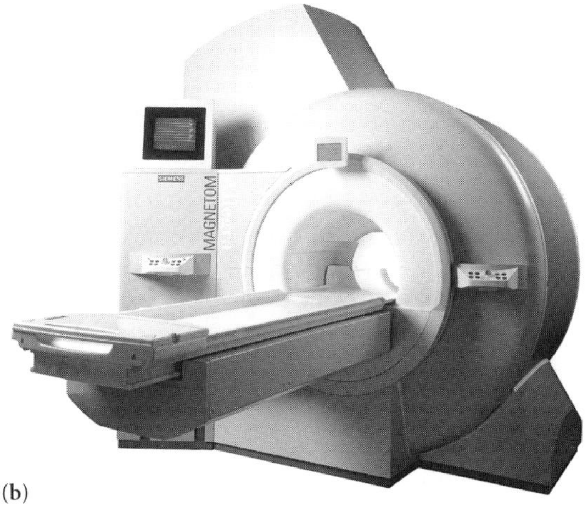


(a) (b)

**Fig. 2.15** (**a**) MRI current passes by superconduction through metal coils to create a magnetic field. The current, once underway, will pass without resistance in an endless circuit as the coils are cooled by a bath of helium. If the helium leaks, the temperature rises and the current flow is resisted. Once a magnet is operating it does not need to be plugged into a supply circuit. (**b**) The magnet.

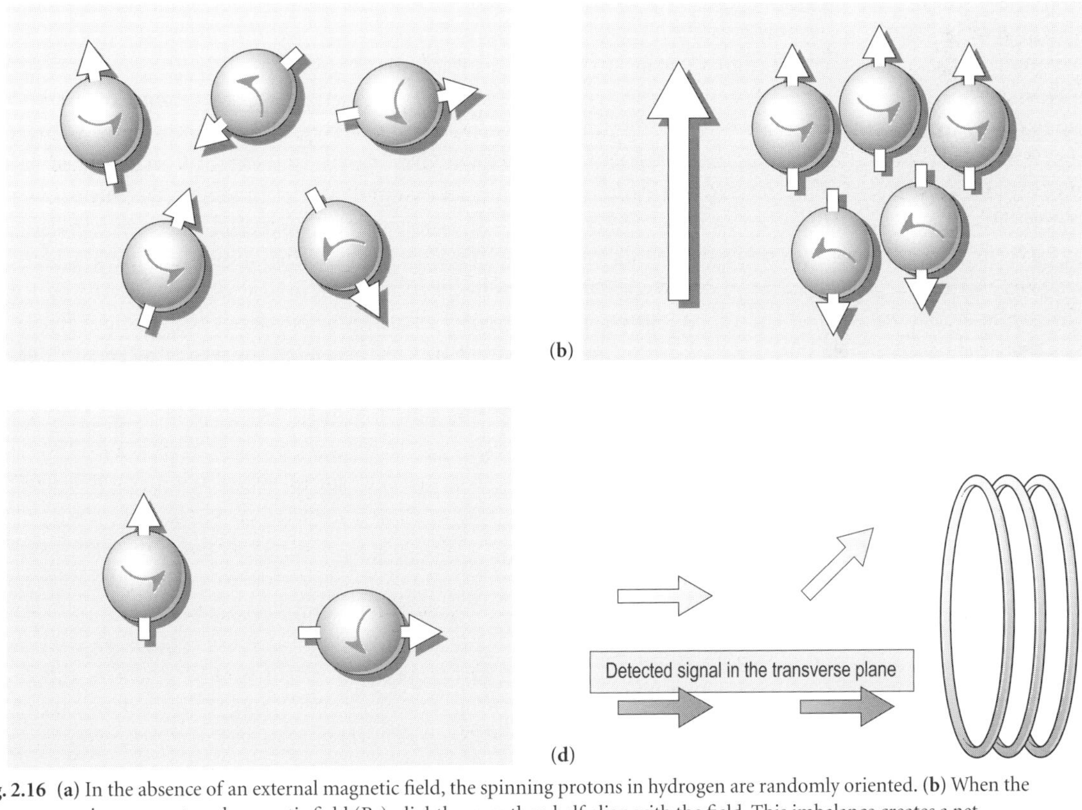

(a) (b) (c) (d)



**Fig. 2.16** (**a**) In the absence of an external magnetic field, the spinning protons in hydrogen are randomly oriented. (**b**) When the protons experience an external magnetic field ($B_o$), slightly more than half align with the field. This imbalance creates a net magnetization of the sample $M_o$. (**c**) When $M_o$ is aligned to the magnetic field $B_o$ it is very difficult to measure as $B_o$ itself is millions of times stronger than $M_o$. $M_o$ may be measured by 'tipping' it perpendicular to $B_o$. (**d**) The RF coils are only capable of picking up a signal in the transverse plane. As $M_o$ returns to $B_o$ the transverse component of the vector $M_o$ reduces.

## The parent magnetic field

A strong magnetic field induces greater magnetism in tissue and hence generates greater image signal following tissue excitation. Permanent magnets commonly employed in dedicated extremity MRI systems are relatively weak (0.2–0.35 T), limiting the recorded image signal and quality. In contrast, superconducting magnets in all-purpose units are stronger (0.5–1.5 T) and generate signal-rich images. Permanent systems are considerably cheaper and incur minimal maintenance costs. Superconducting systems, in contrast, are expensive and incur considerable maintenance costs.

## The applied excitatory electromagnetic pulse

Tissue excitation derived by an applied electromagnetic pulse may be varied in form by the range of frequencies in the excitatory pulse and by the strength, duration and pattern of the delivery pulse. The pattern in which the excitatory pulse is applied is termed the pulse sequence. The *gradient echo pulse sequence* uses a single excitatory pulse that only partially deflects tissue protons before the image signal is sampled; rapid acquisition is achieved at the expense of image signal. The *spin echo sequence* uses an excitatory pulse that deflects spins by 90° followed by a 180° refocusing pulse before the signal is sampled. Such a sequence allows signal-rich image acquisition at the expense of acquisition speed. The *fast spin echo sequence*, which is a modification, and is now the foundation of most modern MRI protocols, uses a 90° pulse followed by a series of 180° pulses, each of which yields an echo or signal. Such a sequence allows the rapid acquisition of high-quality images. Improved image contrast yielded by suppressing the signal from fat may be achieved either by the application of a frequency-selective fat suppression pre-pulse or by the application of an inversion pre-pulse (*inversion recovery sequence*) to any of the above sequences.

*Image contrast* Before tissue excitation, tissue protons align or rotate around the Z-axis of the magnetic field (the parent field) generated by the imaging magnet. Such alignment results in a net magnetization vector in the Z-axis described as longitudinal magnetization. Random rotation around the Z-axis (out of phase) results in neutralization of magnetization in the XY plane, or absence of transverse magnetization.

Following excitation, spins are deflected to the XY plane. Deflected spins now rotate in phase or as a single vector in the XY plane, which results in the presence of transverse magnetization. Magnetic vectors oriented in the XY plane lack longitudinal magnetization.

Following excitation and removal of the excitatory pulse, spins or in-phase magnetic vectors in the XY plane begin to diphase, leading to a loss of transverse magnetization. As protons diphase in the transverse plane, they reorient to the parent field and regain longitudinal magnetization. The recovery of longitudinal magnetization generates a $T_1$ signal; the loss of transverse magnetization generates a $T_2$ signal. If excitatory pulses are applied to tissue repeatedly, the movement of induced magnetic vectors becomes negligible. This is described as the steady state. If the excitatory pulse is applied repeatedly immediately following recovery of longitudinal magnetization (short TR, repetition time), prior to complete loss of transverse magnetization, sequential pulses induce steady-state transverse magnetization and therefore the yielded signal is from the recovery of longitudinal magnetization ($T_1$ weighted) (Fig. 2.17).

In contrast, if sequential excitatory pulses are applied after a delay that allows not only the recovery of longitudinal magnetization but also the complete loss of transverse magnetization (long TR), tissue weighting in the yielded image is a function of the time at which the signal is sampled (TE, echo time). If the signal is sampled early (short TE) it will

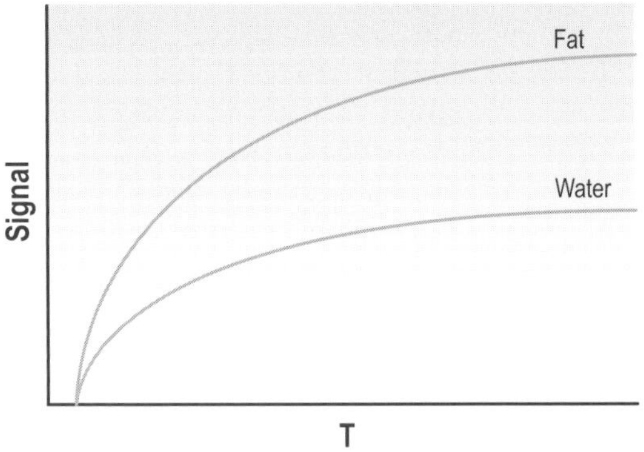


**Fig. 2.17** $T_1$ relaxation as a function of TR.

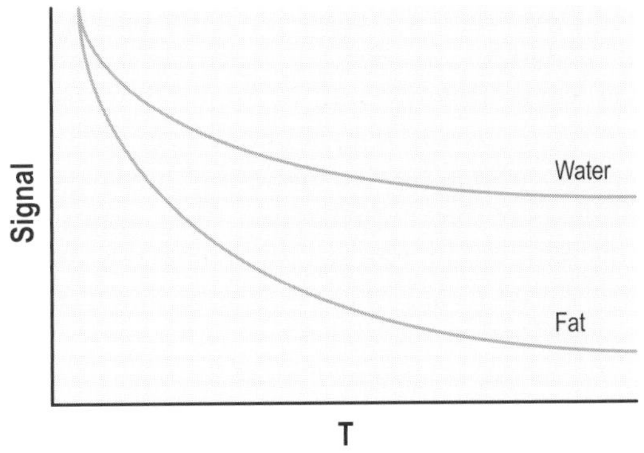


Fig. 2.18 $T_2$ decay as a function of TE.

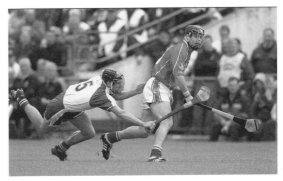

Fig. 2.19 Sports file.

contain both $T_1$- and $T_2$-weighted information (it reflects tissue proton density); if the signal is sampled late (long TE) it will contain predominantly $T_2$-weighted information. On $T_1$-weighted images, fat is hyperintense and fluid is hypointense; on $T_2$-weighted images, fat is hypointense and fluid is hyperintense (Fig. 2.18).

### Receiver coils

The electromagnetic signal generated by the excitatory pulse sequence is sampled by receiver coils, either body or surface coils. The movement of excited protons behaving like bar magnets within these coils generates the image signal.

Surface coils (in contrast to the body coil) are directly apposed to the excited extremity tissues and therefore yield an improved image signal. Simple surface coils may be flexible and conform to the configuration of a joint, thereby improving the image signal, although the field of view or coverage is limited. Variations include the quadrature coil (used routinely to image the knee), which simultaneously samples the signal in two planes to improve image quality. The phased-array coil represents an array of surface coils linked as a single segment, allowing improved coverage without loss of signal.

The ultimate quality of the derived MR image is a function of the type of magnet employed, the method of tissue excitation and the type of coil used to sample the signal.

## Clinical applications

The improved contrast and multiplanar imaging capability afforded by MRI has dramatically altered the understanding of musculoskeletal ailments of the spine and extremities in sports medicine.

## The extremities: intra-articular

### The knee

Magnetic resonance imaging is now routinely employed to evaluate patients with:

- suspected meniscal tears, which are characterized by identification of linear signal abnormality extending to a surface
- suspected cruciate ligament injury, particularly the anterior cruciate ligament, characterized by a primary alteration in the ligament configuration and by secondary signs including contrecoup bone bruises
- collateral ligament injuries, where edema and discontinuity are used as markers of injury.

Less commonly, MRI is used to evaluate the extensor mechanism, e.g. the patella tendon commonly injured in adolescent basketball players and the quadriceps tendon injured in poorly conditioned middle-aged adults. High-resolution imaging affords a detailed evaluation of articular cartilage, particularly at the patellofemoral articulation where a grading system is employed similar to arthroscopy (grades 1–3).

### The shoulder

Multiplanar imaging allows the detailed evaluation of the rotator cuff and the glenoid labrum. Rotator cuff injury, predominantly of the supraspinatus tendon, ranges from degenerative tendinopathy (signal abnormality on $T_1$-weighted scans) to partial (signal abnormality on all sequences particularly $T_2$-weighted scans) and then to full-thickness tears where hyperintense fluid is identified traversing the tendon resulting in communication between the shoulder joint and the subacromial bursa. The labrum is best identified in the axial plane where it is identified as a hypointense structure marginating the osseous glenoid. Most frequently, evaluation of the labrum is undertaken in patients with persistent unidirectional instability complicating dislocation when injury to the anteroinferior labrum is suspected.

Less frequently, MRI is undertaken to evaluate the superior labrum in patients with shoulder pain complicating a fall or throwing patients in whom a superior labral tear is suspected.

### Other joints

Magnetic resonance imaging is now routinely used to evaluate intercarpal ligaments (scapholunate and lunatotriquetral ligaments), the triangular fibrocartilage in the wrist as well as collateral ligaments, and the syndesmosis, long flexor, extensor, peroneal and Achilles tendons in the ankle. MRI is useful in visualizing the labrum in the hip as well as the collateral ligaments, the biceps, and brachialis and the triceps insertions at the elbow.



Intra-articular contrast, introduced either directly (direct arthrography) or by i.v. injection (indirect arthrography), is now commonly used to improve evaluation of joint structures. In this regard, MR arthrography has been shown to improve evaluation of the glenoid labrum and rotator cuff in the shoulder, of recurrent meniscal tears in the knee, of the collateral ligaments in the ankle and elbow, of the intercarpal ligaments in the wrist and the labrum in the hip.

## The extremities: extra-articular soft tissues

### Muscle injury

Muscle injury may follow a direct contusion or laceration, or follow indirect trauma acutely manifested as muscle strain or as delayed-onset muscle soreness (DOMS).

Muscle strains are graded according to severity. On MRI scans, first-degree strains are manifest as focal signal abnormalities without a tear, second-degree tears are seen as a partial tear, and third-degree tears are characterized by full-thickness tears with hemorrhage and retraction. Muscle tears most frequently occur during vigorous exercise and involve muscles that cross two joints, have an abundance of fast-twitch fibers and undergo eccentric contractions such as the gastrocnemii and hamstrings.

DOMS is most frequently identified in muscles with eccentric contractions following chronic overuse. On MRI, DOMS manifests as a local-signal abnormality most frequently at the muscle or fascial attachments, but occasionally at sites remote from the site of tenderness (Fig. 2.20).

## Blood vessels

Both non-contrast 'time of flight' and dynamic gadolinium techniques are used to image vascular injury. In this regard, MRI has been used in the evaluation of post-traumatic arterial laceration and thrombosis of deep veins within the pelvis.

## Infection

The ability of MRI to localize sites of edema identified via signal hyperintensity, particularly on fat suppressed images, allows the non-invasive evaluation of

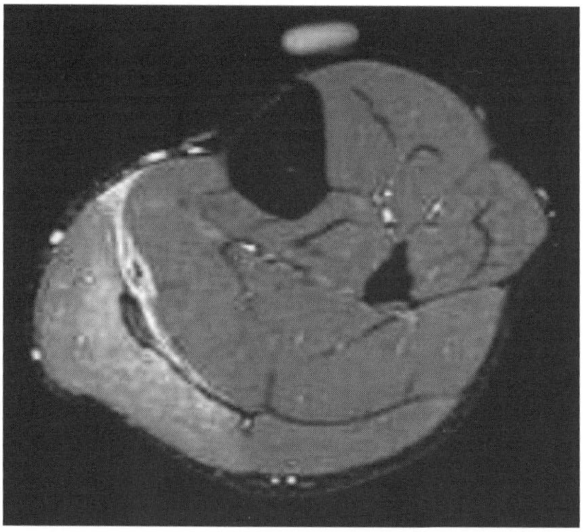

**Fig. 2.20** Axial fat-suppressed image showing hemorrhage and edema following a tear of the medial head of the gastrocnemius muscle.

soft-tissue infection, cellulitis, fasciitis and myositis. Although focal fluid pockets are readily identified on $T_2$-weighted fat-suppressed images, gadolinium enhancement may improve the evaluation of the extent of the inflammatory process.

### Tumors
Improved contrast resolution on MRI affords rapid localization and tissue characterization of soft tissue masses. Features suggestive of malignant masses include a heterogeneous signal within the masses, poorly defined margins, extensive poorly marginated edema within the adjacent soft tissues and dramatic enhancement within the mass following the administration of gadolinium.

### Bone marrow
Unlike conventional radiography, MRI allows the detailed evaluation of bone marrow and specifically allows the detection of marrow edema. Bone-marrow edema may reflect local trauma, the presence of a tumor, hyperemia in infection or inflammation or impaired drainage secondary to venous thrombosis as occurs in avascular necrosis or lymphatic obstruction.

Traumatic bone-marrow edema, termed a bone bruise, varies in pattern relative to mechanism. Impaction injury results in poorly marginated marrow edema; distraction injury results in linear marrow edema perpendicular to the axis of stress and shear injury results in linear bone-marrow edema, usually in oblique orientation.

## The spine

### Degenerative disk disease
The intervertebral disk is composed predominantly of water and mucopolysaccharide accounting for $T_1$-signal hypointensity and $T_2$-signal hyperintensity in health. In adulthood, as the disk degenerates, it loses water and mucopolysaccharide content resulting in morphologic changes, particularly loss of height of the disk and annular bulging.

The precursor to disk degeneration is thought to be tearing of the outer annular fibers anteriorly, laterally or posteriorly. In most cases, these annular tears are not identifiable on MRI. Occasionally, tears are conspicuous on heavily $T_2$-weighted scans as foci of hyperintensity (high-intensity zones or HIZs). secondary to the presence of edema and granulation tissue. Nerve roots apparently exit at the periphery of the annulus and may be irritated, accounting for the correlation between HIZs and low back pain. Disk herniations are well visualized in $T_1$-weighted scans contrasted against epidural fat. On $T_2$-weighted scans the herniated portion is usually slightly hyperintense relative to the rest of the degenerating disk. The compressed nerve root adjacent to the herniated disk may occasionally improve following the administration of gadolinium.

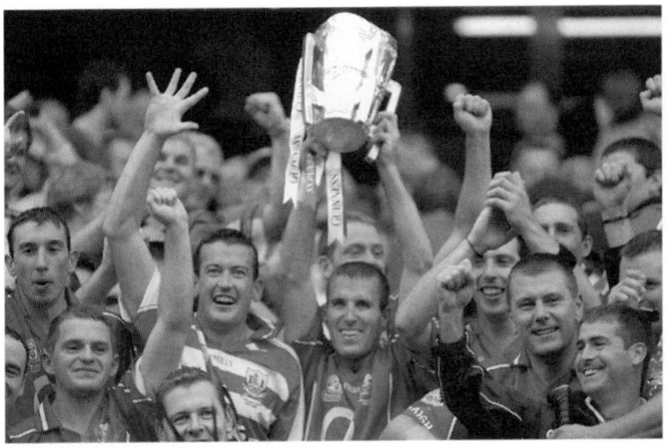

Fig. 2.21 Sports file.

Using MRI, signal abnormalities are identified in the marrow immediately adjacent to the vertebral body end-plate and degenerating disk preceding radiographic evidence of end-plate sclerosis. Early in diskogenic degeneration, end-plate marrow becomes $T_1$ hypointense and $T_2$ hyperintense (type 1 marrow change). Later, the marrow adjacent to the end-plate appears to become fatty and manifests as $T_1$-signal hyperintensity and persistent although slightly less marked $T_2$-signal hyperintensity (type 2 marrow change). In end-stage disease, the marrow becomes replaced by dense bone obvious on radiographs and hypointense on both $T_1$- and $T_2$-weighted scans at MRI. Both type 1 and type 2 marrow changes enhance following the administration of gadolinium and should not be incorrectly interpreted as being due to infection (Fig. 2.22).

### Trauma
Recognizing its ability to visualize soft tissues – including the intervertebral disk and spinal cord – MRI should be considered in patients with neurologic

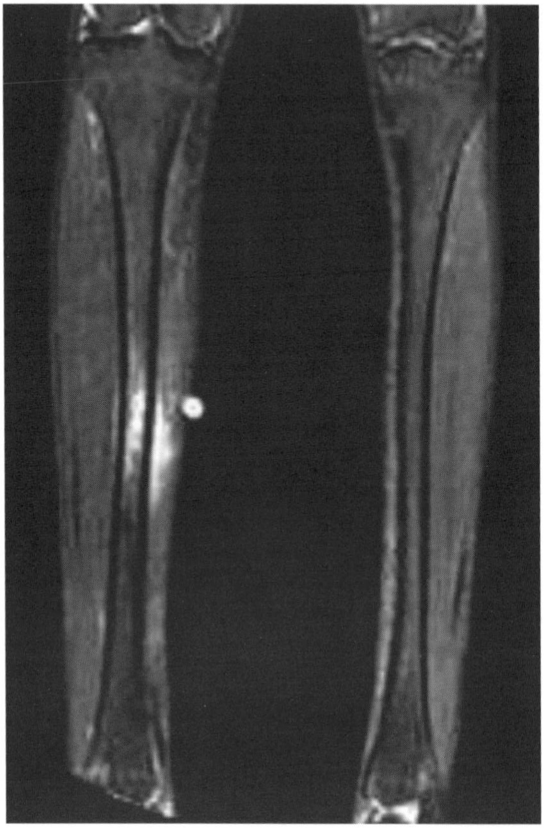

**Fig. 2.22** Fat-suppressed MR image showing right mid-tibia grade 3 medial tibial stress syndrome.



impairment, prior to either a closed or open reduction to determine the integrity of intervertebral disks. The presence of cord enhancement suggests the presence of edema rather than hemorrhage, and the presence of susceptibility artefact suggests cord hemorrhage rather than edema.

## Positron emission tomography (PET)

Positron emission tomography (PET) represents a scintigraphic technique in which an image is generated by recording the distribution of a cyclotron-produced positron emitter following i.v. injection. In general, PET images are generated by recording the distribution of deoxyglucose bound to positron-emitting fluorine-18. The distribution of glucose reflects tissue metabolic activity and hence is avidly consumed by active muscles. Within the skeleton, metabolic activity is maximal within the marrow space where uptake reflects the type of marrow; in effect metabolic activity is more marked within red marrow than within yellow marrow. As the volume of hemopoietic marrow decreases in skeletal maturity and old age, the uptake of $^{18}F$ deoxyglucose by the skeleton tends to decrease with age.

PET scanning is most frequently used in oncology, to stage the spread of primary tumors. In general, tumor cells over-express glut 2 receptors and hexokinase and concentrate glucose following i.v. injection. As a result, tumors cells concentrate the radiotracer and are readily identified as 'hot spots' on acquired images.

The use of PET scanning in sports medicine is (at the time of writing) limited to research studies of muscle function and metabolism (Fig. 2.23).

# ADDITIONAL DIAGNOSTIC STUDIES: MUSCLE COMPARTMENT PRESSURE STUDIES

The soft tissues of the forearm and calf are compartmentalized by thickened fascial bands which essentially support muscle contraction. During exercise or overuse of a specific muscle group, cellular swelling may raise pressure within specific compartments. Such pressure may rise to a critical point which, *although allowing that arterial pulsation impairs capillary perfusion*, leads to an accumulation of lactates. The associated induced acidity leads to further cellular swelling which raises pressures and compresses neurovascular structures to produce pain.

Acute compartment syndrome is uncommon in sports, occurring in patients with tibial midshaft fracture, secondary to direct muscle trauma, or following intense muscular activity.

Chronic exertional compartment syndrome (CECS) is the more common form and reflects muscular overuse, typically in the forearm of oarsmen or the calf of runners.

Measured by needle manometer, the diagnosis is made in a patient with 1-minute recovery compartment pressures of greater than 30 mmHg or the inability of the 5-minute postexercise pressure to decrease to less than 20 mmHg.

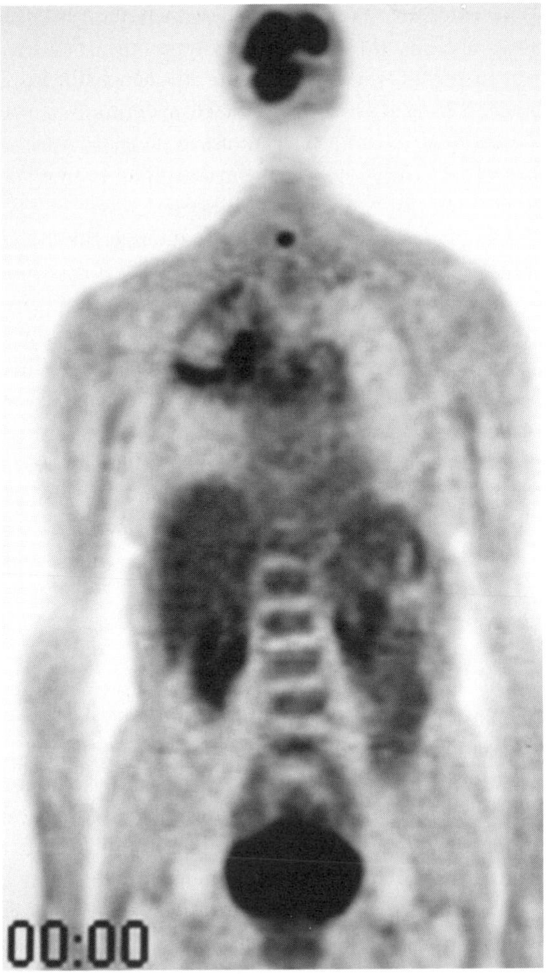


**Fig. 2.23** A whole-body PET scan is a map of glucose or metabolic activity, with high activity in the liver, bowel, brain and genitourinary tract in normality. Additional activity in this patient in the thorax is due to parenchymal inflammatory disease in the right upper lobe.

Recently, demonstration of edema at MRI in patients with compartment syndrome following exercise has been proposed as a non-invasive alternative to needle pressure studies in making this diagnosis.

The management of compartment syndrome may be difficult. Rest and cross-training are recommended in the first instance. Physical therapy, massage and correction of biomechanical factors that contribute to abnormal stress on affected muscle groups are also undertaken. Surgery is undertaken in a minority of patients. Elective fasciotomy allows the rapid compartment pressure decompression but in doing so may weaken the power of muscular contraction within the affected compartment. Following fasciotomy, no exercise should be undertaken for 6–8 weeks.

Preliminary data have suggested that the non-invasive measurement of tissue oxygen saturation using a near infrared spectrometer may obviate the need for invasive pressure measurements and allow the non-invasive diagnosis of compartment syndrome, manifested by a recorded reduction in tissue oxygen saturation levels.

## ADDITIONAL DIAGNOSTIC STUDIES: ISOKINETICS

The accurate assessment of human muscle performance has been the objective of exercise scientists and rehabilitation therapists for many decades. Exercise scientists interested in comparing the effects of various strength and conditioning programs seek to measure muscle force accurately. Practitioners of rehabilitation medicine want to document the efficacy of therapeutic exercise in helping patients, who are recovering from injury to the musculoskeletal system, to regain their strength. Athletic trainers and sport physical therapists emphasize injury prevention by identifying underlying deficits in strength and in bilateral and reciprocal muscle group strength relationships. Underscoring all these objectives is the valid and reliable quantification of human muscle capacity to produce force.

### Assessment of human muscle performance

The capacity of muscle to produce force can be assessed through either a static or dynamic contraction.

Isometric (static) assessment reveals the amount of tension a muscle can generate against a resistance permitting no observable joint movement.

Isotonic (dynamic) strength – the application of force through all or part of a joint's range of motion – can be assessed via a concentric (shortening) or eccentric (lengthening) mode of contraction.

## Isometric assessment

Isometric strength assessment measures a muscle's maximum potential to produce static force. Early objective testing of isometric strength was performed with cable tensiometry and hand-grip and back-lift dynamometry. The cable tensiometer, originally designed to measure the tension of aircraft control cables, was proposed and refined as a tool for measuring the strength of human muscle groups. Accurate measurement by this method depends on a number of factors, including body position, correct joint angle (i.e. that capable of generating the greatest force) and the correct location of the pulling strap on the body part serving as the fulcrum. Cable tensiometry is relatively inexpensive and capable of assessing most major muscle groups. The primary advantage of isometric resistance is that it can be used to assess strength in, or to exercise, a muscle group around a joint limited in motion by either pathology or bracing.

## Isotonic assessment

Isotonic strength can be measured dynamically with dumbbells, barbells and various commercial devices. The strength of a particular muscle group is commonly determined by testing the maximum amount of weight that can be lifted through a joint's range of motion for either one repetition (1 RM) or 10 (10 RM). The limitations of the RM tests include the inability to control test velocity and the amount of contribution from accessory muscle groups. Moreover, isotonic resistance is limited as an exercise modality in the sense that a muscle can be overloaded only by the amount of weight that can be lifted through the weakest part of the exercised range of motion.



Variable resistance equipment was designed to address this limitation; it accommodates the variations in strength by using an elliptical cam. The cam provides the least resistance where the ability to produce force is correspondingly lower (early and late in the range of motion) and the greatest resistance where the muscle is at its optimal length–tension and mechanical advantage (usually mid-range).

A distinct advantage of isotonic resistance is that it permits the exercise of multiple joints simultaneously. For example, the leg press exercises the quadriceps as a knee extensor and the hamstrings as a hip extensor. The resulting co-contraction may be advantageous in controling anterior shear or displacement of the tibia, which would result from isolated contraction of the quadriceps muscle group.

Another advantage of isotonic exercise of the lower extremity muscle groups is that it may be performed in a weight-bearing or 'closed kinetic chain' position. The squat exercise may be more transferable to functional weight-bearing activities of daily living and athletic participation. Clinicians also use techniques of manual muscle testing for a gross measure of a muscle group's ability to produce force through either a static or dynamic contraction respectively. For isometric assessment, the examiner places the joint to be tested in its mid-range of motion, evenly matches the force produced by the patient and subjectively grades the strength of the muscle group in question. Isotonic assessment may be performed by noting strength as the limb moves through its available range of motion.

## Isokinetic assessment

The concept of isokinetic exercise was developed by James Perrine and introduced in the scientific literature in 1967 by Hislop and Perrine. Isokinetic devices allow individuals to exert as much force and angular movement as they can generate – whether large or small – up to a predetermined velocity. When a limb's angular rate of movement equals or exceeds the preset velocity limit, the dynamometer produces an equaling counterforce to ensure a constant movement rate. Note that the limb, rather than the muscle, is moving at a constant rate. Mathematical evidence has been presented that demonstrates that a constant rate of angular limb movement is not accompanied by a constant rate of muscle shortening.

Isokinetic resistance has several advantages over other exercise modalities. One advantage is that a muscle group may be exercised to its maximum potential throughout a joint's entire range of motion. For example, at the mid-range of joint motion (where a muscle is at its optimum length–tension relationship for the binding of actin and myosin and has its greatest mechanical advantage) the isokinetic dynamometer will maintain its preset velocity, and thus more force will be produced. Conversely, at the extremes of joint motion (where a muscle is at a physiologic and mechanical disadvantage) the dynamometer will still maintain its preset velocity but less force will be produced. Because there is no fixed resistance to move through the weakest point in a given arc of motion (as with isotonic exercise), isokinetic exercise facilitates a maximum voluntary force to be produced throughout the entire range of motion.

Isokinetic resistance may also provide a safer alternative to other exercise modalities during the process of rehabilitation. Isokinetic exercise is inherently safer than isotonic because the dynamometer's resistance mechanism essentially disengages when pain or discomfort is experienced. An isokinetic apparatus may also be adapted to the particular rehabilitation challenge at hand. For example, exercise may be submaximal and easily set through pain-free ranges within the total available range of joint motion, and exercise velocities may be selected that have the least potential for joint insult. Isokinetic exercise may be used to quantify a muscle group's ability to generate torque or force, and it is also useful as an exercise modality in the restoration of a muscle group's preinjury level of strength.

A comparison of isometric, isotonic and isokinetic exercises is presented in Table 2.2.

## ADDITIONAL DIAGNOSTIC STUDIES: GAIT ANALYSIS

The gait cycle has been divided into different phases: stance and swing phases with associated impact on relevant lower limb weight-bearing joints. In the foot the biomechanics are complex involving the integrated motion of 57 articulating surfaces. During the gait cycle impaction forces are distributed to either one or both feet. The weight-bearing cycle is divided into heel strike, planted foot (Fig. 2.24) and toe-off phases (Fig. 2.25). On heel strike the hindfoot is

**Table 2.2** Comparison of isometric, isotonic and isokinetic exercises

| Exercise | Advantages | Disadvantages |
|---|---|---|
| Isometric | Useful when joint motion is contraindicated | Strength increases specific to exercised joint position |
| | Requires minimal or no equipment | Absence of feedback from objective increases in strength |
| Isotonic | Includes a natural component of concentric and eccentric resistance | Amount of resistance limited to weakest point in range of motion |
| | Positive reinforcement from progressive increases in resistance | Inability to quantify torque, work and power |
| | Permits exercise of multiple joints simultaneously | Stronger muscles may compensate for weaker muscle groups during closed kinetic chain exercise |
| | Is easily performed from weight-bearing closed kinetic chain positions | |
| Isokinetic | Permits isolation of weak muscle groups | Reliable assessment is limited to isolated muscle groups through cardinal planes of motion |
| | Accommodating resistance provides maximal resistance throughout the exercised range of motion | Exercise occurs primarily from non-weight-bearing open kinetic chain positions |
| | Accommodating resistance provides an inherent safety mechanism | Cost of equipment may be prohibitive for some settings |
| | Permits quantification of torque, work and power | |

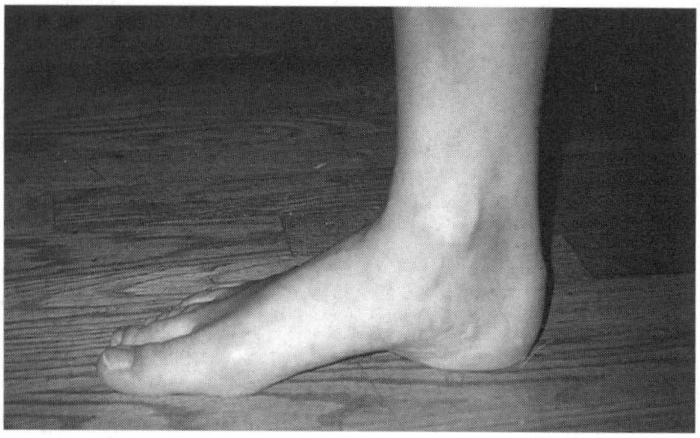

**Fig. 2.24** Planted foot phase.

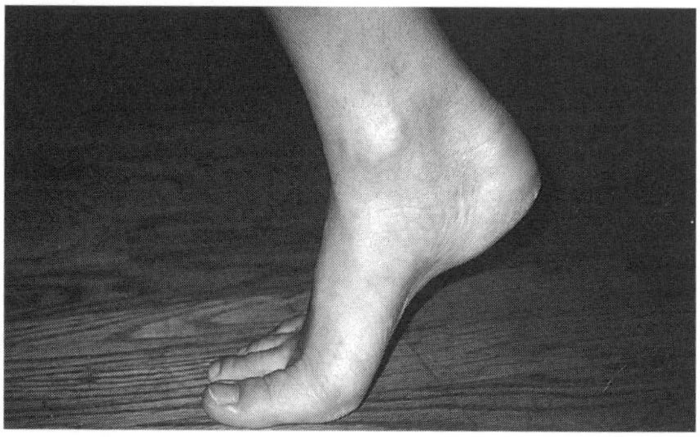

**Fig. 2.26** Toe-off phase. All the weight is transmitted through the base of the great toe.

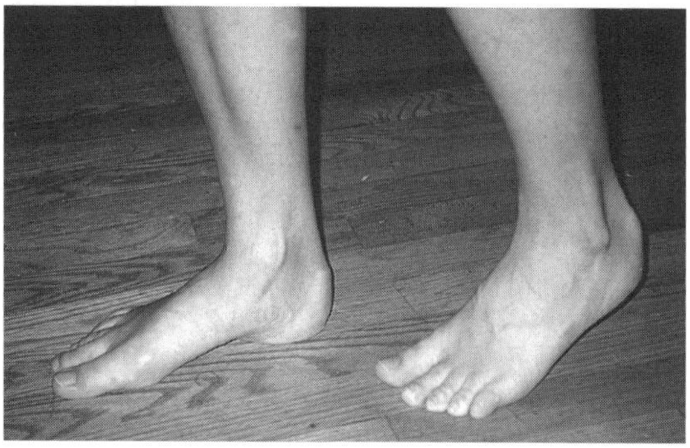

**Fig. 2.25** Toe-off phase on left, planted foot phase on the right.



everted, and the midfoot articulations are aligned and mobile, allowing the even distribution of impaction forces. As the foot is planted the long flexors of the calf begin to contract, elevating the medial longitudinal arch and drawing the calcaneus into neutral or varus. Such movement disrupts the alignment of the midfoot articulations and the foot becomes rigid or locked in preparation for the final toe-off phase in which all forces are transmitted to the base of the first toe propeling the foot forward (Fig. 2.26). Injury to bones, collateral ligaments, and both intrinsic and extrinsic muscle groups will manifest in alterations in this normal pattern, affect the gait and produce abnormal stresses on adjacent soft-tissue or osseous structures.

Any pathology affecting the lower limb can alter the gait in a specific way. The corollary of this is that a specific gait pattern abnormality can reflect a specific underlying pathology. Because there is so much happening during the gait cycle, sophisticated techniques have evolved to analyze gait patterns and abnormalities.

Movement analysis for the gait cycle and to assess other movements, e.g. golf swing assessment, is used in sports to avoid injury or improve performance, e.g. to study the technique of high sporting achievers or compare the same individual before and after a training module to allow assessment and feedback.

## Observational analysis

This is the most basic form of gait analysis and involves clinical assessment of the gait pattern while observing the patient walking from the side (sagittal plane) and from the front and back (coronal plane). This examination can distinguish different gait abnormalities such as antalgic (which is a painful limp with a shortened stance phase on the affected side), Trendelenburg (which reflects dysfunction of the abductor mechanism), short-leg gait and other patterns. The experienced clinician can identify pathologic gait patterns; however, it is subjective and not possible objectively to record the abnormality (qualitative analysis) or quantify the degree of abnormality to allow the assessment of progression or comparison of pre- and post-intervention patterns (quantitative analysis).

## Photography and video analysis

This involves studying serial photos or frame-by-frame analysis. Stride length and basic kinematics can be measured and the phases can be measured.

Modern video recording allows high-quality freeze-frame analysis from multiple angles and these fields of video can be digitized and assessed on computer.

## Opto-electronic movement analysis

These systems use a marker placed at specific anatomic locations on the subject. A very sensitive sensor can detect alterations in the position of the markers in three dimensions. The displacement of the markers in all three planes gives a large amount of information on displacement and kinematics. The data are processed rapidly and presented for analysis in a user-friendly image. Accuracy clearly depends on the precise placement of the markers and minimal movement of the skin relative to the deeper structures.

## Electromyography

This records electrical activity in the muscle. The electrodes are surface or fine-wire indwelling. Electromyography objectively assesses if a muscle is firing and the sequence of firing. The interaction of agonists and antagonists gives useful biomechanical information for sports and movement analysis.

## Force plate analysis

A force plate measures the force applied to it. It is different to a pressure platform, which shows the pattern of applied force across the surface. Force plates measure ground contact force of the whole body, for example at heel-strike and the changes in ground reaction force throughout the stance phase till toe-off. These data, which are kinetic, is usually combined with movement analysis data, which are kinematic.

# ADDITIONAL DIAGNOSTIC STUDIES: ELECTROMYOGRAPHY

## Neurologic injuries in athletes

A relatively small but significant number of sports injuries involve the peripheral nervous system.

At times these lesions are difficult to differentiate clinically from the more commonly encountered abnormalities of bone or soft tissue. In most cases the electromyography (EMG) examination can be of considerable assistance in making such distinctions as it is the premier laboratory diagnostic procedure for assessing the peripheral neuromuscular structures. It is useful not only for demonstrating the presence of these lesions but also for determining their location, pathophysiology and severity; the last two factors assist in accurate prognostication.

From the clinician's viewpoint, three distinct scenarios can ensue whenever a patient is referred to the EMG laboratory with the possibility of a neurogenic sports injury. First, the study may confirm that such a lesion is present and provide valuable data about it. Second, the examination may confirm that a neurogenic lesion is present but demonstrate that it is not the one suspected clinically; it may or may not prove to be a sports-related injury. Thus many patients are ultimately shown to have proximal mononeuropathies of the upper extremities, e.g. axillary or suprascapular mononeuropathies, having been referred to the EMG laboratory with the clinical diagnosis of brachial plexopathy. Moreover, occasionally the EMG examination reveals evidence of a neurogenic lesion that was erroneously attributed to a sports injury, e.g. an acute brachial neuropathy which develops in an athlete. Third, the EMG examination may reveal no evidence of a neurogenic lesion. If obvious clinical findings are present, such as muscle wasting, then these results point toward some musculoskeletal disorder causing disuse atrophy, which does not produce electrical abnormalities, e.g. patients with rotator cuff tears are often referred to the EMG laboratory with a diagnosis of axillary or suprascapular mononeuropathy, or of an upper trunk brachial plexopathy. Alternatively, if the physical examination is normal or inconsistent with the clinical presentation, then the accompanying normal EMG examination will encourage the clinician to consider that other than organic factors may be involved.

## The EMG examination

The EMG examination is not a standardized procedure from one laboratory to another. Nonetheless, in almost all EMG laboratories the study is a two-part process, composed of nerve conduction studies (NCS), and the needle electrode examination (NEE). Although most of these use much the same EMG equipment, they are independent entities, typically performed sequentially on each patient solely because they complement one another so well.

## Nerve conduction studies

The NCS comprise the newer portion of the EMG examination, having come into clinical use in the 1950s. They are customarily subdivided into 'basic' studies (e.g. motor, sensory and, to a lesser extent, mixed) and various 'special' studies (e.g., H-responses, F-waves and repetitive stimulation studies). The latter, generally, are of limited if any value with sports injuries and so will not be discussed here.

During motor NCS the nerve being assessed is stimulated percutaneously at one or two points along its course, while the response this elicits from one of the muscles it innervates is recorded with surface recording electrodes. The parameters measured during the motor NCS include the maximal amplitude of the compound muscle action potential (CMAP) evoked by nerve stimulation and reported in millivolts, which is a semiquantitative measure of the number of nerve fibers capable of conducting impulses between the stimulation point and the recording point.



For sensory NCS usually only one stimulation point is used and the tune of impulse transmission for the average, rather than the fastest, conducting fibers is determined, by measuring the interval between the shock artifact and the peak of the sensory nerve action potential (SNAP), as opposed to measuring to the onset of the response, which is done for the motor distal latency. Thus the parameters recorded for the typical sensory NCS are an amplitude in microvolts, and a 'peak latency' in milliseconds. The amplitude of the sensory NCS response is approximately 1/100 the amplitude of the motor NCS response because it represents a recording of a summated nerve action potential rather than a compound muscle action potential.

Of the *various* motor NCS parameters, the conduction velocity is the most widely known; many physicians erroneously assume the term 'nerve conduction velocity' is synonymous with 'nerve conduction studies'. In spite of its reputation, however, the conduction velocity is probably the least important of the measurements obtained during the NCS; the amplitude of the response is far more informative. This is because the conduction rates (both distal latencies and conduction velocities) are materially affected in most patients studied in the EMG laboratory only by certain demyelinating lesions (those causing focal slowing) occurring along the segment of nerve being assessed. In contrast, the amplitudes of the responses are affected not only by some demyelinating lesions (those causing conduction block or differential slowing) located along the nerve between the stimulation and recording points but also by axon lesions affecting the nerve fibers at any point at, or distal to, their cell bodies of origin, i.e. the anterior horn cells for motor fibers and the dorsal root ganglia (DRG) for sensory fibers. Thus NCS performed solely on a more distal portion of nerve fibers can detect evidence of axon loss that has occurred along their most proximal portion. For example, the ulnar sensory and motor NCS amplitudes, obtained by stimulating the ulnar nerve at the wrist while recording from the fifth finger and hypothenar eminence, respectively, are diminished by axon loss lesions located along the lower trunk of the brachial plexus. In addition, the SNAP amplitudes are more sensitive than the CMAP amplitudes for any given degree of incomplete axon loss, i.e. their amplitudes are typically decreased by milder degrees of axon loss than the motor amplitudes are, and when the lesion is of sufficient magnitude to affect both sensory and motor amplitudes, the former are relatively reduced. For these reasons, the SNAP amplitudes are the single most important NCS result when assessing for axon loss plexopathies and mononeuropathies. The sensory NCS are not affected by axon loss lesions occurring proximal to the DRG, e.g. at the root or spinal cord level, regardless of severity.

## Needle electrode examination

The needle electrode examination (NEE) is the older portion of the EMG examination, having achieved some clinical usefulness by the 1940s. The term 'EMG examination' in strict usage applies only to the NEE, although it has become a convenient label for the entire electrodiagnostic evaluation.

During the NEE a needle electrode is inserted into a muscle and the electrical activity generated within that muscle is assessed during three segments: needle movement; at rest; and voluntary muscle activation. Fibrillation potentials are one type of 'spontaneous activity' that can be seen when the muscle is at rest. They are repetitive action potentials generated by individual muscle fibers that (at least in the context of neurogenic disorders) have lost their nerve supply; they can neither be generated nor suppressed voluntarily. Fibrillation potentials are the cardinal NEE evidence of denervation. Unfortunately, they typically do not appear, or at least become fully established in the muscle, until about 21 days after nerve fiber injury. In contrast to fibrillation potentials, which are observed when the muscle is relaxed, voluntary motor unit potentials (MUPs) are seen when the patient contracts the muscle. A motor unit is composed of one anterior horn cell and all the muscle fibers innervated by it via its axons and neuromuscular junctions. Alterations in the firing pattern and external configuration of the MUPs are the predominant changes seen with neurogenic lesions. When an appreciable number of nerve fibers are not conducting impulses to the muscle, caused by either conduction block or axon loss (either acute or chronic), the MUPs during maximal effort fire in decreased numbers at a rapid rate. This is referred to as a 'neurogenic' MUP firing pattern. In contrast, with both upper motor neuron lesions and poor voluntary effort, the MUPs fire in similarly decreased numbers but at a slow to modest rate. During early reinnervation, the MUPs are of increased duration, low amplitude and highly polyphasic in configuration; these are called 'reinnervation' MUPs. With chronic neurogenic lesions collateral sprouting occurs, causing the surviving motor units to contain more than the usual complement of muscle fibers. As a result, the MUPs seen on NEE are of increased duration and sometimes increased amplitude; these are termed 'chronic neurogenic MUP changes'.

The NEE has several major disadvantages when compared with nerve conduction studies in that it is far more uncomfortable for the typical patient, it only assesses motor nerve fibers and it is very insensitive for detecting demyelination. Demyelinating lesions causing focal slowing along nerve fibers do not materially affect the NEE regardless of the degree of slowing, whereas demyelinatiug conduction block lesions register only when they are quite severe, by causing a neurogenic MUP firing pattern. These limitations, in many instances, however, are more than compensated for by the major benefits the NEE provides. In the first instance, it is extremely sensitive to motor axon loss. Each motor axon comprising a peripheral nerve supplying a limb muscle typically innervates several hundred individual muscle fibers.

### Limitations of the EMG examination

Even when both portions of the EMG examination are performed, certain significant limitations are encountered. One of these, too frequently unappreciated by the clinician, is the time that must elapse between when the lesion is sustained and when the EMG examination is performed.



## Further reading

De Lee JC, Drez, Jr D, Miller MD. Orthopaedic sports medicine, 2nd edn. Philadelphia, WB Saunders, 2003.

Eustace S. MRI of orthopaedic trauma. Philadelphia, Lippincott Williams & Wilkins, 1999.

Fitzgerald RH, Kaufer H, Malkani AL. Orthopaedics. Oxford, Mosby/Elsevier, 2002.

Greenspan A. Orthopedic radiology: a practical approach. Philadelphia, JB Lippincott, 1988; 7.1–7.34.

Horowitz AL. MRI physics for radiologists: a visual approach, 2nd edn. New York, Springer Verlag, 1992.

Stark DD, Bradley WG eds. Magnetic resonance imaging, Vols 1, 2, 2nd edn. Chicago, Mosby, 1992.

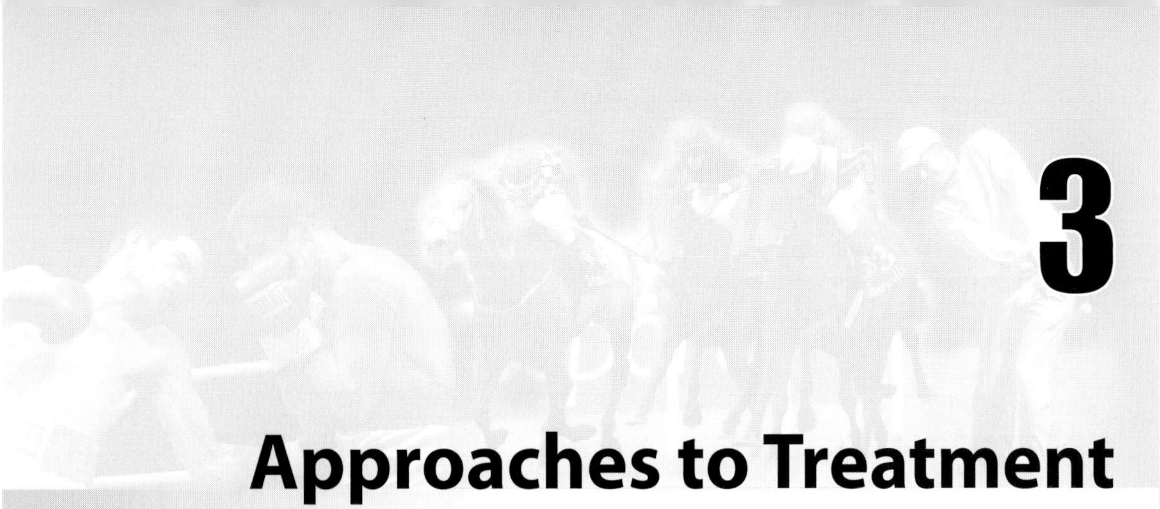

# 3 Approaches to Treatment



## THE MANAGEMENT OF PAIN AND INFLAMMATION IN ATHLETES

Sports and athletic injuries are characterized in two broad categories: acute macrotrauma and chronic microtrauma due to repetitive motion and overuse. Both the acute and chronic injuries initiate a human tissue response. Specifically, three phases of human tissue response are identified:

- acute vascular inflammatory phase
- repair–regeneration phase
- maturation phase.

Inflammation is one facet of the body's orderly progressive and interdependent biological repair process. Any treatment plan introduced by a sports medicine physician attempts to stimulate, enhance

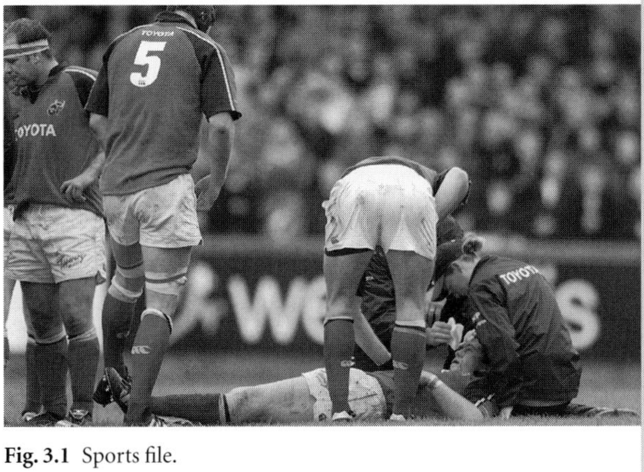


**Fig. 3.1** Sports file.

or expedite this process. Inflammation is histologically characterized by the following:

1. Dilatation of the vascular components, i.e. arterioles, capillaries and venules. There is also an associated increased permeability and blood flow.
2. Exudation of fluids.
3. Activation and release of immunologically active initiators.
4. Activation of hormonal response mechanisms.
5. Leukocyte migration to the inflammatory focus.

Neutrophilic activation leads to the formation of oxygen-free radicals, which lead to generation of arachidonic acid metabolites. This occurs via the breakdown of phospholipase structure through lipid peroxidation leading to the dissolution of the cell membrane. The initiation step in the inflammatory process is vascular injury. Factors in the inflammatory initiation include vasoactive substances, chemotactic factors, prostaglandins, and agents causing cell and tissue damage. This process in its entirety is initiated by vascular injury.

Vasoactive substances include vasoactive amines (histamine and serotonin), anaphylatoxins (C3a), and kinins (bradykinin). These cause vasodilatation and increase vascular permeability. Chemotactic factors include elements of the complement system kallikrein, peptides from fibrin and collagen, and bacterial products. These increase cell mobility and initiate and enhance directed cell movement. Prostaglandins, such as $PGE_2$ and $PCI_2$, are mediators of inflammation. $PGE_2$ also stimulates monocytes and enhances collagenase induction. Agents causing cell and tissue damage include collagenase, elastase and cathepsin G. These substances have a destructive effect on structural components such as collagen and elastin.

An understanding of the pathophysiology of pain and inflammation is critical if one is to understand the role of non-steroidal antiinflammatory drugs (NSAIDs) and corticosteroids as modulators of pain and inflammation resulting from sports injuries.

## NON-STEROIDAL ANTIINFLAMMATORY DRUGS

### Mechanism of action

There has been a recent interest in the mechanisms through which NSAIDs produce their effects. It is generally accepted that this class of medications has antiinflammatory, antipyretic and analgesic properties of varying degrees depending on the individual and the dose. Classically, the ability of NSAIDs to limit prostaglandin synthesis was believed to be the main mechanism responsible for the antiinflammatory effects. Recent studies have suggested that other mechanisms may be equally important (Box 3.1).

### Prostaglandin-related effects

The NSAIDs, as a class, have the ability to inhibit the production of prostaglandins, which are pro-inflammatory mediators. In 1971, Sir John Vane proposed this ability to be the primary mechanism of reducing inflammation. These drugs inhibit the enzyme cyclooxygenase (COX), which is responsible for the conversion of arachidonic acid to terminal prostaglandins. These terminal prostaglandins promote the inflammatory process and can excite or sensitize various neurons in producing pain.

There are at least two forms of COX enzymes present in humans. These distinct enzymes account for different roles in the normal physiologic processes. COX-1 (or PGH synthetase-1) is a constitutive enzyme present in most human tissues. COX-1 is essential for maintaining certain physiologic autoregulation processes. Regulation of the gastric mucosa, renal parenchyma and platelets depends somewhat on the prostaglandins produced by COX-1. Most untoward effects of NSAIDs are a result of the inhibition of COX-1. COX-2 (or PGH synthetase-2) is an inducible form of this isoenzyme and is only present in small amounts in tissues. The expression of COX-2 increases dramatically during inflammation due to mitogenic stimuli. Its expression has been shown to increase anywhere from 10- to 80-fold during inflammation. NSAIDs' ability to inhibit COX-2 is expected to be the major effector in decreasing inflammation.

Prostaglandins also play a large role in the production of painful stimuli. Hyperalgesia is commonly associated with the effects of $PGE_2$ on the PP receptor and $PGI_2$ on the IP receptor. Prostaglandins have also exhibited the ability to excite sensory neurons by increasing membrane Na and Ca permeability. The ability of NSAIDs to reduce painful stimuli has been beneficial in improving the rehabilitation of musculoskeletal injuries.

**Box 3.1 Classes of non-steroidal antiinflammatory drugs (NSAIDs)**

Salicylic acid derivatives
Arylpropionic acids
Acetylsalicylic acid
Ibuprofen
Sodium salicylate
Naproxen
Choline magnesium trisalicylate
Flurbiprofen
Salicylate
Ketoprofen
Diflunisal
Fenoprofen
Salicylsalicylic
Oxaprozin
Sulfasalazine
Fenamates
Indole and indene acetic acids
Mefenamic acid
Indomethacin
Meclofenamic acid
Sulindac
Enolic acids
Etodolac
Oxicams
Heteroaryl acetic acids
Piroxicam
Diclofenac
Tenoxicam
Ketoralac
Pyrazolidinediones
Tolmetin
Phenylbutazone
Oxyphenthatrazone
Alkanones
Nabumetone

There has been recent interest in the idea of other mechanisms accounting for the antiinflammatory effects of NSAIDs. It has been shown that certain nonacetylated salicylates are only weak inhibitors of COX *in vitro*. However, they demonstrate decreased clinical evidence of inflammation as well as other NSAIDs. This leaves open the question of what other mechanisms may be involved in limiting inflammation.

## Non-prostaglandin effects

NSAIDs have the inherent ability to inhibit a number of membrane-associated processes. These drugs have the physiochemical ability to intrude into biological membranes and disrupt protein–protein interactions, which are needed for cell function. NSAIDs have also been observed to interfere with neutrophil–endothelial cell adherence. This is critical in the organism's response to inflammation. A variety of other membrane-associated processes are affected by NSAIDs. NSAIDs inhibit the NADPH (nicotinamide adenine dinucleotide phosphate) oxidase of neutrophils in a cell-free system, which reduces superoxide anion generation. The uncoupling of oxidative phosphorylation and the inhibition of phospholipase C activity has also been observed. Glycosaminoglycan synthesis by articular cartilage is also apparently inhibited by certain NSAIDs. This suggests that the antiinflammatory properties of NSAIDs are not restricted to the inhibition of prostaglandin synthesis.

## NSAIDs in sports injury

There is little doubt of the ability of NSAIDs to decrease the production of inflammatory mediators at sites of injury to limit pain. Their use in treating soft-tissue injuries has been common in sports medicine. Questions have been raised as to whether or not this use is truly of benefit. The antiinflammatory effect may be inconsequential to adequate healing. There is also some thought as to where a reduction in inflammatory response may actually lengthen healing.

An inflammatory response clearly develops in response to soft-tissue injury. Animal models have demonstrated this response within 48 hours. This is accompanied by significant muscle weakness, which is most pronounced at 48–96 hours after injury. This same type of response has been demonstrated in muscle strains in human studies. The inflammatory response results in the liberation of mediators responsible for pain, swelling and the limitation of activity. Thus, one of the proposed benefits of NSAID use in this setting is that by limiting these events, there is an earlier return to activity. This inflammatory response, however, may be somewhat beneficial by removing cellular debris from sites of injury to allow quicker healing. The use of NSAIDS in acute soft-tissue injury has proven beneficial in a number of clinical studies. An interesting trial conducted by Dudley and colleagues examined the efficacy of the NSAID naproxen sodium on exercise-induced muscle injury and soreness. In this double-blind, crossover study, healthy adult males were exercised for 10 sets of 7 to 10 eccentric quadriceps femoris muscle contractions at 85% of their one repetition maximum. They were then treated with naproxen sodium or placebo for 10 days. Naproxen sodium appeared to improve recovery after this form of exercise. This recovery from muscle soreness and injury was believed to be due to the attenuated expression of the inflammatory response to injury.

Beneficial effects have also been documented in other studies. A large review of NSAID use in acute ankle sprains for the most part revealed positive effects. Placebo-controlled studies with diclofenac have shown significant improvement in pain relief and inflammation in ankle injuries. Another study review demonstrated that ibuprofen was effective in improving the progress of rehabilitation of ankle injuries. In all of these studies, there was no significant difference in the ultimate outcome of these injuries.



On the other hand, there has been evidence to show no clinical benefit or even the possibility of delayed healing in injuries treated with NSAIDs. Labelle and Guibert examined the treatment of lateral epicondylitis with diclofenac along with immobilization. This was a double-blind, randomized, placebo-controlled trial of 4 weeks' duration. The experimental group was given diclofenac sodium (150 mg) daily, whereas the control group received a placebo. Both groups were treated with cast immobilization for 2 weeks. There was a decrease in reported pain in the diclofenac group that was significant. There was no clinically significant improvement, however, in grip strength or function. Side-effects such as diarrhea and abdominal pain were more frequent in the experimental group.

Almekinders and Gilbert raised the question of delayed muscle regeneration as a result of anti-inflammatory treatment. Using an experimental animal model, they demonstrated that muscle strains continue to weaken in the early postinjury period. Histologic examination of the muscle strains revealed delayed inflammatory reaction and delayed muscle regeneration in a group treated with piroxicam. Both groups, however, showed muscle regeneration by day 11 of the study. This possibility of delayed muscle healing in minor stretch injuries must be considered.

Another trial evaluated acute hamstring injuries treated with NSAIDs. This treated both treatment and placebo groups with the same physiotherapy regimen. Meclofenamate and diclofenac were the drugs used for this trial. The reduction of pain and swelling, and a return to normal strength, was no better with or without NSAIDs. Surprisingly, in the group with severe strains, the reduction of pain was better in the placebo group. As a result, this study did not advocate the use of NSAIDs in acute hamstring strains.

Clearly, there is no consensus of opinion of the true place NSAIDs have in the treatment of acute soft-tissue injuries. More studies need to be performed for specific injuries to give clinicians more information to better evaluate their usefulness.

## New advances

The most common side-effect of NSAID use is the toxicity to the gastrointestinal (GI) tract represented by dyspepsia, gastritis and ulceration. A third to a half of all patients who die of ulcer-related complications have recently been on NSAID therapy. Studies have shown the current use of NSAIDs to be linked with a 4- to 30-fold increase in the risk of ulcer disease. This aspect of NSAID use presents a real danger that must not be underestimated. Attempts at reducing this risk should be advanced in the future. The predominant mechanism resulting in GI toxicity is the inhibition of prostaglandin synthesis. Prostaglandins normally have a protective effect on the gastric mucosa by inhibiting acid secretion, raising bicarbonate levels, increasing mucus secretion, maintaining mucosal blood flow and altering mucosal permeability to $H^+$ ions. The NSAID-induced reduction in prostaglandins compromises the physiologic defense mechanisms of the gastric mucosa. Compensatory regulation mechanisms of the kidney are also disrupted.

As mentioned above, the inhibition of prostaglandin production is the result of inhibiting COX enzymes. There has been a considerable amount of interest in developing NSAIDs that will selectively inhibit COX-2 while sparing COX-1. Essentially, this type of product could be devoid of GI and renal adverse effects. Recent studies have shown that such a reduction in GI and renal adverse effects may be at the expense of the rare spurious complication of venous thrombosis and stroke, currently resulting in the removal of a number of commonly prescribed COX-2 inhibitors from the clinical market.

Two of the newer NSAIDs appear to be more COX-2 selective than previous drugs. Nabumetone is a once-daily NSAID whose active metabolite *in vivo* is 6-methoxy-2-naphthylacetic acid. Fluorobiprofen, ibuprofen and meclofenamate were found to be equipotent inhibitors of each COX isoform. Although piroxicam, indomethacin and suldinac inhibited COX-1 10 to 30 times as powerfully as COX-2, not all studies have given evidence of this COX-2 selectivity. In some human models nabumetone at adequate dosage inhibited both isoforms of COX equally.

Etodolac is another newer antiinflammatory agent that appears to demonstrate some degree of COX-2 selectivity. In an *in-vitro* study with human cells, etodolac had ten times more inhibitory effect on COX-2 than COX-1. However, COX-1 inhibition increased as dosages increased. Neustadt showed etodolac to be equally effective, if not superior, to ibuprofen in clinical response and had fewer side-effects of dyspepsia. Currently, none of the NSAIDs specifically inhibit the inducible COX isoenzyme. The development of such a drug would possibly greatly decrease the adverse effects.

## Topical NSAIDs

Altering the drugs specificity for COX is not the only way to try to reduce side-effects. Topical preparations which could potentially spare the gastric mucosa, as well as renal parenchyma, have been used quite frequently in Europe. The pharmaceutical compounding of NSAIDs in the USA has also become common. This has made topical preparations an alternative in acute soft-tissue injury.

Topical application does appear to lessen the presence of GI side-effects. This is probably because of a decrease in blood concentrations compared with an oral or intramuscular (i.m.) dose. Blood concentrations after topical administration will reach less than 10% of levels after oral or i.m. administration. NSAID levels are found in muscle and subcutaneous tissue after topical use. The result is much less frequent GI and renal adverse effects and fewer drug interactions; the most prevalent side-effect is a local rash at the site of application. Their efficacy in treating soft-tissue injury has also been studied. One of the largest studies of this type was carried out by Russell. Use of piroxicam 0.5% gel was associated with an improvement in pain scores, improved joint motion and decreased tenderness versus placebo. These improvements were significant in tendinitis but not in sprains. Naproxen gel also had superior ratings in subjective complaints by patients after injury. Interestingly, in this study there was no improvement in physician-measured treatment response. The same type of results were also found in two other studies using ketoprofen and indomethacin.

The use of these topical preparations may have a role in the treatment of sports injuries. Even without significant evidence of objective benefit, there is good proof of improvement in objective symptoms.

There are also data to suggest fewer gastric and renal effects. The improvement in symptoms can be valuable in improving rehabilitation.

## Prevention of gastrointestinal toxicity

Along with the previously mentioned attempts at COX specificity, there has been interest in the prophylaxis of GI pathology. Treatment with prostaglandin analogs has been studied to a certain degree. This type of therapy has proven to be beneficial in the at-risk population.

Misoprostol is a $PGE_1$ analog, which is a well-established drug in preventing NSAID-induced ulcerations. The use of misoprostol has been effective in preventing gastric and duodenal ulcerations. The recent misoprostol ulcer complication safety assessment (MUCOSA) study revealed a 40% reduced risk of gastric pathology compared with the placebo. Misoprostol as a twice-daily dosage was also beneficial in lowering the incidence of ulcerations. This dosage is half of the normal dosage and accounted for less complaints of diarrhea.

The hydrogen–potassium pump inhibitor omeprazole has not been studied thoroughly in the prevention of NSAID-induced gastropathy. One study conducted for 3 months concluded that omeprazole provided adequate prevention of gastric ulceration and dyspepsia. The $H_2$-blockers have not proven to be as effective as misoprostol in the prophylaxis of gastric ulcerations but they may be effective in duodenal ulceration.

### Bromfenac

Bromfenac sodium is a peripherally acting analgesic of the NSAID class. It is newly approved by the US Food and Drug Administration and has indications for the short-term management of pain. It is not indicated for chronic management of osteoarthritis or rheumatoid arthritis. As such, there is potentially a place for bromfenac in the treatment of pain and inflammation associated with acute sports-related musculoskeletal injury. There are currently no available studies evaluating its use for this specific indication.

In clinical studies cited in its package insert, a 25-mg dose of bromfenac was comparable to 550 mg of oral naproxen sodium and 400 mg of ibuprofen in postsurgical pain relief. It has also shown to be effective in treatment of pain associated with dysmenorrhea. Another postorthopedic surgery study proved bromfenac to be 11 to 16 times more potent an analgesic than ibuprofen. Adverse events seen with bromfenac are similar to those with other NSAIDs. Cohen examined GI blood loss induced by bromfenac, aspirin and placebo. This 22-day randomized study showed fecal blood loss with bromfenac and aspirin to be higher than with placebo; however, the bromfenac-treated group had less blood loss than the aspirin group. The dose of bromfenac in this study was three times that normally recommended. There does not appear to be a need for dosage adjustment in patients with renal dysfunction. Elderly patients of either gender do not appear to require adjusted doses.



### Ketoralac tromethamine

Ketoralac tromethamine is another peripherally acting analgesic of the NSAID class. It is indicated for short-term management of moderately severe pain. It is a potent NSAID analgesic and should not be used for chronic pain owing to its side-effect profile when used longer than 5 days.

### Leukotriene inhibitors

A new class of antiinflammatory medications recently entered the marketplace. These medications work through the modulation of leukotrienes, which are proinflammatory mediators produced from arachidonic acid by the enzyme 5-lipoxygenase. There are two drugs that work through different pathways: zileuton and zafirlukast. These drugs are indicated for the treatment of chronic asthma. There has been some interest in their effects on inflammation in soft tissues. Zileuton is an inhibitor of leukotriene synthesis. It acts by directly inhibiting the enzyme 5-lipoxygenase. It has been proved clearly useful in the treatment of the inflammation associated with chronic asthma. Zafirlukast produces similar effects by working through a slightly different mechanism. It is a leukotriene receptor antagonist. It does not have an effect on the production of leukotrienes but blocks their action on peripheral receptors.

Though effective in asthma, their use in soft-tissue inflammation outside of the respiratory tract is of interest. Weinblatt and associates performed a clinical study of zileuton in patients with rheumatoid arthritis. It was documented *in vitro* that there was a decrease in levels of leukotriene $B_4$. But, *in vivo*, there was no significant difference in joint swelling, patients or investigators assessment, or number of swollen or painful joints between zileuton or placebo.

Another study assessed the efficacy of leukotriene synthesis inhibitors with or without NSAIDs as treatment options for rheumatoid arthritis.. In this study, there was a significant decrease in inflammation seen when naproxen was used with either leukotriene synthesis inhibitor. As a result of this study, it is reasonable to believe that combinations of NSAID and leukotriene inhibitor may prove effective in soft-tissue inflammation.

## CORTICOSTEROIDS

The use of corticosteroids in the treatment of sports injuries is quite widespread and controversial. Inconsistency in the studies on corticosteroid use does not lend adequate support or direction to the sports medicine clinician in their use. There are many reasons the research is perceived as inconsistent. One is the lack of a reproducible animal model of overuse. Second, animal studies are usually carried out on healthy, not diseased or injured tissue. Additionally, extrapolation from animal models to human application is difficult. Also, studies of cell monolayers may be helpful in the studies of NSAIDs but not of the effect of corticosteroids on the three-dimensional collagen matrix.

The mechanism of antiinflammatory action that corticosteroid has is understood at this time primarily to be the following:

1. *Through the direct inhibition of phospholipase* This disrupts the inflammatory arachidonic acid cascade and limits the production of mediators of inflammation by both the COX and lipoxygenase pathways.
2. *Through the redirection of lymphocyte traffic* This effectively causes white blood cells to be retained in the lymphatic system, which prevents the movement of white blood cells to the area of injury. The chemotactic or chemoattractant process is greatly limited.
3. *Through the inhibition of cytokine expression e.g., interleukin-1 (IL-1) and tumor necrosis factor (TNF), both part of the cell-mediated immune response to injury*, IL-1 is produced primarily by monocytes and macrophages. Also involved are various parenchymal cells, such as synovial cells, epithelial cells, fibroblasts, endothelial cells, mesangial cells and several tumor cell lines. IL-1 induces both immune and inflammatory reactions. It induces the production of several proteins by endothelial cells, thus modulating thrombus formation and the activation of the immune/inflammatory cells. Other proteins induced by IL-1 include procoagulant proteins and adhesive factors for neutrophils, monocytes and lymphocytes. IL-1 also stimulates endothelial cell arachidonic acid metabolism and the synthesis of $PGE_2$ and $PGI_2$. TNF has similar effects by stimulating the production of procoagulant neutrophil chemotactic factors, and adherence proteins for granulocytes. Corticosteroids modulate inflammation through an effect on not only the prostaglandin production but by modulating the cytokine activity in the parenchymal tissue as well as the cellular components.
4. *Through the stabilization of the cell membrane* This effect involves the cell membranes of the vascular elements as well as other cellular components. By stabilizing vascular structures, capillary permeability is diminished thus decreasing the displacement of fluid and cellular components from the intravascular space. Membrane stabilization is also helpful in preventing the release of lysosomal enzymes. Neutrophils are also prevented from releasing their degrading enzymes.

Although side-effects cannot be extensively discussed in this chapter, some are worth mentioning. Impaired wound healing is the most common and consistent side-effect of corticosteroid use. Corticosteroids effectively abolish collagen synthesis in granulation tissue and inhibit fibroblastic function in cell culture. Immune suppression, osteoporosis and osteonecrosis are other complications. Side-effects may also vary in different individuals; it appears to depend on individual differences in plasma protein binding. The route of administration (i.e. oral versus injection) also determines (to some degree) the side-effects that are expressed.

There is a lack of peer review studies on the clinical use of corticosteroids. Their use, both when to use and the dosage to use, has been very arbitrarily determined. Some studies have indicated clinical improvement in patients with lumbar disk disease with short-term use of oral corticosteroids. Holt and associates showed that clinical improvement and return to sport was expedient in athletes with osteitis pubis who were treated with corticosteroids injected into the pubic symphysis. It is generally agreed that injections around tendons should be approached with caution owing to the effect of corticosteroids on ligament and tendon-type tissue. In addition, the number of injections should be limited but this number is still quite arbitrary. Some clinicians have indicated a reluctance to use injections whereas others may consider up to four or five injections if the condition is improving.

There is also some debate concerning a restricted activity period for the anatomic area injected. Recommendations generally range within the 10- to 14-day time frame. The frequency of injection is also quite arbitrary. Although most clinicians would recommend injections no more frequently than 2 to 4 weeks, there is not a peer review, double-blind study to establish this as protocol.

In selecting an injected corticosteroid, one has to consider the desired duration of action. The shorter-acting corticosteroids are more soluble and theoretically have less potential for complications, especially when injected around tendons.

One also has to be aware of other active ingredients in the injectable preparations. Contents, such as phenol or benzoyl alcohol, may be very caustic to soft tissue. Compounds such as sodium bisulfite may be responsible for anaphylactic reactions seen in sensitized patients.

Corticosteroids may also be delivered with phonophoresis or iontophoresis. The literature is also unclear concerning the efficacy and potential side-effects when corticosteroids are used in this way. These are common physical therapy modalities especially used to treat some of the more chronic problems in athletics, such as tendinitis or bursitis.

Given orally, corticosteroids also exert an intense antiinflammatory effect. Medrol dose pack is a common oral form used. Many different 'customized' prescriptions of prednisone have been touted as a regimen for treating chronic or acute injuries in athletes. If given for more than a few days, a definite tapering protocol should be followed.

So how should the sports medicine clinician approach the usage of corticosteroids? Since the early part of the 20th century, they have been recognized as our most potent inhibitors of inflammation; one would want them in their treatment armamentarium. Conversely, they have some significant side-effects that have to be monitored closely when used in a clinical setting.

As one reviews the literature, it is clear that most of the information published is anecdotal, containing case reports, retrospective studies and studies that are largely uncontrolled. The clinician is largely left to determine his or her own regimen or protocol for use of corticosteroids but this should be done with caution until better studies are available. The sports medicine clinician does have at his or her disposal an incredible armamentarium of drugs in the non-steroidal antiinflammatory class. There are also multiple choices among injectable corticosteroids drugs. It is clear when reviewing the literature that a much better understanding of the use of these drugs is needed. Thought and consideration needs to go into choosing the NSAID or the injectable cortisone drug as it applies to each individual situation (Box 3.2).

**Box 3.2 Local and systemic complications with local injections of corticosteroids**

**Local**

Subcutaneous atrophy

Pigmentation abnormalities

Tendon/ligament rupture

Flare reactions

Infections/sterile abscess

Peripheral nerve injury

Muscle damage

Vascular injury

**Systemic**

Significant transient hyperglycemia

Vasovagal symptoms/syncope

Psychologic problem

Systemic allergic reactions

Hypothalamic–pituitary–adrenal axis suppression

Avascular necrosis

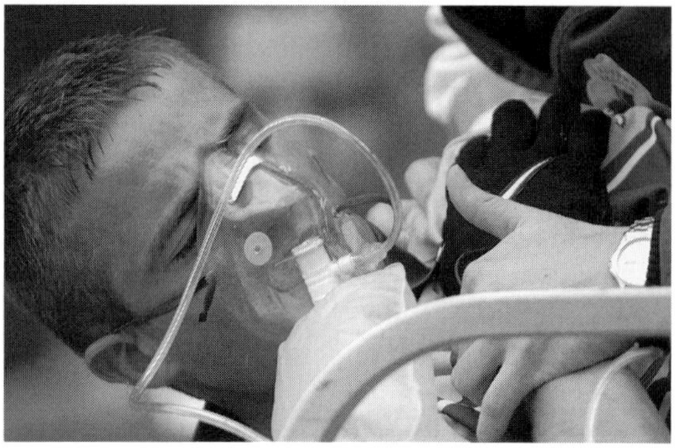

**Fig. 3.2** Sportsfile.

## LITHOTRIPSY

Extracorporeal lithotripsy was initially introduced as a treatment for renal calculi. Focused sound waves generated by the induced movement of crystals by an applied current source to a delivery probe are aimed at a localized region. These focused waves produce a local pressure wave, capable of providing a dramatic pressure shock that can fragment calculi.

More recently, a similar technology has been applied to fragment calculi and soft-tissue calcifications occurring in the rotator cuff in the shoulder in patients with calcific tendinitis, and in the common extensor and flexor tendons at the elbow in patients with tennis elbow, in the patella tendon, and in the treatment of chronic inflammation in patients with plantar fasciitis. In each setting, lithotripsy or shock-wave therapy is combined with a period of immobilization and/or local steroid injection therapy. The mechanism of action of the treatment is unclear although it is postulated that the shock waves promote local hyperemia and subsequent improved healing, and that it induces neuropraxia in nerves decreasing induced pain. There is limited scientific assessment of the therapy although preliminary studies have cast doubt on its use on tennis elbow, while supporting its use in the treatment of plantar fasciitis. Beneficial effects are often recorded immediately following therapy though secondary to neuropraxia, while more delayed effects at 2–4 weeks are attributed to the enhanced tissue-healing effects.

Beyond soft-tissue treatments, lithotripsy has been employed to promote healing at the site of non-union fractures and has been employed as an alternative to core decompression in the treatment of stage 1 avascular necrosis of the femoral head. When employed in the setting of avascular necrosis, lithotripsy is thought to induce microfractures and hemorrhage with local delivery of new stem cells. Improvement in this setting is delayed and occurs as late as 3 months following treatment, reflecting the healing of bony trabeculae and neovascularization.

No adverse effects have been reported.

## SONOTHERAPY

Sonotherapy comprises sound waves delivered from a crystal source at 1 Mhz, which, when delivered in a continuous form, result in mild heating of both deep and superficial soft tissues. The induced hyperemia is thought to improve collagen synthesis and induce improved mechanical strength.

## CRYOTHERAPY

In practice, the application of ice or cold therapy is the most common method used by clinicians treating sports injuries. Cryotherapy can be administered with ice packs, customized cold packs, ice massage or cold whirlpool baths. Clinically, the primary goal is the prevention of swelling by blocking the histamine response and impeding edematous fluids from building up at the injury site as well as any secondary injury that may have occurred due to surrounding tissue hypoxia. The body's response to cryotherapy application includes vasoconstriction, decreased cellular metabolism and temperature, decreased peripheral nerve conduction, and a decrease in pain. These effects are commonly useful during an acute injury or in the immediate post-operative period in which a localized inflammatory response has occurred with resultant swelling and pain.

Cryotherapy can also reduce spasticity in neurologic conditions through a decrease in muscle spindle activity. The normal sensation experienced by the patient receiving cryotherapy is a sequence of cold, burning, aching and finally numbness.

Typically, cold packs are applied for 20 minutes with periodic skin checks to prevent blister and frostbite formation. Ho and others studied the effects of icing time on skeletal blood flow, bone metabolism and knee temperatures. The results indicated that the optimal time of icing a knee is 25 minutes, which resulted in a three- to fourfold increase in the desired effects. Cold application will also decrease nerve conduction speed through the 'gate' theory mechanism and prevent or slow pain impulses from reaching the brain. Therefore occasional ice or cold massage may be used prior to range of motion or stretching such as cold spray and stretch. Clinical trials conducted by Osbahr and others reported the effects of continuous commercial cold therapy to the shoulder joint following rotator cuff repair surgery The investigators reported that the continuous cold group exhibited significantly cooler subacromial space temperatures as compared to the control group. Martin and others

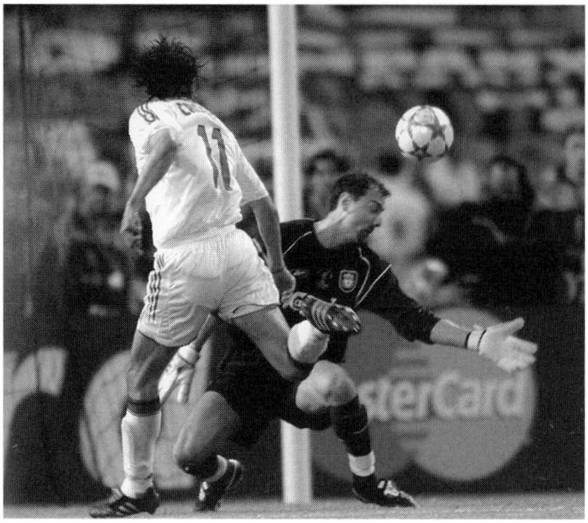

Fig. 3.3 Sports file.

determined a statistically significant decline of 2°C in the knee's intra-articular temperature with the application of cryotherapy and compression after routine knee arthroscopy. The contraindications to cryotherapy are cold allergy, hypersensitivity skin irritation, compromised circulation and cold intolerance. Continuous cold therapy over nerve tissue, for example the peroneal nerve, should be avoided.

Reports comparing cold whirlpool baths to ice packs suggest that cold whirlpool therapy allows more prolonged deep soft-tissue temperatures than ice packs, although similar temperatures are achieved in the deep compartments. Ice therapy, in contrast, has been shown to lead to more marked temperature reduction within the near-field superficial soft tissues.

Although one can find studies for and against cryotherapy, the weight of opinion suggests a beneficial impact on reducing inflammation and pain within soft tissues following injury and surgery.

No adverse effects have been reported.

## HEAT THERAPY

Hot packs are a form of superficial therapeutic heat. They are frequently used to assist in the treatment of a variety of injuries. Through conduction, moist heat is capable of reaching subcutaneous tissues to a depth of up to 1 cm. The application of heat causes vasodilatation with resultant increases in local circulation, thus increasing the delivery of oxygen and nutrients to the area. Generally these packs are stored in a hydrocollator unit maintained at a temperature of 170°F (76.7°C).When hot packs are in contact with skin, the temperature is raised by a few degrees (to 104°F, which is 40°C) and maintained for only a very short period. The topical application of heat may aid in relieving pain by the stimulation of cutaneous thermoreceptors, which may block the pain impulses in the central system ('gate' theory) before they are transmitted to the brain.

Pain due to joint capsule tightness or muscle spasms may be relieved by increasing tissue extensibility or reducing muscle tone. Much controversy still exists on the exact mechanism of action of superficial heat but clinical application continues to be very successful in relieving painful symptoms. Lentell and colleagues reported that the use of superficial heat with concomitant low-load, long-stretching techniques to improve shoulder external rotation was extremely beneficial compared to non-thermal agents or ice.

## WHIRLPOOL BATHS

Whirlpool baths, or whirlpools, have been a mainstay in athletic training rooms for years and continue to be used for various reasons. Their uses can be classified as a deep or superficial heating modality to treat chronic or acute injuries.

Whirlpools range in size from being able to submerge an extremity to Hubbard tank size, which allows full body submersion. Water in the tank is generally at 98–104°F (37–40°C) but varies based on the desired effects. Turbines are used to agitate the water, serving several purposes: they provide phasic stimulation to reactive skin afferents; increase hydrostatic pressure; apply resistance/assistance for exercise; remove necrotic tissue; and decrease the thermal gradient to keep the temperature stable. The usual temperature ranges are very hot (104–110°F; 40–43°C), hot (99–104°F; 37–40°C), warm (96–99°F; 36–37°C), neutral (92–96°F; 33–36°C) and tepid (80–92°F; 27–33°C).

One common use of the whirlpool in sports medicine is for wound lavage. The addition of solutions such as povidone-iodine or a bleach solution to the water will help reduce the bacterial load in addition to the agitation, which acts as a means of mechanical debridement. Immobilized joints are also frequently treated in a whirlpool by taking advantage of the water's buoyancy properties, which facilitate regaining range of motion while using the heating properties to increase tissue extensibility. Warm to hot whirlpools, as is the case with any other heating modalities, should not be used when edema is present. The effects of heat on the edematous area may increase blood supply resulting in increased swelling.

Whirlpools can also be used for intermittent contrast (hot/cold) therapy. Often contrast baths are used by submerging the injured area into a warm whirlpool then a cold whirlpool, resulting in vasodilatation/vasoconstriction. This may be beneficial to reduce chronic types of swelling or edema.

## ULTRASOUND

Therapeutic ultrasound is a deep-heating modality which penetrates tissue deeper than a superficial hot pack or warm whirlpools. Heat is generated by the molecular motion transmitted by a continuous sound wave of 0.8–3.0 MHz that penetrates to depths of 5 cm or more. Continuous ultrasound intensities of 1.0–2.0 W/cm$^2$ for 5–10 minutes are necessary to achieve tissue temperatures that range from 104–113°F (40–45°C). Sound waves are absorbed by various tissues, causing the production of heat. The greatest rise in temperature occurs in tissues with high protein content such as muscle, tendon and nerve.

Relatively little increase in adipose tissue temperature occurs with ultrasound treatment. In order for the sound waves to travel from the sound head to the skin, a coupling agent such as commercially prepared gels or water is required. The sound head is constantly moved in a circular motion with overlapping strokes and should not be held stationary over one area for a prolonged time. This will cause a rapid rise in temperature and create a 'hot spot' and burning sensation for the patient.

Ultrasound increases tissue temperature by vasodilatation and increased blood flow to the area. Other effects are increased collagen extensibility, changes in nerve conduction velocities and the inhibition of muscle spindles.

## ELECTRICAL MUSCLE STIMULATION (EMS)

The electrical stimulation of muscle unit contraction is employed to maintain muscle bulk and strength during rehabilitation following muscle injury. In this setting, electrical stimulation can be provided by a battery or console source (although the latter is favored) with electricity delivered at differing burst rates per second and at differing maintenance frequencies (70–90 bps at 2500, 5000 or 10 000 Hz). It is thought that such an effect maintains muscle bulk and strength despite limited use during a period of relative inactivity as occurs during the recovery period following injury.

## TRANSCUTANEOUS ELECTRICAL NERVE STIMULATION

This therapy, TENS, is employed to alter the pattern and frequency of nerve action potentials transmitted towards the central nervous system along the stimulated nerve fibers. In so doing it is thought that TENS units close a theoretical gate to nociceptive impulses associated with tissue injury and promote the release of endogenous endorphins from the brainstem. Reflective of pain reduction, TENS units often reduce the requirement for high-dose analgesia and facilitate more rapid recovery following musculoskeletal injury in sport or following surgery.

## HIGH-VOLT PULSED CURRENT (EDEMA CONTROL)

In this therapy, current is employed at levels sufficient to produce motor contraction and has been shown to reduce edema once it has been formed. In contrast, current applied at the sensory level has been shown to alter microvascular permeability and hence decrease capillary leakage and edema formation.

High-voltage stimulation involves delivering a short monophasic pulse of short duration with known charge across the skin and into acutely edematous tissue. Edema is comprised of negatively charged plasma proteins, which leak into interstitial space. By placing a negative electrode over the edematous site and a positive electrode at a distant site, the monophasic high-voltage stimulus applies an electrical potential, which disperses the negatively charged proteins away from the edematous site, thereby helping to reduce the edema.

## IONTOPHORESIS

The concept of iontophoresis involves the delivery of a electrical current to assist in the transudation of medication through the skin to underlying tissues. When employed to deliver dexamethasone and lidocaine, iontophoresis has been shown to reduce pain and inflammation in soft tissues and joints when compared to placebos.

## ACUPUNCTURE

Needle placement in acupoints (the number described ranges from 365 to 2000) is thought to produce repetitive neuronal firing thereby altering the anatomic structure, the release of chemical modulators and the chemicals controling physiologic responses. Scientific validation in the traditional West has not taken place but it is recognized that acupuncture may be valuable as a therapeutic modality. More scientific validation is encouraged.



## MAGNETIC FIELD THERAPY

Altered magnetic fields are thought to reduce pain and inflammation by an action on the cell membrane potentials and associated ionic fluxes producing a local change in microenvironment, promoting local tissue growth and repair.

## BIOFEEDBACK

This technique provides a way of monitoring and amplifying the physiologic responses that are not within the patient's awareness or control.

Biofeedback in the training room involves the objective or subjective monitoring of some physiologic event which can be used to alter or enhance performance. Many different instruments are used; the most common one is electromyographic biofeedback, in which skeletal muscle electrical activity is detected by surface electrodes and converted into a visual or audible signal. For example, if the goal is to re-educate a postoperative atrophied muscle, the biofeedback unit may be used to indicate electrical activity associated with that muscle contraction. Further intensification of the feedback signal would indicate a stronger relative contraction. Research has demonstrated positive effects through the use of electromyographic biofeedback versus exercise alone especially following anterior cruciate ligament reconstruction. Biofeedback may be contraindicated if a muscular contraction exacerbates a pathologic condition or further damages the injured tissues.

## MASSAGE THERAPY

Beneficial effects of massage are only seen in patients who follow the therapy with a period of active recovery rather than passive recovery.

## LASER THERAPY

While relatively new in the USA, cold-laser (i.e. low-power) therapy has been used in Europe and Canada for 20 or 30 years. Cold lasers are less powerful than hot lasers, which may be used for surgery. Cold-laser therapy reduces pain and inflammation, while the influence on cell metabolic activity increases healing. The laser beam is neurochromatic and is usually concentrated into a microscopic beam width. It is non-invasive and is generally used for localized lesions. There is limited objective documentation of the effectiveness of cold-laser therapy.

## HYPERBARIC OXYGEN THERAPY

By definition, hyperbaric oxygen therapy is the inhalation of 100% oxygen while the treatment chamber is pressurized at more than 1 atmosphere absolute. When breathing under normal conditions, 98.4% of the available oxygen is bound to hemoglobin while the remaining portion is dissolved in plasma. Normally, hemoglobin is 97% saturated by inspired air; thus changing to breathing a source of pure oxygen can increase the hemoglobin-delivered oxygen by only 3%. The remaining oxygen will be dissolved in the plasma. For each additional atmosphere of pressure, the amount of additional oxygen dissolved in plasma is 2.3%. Normal peripheral oxygen tension, measured through the skin, is approximately 40 mmHg. At hyperbaric oxygen treatment levels, this can be raised to over 2200 mmHg.

Previously authors have demonstrated that following a traumatic crash injury, there was a preservation of ATP in post-ischemic muscle with a reduction of edema by 50% after treatment with hyperbaric oxygen. Others have demonstrated a reduction in ischemia-induced skeletal muscle injury in a rat model treated with hyperbaric oxygen. It is proposed that hyperbaric oxygen treatment demonstrated these positive effects for at least 48 hours after a fairly severe ischemic injury by raising the levels of high-energy phosphate compounds.

Hyperbaric oxygen therapy has also been shown to promote neovascularization, enhance fibroblastic proliferation and increase collagen formation. Researchers have demonstrated that the quantity and size of blood vessels in skin flaps in an animal model were significantly greater when treated with hyperbaric oxygen as compared with controls.

At present there is no scientific support for the use of hyperbaric oxygen therapy in sports.

## Further reading

Abrahamson SB. Nonsteroidal antiinflammatory drugs: mechanism of action and therapeutic considerations. In: Leadbetter WB, Buckwalter JA, Gordon SL eds. Sports-induced inflammation: basic sciences and clinical concepts. Park Ridge 111, American Academy of Orthopedic Surgeons, 1990.

Behrens TW, Goodwin JS. Oral corticosteroids. In: Leadbetter WB, Buckwalter JA, Gordon SL eds. Sports-induced inflammation: basic sciences and clinical concepts. Park Ridge 111, American Academy of Orthopedic Surgeons, 1990.

# 4

# Acute Injury Management



## HEAD INJURY

### Unconscious with compromised airway

The unconscious athlete with a compromised airway must be approached with the expectation that there may be an underlying cervical spine injury. Accordingly the head and neck should be immobilized. If the airway is compromised using in-line immobilization, the athlete should be carefully and in a controlled manner rolled into a supine position. A jaw-thrusted chin lift should be performed to clear the upper airway. If there are sufficient personnel, a Guedel airway can be inserted.

A Laerdal mask can be applied over the Guedel airway. A carefully measured cervical collar should

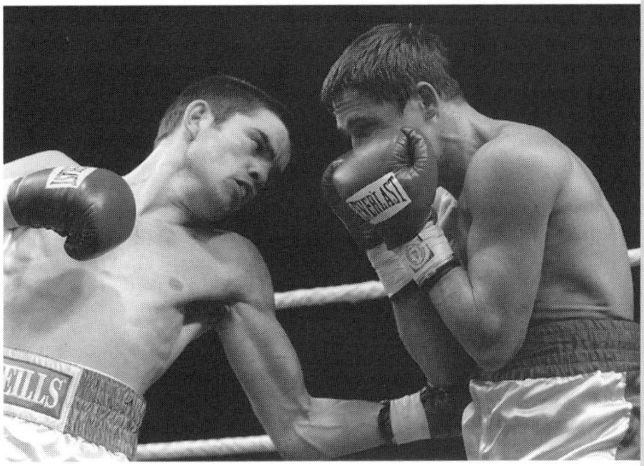

**Fig. 4.1** Sportsfile.

be applied to the neck. Following these initial maneuvers and immobilization the athlete should be transported as quickly and safely as possible.

## Concussion

This is defined by the American Academy of Neurology as 'the trauma-induced alteration in mental status that may or may not involve loss of consciousness.' Many guidelines have been produced but most would incorporate the following guidelines:

1. If any symptoms are present on static testing or during play the athlete should discontinue participation.
2. If there is evidence of loss of consciousness or postconcussive symptoms that persist beyond 20 minutes after the injury, then the athlete should not participate any further on that day and should undergo further assessment.
3. An athlete with mild concussion, which fully resolves within 15–20 minutes and with no evidence of loss of consciousness, who finds that resumption of activity does not provoke any further symptoms may be allowed to continue to play.
4. All the above clinical scenarios require regular re-evaluation involving history taking and physical examination.



# NECK INJURY

Neck injuries are infrequent. However, if severe they can have catastrophic sequelae. An athlete who has sustained a high-impact injury and is complaining of neck pain should be immobilized with full spinal precautions and transferred to a suitable facility where further imaging and evaluation can take place before the spine can be regarded as 'clear'.

A patient who is complaining of any neurological symptoms or exhibits any signs of neurological deficit should be immobilized using full spinal precautions and transferred to a suitable facility.

Patients who have sustained a neck injury but have absolutely no neck pain or neurological symptoms and absolutely normal examination may return to play. It is essential that the athlete confirms that they have no neck pain before they are asked to perform an active range of motion. The athlete should demonstrate full free active range of motion of the cervical spine with no neurological a symptoms or signs. In this instance it is reasonable to allow the athlete to continue to play.

# LACERATIONS

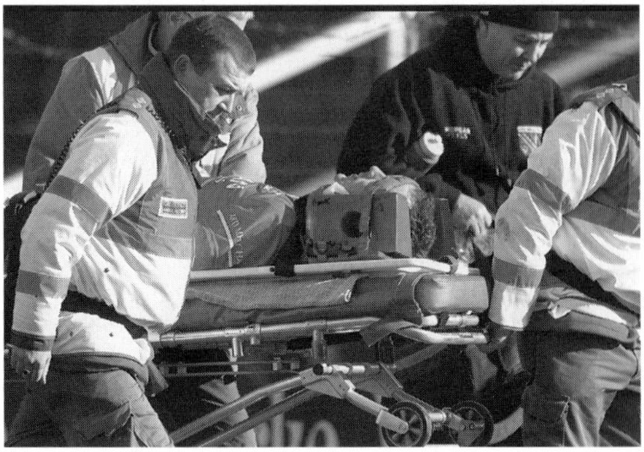

**Fig. 4.2** Sportsfile.

Lacerations around the head and neck are not uncommon in contact sports. Those requiring on-field management include scalp laceration, which can bleed copiously and require apposition of wound edges and control of bleeding. It is important to realize that certain areas require specialized treatment. Any laceration involving the eyelid or nasolacrimal duct should be assessed by an ophthalmologist. Any laceration that is full thickness involving the lip and surrounding skin should be very carefully assessed and repaired.

Lacerations should be carefully assessed and cleaned. Methods for repairing lacerations include steristrips, skin glue, skin clips and suture material. Any laceration that is treated during a competition should be carefully covered and sealed. Any laceration treated like this should be very carefully assessed at the end of the competition and, if necessary, reviewed by a specialist.

## RESUSCITATION

Resuscitation may be required at sports events to treat both the participants and the spectators. For this reason medical and paramedical staff involved in such events need to be trained in the emergency resuscitation of both adults and children. This includes the provision of basic life support and advanced interventions such as airway management and defibrillation.

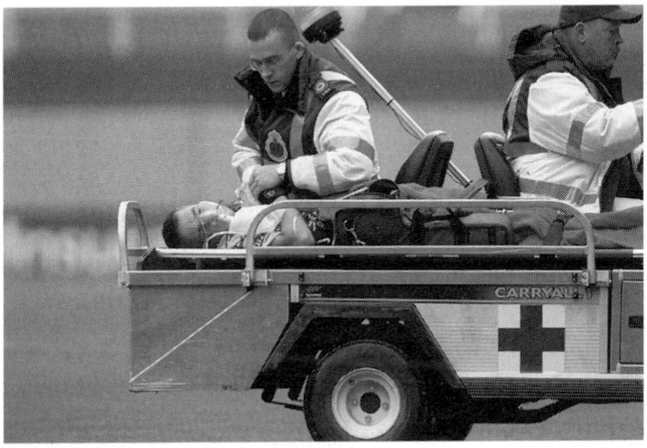


**Fig. 4.3** Sportsfile.

# Adult resuscitation

The European Resuscitation Council published the most recent guidelines in 2000. These follow consensus meetings of the Liaison Committee on Resuscitation. The key elements remain the provision of basic life support and early defibrillation. All resuscitation starts with basic life support; if this is not provided, advanced techniques are less likely to succeed. There is an urgent need to promote more and better cardiopulmonary resuscitation (CPR), which is complementary to, and does not replace, policies aimed at providing earlier defibrillation. The guidelines describe a stepwise sequence to be followed in all cardiac arrest situations. The international consensus group ILCOR recently recommended that basic life support should become part of the school curriculum. Good basic life support prevents the deterioration of ventricular fibrillation to asystole. Survival rates deteriorate, in cardiac arrests, by 7–10% for every 1 minute that defibrillation is delayed.

The first steps ensures the safety of both the rescuer and the injured person and are known as the SAFE approach.

### The SAFE approach

**S**hout for help
**A**pproach with caution
[Area] **F**ree from danger
**E**valuate.

### Evaluate

Assess or evaluate the patient by gently shaking their shoulders and shouting 'Are you all right?' (The cervical spine should be immobilized if there is a possibility of neck injury.)

If the patient responds, leave them in the position in which you found them and get help. If the patient does not respond, shout for help, place them on their back and open the airway.

### Airway and breathing

Airway management is essential and is often poorly performed as it is a more difficult skill to perform compared to chest compressions.

To open the airway, place your hand on the patient's forehead and gently tilt the head back. Remove any visible obstructions. Lift the chin to open the airway. The jaw-thrust maneuver can also be used and is performed by placing the index or little fingers behind the angle of the jaw and lifting the jaw upwards. These maneuvers lift the soft tissue away from the palate and maintain a patent airway.

If the patient is not breathing give five rescue breaths or two effective breaths. The breaths should be given slowly by mouth, or bag and mask if available, and the chest seen to rise. The breaths should be given over 2 seconds. If the rescue breaths are unsuccessful, it is essential to recheck the patient's head position to ensure that the airway is opened, i.e. the head is extended and chin lifted and that there is no visible obstruction.

### Circulation

The current guidelines recommend moving on to checking circulation even if rescue breaths have been unsuccessful. If trained, a pulse check should be performed feeling for a carotid pulse for no more

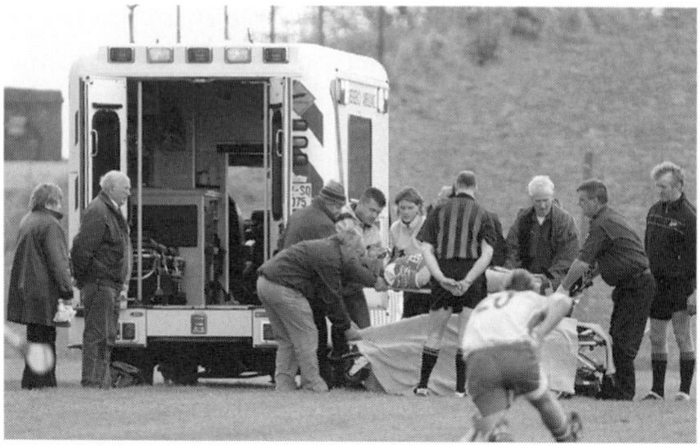

Fig. 4.4 Sportsfile.

than 10 seconds. Otherwise look for signs of circulation such as breathing effort or movement by the patient.

If signs of circulation are detected continue rescue breaths; if not commence chest compressions.

Chest compressions are performed by placing the heel of your hand one finger's breath above the xiphisternum, place the heal of the other hand on top of the first and interlock the fingers of the hands. Position yourself directly over the patient and while keeping your arms straight press down on the sternum to a depth of 4–5 cm. Release the pressure and allow the chest to rise and repeat at a rate of about 100 compressions per second.

After 15 compressions give two effective breaths.

Remember to recheck your hand positions when repositioning them after giving the breaths. Continue at a ratio of 15:2 until help arrives or the patient shows signs of circulation (Fig. 4.5).

## ADVANCED LIFE SUPPORT

Advanced life support is usually carried out in a hospital setting and includes the administration of drugs and definitive airway management (intubation). It does not replace effective basic life support and is used when a patient fails to respond to initial resuscitation and defibrillation.

Following the initial defibrillation, intravenous (i.v.) adrenaline (epinephrine) 1 mg is given once i.v. access is established, or 2–3 mg via an endotracheal tube if it is present and i.v. access is not established.

No antiarrhythmic agent has been shown to improve outcome following cardiac arrest. The current guidelines recommend that amiodarone should be considered following adrenaline in resistant ventricular fibrillation or pulseless ventricular tachycardia.

The airway should be secured by intubation with an endotracheal tube. Where this is not possible bag-mask ventilation is acceptable and the use of the laryngeal mask is increasing.

Increasingly, paramedics are carrying airway equipment and drugs such as adrenaline and atropine so it will be possible to perform advanced life support at

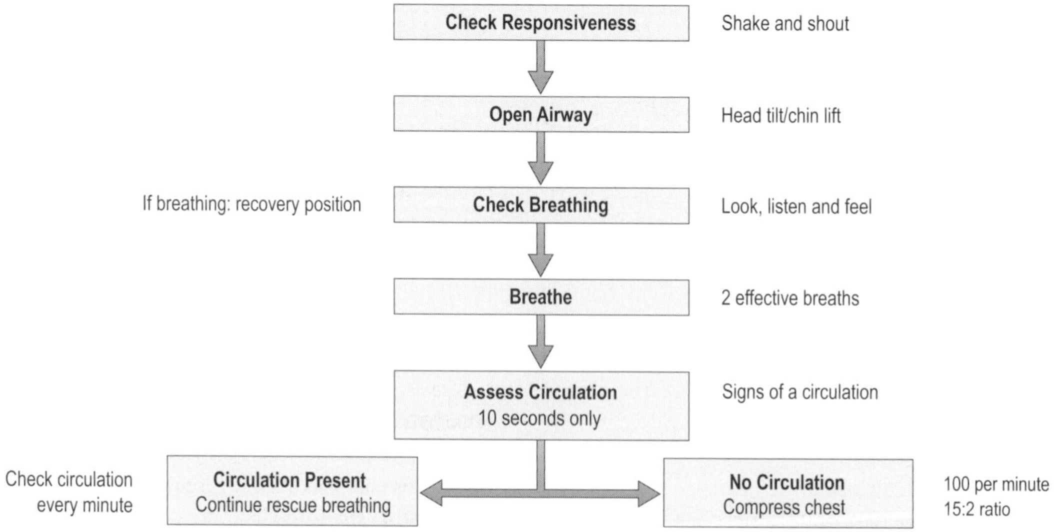


Fig. 4.5 Algorithm for adult resuscitation.

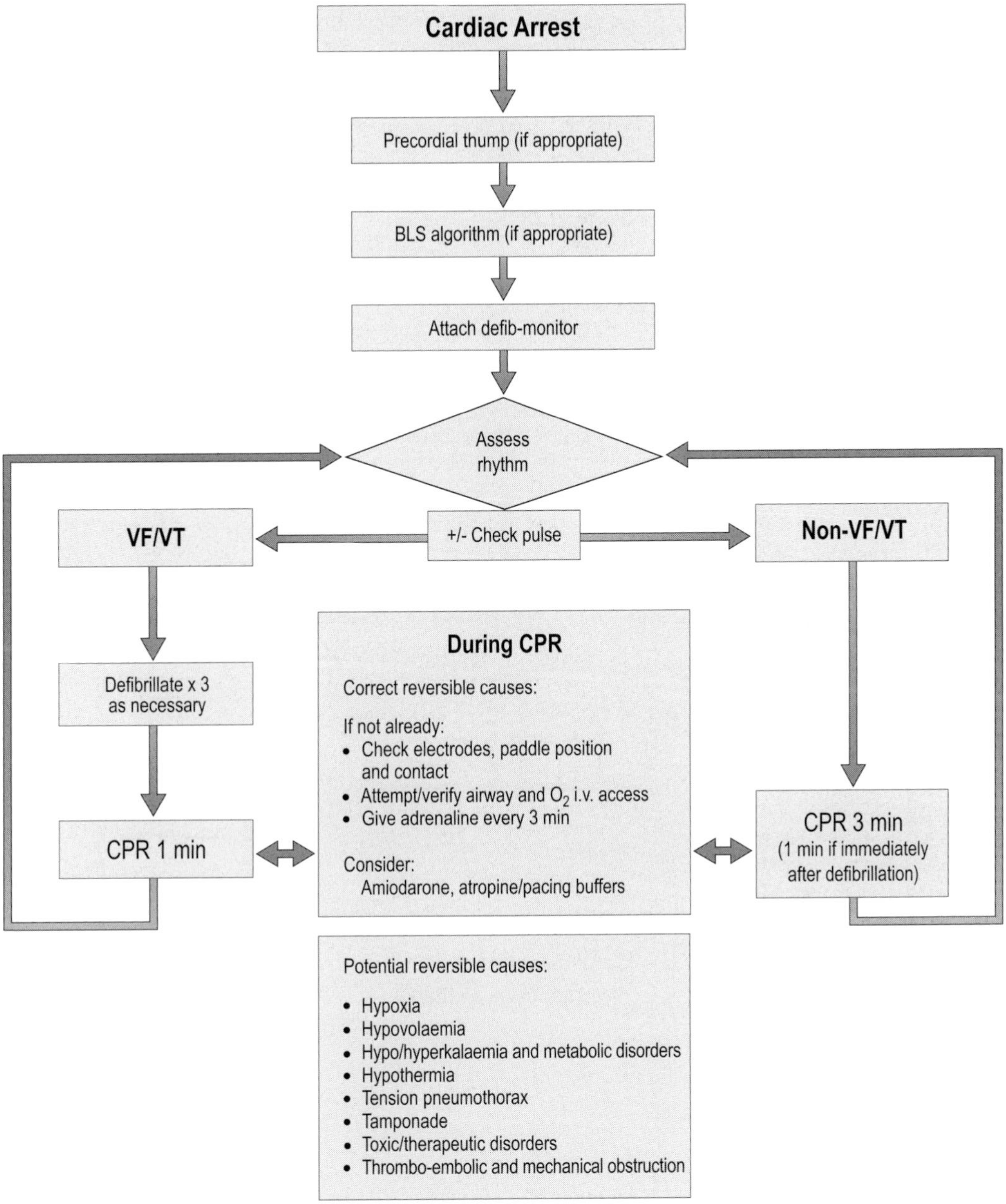


**Fig. 4.6** Algorithm for adult advanced life support following cardiac arrest.

the scene of cardiac arrest with aim of increasing survival (Fig. 4.6).

## Automatic external defibrillators

An automatic external defibrillator (AED) is a device that incorporates a rhythm analysis system and a shock advisory system for victims of cardiac arrest. The device analyzes the patient's rhythm and advises whether to shock or not to shock. The final decision to deliver the shock must be given by the operator. The AED makes the delivery of early defibrillation simpler, which is a key element in the chain of survival. Survival rates as high as 90% have been described when defibrillation has been given within

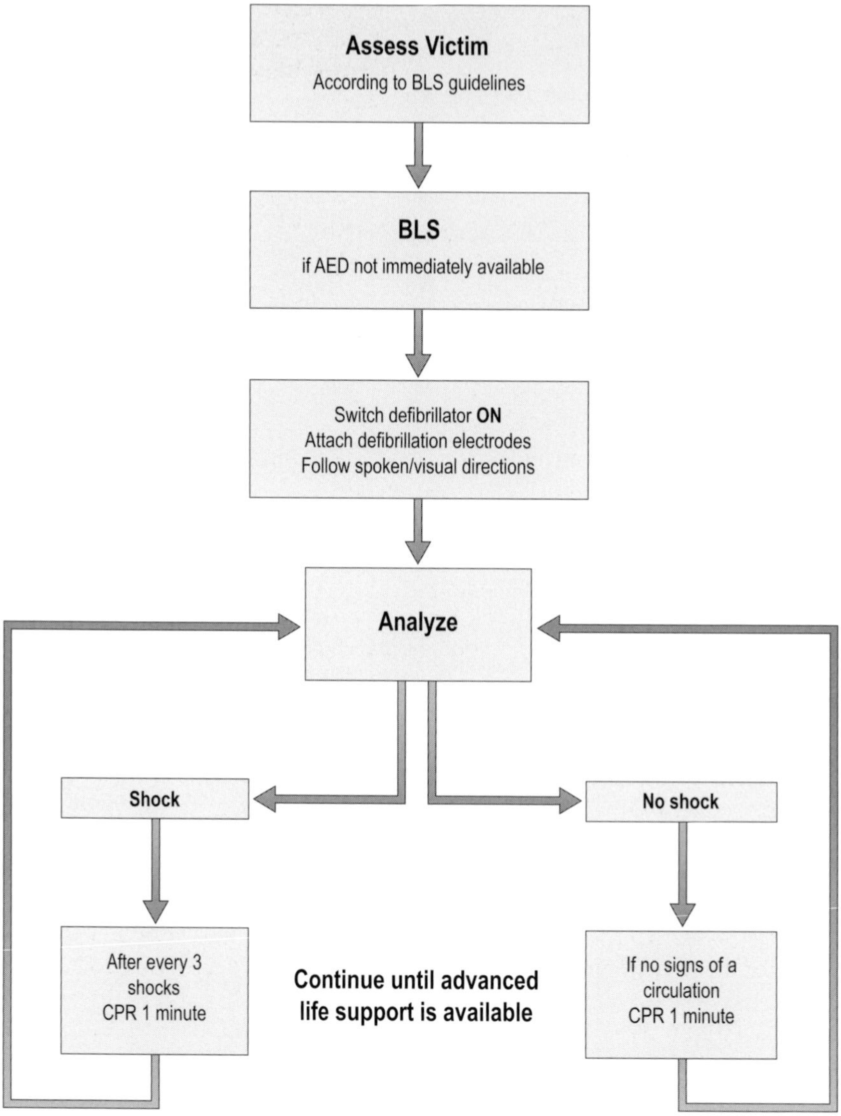


**Fig. 4.7** Algorithm for using an AED on an adult.



the first 60 seconds. It is now recommended that AEDs should be available in health/sports facilities and staff trained in basic life support and their use. The American Heart Association in 2003 advised that AEDs are now safe to use in children over 1 year old.

## How to use AEDs

The initial management of the patient is the same as before with assessment of responsiveness, breathing and circulation (Fig. 4.7). If no respiratory effort is being made call for help, send for the AED and give two rescue breaths.

If there are no signs of circulation, switch on the AED, apply the electrodes and follow spoken/visual prompts.

If shock is indicated, push the shock button as indicated making sure everyone is clear of the patient. Give three shocks if indicated.

After the shocks (or if no shock is indicated), check for signs of circulation. If no signs of circulation are present perform CPR for 1 minute. After

1 minute stop CPR to allow rhythm analysis. Continue following instructions from the AED until advanced life support is available.

## PEDIATRIC RESUSCITATION

Children are different from adults – they are not just scaled-down versions. Therefore there are significant differences in the resuscitation of children as compared to adults, although the aims and sequence of interventions is similar. Hypoxia is a more common cause of cardiac arrest in children as cardiac disease is rare in this age group. For this reason airway management is essential in pediatric cardiac arrests.

The guidelines discussed are from Advanced Paediatric Life Support, 3rd edition (APLS). The fourth edition is about to be published but is unlikely to have significant changes to basic life support in children. Other pediatric courses derived from the APLS including the one-day Paediatric Life Support and Pre-Hospital Paediatric Life Support for the prehospital provider.

The sequence of resuscitation is similar to that in adults; the major differences occur in relation to airway management. The position used to open the pediatric airway is different. In infants the head is placed in the neutral position; if the neck is overextended the airway will become occluded. In older children the airway is maintained in a similar position to adults (the 'sniffing' position).

The hand position for chest compression also varies with age. The rate of chest compressions is faster in children: a rate of 100 compressions per minute is recommended. The ratio of chest compressions to breaths is 15:2 (Table 4.1).

Recent advances in AEDs allow their use in children and simplify defibrillation in children. These include pediatric-sized electrode pads with cables that reduce the adult-size shock to a level more suitable to children aged 1–8 years.

## SUDDEN ADULT DEATH SYNDROME

Sudden adult death syndrome or sudden arrhythmic death syndrome (SADS) describes any cause of unexplained death with normal toxicology and normal cardiac morphology. In a national epidemiologic survey undertaken by the SADS study investigators, the incidence of unexplained sudden cardiac deaths in England in healthy people aged 16–64 years was estimated at 11 per 100 000 (3500 deaths) per year; 4.1% of these deaths were still unexplained after investigation and felt to be due to SADS. Potential causes include genetic conditions, such as long QT syndrome, which produces cardiac electrophysiologic dysfunction without structural disease. Other possible causes include hypertrophic cardiomyopathy and catecholaminergic polymorphic ventricular tachycardia. Most people who die from SADS are young males who die while inactive or asleep (Fig. 4.8).

These conditions could increase the risk of sudden cardiac death for the relatives of the patients and screening of relatives is recommended.

The availability of prompt and effective basic life support and early defibrillation are the key to victims surviving near SADS particularly with witnesses such as at sporting events.

**Table 4.1** Summary of resuscitation head and hand positions in children

| Age | Head position | Hand position |
|---|---|---|
| Infant | Neutral | One finger breadth below nipple line |
| Young child | Sniffing | One finger breadth above xiphisternum |
| Older child | Sniffing | Two finger breadths above xiphisternum |

## ARRHYTHMOGENIC RIGHT VENTRICULAR DYSPLASIA

Although uncommon, arrhythmogenic right ventricular dysplasia has become a more frequently recognized cause of SADS in sports persons. The disorder may be mild, characterized by subtle myocardial dysplasia through to marked fatty replacement of the right ventricular wall muscle and in severe cases by the development of right ventricular aneurysms. Secondary arrhythmias in affected persons account for sudden unexpected death.

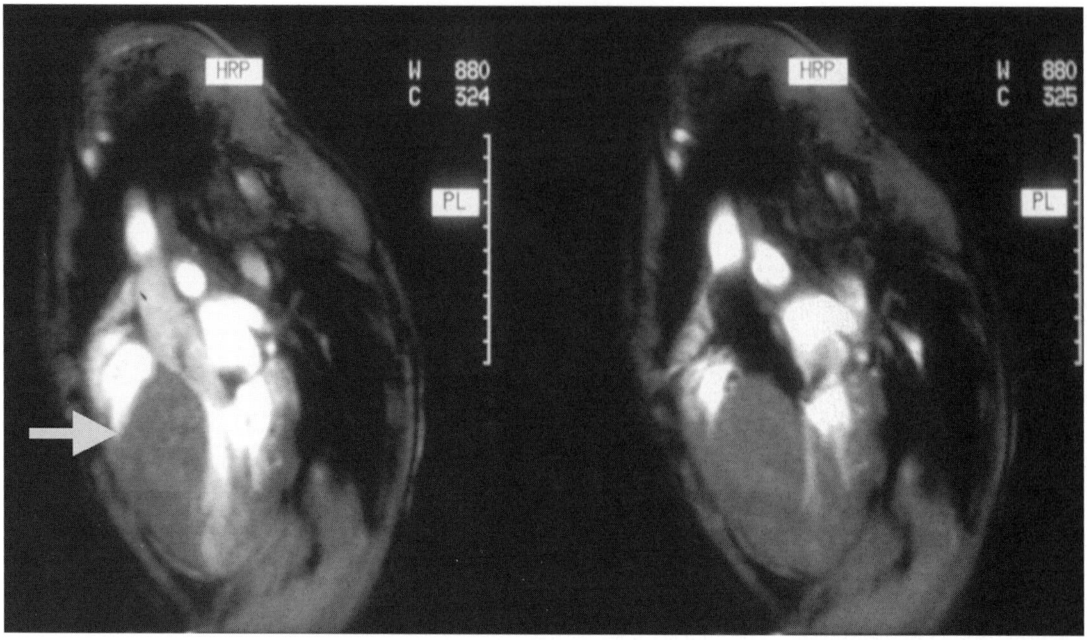


**Fig. 4.8** Sagittal MR images showing gross muscular thickening of the ventricular septum secondary to hypertrophic obstructive cardiomyopathy.



A screening ECG may reveal a spectrum of cardiac arrhythmias. Following normal echocardiagrams and catheter studies these patients are often referred for MRI, which allows definitive diagnosis by revealing right ventricular wall changes, dysplasia, fatty replacement, wall motion dyskinesia and even right ventricular aneurysms (Fig. 4.9).

## CONCLUSION

Everyone involved in the provision of medical cover at sports events should be proficient at basic life support and the use of defibrillators and AEDs. A reduction in the time from cardiac arrest to defibrillation is the key to improving outcome.

## TEAM PHYSICIAN'S MEDICAL BAG

The medications and equipment included in the team physician's medical bag will in some ways determine what type of emergency treatment he (or she) can render on the field. Because of limited space available in the hand-carried bag, he/she must carefully discriminate and select only equipment and medications that are frequently used or essential for emergencies. When a physician travels with the team, the bag itself must be sufficiently small to be carried on a bus, train or aircraft. A team physician who does not travel with the team may wish to limit the medical bag content to emergency items only. Frequently, the team physician will be evaluating the players or athletes late in the day or on weekends after normal working hours and may wish to have medications available so that he or she may initiate treatment for urgent but non-emergency conditions without delay. Most physicians do, or at least should, know how to perform CPR; as a practical reality this skill is infrequently used by most after departing graduate or residency medical training excepting emergency/critical care physicians, trauma specialists and cardiac specialists. In most circumstances, readily available paramedic units will be better able, from a skill and equipment standpoint, to perform CPR. Although this does not excuse the team physician from learning and updating the requisite skills to be certified in CPR + BLS ATALS, it does mean that he/she may not need to include all the equipment and medication necessary for CPR in his or her medical bag. The team physician, physiotherapist,

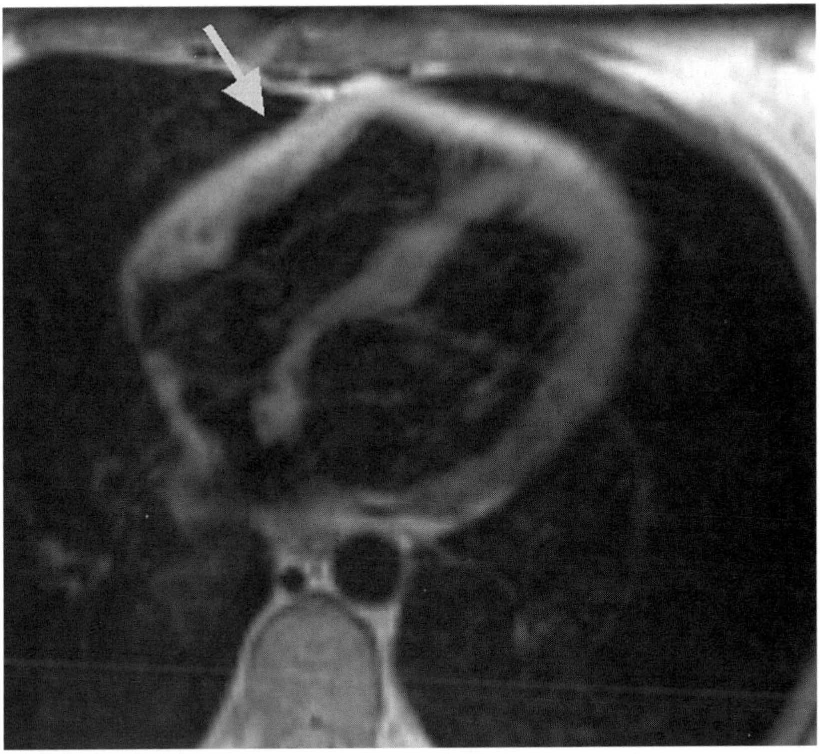

**Fig. 4.9** Axial MR image shows fatty replacement of the anterior wall of the right ventricle, which is characteristic of right ventricular dysplasia.



sports therapist and athletic trainer must, in any situation, know how they can readily access paramedic units. In a situation such as a training-grounds camp in a rural or inaccessible area, where paramedic units are not readily available, they must be prepared to perform CPR.

Circumstances will determine which medications and equipment are necessary in the medical bag. For example, in warmer climates, more i.v. solution would be required. Specialized medications may be included for known medical conditions of players and athletes, special needs athletes or players, coaches or team officials. The team physician will tend to choose those medications that he/she is familiar with and can use safely and confidently. The following is a list of medications and equipment.

# Medications

## Antibiotics

Penicillin 500 mg, tablets or injectable
Erythromycin 500 mg, tablets
Cloxacillin 500 mg, tablets
Ampicillin 500 mg, tablets.

The team physician must be alert to the possibility of a streptococcal pharyngitis epidemic in a group of young people when traveling in close company and initiate treatment right away based on clinical findings. Penicillin remains the first choice for group β hemolytic streptococcus; erythromycin should be available for individuals allergic to penicillin. Cloxacillin is useful for staphylococcal skin infections. Ampicillin is useful for ear infections. Expensive second- and third-generation antibiotics need not be included as not only are they unlikely to be used but their use should be limited to serious sepsis or culture-proven infections.

## Antiinflammatories

Ibuprofen 600 mg, tablets
Betamethasone suspension 5 mL, vial.

Many choices of NSAID and injectable corticosteroids are available. The one that is chosen depends on the team physician's preferences. Ibuprofen is well tolerated by most people and can also be used for menstrual cramps. Some physicians recommend including dexamethasone for spinal cord injury. However, its use is somewhat controversial and should be discussed with the team neurosurgical consultant. The use of aspirin is discouraged because of its known effects on platelets, causing an increased bleeding tendency.

## Anti-allergic and asthmatic medications

Diphenhydramine 25 mg, capsules, and 50 mg, prefilled syringe
Adrenaline (1:1000) 0.3 mg, autoinjector
Alupent inhaler.
Allergic reactions can occur from many causes, including medications administered by the team physician. The availability of adrenaline can be life saving in the face of an anaphylactic reaction. Most asthmatic individuals will bring their own medication but having back-up medication available in the medical bag is important.

## Cardiac medications

Atropine 2 mg, prefilled syringe
Dextrose 5% water, 250 mL bag
Adrenaline (1:10 000) 2 mg prefilled syringe
Lignocaine 100 mg, vial
Nitrostat 0.4 mg, tablets
Sodium bicarbonate 50 mEq, ampoules.
This list of medications should provide the necessary means to begin effective CPR. Their use, of course, requires appropriate skill and monitoring equipment. Some physicians also recommend frusemide 40 mg ampoule for i.v. use but the likelihood of acute pulmonary edema in most circumstances is quite small.



## Gastrointestinal medications

Antacid tablets
Lomotil tablets
Trimethobenzamide HCl 200 mg prefilled syringe.
Antacid tablets take up much less space than liquids and are lighter to carry. An injectable anti-emetic combined with i.v. fluids can ameliorate the effects of acute viral gastroenteritis quite rapidly.
Protein pump inhibitors
Metoclopramide
$H_2$ receptor antagonists

## Intravenous fluids

Lactated Ringer's solution, ampoule, 1000 mL bags
Dextrose 50% solution ampoule
Solution tubing
Assorted Intracath needles, especially 16 or 18 gauge.
The primary use for i.v. solutions is for rapid rehydration as a result of heat illness or gastroenteritis. Large i.v. needles are necessary for rapid administration. Dextrose 50% solution can he used to reverse insulin shock in insulin-dependent diabetic patients.

## Local anesthetics

Lignocaine 1%, 20 mL vial
Lignocaine 1% with adrenaline, 20 mL vial
Bupivacaine 0.5%, 50 mL vial.
Bupivacaine is a long-acting local anesthetic that can provide sustained pain relief in a sutured area.

## Muscle relaxants

Parafon Forte tablets
Diazepam 10 mg (Valium), prefilled syringe.
Muscle relaxants have limited usefulness but can he helpful with muscle cramps. The use of oral diazepam as a muscle relaxant has the risk of side-effects and addiction. Intravenous diazepam is used for grand mal seizure.

## Ophthalmic injury kit

Eye patch
Fluorescein strips
Mirror
Neosporin ophthalmic solution
Prednisone 1% ophthalmic solution
Sodium ophthalmic solution
Ultraviolet pen-light.
A selection of medications for the initial treatment of eye injuries and infections should be coordinated with the consulting ophthalmologist for the team.

## Pain-relieving medications

Paracetamol tablets
Paracetamol with codeine
Pethidine 100 mg, prefilled syringe
Morphine sulfate 15 mg, prefilled syringe
Naloxone HCl 0.4 mg, prefilled syringe.
The use of narcotic analgesics should be kept to a minimum because of the potential for abuse and addiction and, therefore, the number and amount in the team physician's medical bag should be small. Choice for oral narcotic analgesia is paracetamol with codeine. Because they are known to be drugs of

abuse, with a high street value and a high addiction potential, we recommend against using oxycodone or hydromorphone as an oral pain medication. Keeping these medications in the medical bag can make it a target for theft. Pethidine has a relatively short duration of action (1–2 hours) and is particularly useful intravenously for the reduction of dislocations. Morphine appears to be a more powerful analgesic but has a longer duration of action (3–4 hours). Morphine is particularly useful when an injured athlete has to be transported over a long distance and it can also be useful as a cardiac medication. Naloxone must be available if narcotic analgesics are being used to reverse their effect if respiratory depression occurs. All narcotic medication should be handled with extreme care, dispensed only with a physician's order and accounted for accurately.

### Topical agents

Betadine solution
Corticosteroid cream
Neosporin ointment
Myeolog ointment.

Any of a number of antibiotic ointments may be selected by the team physician. Contact dermatitis is a common problem in athletes and can be treated with a corticosteroid cream.

The medical bag itself should be large enough to accommodate the necessary medications and small equipment but not so large as to be difficult to transport. Multiple compartments, which can be labeled, make finding the equipment in an emergency easier. Being able to lock the bag will discourage theft or use of the emergency equipment for routine problems. In the latter circumstance, the medical bag could he depleted of supplies and medications that will then be unavailable for an emergency. Several physicians have suggested the use of a large fishing tackle box or toolbox. The medical bag must be checked on a periodic and regular basis to make sure all the medications and supplies are present and not outdated.

## Emergency equipment

The team physician will need various types of equipment available to him (or her) for handling emergency problems. Not all of the equipment, of course, can literally be kept in the medical bag but this equipment, as much as medication, is a key part of the emergency armamentarium. The equipment selected will depend on the expertise of the physician. Whether these items are supplied by the physician, school or local ambulance service will be determined by individual circumstances. The following lists of equipment are categorized by function. They represent only our recommendations and are not meant to be inclusive. Sizes are suggested but can be revised if athletes are very small or very large.

### Airway maintenance

Airways, nasal, sizes 26, 28, and 30 mm (two each)
Airways, oral, sizes 3, 4, 5, 6 (two each)
Bag valve mask F
Endotracheal tubes, sizes 6.5, 7.0, 7.5 and 8.0 mm
Endotracheal tube holder
Laryngoscope with assorted blades and stylet
Magill forceps
Oxygen, size D tank with demand valve, simple mask and nasal canula
Syringe, 10 mL
Surgitube (three packs).

The team physician should be prepared to maintain an airway on the rare occasion of a catastrophic injury or cardiac arrest. The local ambulance service may have this type of equipment available.



### Diagnostic equipment

Chemsticks with finger lancet for blood glucose level
Labsticks for urine
Ophthalmoscope F
Otoscope
Sphygmomanometer with appropriately sized cuffs
Stethoscope
Thermometer
Vacutainer tubes, holder and needles.

Diagnostic equipment can he useful for emergencies and for routine evaluation when away from the office or clinic.

### Pocket equipment

Airway, common size
Knife for cutting a face-mask
Pen-light
Pocket mask for resuscitation
Reflex hammer
Scissors
Bandage.

This type of equipment is particularly useful for immediate on-field examination and for obtaining an airway.

### Splints

Ace bandages, 3, 4 and 6 inch (two each)
Air splints (one complete set)
Aluminum foam splints, $\frac{1}{2}$ inch size for fingers
Cervical collar, stiff-neck (*foam-type collars are unacceptable*)
Cotton cast padding, 4 inch (three packs)
Crutches
Knee immobilizer
Plaster, 4 and 6 inch, for posterior and gutter splints
Slings (two)
Spine board, long, with cervical immobilization device and three straps
Wrist and forearm splint, universal size, one for each extremity.

Effective splinting or casting allows the safe immobilization of injured parts to relieve pain and prevent further damage in transportation. Plaster of Paris remains the most versatile material for splinting and casting and, unlike fiber-glass, can he removed without a cast saw. Effective splinting can enable an injured athlete to be returned home on, say, the team bus or airplane rather than being taken to a local hospital and, as a result, left behind for treatment.



### Surgical equipment

Alcohol swabs (12)
Betadine swabs (12)
Gloves, sterile (two pairs)
Needles, 18, 22 and 25 gauge (six each)
Scalpels, disposable, 10 and 11 (two each)
Sterile saline for irrigation, two 25-mL plastic bottles
Steristrips, $\frac{1}{4}$ and $\frac{1}{8}$ inch (six each)
Sutures, assorted sizes and types
Syringes TB 3, 5, 10 and 50 mL.

**The ability to suture lacerations in the locker room can avoid time-consuming trips to the emergency room.**

### Miscellaneous

Adhesive tape, 1 and $1\frac{1}{2}$ inch (two rolls each)
Band-Aids (plasters), assorted sizes (six each)
Benzoin tincture
Gauze pads sterile, 4 × 4 and 2 × 2 (six to ten each)
Ice (amount dependent on environment) – on a hot, humid day 500 g is not unreasonable
Ice bags (ten)
Kling, 3 inch (four to six rolls)
Paper bag, for hyperventilation
Q-tips (six)
Tape measure, for girth measurements
Tongue blades.

## Ambulance availability

The need to have an ambulance on standby at an athletic event will depend on the injury potential of the sport and the availability of the local emergency medical service (EMS). An ambulance on the scene will provide the physician with a cardiac monitor, defibrillator, suction equipment, splints, spine hoard and stretcher. The team physician should confer with the medical director of the local EMS to determine its capability and how the medical requirements of the sporting event may best be served. Reliable and efficient communication such as mobile/cell phone or radio is a must for the physician, if an ambulance is not on site, for the physician must be able to summon one without delay. Use of a pay telephone can be unreliable and use of a locker room or school office phone may cause an unacceptable delay. Portable radios are subject to atmospheric and geographic limitations to a greater extent than mobile phones. Note that the popularity of scanners means that the information communicated by radio will not be confidential. Improvements in cellular telephone technology makes a mobile phone the best means for effective communications.

## Conclusion

When a team physician and athletic trainer prepare their medical bag, they are, in a sense, preparing themselves for any medical emergency they might face. The thought and effort that is placed in this preparation will be manifest in the successful management of emergencies by the physician and athletic trainer. Our role is to plan for all types of emergency that may be reasonably encountered in the athletic area, even though some of the treatment or equipment may be provided by others such as the paramedic units. We have presented a list of medications and equipment that we have found to be necessary or useful in the relevant emergency situations. This guide is designed to serve as a starting point for the team physician and athletic trainer as they prepare themselves and the medical bag.

## Further reading

Advanced Life Support Group. Advanced paediatric life support: the practical approach, 3rd edn. London, BMJ Books, 2001.

Balady GJ, Chaitman B, Foster C et al. Automated external defibrillators in health/fitness facilities. Circulation 2002; 105: 1147–1150.

Behr E, Wood DA, Wright M et al. and the Sudden Arrhythmic Death Syndrome (SADS) Steering Group. Cardiological assessment of first-degree relatives in sudden arrhythmic death syndrome. The Lancet 2003; 362: 1457–1459.

De Latorre F, Nolan J, Robertson C et al. European Resuscitation Council Guidelines 2000 for Adult Advanced Life Support. Resuscitation 2001; 48: 211–221.

Handley AJ, Monsieurs KG, Bossaert LL. European Resuscitation Council Guidelines 2000 for Adult Basic Life Support. Resuscitation 2001; 48: 199–205.

Monsieurs KG, Handley AJ, Bossaert LL. European Resuscitation Council Guidelines 2000 for Automatic External Defibrillators. Resuscitation 2001; 48: 207–209.

Philips B, Zideman D, Garcia-Castrillo L et al. European Resuscitation Council Guidelines 2000 for Basic Paediatric Life Support. Resuscitation 2001; 48: 223–229.

5

# The Pelvis, Hip and Groin



## CLINICAL EXAMINATION

### Clinical history

Clinical history must include sport played, mechanism of injury, onset of symptoms, aggravating and relieving factors, location and type of pain, and chronicity. This will frequently identify the likely injured structure. For example, groin pain on sideways kicking in soccer localized to the medial groin will usually be related to adductor longus tendon dysfunction. Diffuse groin or perineal pain may be related to osteitis pubis. Progressive pain and stiffness may indicate degenerative change in the hip joint. Essentially, the distinction should be made between intra-articular hip pathology and periarticular/soft-tissue pathology. Other more rare causes of hip pain, e.g. intrapelvic and spinal lesions, should also be considered.

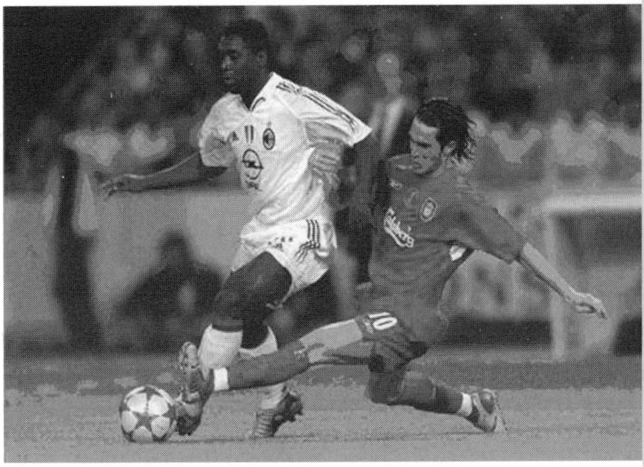

**Fig. 5.1** Sportsfile.

# Physical examination

## Inspection

### Gait

Is the patient using a crutch? If they can walk, they should be asked to do so. Look for the following features:

1. *Antalgic gait* – this is a painful limp and the stance phase is shortened on the affected side.
2. *Short leg gait* – this may be real or apparent and is identified by the pelvis on the *affected* side dropping during stance on the affected side.
3. *Trendelenburg gait* – this reflects failure of the abductor mechanism on the affected side and is identified by noting the pelvis on the *opposite* side dropping during the stance phase on the affected side. This can be difficult to identify clearly during walking and Trendelenburg's test should be performed.

### Trendelenburg's test

The patient is requested to stand on the affected lower limb and flex the opposite knee. Normally the unaffected pelvic side will remain higher than the affected side. If the unsupported/unaffected side sags, this is a positive test indicating neurological or mechanical dysfunction. Traditionally, this is observed from behind, comparing the skin dimples at the posterior superior iliac spines but in practice the examiner frequently stands in front of the patient while gently palpating both anterior superior iliac spines.



### Palpation

The patient lies supine and the attitude of hip is inspected. Any previous incisions or scars are noted. Limb length should be measured from the anterior superior iliac spine to the medial malleolus. If there is a discrepancy, ensure that both lower limbs are in a comparable position. If a true discrepancy is identified, flex the knees to 90° with the feet flat on the table and identify if the longer side shows a knee that appears higher or more anterior to the opposite side. To identify if the shortening is above or below the greater trochanter, we use Bryant's triangle and Nelaton's line.

### Bryant's triangle

The patient lies supine. A vertical line is dropped from the anterior superior iliac spine towards the couch. A horizontal line is drawn from the tip of the greater trochanter to the vertical line. The length of this line is compared with the opposite unaffected side.

### Nelaton's line

The patient lies on the unaffected side. A line between the anterior superior iliac spine and the ischium is drawn. The greater trochanter should lie on or below this line.

### Movement

The active range of motion should be assessed before the passive range while always checking the patient for discomfort. It is important to distinguish true hip joint movement from pelvic movement. Abnormalities of movement may reflect articular or periarticular pathology.

### Flexion

While supine, the patient should bring the knees almost to the anterior chest wall with normal values between 100° and 135°. The ileopsoas muscle is the main hip flexor.

### Abduction

This can be measured with the patient standing and spreading their legs, or supine with attention paid to ensuring that the movement is truly occurring at the hip joint by stabilizing the pelvis. Abductor power has been tested during gait and Trendelenburg's test. The ileotibial band acts as a secondary hip abductor and, to neutralize its effect, the active hip abduction can be tested with the knee flexed. Normal abduction is 45°.

### Adduction

Stabilize the pelvis and cross the examined leg over the fixed opposite leg: 20° is normal although bulky thighs can affect the measurement.

### Extension

This can be measured in the prone position with the knees flexed slightly to relax the hamstring muscles.

### Thomas's test

This detects fixed flexion deformity and can be assessed during flexion measurement. The patient lies supine. Place your hand under the lumbar spine. The patient flexes the hip until the thigh is against the abdominal wall. At this point, the lumbar lordosis will be obliterated as evidenced by pressure of the lumbar spine on the examiner's hand. The pelvis is now stabilized. Now inspect the opposite hip, which should be able to lie supine on the couch. If it is elevated, it indicates a flexion contracture of that hip joint. The angle subtended between the thigh and the couch is the degree of fixed flexion deformity.

### Rotation

Internal rotation is from 0° to 35° and external rotation is from 0° to 50°. This can be measured with the patient supine and the hips in extension with the legs hanging over the end of the couch. Rotation should also be measured with the hips flexed either with the patient supine and the hips and knees flexed or with the patient seated and legs hanging over the side of the couch.

Test for non-articular causes of pain. The examination of periarticular causes of pain can be divided into anatomical areas.

### Anteriorly

**Labral tear** The hip is flexed, adducted and internally rotated. This is to cause a gentle impingement of the anteverted femoral neck against the anterior labrum. This is performed as a passive test. Alternatively, and particularly in the dysplastic acetabulum, extension and external rotation increases the pressure on the anterior labrum and capsule, which can provoke discomfort if this area is injured.

**Rectus femoris injury** A chronic avulsion-type injury or contracture can be identified by pain on resisted flexion of the hip. Tightness can be identified by Ely's test, which involves passive flexion of the knee while the patient is prone. If the rectus tendon is tight, the hip will rise on that side. If the tendon ruptures, a defect and tenderness may be noticed on deep palpation.

**Iliopsoas dysfunction** This includes iliopsoas tendon or iliopsoas bursa pathology. Painful flexion of the hip against resistance implies tendon dysfunction. An inflamed bursa may be painful on passive flexion or deep palpation anteriorly.

**Hernia** These include inguinal hernias, femoral hernias and miscellaneous anterior abdominal wall weaknesses. Examination of the abdominal wall for defects or pain with increased intra-abdominal pressure can identify these tensions.

**Medial** *Adductor muscle* This is one of the commonest lesions. Tenderness can be identified on direct deep palpation and pain can be provoked by the examiner placing a clenched fist between the patient's knees and asking the patient to squeeze the knees together against the fist.

Flexing the knees and hips, placing the feet flat on the couch and asking the patient to allow the knees to 'fall out' may also demonstrate tightness and discomfort.

Rupture of the adductor muscles can be identified by a defect at the site of the injury.

**Osteitis pubis** The location of pain is diffuse. The symphysis pubis may be tender and passive abduction of the hip may reproduce the pain.

### Laterally

**Trochanteric bursitis** This can affect the superficial or deep bursa and is aggravated by deep palpation or passive adduction of the hip in flexion.

**Iliotibial band contracture** Ober's test identifies fixed abduction of the hip while the patient lies on the unaffected side.

### Posteriorly

**Piriformis discomfort** This can be compression of the sciatic nerve by piriformis. Patients have pain on flexion and internal rotation. Direct palpation on internal rotation in extension can reproduce the pain.

**Pace's sign** Pain and weakness on resisted abduction and external rotation.

**Hamstring syndrome** Exquisite tenderness at the ischial tuberosity and resisted leg extension causing pain suggest this diagnosis.

- Knee pain may be hip pathology especially in slipped upper femoral epiphysis in adolescents.
- Other causes of hip/groin pain include pelvic tensions, sacroiliac (SI) and spinal pathology, stress fractures and traumatic fractures, and dislocations (Figs 5.2–5.5).

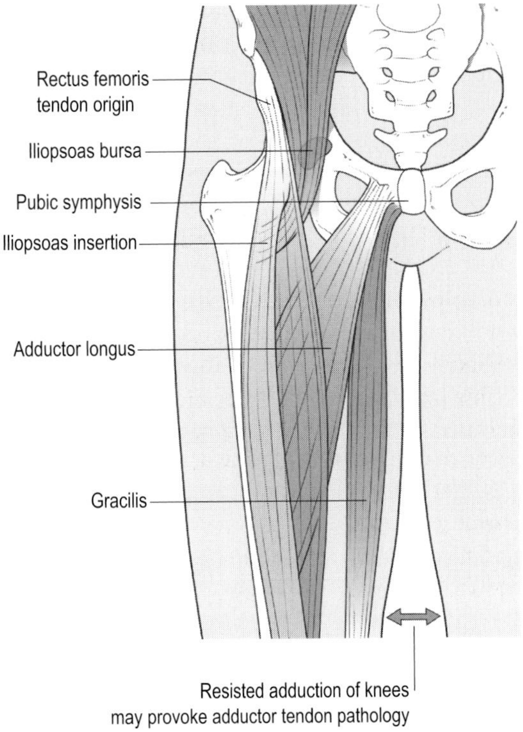


**Fig. 5.2** Anterior and medial soft-tissue pain sources.

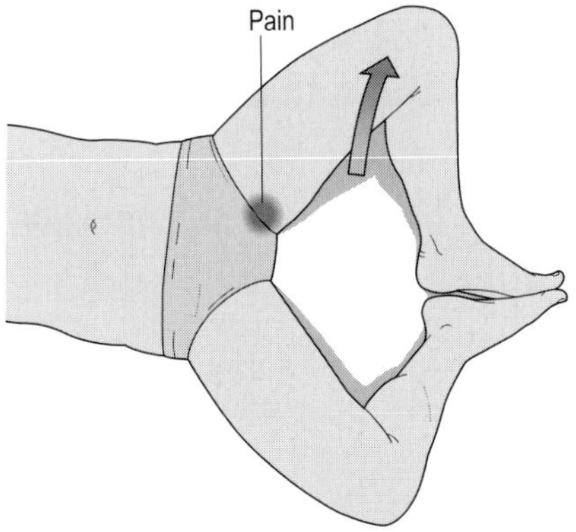


**Fig. 5.3** The patient is supine with the feet together and the knees and hips flexed, and allow the knees to 'fall out'.

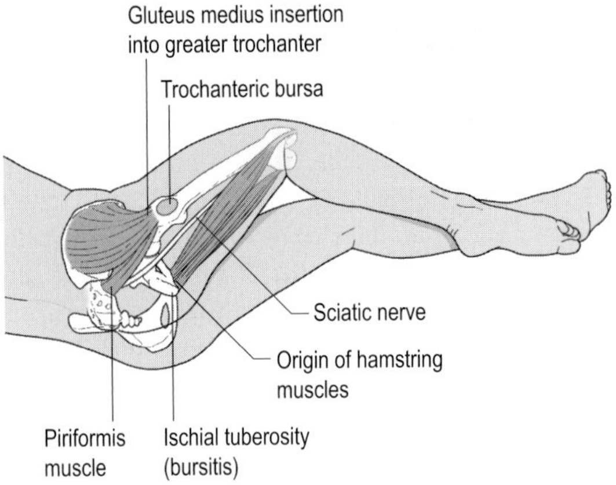


**Fig. 5.4** Posterolateral and potentially painful structures.

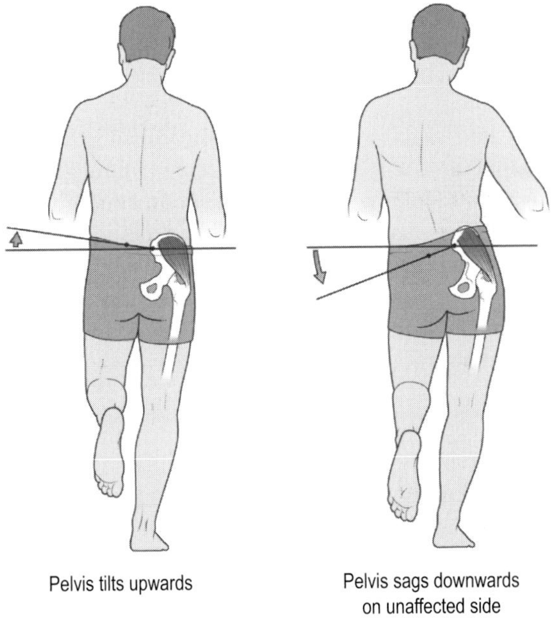


**Fig. 5.5** Trendelenburg test.

# INJURIES AND PATHOLOGIES

## Labral tears

### Anatomy

- The acetabular labrum represents a discontinuous semilunar ring of fibrocartilage covering the anterior, superolateral and posterior columns of the acetabulum. (The inferior margin is bridged by the transverse acetabular ligament.)
- It is triangular in cross-section, most frequently inverted in orientation and is usually thicker posterosuperiorly than anteroinferiorly (reflecting its function to provide stability and prevent subluxation).
- The synovial lined capsule of the hip joint arises from bone adjacent to the outer attachment of the labrum. In this way, a sulcus – the paralabral sulcus – is created between the labrum and the capsule. It is lined by synovium and from which vascularity to the labrum is derived.
- Articular hyaline cartilage extends to the inner or medial margin of the labrum but does not extend between the labrum and underlying bone. (The junction of the articular cartilage and the fibrocartilage may be mistaken for a partial tear.)
- Superior tears more common.

### Mechanism of injury

- Labral tears may follow significant injury, especially posterior hip subluxation or dislocation.
- Acute traumatic tears are common in sports with extreme hip rotation and flexion; runners and athletes whose sport involves repeated twisting are most at risk.
- Patients with pre-existing hip pathology (e.g. Perthes' disease, congenital dislocation of the hip: CDH) are more at risk (Fig. 5.6); these entities contribute to femoroacetabular impingement syndrome.



### History and clinical findings

- A sharp, catching pain radiating to the groin, worsened by pivoting and gradually increasing in severity.
- Clicking frequently present and the hip may give way.
- Pain on axial compression of the affected leg.
- Apprehension on impingement provocation test (flexion, adduction and internal rotation for anterosuperior tears and hyperextension, abduction and external rotation for posteroinferior tears).

### Imaging findings

#### Radiography

- The patient may show a pre-existing condition predisposing to labral tear (e.g. CDH) or sequelae of a tear (arthritis).

#### Arthrography

- Diagnostic and therapeutic.

#### Computerized tomography

- Complete detachment of the labrum may be identified at CT (particularly when associated with posterior column avulsed fractures) ± acetabular subchondral cysts.

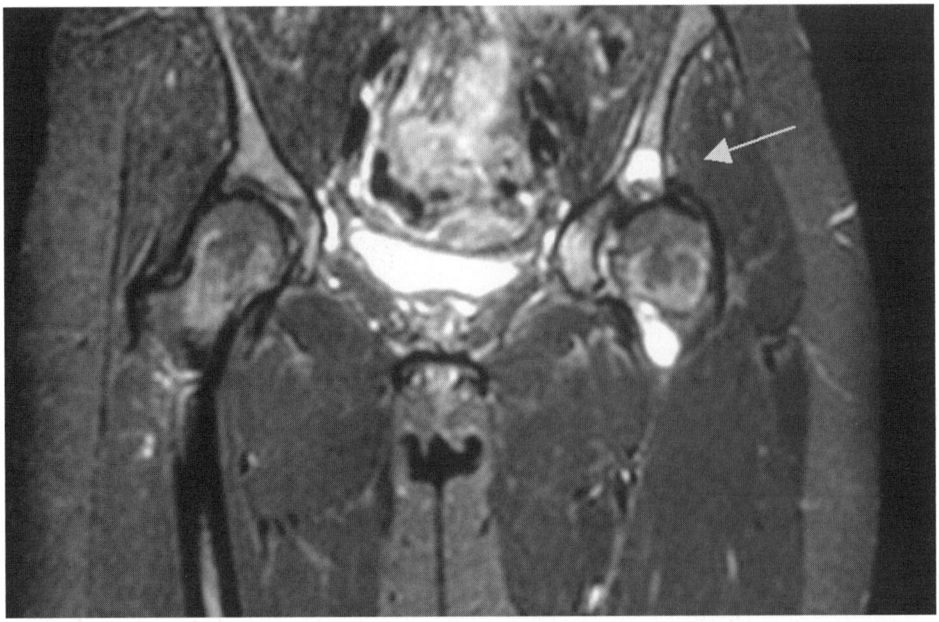

(a)

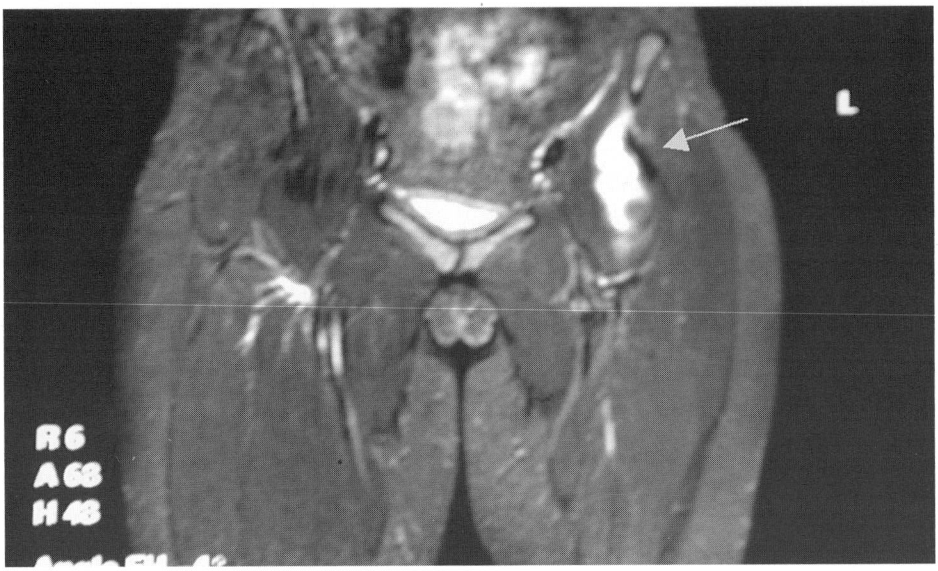


(b)

**Fig. 5.6** (**a**, **b**) Coronal images showing superior subluxation of the femoral head with degenerative tear of the superior labrum in a patient with acetabular dysplasia complicated by the formation of a superior labral ganglion cyst.



## Magnetic resonance imaging

- MRI may be performed with or without intra-articular contrast.
- Under ideal circumstances, MRI is performed with a dedicated phased array flexible surface coil allowing signal-rich high-resolution images with a 14- to 18-cm field of view. Following trauma, examination is usually with a larger field of view, as injury to the hip is often accompanied by further injuries to the pelvis.

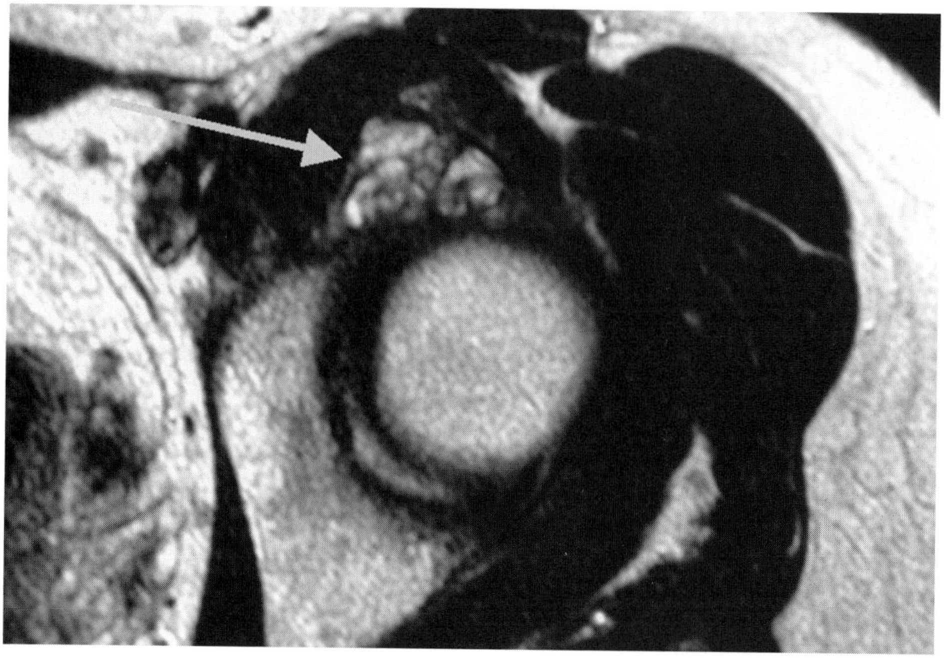

**Fig. 5.7** Axial image of the left hip showing a lobulated, ganglion cyst arising from a tear of the anterior margin of the acetabular labrum.

- Without intra-articular contrast, optimum contrast and detection of labral tears is achieved with $T_2$* weighting. In such a way, any joint fluid is hyperintense, articular cartilage is isointense and labrum is dark or hypointense. Tears are diagnosed on the basis of signal abnormality, linear signal hyperintensity or on the basis of altered morphology, an absent labrum or abnormal labral configuration. The presence of subchondral cystic change adjacent to or below the labrum is often associated with labral abnormality and should trigger additional scrutiny.
- When employed, MRI arthrography is performed using 4–5 cc of a solution containing 0.1 mL of gadolinium DTPA to 5 mL of 1% lidocaine and 15 cc of ionic contrast. Intra-articular contrast improves visualization of the labrum, the conspicuity of which is enhanced by distension of the sublabral sulcus.
- MRI arthrography also facilitates the detection of loose bodies following hip trauma, although CT is often favored when this diagnosis is suspected (Fig. 5.7).

## Management

### Non-surgical

- Non-weight bearing and reduction of flexion and internal rotation.
- Antiinflammatories.
- Intra-articular steroid injection during acute painful episodes.

### Surgical

- Arthroscopic debridement.
- Open arthrotomy and debridement if arthroscopic means are not possible.

# Quadriceps muscle strains

## Anatomy

- The quadriceps muscle is composed of the rectus femoris and vastus muscles (medialis, lateralis and intermedius).
- They converge to a conjoint tendinous insertion on the superior patella.
- Knee extensors and hip flexor (rectus femoris).

## Mechanism of injury

- Muscle strains account for up to a third of sports-related injuries.
- In most cases, quadriceps injury follows minor trauma (e.g. overstretching or overuse) and is characterized by local edema corresponding to a site of focal tenderness; it is frequently seen in kicking sports, less frequently in sprinters.
- Less frequently, injury is more severe and is characterized by partial or complete disruption of muscle fibers:
  - Grade 1 strain is characterized by local muscle edema and hemorrhage without a significant change in morphology
  - Grade 2 strain is characterized by partial tear of up to 50% of tendon fibers
  - Grade 3 strain is characterized by near complete rupture with or without retraction.
- The distal musculotendinous junction is the weakest site.
- The rectus femoris is the most frequently injured muscle.

## History and clinical findings

- History of recent muscle trauma, overuse and improper warm-up.
- Tightness in the thigh, inability to walk properly or fully extend the knee.
- Edema and swelling at the anterior thigh.
- Weakness only in more severe (grade 2 or 3) strains.
- In more severe strains, pressing on the muscle will produce pain.
- Pain on straightening the knee against resistance.
- Palpable defect and asymmetry in grade 3 sprains with retraction.



## Imaging findings

### Radiography

- Usually normal but soft-tissue mass may be seen in more severe strains.
- High-riding patella on lateral view in complete grade 3 sprains with retraction.

### Ultrasound

- This is operator dependent but may show focal hypoechoic tendinosis or muscle tear. Acute hematoma will show as predominantly hypoechoic fluid collection with internal echoes.

### Computerized tomography

- Less useful than MRI.
- May show muscle swelling with focal areas of low attenuation (edema) or high attenuation (hemorrhage).

### Magnetic resonance imaging

- Injury is invariably manifest by the presence of hyperintense local edema on $T_2$-weighted or fat-suppressed images (extent best demonstrated on axial and coronal images).
- Following injury, hemorrhage and edema may become localized with capsular or pseudocyst formation. Hypointense fibrous encasement may occur in chronicity, resulting in a pseudotumor appearance.

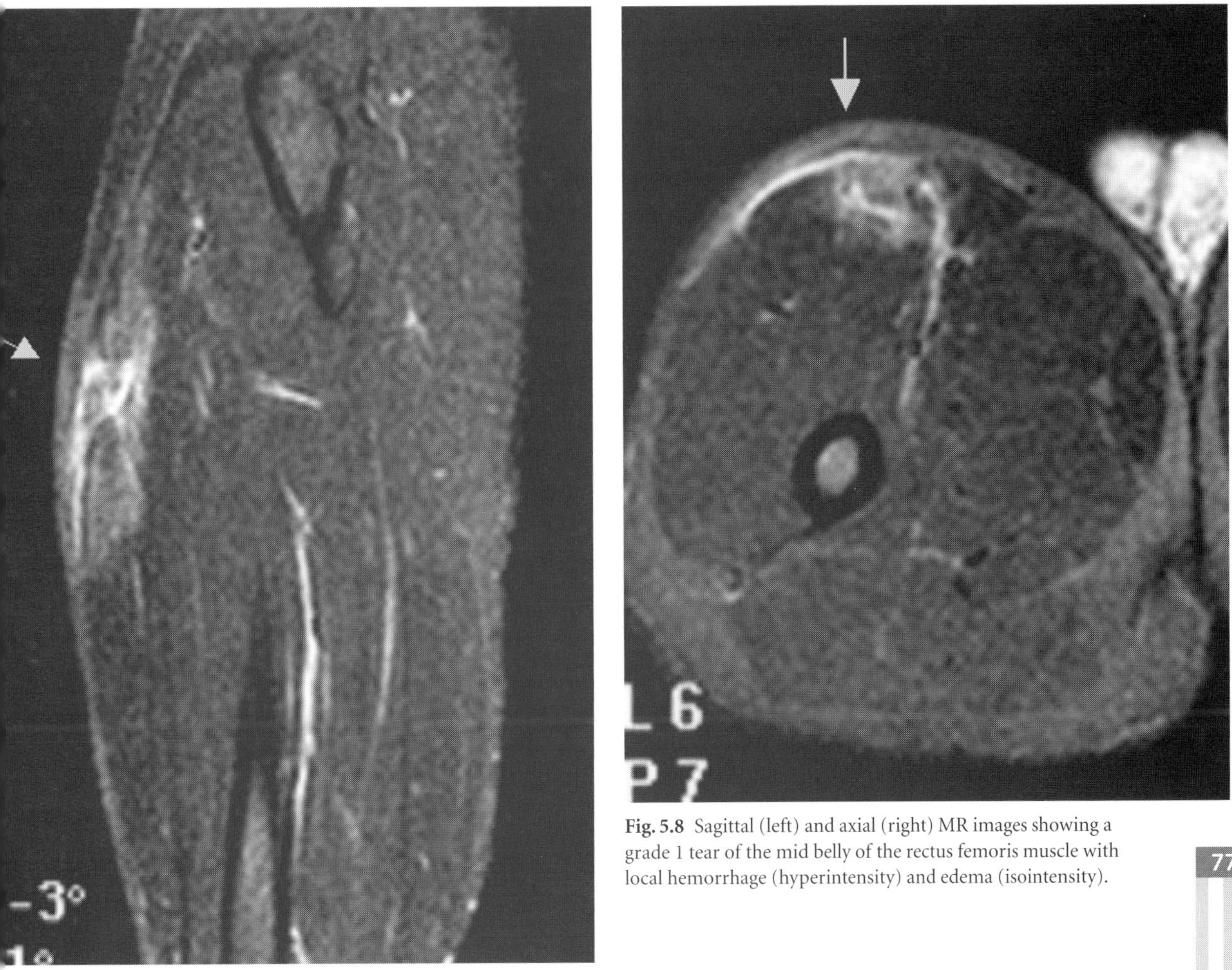


**Fig. 5.8** Sagittal (left) and axial (right) MR images showing a grade 1 tear of the mid belly of the rectus femoris muscle with local hemorrhage (hyperintensity) and edema (isointensity).



- Susceptibility blooming on gradient echo sequences (within the hematoma) and lack of internal enhancement allow differentiation from a true tumor (Fig. 5.8).

## Management

### Non-surgical

- Usually only conservative treatment is required.
- Compression bandage, heat retainer, ice, elevation and rest for grades 1 and 2 sprains.
- Sports massage techniques.
- Ultrasound and electrical stimulation have been successful in promoting healing.
- Rehabilitation program (recovery for grade 1 sprains is 2 weeks, and for grade 2 sprains is 2 months or more).

### Surgical

- Operative repair is rarely needed for grade 3 sprains (if a tendinous attachment has been avulsed or if there is an accompanying detached bone fragment).
- Rarely, decompression is needed for compartment syndrome.

# Hamstring tears

## Anatomy

- Hamstrings consist of three muscles (the semimembranosus forms the bulk, with the semitendinosus medially and the biceps femoris laterally) that run from the hip to the knee and assist with hip extension and knee flexion.
- Main origin is the ischial tuberosity.
- Function primarily to decelerate the extending knee prior to foot strike and to assist with hip extension after foot strike.
- As with other frequently injured muscles, the hamstrings span two joints and are therefore subject to stretching at more than one point.

## Mechanism of injury

- Most hamstring injuries are of a single muscle near the muscle–tendon junction (usually proximal semimembranosus musculotendinous unit).
- Rarely, the hamstring muscle group may avulse from the ischial tuberosity.
- Common in sports that require bursts of speed or rapid acceleration, such as soccer, running, [American] football and rugby.
- Often recurrent and difficult to treat.

## History and clinical findings

- 'Popping' sensation and sudden onset of pain in the posterior thigh in acute strains.
- On examination, ecchymosis and local tenderness over the posterior thigh.
- Pain worse on resisted hip extension and knee flexion.
- In grade 3 tears of an avulsed ischial tuberosity, a palpable defect may be felt.

## Imaging findings

### Radiography



- May demonstrate ischial tuberosity avulsion, especially in younger patients with incompletely fused epiphyses.

### Ultrasound

- Operator dependent but may show focal hypoechoic tendinosis or muscle tear. Acute hematoma will show as predominantly hypoechoic fluid collection with internal echoes.

### Computerized tomography

- May show muscle swelling with focal area of low attenuation (edema) or high attenuation (hemorrhage).

### Magnetic resonance imaging

- Partial tear results in local hemorrhage and edema, which is acutely hyperintense on $T_2$-weighted scans but becomes hyperintense on both $T_1$- and $T_2$-weighted scans when subacute.
- Ischial tuberosity avulsion recognized as hyperintense bone edema with local fluid collection and detached hypointense bone fragment (Figs 5.9, 5.10).

## Management

### Non-surgical

- Initial treatment typically consists of rest, ice, compression, elevation and pain relief.
- Ultrasound and electrical stimulation may aid healing.

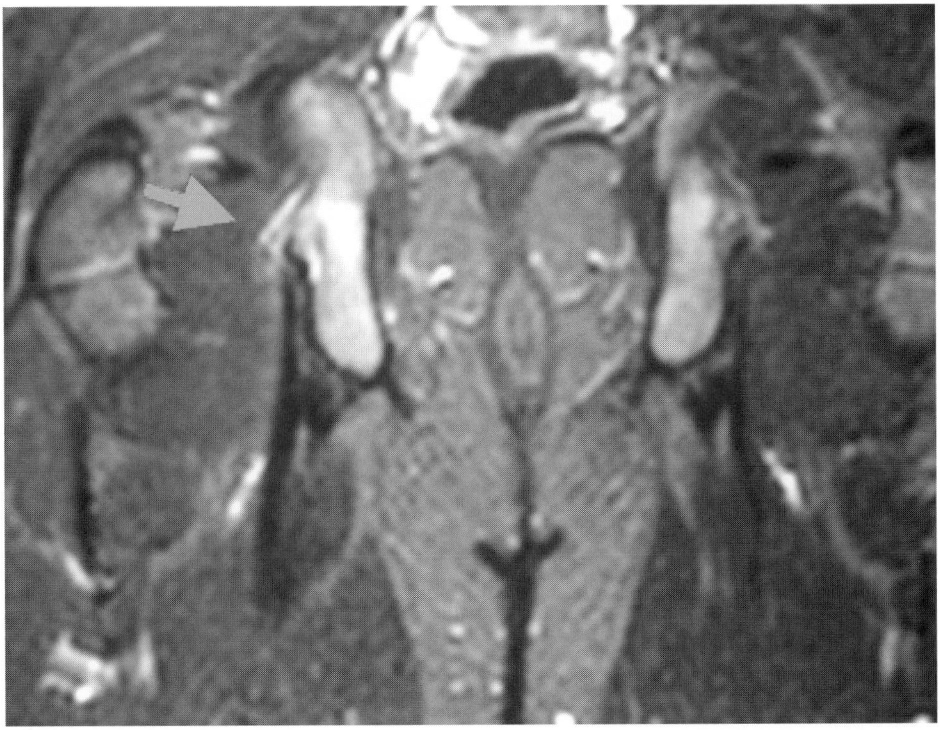

Fig. 5.9 Coronal, fat-suppressed MR image showing an undisplaced avulsion at the attachment of the hamstring to the ischial apophysis on the right.

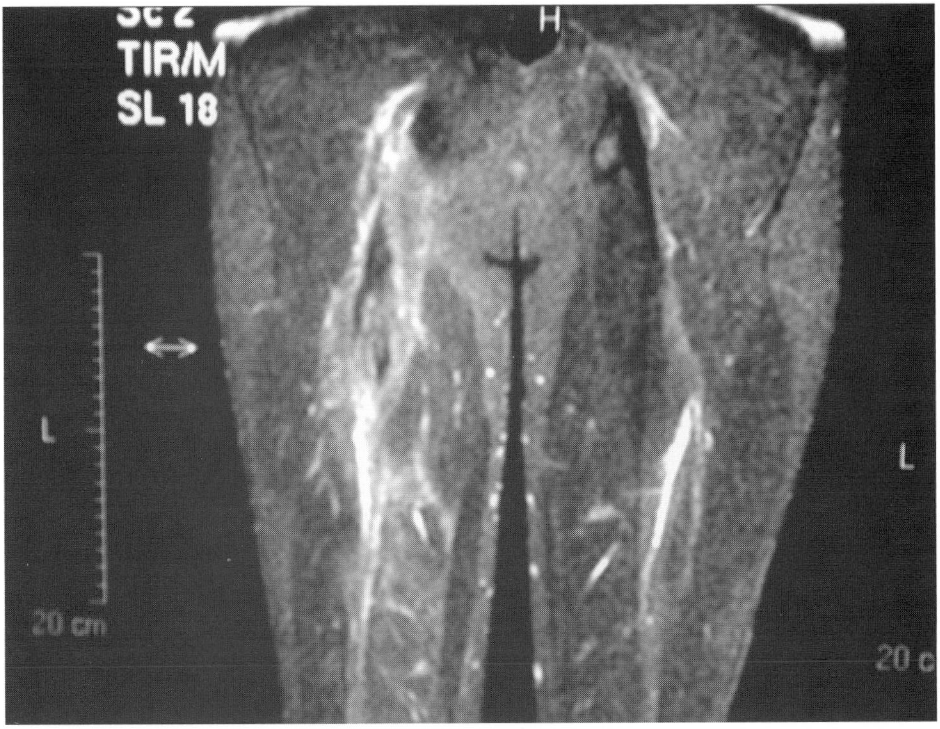


Fig. 5.10 Coronal, fat-suppressed MR image showing a 3-cm retraction at the site of a hamstring avulsion on the right.

- Emphasis on functional exercises with passive stretching and isometric strengthening initially, progressing to concentric then eccentric strengthening.
- Sports massage therapy.
- Recent studies have indicated earlier healing without scar formation by injecting 40 mg of prednisolone to the site of the muscle tear in muscle belly injuries.

Surgical

- For complete avulsion of the hamstring complex at or near the proximal bone–tendon junction, an acute surgical repair is preferred.

# Snapping hip syndrome

## Anatomy

- Variously divided into internal, external and intra-articular forms.

## Mechanism of injury

- Snapping hip syndrome (internal form) is the term used to describe a snapping sensation encountered in the region of the hip as the iliopsoas tendon passes over and catches on the iliopectineal eminence of the pubis, usually associated with iliopsoas bursal inflammation ('anterior deep snapping').
- Infrequently, snapping hip syndrome is attributed to a catching of the iliofemoral ligaments as they slide over the femoral head in flexion extension or to a snapping of the long head of the biceps as it slides over the ischial tuberosity on flexion and extension.

## History and clinical findings

- Snapping associated with hip movements is the reason for this complaint; it mainly occurs with hip abduction and external rotation (the iliopsoas tendon form).
- Usually non-tender and with no specific precipitating event.
- If pressure is applied over the iliopsoas tendon at the level of the femoral head, snapping is eliminated (internal type).

## Imaging findings

### Radiography

- Usually not useful; may show a loose body.

### Fluoroscopy

- With bursography to assess active iliopsoas muscle movement and presence of bursography.

### Ultrasound

- Real-time assessment of iliopsoas muscle and tendon over iliopectineal eminence, femoral head and lesser trochanter.

### Computerized tomography

- Generally not employed; useful for intra-articular loose bodies.

### Magnetic resonance imaging

- Bursitis with high-signal iliopsoas bursal fluid (Fig. 5.11).

## Management

### Non-surgical

- Reassurance and activity modification.
- Does not require treatment if non-tender.
- If tender, administer antiinflammatories progressing to intra-articular steroid injection.

### Surgical

- If the tenderness is troublesome and there is no response to conservative measures, then lengthen or divide the iliopsoas tendon with bursectomy.

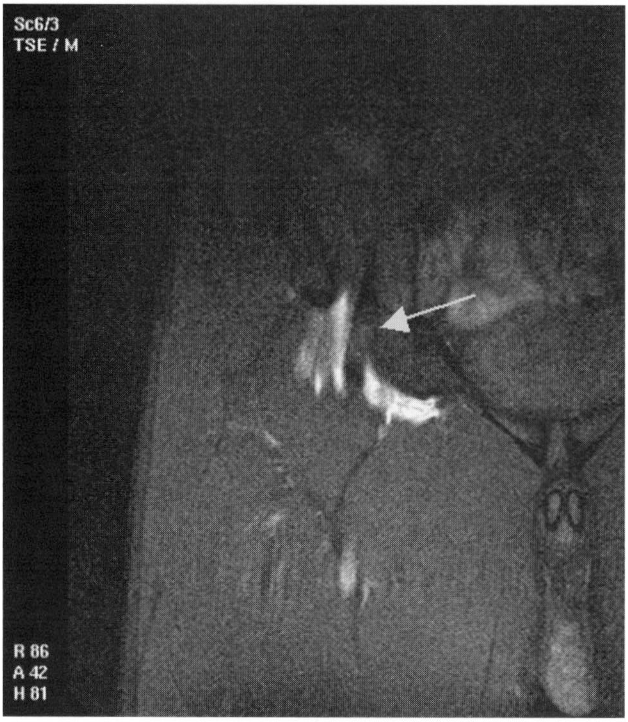


(a)

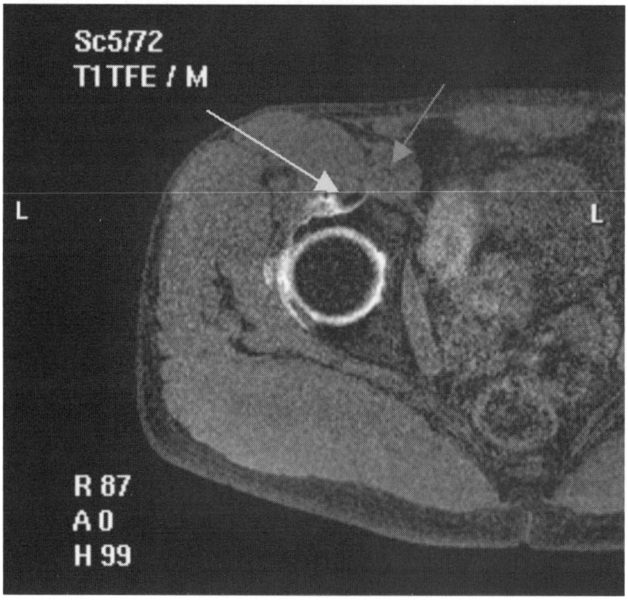


(b)

**Fig. 5.11** (**a**) Coronal fat-suppressed image showing fluid around the iliopsoas tendon within the associated bursa and (**b**) axial image in the same patient showing the iliopsoas tendon limited by a focal bone overgrowth over which the tendon subluxes to produce a snapping sound during hip flexion and extension.

# Trochanteric bursitis

## Anatomy

- Two bursae lie in relation to the greater trochanter: a superficial one between the fascia lata and gluteal tendons, and a deeper one between the gluteus medius tendon and posterior surface of the greater trochanter.

## Mechanism of injury

- Occasionally the trochanteric bursa becomes inflamed by friction and trauma imposed by the repetitive motion of the iliotibial band or tensor fascia lata sliding over the greater trochanter during active sports.
- In chronicity, induced bursal inflammation may result in marked bursal distension.
- Frequently bilateral.

## History and clinical findings

- Pain over the posterolateral aspect of the hip, which is worse during running.
- Symptoms worsen with hip external rotation and adduction.
- Pain and sometimes crepitus on adduction of the leg with the hip flexed.
- Tested by lying with the normal side down and raising the affected leg; pain results from superficial bursal compression and is exacerbated by resistance.

## Imaging findings

### Radiography

- Usually normal; may show a loose body in relation to the greater trochanter.

### Magnetic resonance imaging

- Coronal short tau inversion recovery (STIR) sequences show high-signal fluid/edema adjacent and parallel to the lateral aspect of the greater trochanter (Fig. 5.12).

## Management

### Non-surgical

- Rest, icing, NSAIDs and activity modification if possible.
- Bursal drainage ± steroid injection under fluoroscopy.

### Surgical

- In resistant cases, bursectomy with removal of any loose bodies.

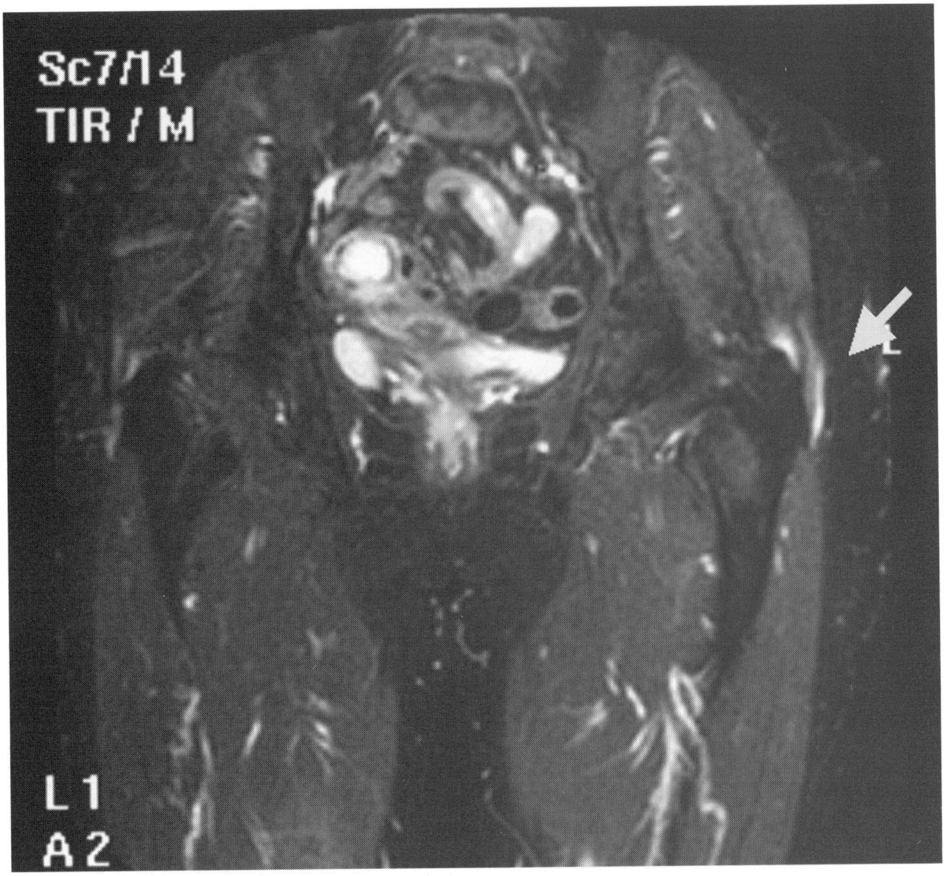




**Fig. 5.12** Coronal, fat-suppressed MR image showing focal inflammation over the greater trochanter in a patient with left trochanteric bursitis.

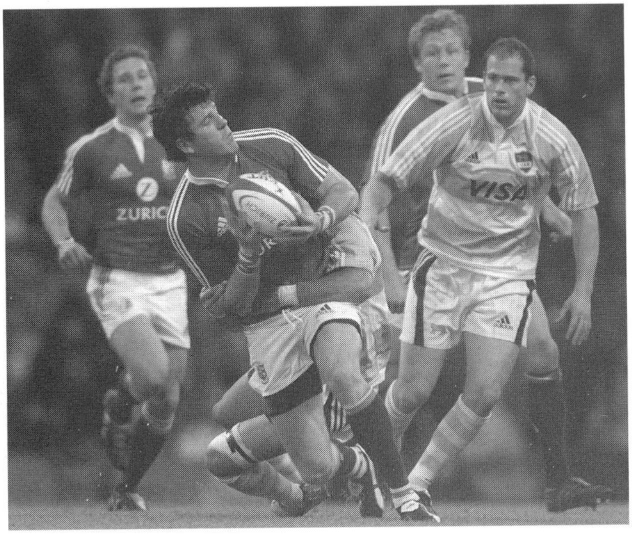


**Fig. 5.13** Sportsfield.

# Unstable pelvic ring fractures

## Anatomy

- The pelvis is a ring structure composed of integrated osseous and ligamentous structures. The osseous ring is composed of the sacrum, the ilium, the ischium and the pubis. Ligamentous stability of the pelvic ring is afforded by the iliolumbar, ventral and dorsal SI, sacrotuberous, sacrospinous and posterior interosseous ligaments.
- The ring configuration affords stability, only being disrupted following acutely applied forces in the vertical plane, lateral or anteroposterior compression (or a combination of all three forces).

## Mechanism of injury

- Fractures of the pelvis are classified, after Tile, as *stable* (in which the ring structure is not disrupted – avulsion injuries – or is only minimally displaced) or *unstable* (in which the inner ring is disrupted and injury is aggravated by persistent weight-bearing).
- Lateral compression results in acute pelvic implosion, with injury to the pelvis both anteriorly and posteriorly; typically, transverse rami fractures and sacral compression fractures concertina in configuration.
- Anteroposterior compression occurs as a result of forces applied anteriorly or as a result of compression applied through impacting lower extremities. Such forces result in symphyseal diastasis with dislocations in the posterior pelvis (Fig. 5.14).
- Vertical forces result in shear to the pelvis with vertical rami fractures, vertical symphyseal diastasis and SI joint disruption. Vertical shear injuries are often associated with soft-tissue injuries including arterial lacerations of the internal iliac vessels (Fig. 5.15).



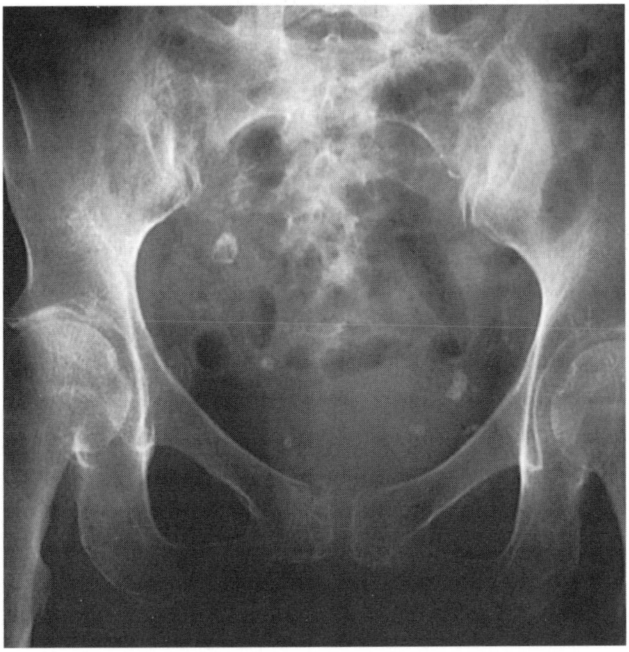

**Fig. 5.14**
Anteroposterior view of the pelvis showing linear sclerosis through the right sacral ala at a site of undisplaced fracture.

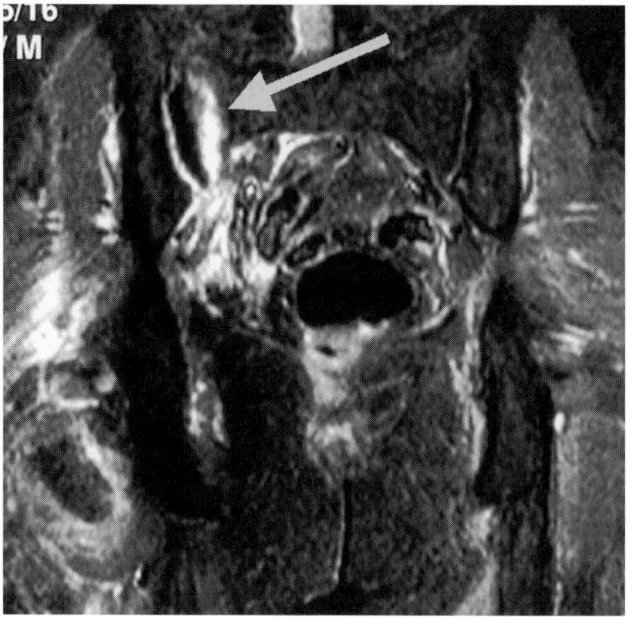


**Fig. 5.15** Coronal, fat-suppressed image showing linear signal hyperintensity through the right sacral ala at a site of fracture following vertical shear injury. Shear forces in the vertical orientation may be complicated by associated shear of pelvic side wall vessels and major secondary hemorrhage.

## History and clinical findings

- Usually history of significant trauma.
- Pelvic, groin, gluteal and thigh pain.
- Destot's sign: superficial hematoma above the inguinal ring at the scrotum or thigh.
- Pelvic stability assessed by bimanual compression, distraction of the iliac wings, and hip abduction and adduction.
- Leg deformity and shortening.
- PR and PV examinations should be performed in the acute setting to assess for internal soft-tissue injury or bone spicules from sacral fractures.



## Imaging findings

### Radiography

- Conventional radiography facilitates the routine evaluation of osseous injury although evaluation of the sacrum and SI joints is often limited.
- Views should include an inlet view (tube angled at 45° caudad) and outlet view (tube angled at 45° cephalad).

### Computerized tomography

- Computed tomography with 3D reformats is routinely employed to supplement evaluation in the axial plane, particularly to improve evaluation of the SI joints.

### Magnetic resonance imaging

- MRI in the axial plane affords a similar evaluation of the sacrum and SI joints although it is currently rarely employed for this purpose.
- Sensitivity to marrow edema (high signal on $T_2$-weighted images) may improve the detection of undisplaced fractures.
- Fracture lines appear hypointense on $T_2$-weighted images.

**Management**

- In the acute injury setting, follow ATLS guidelines with particular care regarding pelvic hemorrhage.

Non-surgical

- Some fractures can be conservatively treated, e.g. protected weight-bearing for unilateral pubic rami and sacral lateral compression fractures.
- Others may be treated with an external fixator, e.g. AP compression fractures with <2 cm symphyseal diastasis.

Surgical

- Open reduction, internal fixation (ORIF), with anterior and posterior stabilization required for higher-grade fractures.
- Patient usually also requires temporary colostomy for fecal diversion.

## Stable pelvic ring injuries: avulsions and coccygeal injuries

**Mechanism of injury**

- The musculotendinous unit is composed of a muscle belly that attaches either directly to bone or indirectly through an inelastic tendon. Trauma may induce injury to any part of the unit: compression resulting in contusion; and tension resulting in eccentric contraction, muscle strain or tear, tendon rupture or avulsion from bone.
- Prior to growth plate closure, the apophysis (attachment of tendon to bone) is the weakest point in the musculotendinous unit and is the most frequent site of injury following acutely applied tensile forces.
- With maturity and growth plate closure, tensile forces result in tearing either at the musculotendinous junction (usually a site of poor vascular perfusion) or in the muscle belly itself.
- Injury to, or weakening of, the tendon following intratendinous steroid injection or as a result of peritendinous inflammation (bursitis) may lead to intrasubstance tendon rupture.
- In the pelvis, apophyses appear later than epiphyseal centers in long bones, and so avulsions tend to occur after adolescence.
- Avulsion fractures represent 1 in 7 pelvic fractures in children.

# Ischial avulsions

## Anatomy

- The ischial tuberosity is the site of insertion of the conjoined tendon of the hamstrings and is the commonest site of pelvic avulsion fracture.

## Mechanism of injury

- Repeated rapid contraction of the muscle belly in athletes (e.g. hurdlers) or an acute contraction as an athlete attempts to maintain stability during sliding or hyperflexion at the hip is transmitted to the ischial apophysis resulting in avulsion.
- Injury as a result of chronic or repetitive trauma may produce local remodeling or osseous overgrowth as repeated attempts at healing are thwarted by further trauma. Callus superimposed on callus may lead to gross bony spur formation at the site of trauma in maturity, occasionally resulting in sciatic nerve compression.

## History and clinical findings

- Pain in the buttocks, which is worse on sitting and running.
- Point tenderness over a tuberosity.
- Limitation of activity involving the hamstring muscle group.

## Imaging findings

### Radiography

- When suspected, displaced avulsions are easily recognized by conventional radiography.
- If the apophysis not yet calcified, radiography will be normal.
- Callus formation at the fracture site.

### Computerized tomography

- Rarely needed; shows fracture fragment and degree of displacement.



### Magnetic resonance imaging

- MRI is of value in undisplaced avulsions; the sensitivity of fat-suppressed sequences to marrow edema allows the ready identification in the coronal, sagittal and axial planes (Fig. 5.16).
- Hyperintense marrow edema on $T_2$-weighted images at the fracture donor site with surrounding high-signal hemorrhage and soft-tissue edema.
- The avulsed fragment appears as a low signal but may be difficult to discern (correlate with plain radiography).

## Management

### Non-surgical

- Acute injury, if undisplaced, usually heals over 6 weeks to 3 months if immobilized.
- Initial rest, ice and antiinflammatories.
- Gradual return to weight-bearing with hamstring strengthening.

### Surgical

- Displaced acute avulsions are usually treated by surgical internal fixation with excellent results.
- In chronic cases with pain or non union, resection of bone fragment with tendon reattachment.

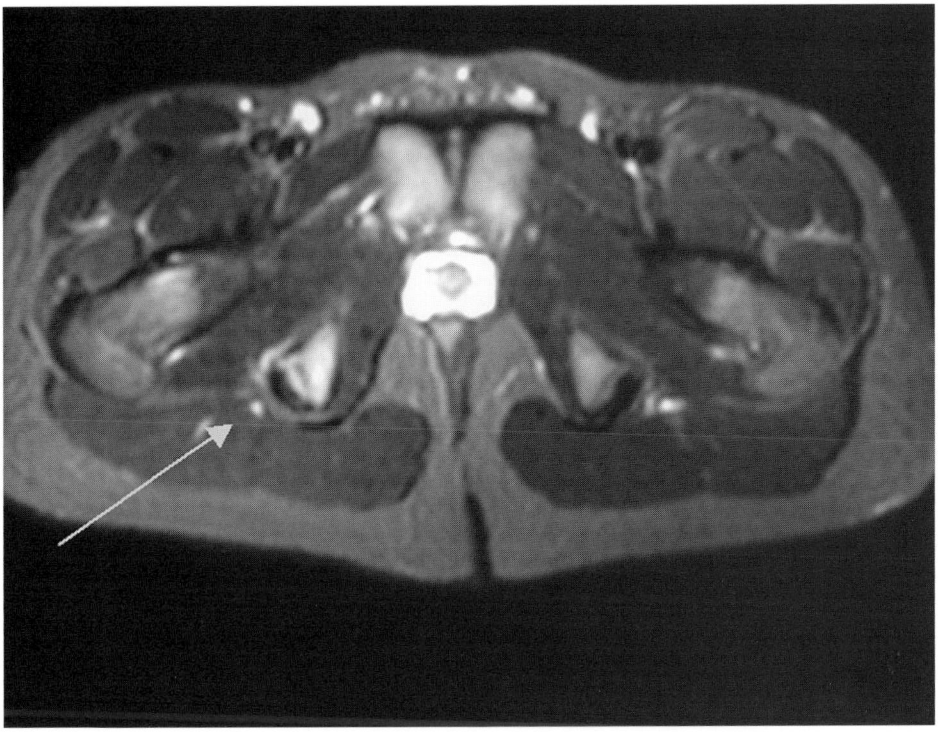

Fig. 5.16 Axial MR image showing an undisplaced avulsion at the hamstring attachment to the ischium.

# Pubic ramus avulsions

## Anatomy

- The adductor longus, magnus and brevis insert on the pubic rami at the junction of the inferior ramus and the symphysis.

## Mechanism of injury

- Repeated or acute traction may result in avulsion with osseous irregularity at this site, e.g. such as occurs following the use of 'Stair Master' exercise equipment.

## History and clinical findings

- Pain on palpation of the affected pubic ramus.
- Pain with stretching of the adductor or gracilis muscles.

## Imaging findings

### Radiography

- Although normally self-evident, osseous irregularity may be misinterpreted as being due to a malignant tumor, most frequently Ewing's sarcoma. Biopsy should not be undertaken without a detailed review as biopsy of marginal callus, secondary to attempted healing, may be misinterpreted as being a malignant osseous sarcoma.

### Isotope bone scan

- Scintigraphy typically reveals a focal accumulation of radiotracer at the site of avulsions, a focal 'hot spot' (Fig. 5.17).



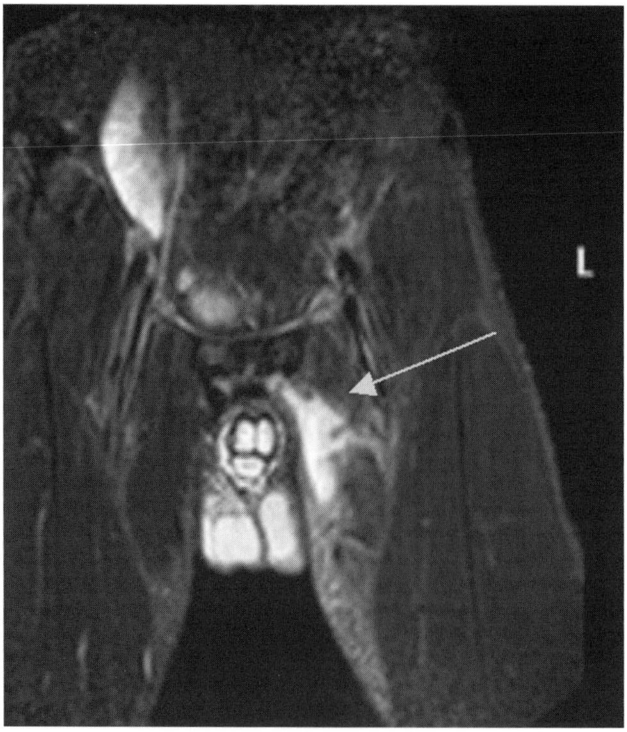


**Fig. 5.17** Coronal, fat-suppressed image showing a complete avulsion of the left adductor longus tendon from the inferior margin of the pubic symphysis in a professional rugby player.

Magnetic resonance imaging

- MRI in this setting may be misleading, revealing extensive edema both within bone and soft tissues.
- Avulsion should be suspected when edema or enhancement tracks along the adductors.
- Although acute avulsions are associated with minimal focal edema in the ramus, repetitive trauma may produce more marked or diffuse bone bruising or edema.

## Management

Non-surgical

- Rest, ice, NSAIDs with an occasional need for crutches.

Surgical

- Generally not required.

# Iliac spine avulsions

## Anatomy

- Iliac spine avulsions occur more commonly superiorly at the insertion of the sartorius and tensor fascia lata, than inferiorly at the insertion of the rectus femoris, which tend to be less symptomatic.

## Mechanism of injury

- Anterior superior iliac spine (ASIS): forceful contraction of the sartorius, e.g. kicking, jumping.
- Anterior inferior iliac spine (AIIS): forceful rectus femoris contraction, e.g. kicking sports.

## History and clinical findings

- Localized pain with point tenderness.
- Swelling after activity.

## Imaging findings

### Radiography

- AP pelvic films may show slight displacement of the ASIS (displacement limited by fascia lata) or distal displacement of the AIIS with or without callus formation.

### Computerized tomography

- For osseus detail.

### Magnetic resonance imaging

- Hyperintense marrow and soft-tissue edema on $T_2$-weighted images (Fig. 5.18).



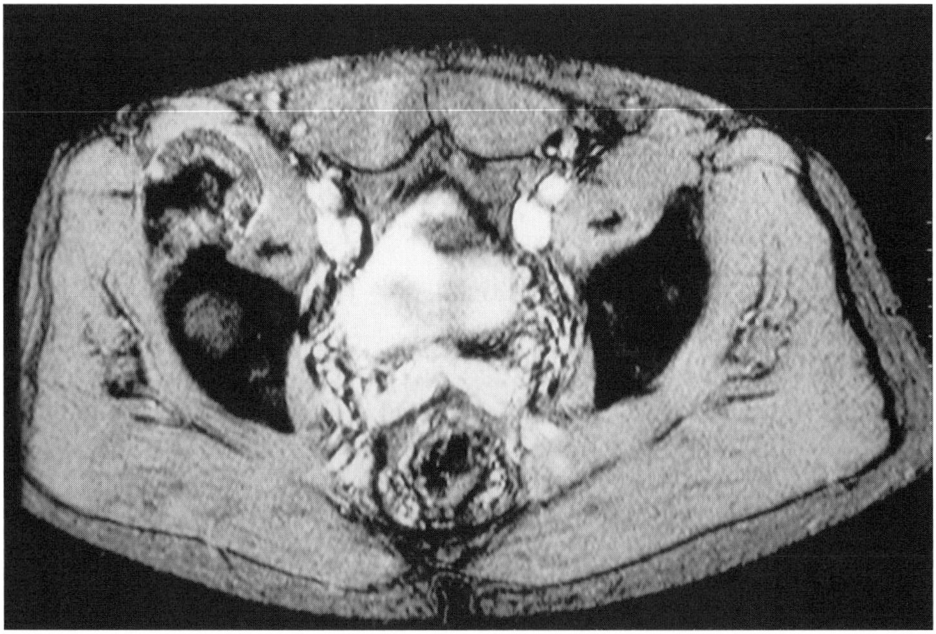

**Fig. 5.18** Axial MR image showing a minimally displaced avulsion at the attachment of the rectus femoris muscle to the anterior inferior iliac spine on the right side.

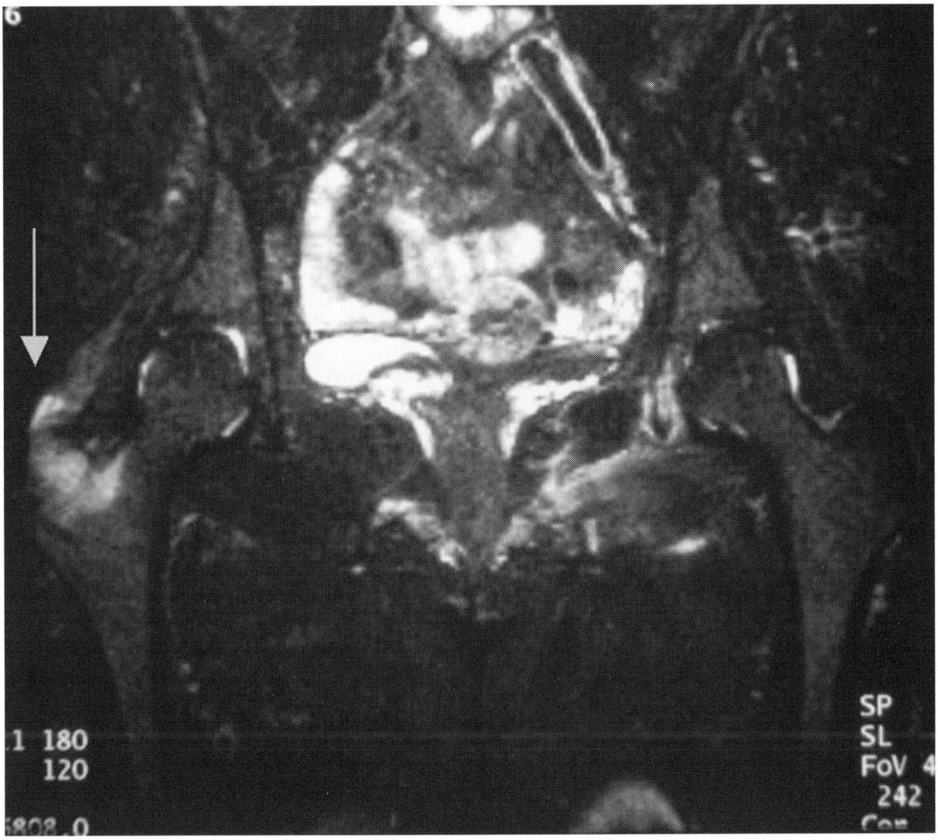


Fig. 5.19 Coronal MR image showing an undisplaced avulsion at the attachment of the abductors to the greater trochanter on the right side in a young female due to overuse incurred by daily gymnastic workout on a Stair Master machine.



## Management

### Non-surgical

- Unlike avulsions in the ischial tuberosity reflecting vascularity (red marrow), avulsions of the iliac spine usually heal without intervention (Fig. 5.19).

# Coccygeal injuries

## Anatomy

- The coccyx usually consists of four fused vertebral bodies rudimentary in nature without laminae and with few processes.
- The most cephalad segment articulates via a small disk with the caudad portion of the sacrum and has articulating processes projecting upward to unite with the sacral cornua via ligaments.

## Mechanism of injury

- As a result of position and delicacy, the coccyx is commonly injured following a direct blow as occurs following a fall on the buttocks.

## History and clinical findings

- Pain at the natal cleft, often remote from a history of trauma.

## Imaging findings

### Radiography

- The coccyx is poorly visualized on both AP and lateral conventional radiography as a result of overlying soft tissues.

### Isotope bone scan

- At scintigraphy, focal accumulation of radiotracer may be identified in the region of the coccyx but anatomic resolution is poor.

### Computerized tomography

- Despite tomographic imaging at CT, injuries to the coccyx are poorly evaluated in the axial plane as the orientation of the coccyx is variable.
- Sagittal 3D reformats are more useful.

### Magnetic resonance imaging

- Direct sagittal imaging and the sensitivity of MR images to edema allow optimum evaluation and detection of coccygeal injury, ranging from contusion through fracture to dislocation.

## Management

### Non-surgical

- Although the management of coccygeal injury is usually conservative, accurate diagnosis is often important in the trauma setting as the injury may have medicolegal implications.
- Local anesthetic injection and the manipulation of the sacrococcygeal synchondrosis have both been tried for chronic coccyx area pain.

### Surgical

- Removal of the coccyx has not been greatly successful in symptom relief.

# Acetabular fractures

## Anatomy

- The acetabulum is composed of an anterior column, superior column, posterior column and roof (quadrilateral plate).

## Mechanism of injury

- Most frequently secondary to femoral head impaction.
- Usually involves the posterior column (hip flexed and internally rotated), less frequently the roof.
- Injury to the anterior column is less common but usually complicates extension of a ramus fracture with the hip flexed and externally rotated at the time of injury.
- Letournel's and Judet's classification.

## History and clinical findings

- Pain at the fracture site.
- High-velocity trauma may result in other pelvic soft-tissue injury or solid-organ injury.

## Imaging findings

### Radiography

- Fractures are generally identified on conventional radiography, supplemented by oblique Judet views, on the basis of the integrity of six acetabular lines.
- The six acetabular lines are:
  - iliopectineal line (anterior column)
  - ilioischial line (posterior column)
  - teardrop
  - acetabular dome
  - anterior margin of the acetabulum
  - posterior margin of the acetabulum.
- 45° oblique Judet views show the obturator foramen, iliac crest in addition to columns, iliac (external) oblique view for posterior column and anterior wall obturator (internal) oblique for anterior column and posterior wall.

### Computerized tomography

- CT provides tomographic evaluation of the fracture position and accurately detects the amount of articular margin step-off (greater than 2 mm is generally treated surgically) and evaluates for associated loose intra-articular fragments.
- When fractures are in the axial plane, CT may be misleading. An 'in-plane' fracture phenomenon may lead to fractures actually being obscured. Since they are not visualized in the source data, they are therefore not identified in subsequent reconstructions.

### Magnetic resonance imaging

- The ability to image in multiple planes reduces the likelihood of 'in-plane fracture obscuration', while sensitivity to edema allows the detection of undisplaced injuries.
- High-signal marrow edema and low-signal fracture line on $T_2$-weighted images with hypointense free fragments.
- Better views of cartilage damage and surrounding soft-tissue structures.

## Management

### Non-surgical

- For a minority of fractures, e.g. nondisplaced or minimally displaced fractures.
- Traction for acetabular dome fractures displaced less than 3 mm.
- Significantly displaced fractures that do not involve the weight-bearing portion of the joint are sometimes conservatively managed, e.g. low anterior column.

### Surgical

- Ideally ORIF of acetabular fractures should be performed within 1 week of injury.
- Especially important for posterior fracture/dislocations to avoid posterior hip instability.
- Total hip arthroplasty.

# Fractures of the femoral neck

## Anatomy

- Fractures of the proximal femur are classified as intra- or extra-articular.
- Intra-articular fractures involve the femoral head and neck, typically occurring at the head/neck junction (termed subcapital) or mid neck (termed transcervical).
- Intra-articular fractures may disrupt the vascular supply to the femoral head via the circumflex vessels.
- Extra-articular fractures are classified as intertrochanteric or subtrochanteric.
- The stability of these fractures is dictated by the obliquity or axis of the fracture.

## Mechanism of injury

- In younger patients, fractures of the femoral neck are usually secondary to a fall on the hip, e.g. when skiing.
- Direct trauma is much less common.

## History and clinical findings

- Garden's classification (Box 5.1) is widely employed to grade femoral neck fractures. It describes the relative displacement of fracture fragment and hence the relative risk of subsequently developing avascular necrosis (AVN) of the femoral head.
- Pain in the hip, groin, anterior thigh or knee, which is worse with exertion.
- Limitation of hip internal rotation with the leg shortened and externally rotated.
- Pain on axial compression or with tapping over the greater trochanter.

## Imaging findings

### Radiography

- AP and lateral views to locate the fracture line and identify the fracture fragment positions.
- Supplementary Judet (oblique) view for acetabular surface.
- Undisplaced (Garden's types I and II) fractures may remain occult and may be particularly difficult to detect in elderly osteopenic patients where minor alterations in trabecular alignment resulting from fracture may be harder to perceive (Fig. 5.20).

### Isotope bone scan

- In the past, this was used to detect radiographically occult fractures on the premise that an early osteoblastic reaction at fracture margins results in a focal linear accumulation of radiopharmaceutical at that site.
- An osteoblastic response at fracture margins is seen in 80% of patients within 24 hours of trauma but may be delayed in the elderly and only begin to occur as late as 72 hours following injury.

**Box 5.1 Garden's classification**

Garden I: incomplete or impacted

Garden II: complete but not displaced

Garden III: complete with partial displacement

Garden IV: complete fracture and total displacement

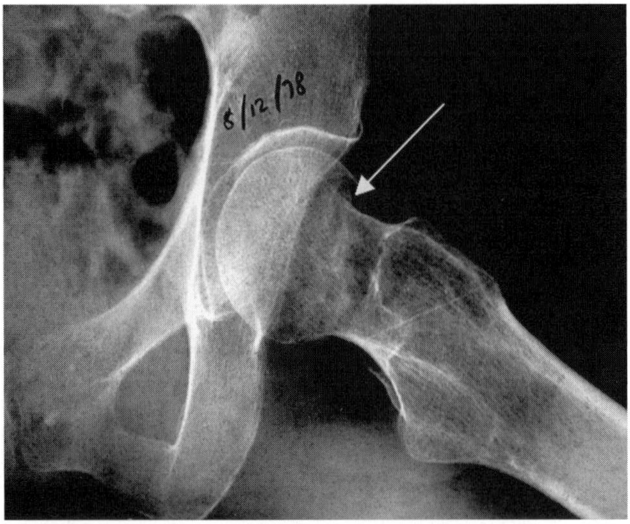


**Fig. 5.20** Radiograph showing an undisplaced subcapital femoral head fracture on the left.

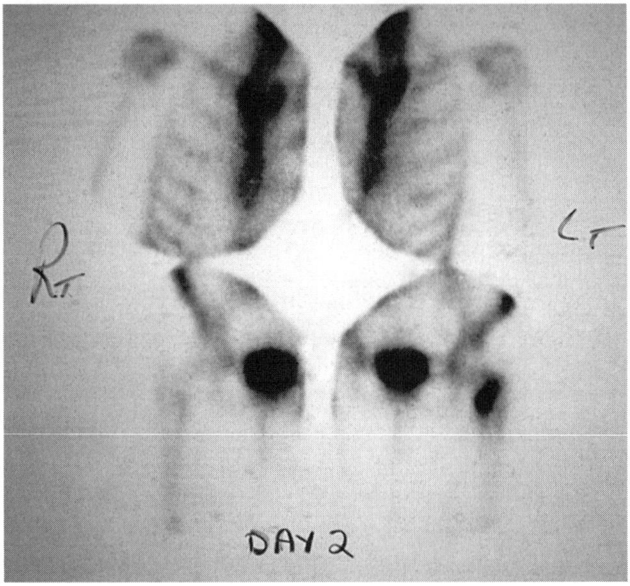


**Fig. 5.21** Isotope bone scan showing the concentration of radiotracer in the left intertrochanteric ridge at a site of undisplaced fracture.



- In addition, bone scintigrams may remain positive for up to 2 years as a result of post-traumatic vascular recruitment (Fig. 5.21).

## Computerized tomography

- Used prior to surgical planning for fragment number and position; best for bone detail, especially post fracture/dislocation.
- Coronal reformats useful.
- Determining extent of union postoperatively.

## Magnetic resonance imaging

- MRI facilitates the immediate detection of undisplaced fractures, manifest as a hypointense fracture line surrounded by adjacent edema (Fig. 5.22).
- MRI not only allows specific characterization of the fracture type but also the axis of the fracture, allowing optimal surgical planning.

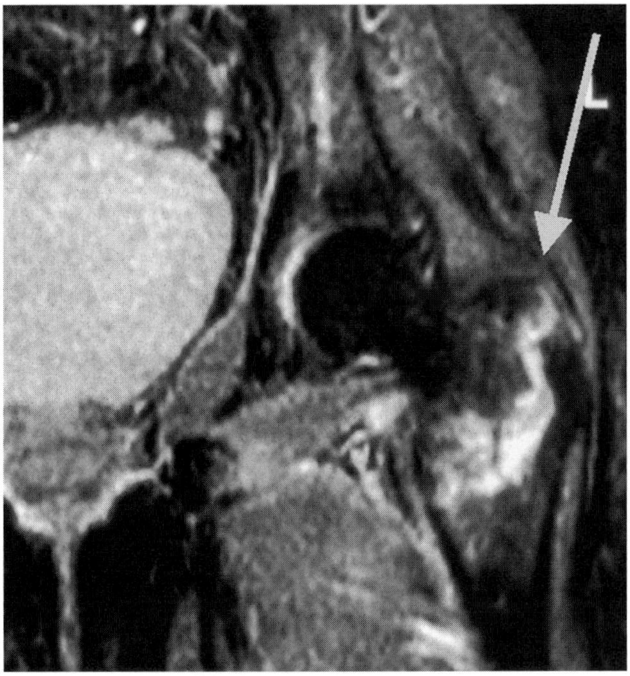


**Fig. 5.22** Coronal, fat-suppressed image showing linear signal hyperintensity through the intertrochanteric ridge at the site of an intertrochanteric fracture.

- Although the American College of Radiology recommends a single coronal $T_1$-weighted scan to evaluate patients with suspected femoral neck fractures, additional coronal $T_1$-weighted and fat-suppressed images (e.g. STIR) are frequently performed.
- A fracture line appears hypointense on $T_1$-weighted images. Cartilage injury is also well appreciated on $T_1$-weighted images as a discontinuity in the intermediate signal hyaline cartilage.
- Accompanying bone edema, hemorrhage, effusion and muscle strains are better appreciated as hyperintense on $T_2$-weighted images.

## Management

### Non-surgical

- Management is usually surgical.

### Surgical

- Patients with recognized undisplaced femoral neck fractures require acute admission from the emergency room and early screw fixation in most cases.
- With unrecognized fractures that progress to displaced fractures with continued activity, AVN or non-union commonly develop following delayed operative intervention.
- Screw fixation/pinning of the hip to anchor the femoral head to the shaft (when there is a low risk of developing AVN so that the native joint can be saved).
- Hemi- or total arthroplasty if there is a high risk of subsequent AVN (Figs 5.23 and 5.24).

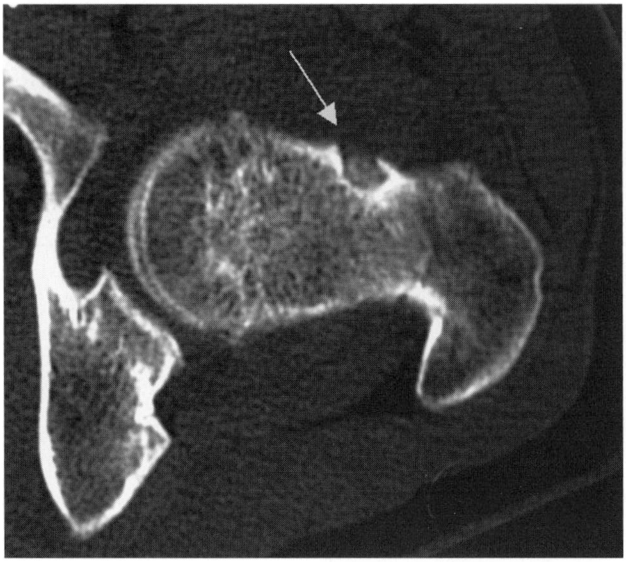

(a)

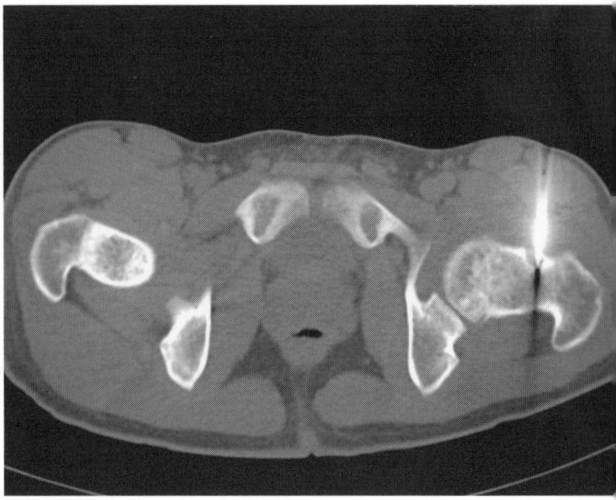

(b)

**Fig. 5.23** (**a**) Axial CT scan showing an osteoid osteoma within the left femoral neck presenting in a young male sportsman with a 3-month history of night pain relieved by aspirin, initially incorrectly attributed to a sports-related hip injury. (**b**) Axial CT scan showing a radiofrequency probe within the nidus of the osteoid osteoma at the time of image-guided ablation.

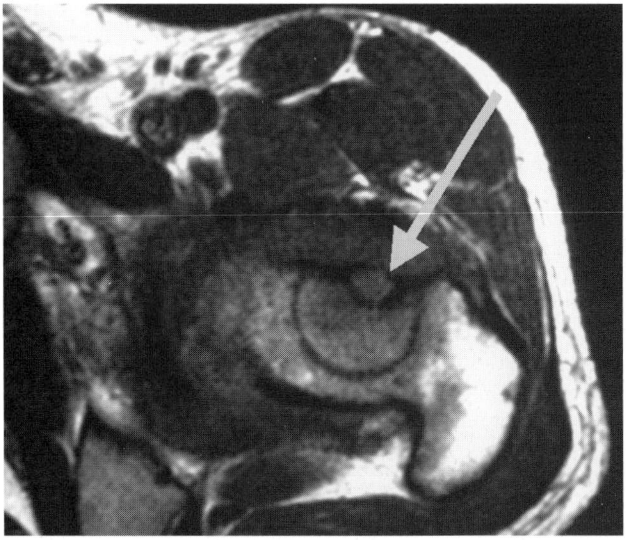

**Fig. 5.24** Post-radiofrequency ablation axial MR image showing circumferential rind of marrow change around the nidus of the treated osteoid osteoma.

## Stress fractures: fatigue versus insufficiency

Stress fractures are either due to *fatigue* (as a result of abnormal stress on normal bone) or *insufficiency* (as a result of normal stress on abnormal bone). In general, the term 'stress fracture' is used to describe fatigue fractures rather than insufficiency, and although they occur as a result of chronic stress they often present as a result of acute fracture to a site weakened over time.

# Femoral neck fatigue fractures

## Anatomy

- The femoral neck lies between the femoral head and intertrochanteric line.
- Weight-bearing forces are transmitted to the inferior aspect; the superior aspect is subject to more tension-like forces.
- There is a high risk of disruption to the femoral head blood supply and subsequent AVN development.

## Mechanism of injury

- Femoral neck stress fractures are not uncommon, occurring in long-distance athletes and military recruits, who present with persistent groin pain exacerbated by exercise.
- Compression stress fractures (inferior femoral neck) are common in younger patients.

## History and clinical findings

- Deep pain at the hip, groin or thigh.
- Pain is worse during loading of the hip joint and after exercise, increasing in severity over weeks if activity continues.
- Antalgic gait on examination with the pain worse when standing on the affected leg.
- Limitation of internal and external rotation.

## Imaging findings

### Radiography

- AP and 'frog leg' views.
- Femoral neck stress fractures are occult on plain radiography in up to 50% of cases.
- In chronicity, they are manifest by a focal periosteal reaction, cortical break or band of sclerosis.



### Isotope bone scan

- Reflecting induced osteoblastic activity, stress fractures appear as a linear band of uptake perpendicular to the long axis of the shaft. A normal bone scan essentially excludes the diagnosis of stress fracture.

### Magnetic resonance imaging

- A low-signal band perpendicular to and continuous with the cortex of the medial femoral neck is seen on all pulse sequences, secondary to osteoblastic activity and bony sclerosis.
- Within 3 weeks of the onset of symptoms, note is often made of adjacent edema and hemorrhage, manifest as signal hyperintensity on $T_2$-weighted and fat-saturated sequences (STIR).
- After 3 weeks, following the resolution of edema, hypointense sclerosis at sites of fractures may be obscured adjacent to hypointense fat on both inversion recovery and frequency selective sequences. The evaluation of a suspected stress fracture is therefore best achieved using a $T_1$-weighted spin echo sequence in which the hypointense line is contrasted against hyperintense marrow fat.

## Management

### Non-surgical

- Usual mode of treatment for inferior (compression) side fractures.

- Rest with use of crutches until complete healing has occurred (usually 5–8 weeks but it can take longer).
- Ice and antiinflammatories to ease pain.
- Dietary review regarding calcium intake/need for supplements.

Surgical

- For superior (tension) side fractures, especially when displaced.
- Internal screw fixation for fractures of the upper lateral femoral neck due to the high incidence of completion to total fracture if not fixed.

# Insufficiency fractures

## Anatomy

- Pelvic insufficiency fractures occur in osteoparotic or osteomalacic bone.
- The pubic rami, femoral neck and sacrum, where they occur parallel to the SI joints, are common locations.

## Mechanism of injury

- In contrast to fatigue fractures, where margins are grossly sclerotic and hypointense, an absent healing response in abnormal bone accounts for the poorly identified marginal healing response.
- Runners and contact sports participants are susceptible.

## History and clinical findings

- Hip, buttock or groin pain.
- Pain on weight-bearing or walking.
- No significant history of trauma.
- Examination unremarkable; may have point tenderness, e.g. over the sacrum.
- May have gait abnormality or reduced range of motion.
- Symptoms out of proportion to clinical findings.

## Imaging findings

### Radiography

- A lack of healing response accounts for the difficulty in detecting insufficiency fractures by radiography.
- Osteopenia is a frequent finding but non-specific.

### Isotope bone scan

- Increased radiotracer uptake.
- Honda sign with bilateral sacral alar fractures with transverse component.



### Computerized tomography

- Not generally used; the fracture line is vertically orientated along the sacral ala parallel to SI joints.
- Sclerosis at the fracture line margin.

### Magnetic resonance imaging

- Commonly observed are signal hyperintensity and edema at the site of injury on $T_2$-weighted images.
- Fatigue fractures are best visualized on fat-suppressed sequences such as STIR.
- Sacral insufficiency fractures are best visualized in the coronal plane oblique to the axis of the sacrum off a sagittal localizer.
- 'Honda' sign in bilateral sacral alar fractures on $T_2$-weighted images.

## Management

### Non-surgical

- This is for the majority of patients but healing may take months.
- Rest and reduced weight-bearing to prevent progression to complete fracture.
- Pain relief.
- Muscle strengthening exercises with gait training.

### Surgical

- Sacroplasty (akin to vertebroplasty with injection of polymethylmethacrylate) for pain relief.

# Hip dislocations

## Anatomy

- The hip joint is extremely stable under normal conditions due to its ball-and-socket configuration and supporting ligaments.
- 75% of hip dislocations are posterior.

## Mechanism of injury

- This is rare in sport but does occur in high-energy impact sports, e.g. water skiing and rugby, when the knee is flexed and the hip flexed and adducted.
- More commonly accompanies high-velocity trauma, e.g. a motor vehicle accident involving a dashboard injury. Impaction against the dashboard is transmitted through the patella and femur to the posterior column of the acetabulum.
- In severe injury the femoral head either subluxes or dislocates posteriorly, with or without fracture of the posterior column of the acetabulum and/or of the femoral head.
- The incidence of AVN complicating posterior dislocation is high as both circumflex vessels and the ligamentum teres are disrupted; AVN occurs in almost 100% of cases if reduction is delayed for over 24 hours.

## History and clinical findings

- Severe hip pain with radiation to the knee or back.
- Numbness/tingling in the leg due to sciatic nerve neuropraxia (as the sciatic nerve runs posterior to the hip joint).
- Reduced hip movements and an inability to walk.
- In posterior dislocation, the hip is shortened, internally rotated and adducted.
- Possible vascular damage, sciatic nerve injury and coexistent knee injury.

## Imaging findings

### Radiography

- AP, lateral views with supplementary internal and external oblique views.
- Dislocation is readily evaluated by conventional radiography and infrequently requires additional imaging.
- Post-reduction films are required to check for alignment and any loose bone fragments.

### Computerized tomography

- Used for failed closed reduction, asymmetry between joint spaces post-reduction, loose body location and coexistent acetabular fractures.

## Management

### Non-surgical

- Closed reduction should be performed as soon as possible post-injury to minimize the risk of AVN using the Allis, Stimson or Bigelow maneuvers.
- Post-reduction traction for 1–2 weeks if reduction is successful.
- Rest and antiinflammatories.
- If instability is present, use short leg cast in external rotation.
- Gradual reintroduction of activity.

### Surgical

- If closed reduction is unsuccessful, bone fragments are present in the joint or the joint remains unstable.
- Open reduction via posterior approach with internal screw fixation.

# Avascular necrosis of the femoral head

## Anatomy

- The vascular supply to the femoral head is predominantly through perforating branches of the circumflex femoris artery (superior retinacular artery), with additional supply through the ligamentum teres artery.

## Mechanism of injury

- Trauma is the most common cause of femoral head AVN.
- Femoral neck fractures result in the disruption of retinacular and sinusoidal vessels markedly reducing perfusion following injury.
- Post-traumatic ischemia generates marrow and impaired vascular drainage, secondary to raised intramedullary pressure.
- In undisplaced fractures, vascular recanalization frequently occurs and the subsequent development of bone necrosis is uncommon.
- In practice, evidence of osteonecrosis is identified in 10% of undisplaced fractures, and in up to 35% of displaced fractures.
- Since both the retinacular vessels and the artery of the ligamentum teres are injured following posterior dislocation of the hip, the incidence of AVN in this group is even higher at up to 50%, particularly in patients with fracture dislocation. Delayed reduction following hip dislocation over 24 hours increases the rate of AVN to almost 100%.
- The anterolateral femoral head is the most common location (due to weight-bearing).

## History and clinical findings

- Can be asymptomatic initially.
- Gradual onset of pain over the groin or hip, which may radiate to the gluteals, thighs or knees.
- Pain is worse with activity and eased by rest.
- Hip 'clicking' on external rotation or rising from sitting.
- Decreased range of motion (flexion, abduction, internal rotation) with or without a limp.



## Imaging findings

- An international staging system using radiographic findings has been developed by Ficat (Box 5.2) and Arlet and has been used widely for treating AVN. This has been supplanted by the classification system of Steinberg which incorporates MRI and scintigraphic findings.

### Box 5.2 Ficat classification

Stage 0: osteonecrosis on bone biopsy, normal imaging

Stage 1: positive bone scan ± MRI (early resorptive stage)

Stage 2: mottled femoral head with sclerosis, cystic change, demineralization on radiograph, and positive bone scan and MRI (reparative stage)

Stage 3: crescent sign lesion and depressed femoral head articular surface (early collapse)

Stage 4: flattened articular surface, joint space narrowing and secondary acetabular changes (degenerative)

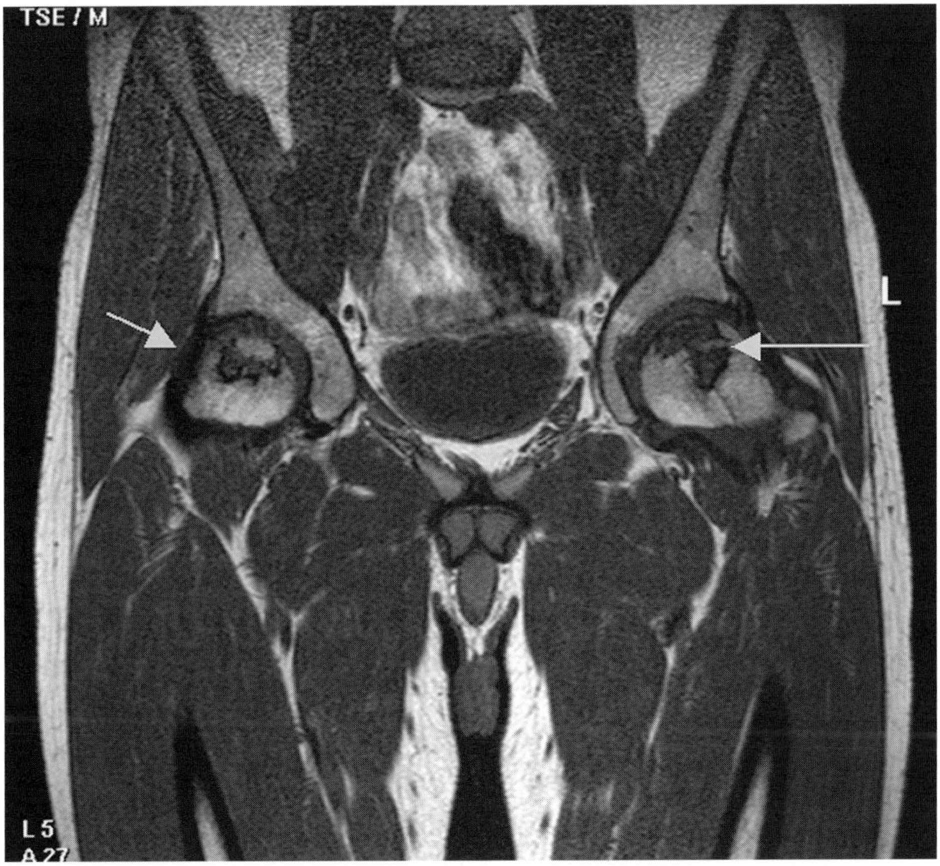


**Fig. 5.25** Coronal MR image showing well-demarcated serpiginous areas of marrow change within the right and left femoral heads indicating bilateral avascular necrosis.



## Radiography

- AP and frog lateral views.
- Ficat classification (Box 5.2).
- Not sensitive for lower stages 1 and 2; a delay of 1–5 years can occur between the onset of symptoms and the appearance of radiographic abnormalities.
- Femoral head sclerosis and subchondral collapse are late features.

## Computerized tomography

- Sensitivity greater than with plain films but less than with MRI.
- Only as sensitive as nuclear medicine in the early stages.
- CT is better able to help define the extent of disease at stage 2 and higher than MRI and plain film.
- For the detection of subchondral or cancellous fractures and collapse, especially with multiplanar reconstruction pretreatment.

## Magnetic resonance imaging

- Allows the earliest detection of AVN; the coronal plane is the most useful (Fig. 5.25).
- Dynamic gadolinium-enhanced techniques allow the earliest evaluation of vascular integrity. Using a fat-saturated $T_1$-weighted fast field echo sequence,

with sequential keyhole acquisitions, relative enhancement of the femoral head may be determined. Early identification of ischemia might prompt prolonged immobilization and hence even greater vascular reperfusion.

- As AVN progresses, the zone of ischemia becomes marginated by a serpiginous dark outer and a bright inner band, the so called 'double line' sign (seen in 80%), evident up to 6 months pre-detection of abnormality on conventional radiography.
- This sign is thought to reflect vascular ingrowth from the viable margins to the infarcted segment, hypointense sclerosis or new bone being laid down behind the hyperintense fluid-rich tissue as vascular ingrowth occurs.
- In established ischemia, subchondral bone becomes necrotic and collapses to produce the radiographic crescent sign. Loss of subchondral biomechanic integrity is followed by articular margin collapse and eventually joint space osteoarthritis.

### Isotope bone scan

- Planar scanning with pinhole collimator has a sensitivity of 55% for early AVN.

### Single photon emission computed tomography (SPECT)

- Initially, SPECT images reflect vascular integrity. Early in the disease, scans may demonstrate an avascular focus.
- Sensitivities approach MRI.

## Management

### Non-surgical

- Non-operative treatment usually results in a poor prognosis.
- Protected weight-bearing is associated with a greater than 85% rate of femoral head collapse.



### Surgical

- Bone marrow decompression (core decompression) is proposed to decrease vascular engorgement and inflammation and to relieve the increased intramedullary pressure. It should be performed before the onset of subchondral fracture. Bone marrow decompression is more effective when less than 30% of the femoral head is involved.
- Other options include bone grafting, osteotomy, joint fusion and total hip arthroplasty.
- Angular or rotational osteotomies are useful for the treatment of stage 3 disease and can help delay the time for total joint replacement.
- Bone grafting may become useful in treating severe stage 2 pre-collapse lesions, early stage 3 lesions or hips that have been treated unsuccessfully using core decompression.
- Femoral head collapse diminishes the success of operative procedures. Most patients proceed to femoral head replacement.

# Traumatic myositis ossificans

**Anatomy**

- This problem may occur in any muscle post-injury, commonly the thigh muscles.

**Mechanism of injury**

- Heterotopic bone formation within para-articular soft tissues is a well-recognized complication of contact sports.
- Although occasionally identified in the absence of trauma, there is a history of isolated or repeated hip trauma in two-thirds of cases.
- Following muscle trauma, mesenchymal cells proliferate at the site of tissue damage and become mineralized as they differentiate into osteoblastic components and subsequently into mature bone.

**History and clinical findings**

- History of precipitating trauma.
- Local pain at the site of injury with reduced movement in an adjacent joint if extensive.
- Active contraction of the affected muscle causes pain.

## Imaging findings

Radiography

- Early examination may be negative.
- Floccular calcification seen from 3 weeks with or without soft-tissue mass.
- Matures by about 6 weeks.
- Can be separate from adjacent bone but in 50% of cases adheres to adjacent bone.
- Differentiated from osteosarcoma by a history of trauma, diaphyseal location (vs. metaphysis in osteosarcoma) and progression of calcification from periphery inwards (opposite to osteosarcoma).



Isotope bone scan

- Mineralization may be seen in damaged soft tissues as early as 11 days, characterized by focal accumulation of radiotracer (technetium 99m methylene diphosphonate) at scintigraphy.

Computerized tomography

- For early detection prior to radiographic evidence.
- For site and size of new bone mass and associated soft-tissue asymmetry.

Magnetic resonance imaging

- Not as useful as CT.
- Once identified, imaging is used both to determine the true extent but also the maturity of the process.
- Early soft-tissue mineralization is characterized by the focal accumulation of edema and signal hyperintensity at $T_2$-weighted imaging, usually with a soft-tissue mass.
- With maturity, lesions appear as inhomogeneous masses with fat-signal intensities on both $T_1$- and $T_2$-weighted images.

## Management

Non-surgical

- Most episodes can be managed conservatively.

- The reduction of swelling and hematoma formation by compression at the time of injury may limit the subsequent development of myositis ossificans.
- Gradual introduction of an exercise program to increase range of motion.
- Progressive mineralization may be limited by immediate radiation therapy in patients following its identification.

Surgical

- If there is restricted function despite optimal conservative treatment.
- Surgery prior to completed ossification may result in incomplete resection and recurrence.
- No change in the extent on three consecutive radiographs, markedly reduced concentration of radiotracer at scintigraphy (similar uptake to adjacent mature bone) and absence of edema surrounding heterotopic bone at MRI are used as markers of mature heterotopic bone.

## Osteitis pubis

**Anatomy**

- This occurs in the fibrocartilagenous disk between bodies of two pubic bones (Figs 5.26–5.28).

**Mechanism of injury**

- Painful, non-infectious inflammation of the pubic symphysis.
- Results from repetitive abnormal shearing-type stress to the pelvis.
- Common in sports with repetitive kicking.
- Frequently associated with adductor origin microtear.

**History and clinical findings**

- Gradual onset pain localized over the symphysis, which may radiate to the groin, medial thigh or abdomen.
- Pain is exacerbated by activities such as running, twisting and kicking, and by lying on the side; pain can be relieved by rest.
- The patient may experience a sensation of 'clicking' or grinding when rising from a seated position or walking on uneven ground.

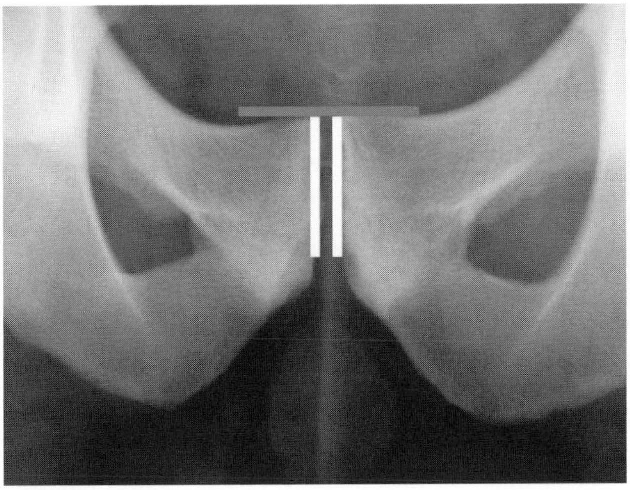

**Fig. 5.26** Radiograph showing superior congruity of the symphysis pubis with parallel articular surfaces.

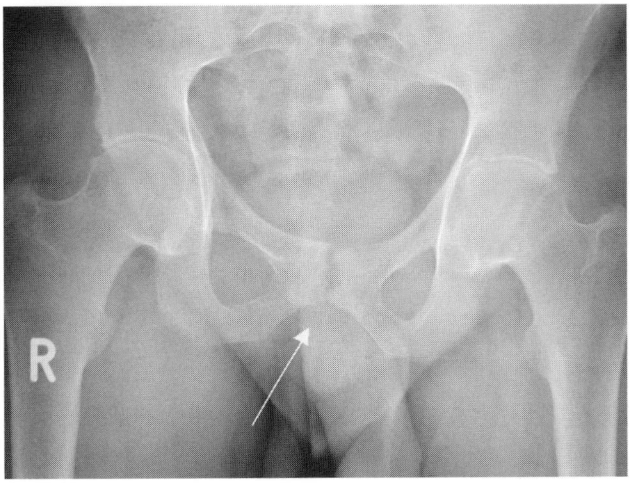


**Fig. 5.27** AP view of the pelvis showing a loss of symphyseal superior congruity with articular surface irregularity and erosion secondary to symphyseal laxity in a patient with osteitis pubis.

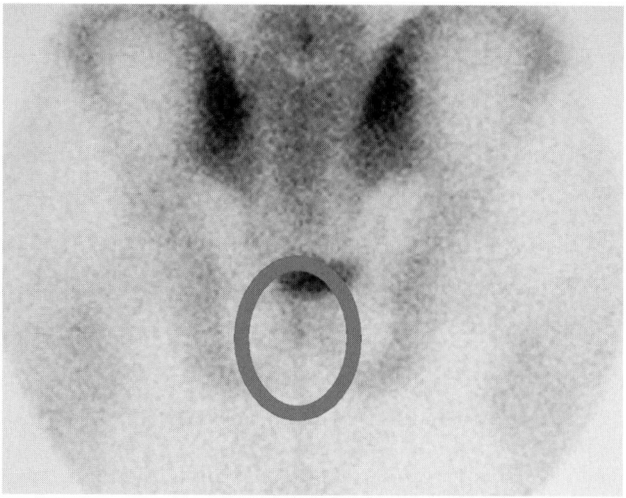

**Fig. 5.28** Bone scan showing no significant activity in the healthy symphysis pubis.

- Rarely, there is leg weakness (especially in the hip adductors) and difficulty walking.
- Pain on direct palpation of the pubic symphysis, and symphyseal pain induced by compressing the iliac blades.
- Rarely, adductor muscle spasm and abnormal gait, e.g. antalgic gait.

## Imaging findings



### Radiography

- Findings are non-specific and may not be radiographically apparent normally until 4 weeks after symptom onset.
- Plain radiography may demonstrate sclerosis or cystic change and irregularity at the pubic symphysis (osteolysis) and perisymphyseal osteopenia.
- Instability: >2 mm of cephalad translation of the superior pubic ramus on each side with the patient standing ('flamingo view' radiography).
- Widening of the cleft (>10 mm is abnormal).

### Isotope bone scan

- This shows increased radiotracer uptake in a perisymphyseal distribution (Fig. 5.29).

### Ultrasound

- Has been employed with varying success to show a widened cleft.

### Computerized tomography

- Used for the evaluation of the pubis symphysis and the posterior pelvic ring.

### Magnetic resonance imaging

- Hyperintensity in a perisymphyseal location reflecting microtrabecular trauma and edema.
- Symphyseal irregularity with cartilage disruption and symphyseal widening on coronal $T_1$-weighted images.
- Sclerosis appears as a low signal on all sequences (Fig. 5.30).

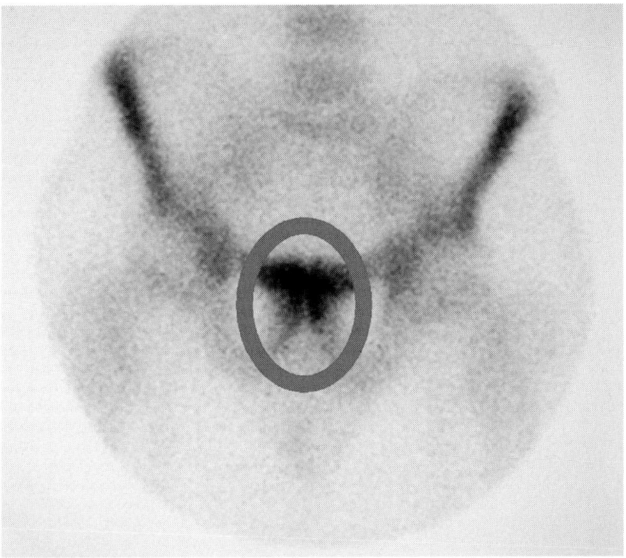

**Fig. 5.29** Bone scan showing a concentration of radiotracer activity at the symphysis pubis in a patient with increased marginal osteoblastic activity due to osteitis pubis.

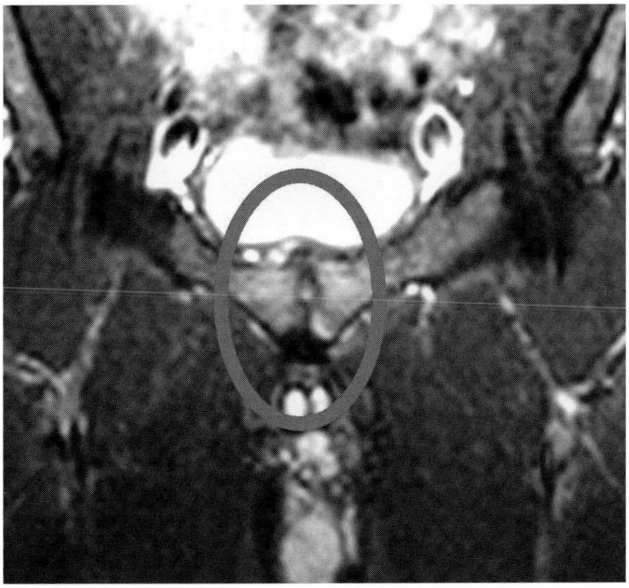

**Fig. 5.30** MR image showing symphyseal inflammation, para-articular bone edema and articular surface irregularity in a patient with osteitis pubis.



## Management

### Non-surgical

- Rest, ice or hot-pack application.
- Exercises to reduce the load on the pelvis.
- Antiinflammatories.
- Therapeutic ultrasound and electrical stimulation have been employed with success.
- Image-guided local anesthetic and steroid injection to the symphyseal cleft.

### Surgical

- Wedge resection of the pubic symphysis is rarely performed in refractory cases.
- Stabilization or fusion procedure more commonly performed.

# Adductor dysfunction

## Anatomy

- Hip adductors include the adductors longus, magnus and brevis, and pectineus.
- Adductor longus, which originates at the anterior surface of the pubic ramus and inserts into the posterior femoral mid diaphysis (linea aspera), is most commonly injured with pain at the pubic symphysis radiating to the groin (Figs 5.31 and 5.32).
- The adducor tendon attachment is intact.

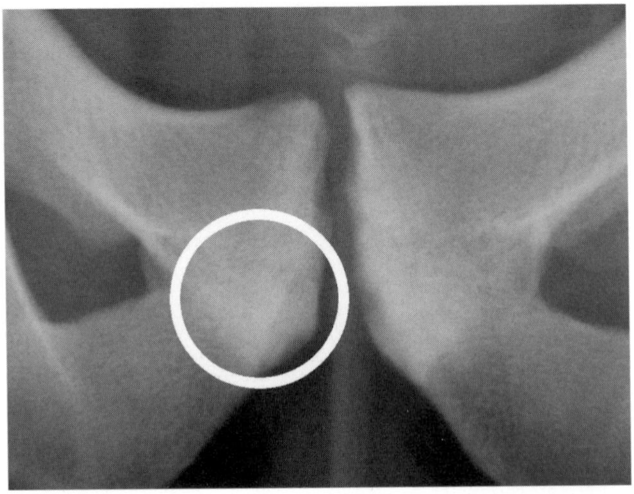

**Fig. 5.31** Radiograph showing focal sclerosis due to excess traction at the adductor attachment bilaterally in a soccer player with bilateral groin pain.

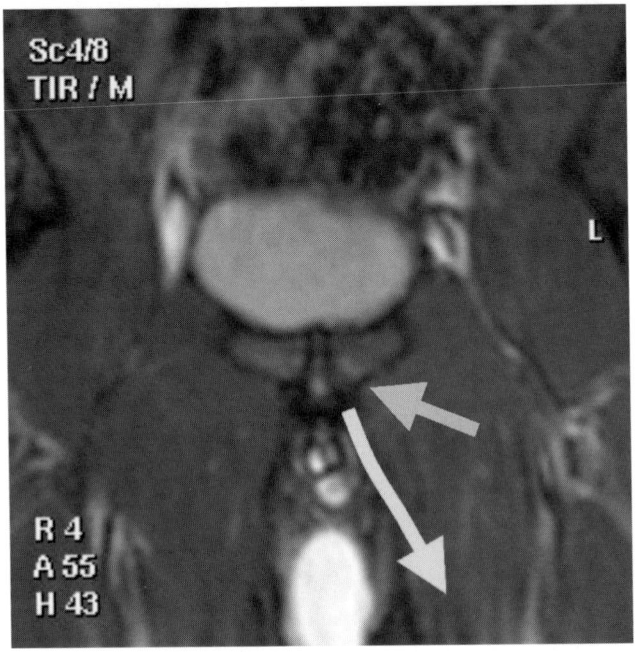


**Fig. 5.32** MR image showing focal bone edema secondary to abnormal traction effect at the adductor attachment on the left in a soccer player with recent-onset left groin pain.

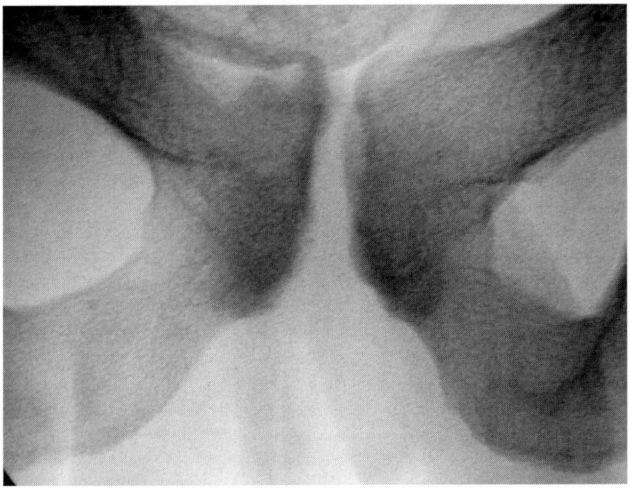

(a)

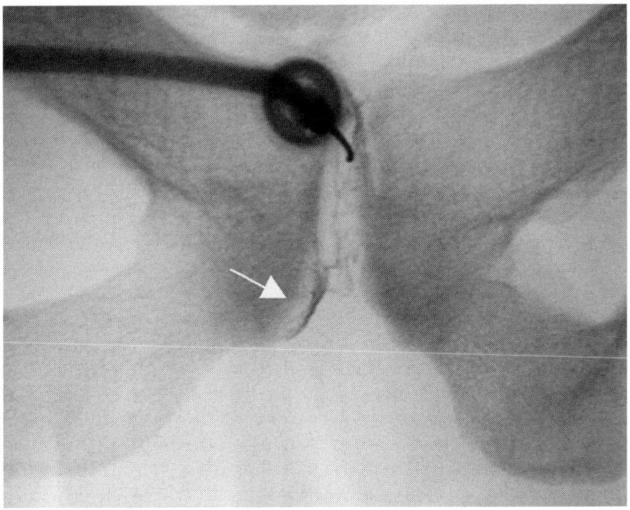

(b)

**Fig. 5.33** (**a**) Radiograph showing sclerotic changes at the adductor attachments in a soccer player with right groin pain. (**b**) Contrast injection to the symphysis (symphysography) in the same patient as in (a) showing contrast filling of an accessory cleft on the right at a site of microtear at the right adductor attachment accounting for right groin pain. Symptom relief in this patient was yielded by subsequent injection of steroid and bupivacaine hydrochloride to the symphysis and secondary accessory cleft.



## Mechanism of injury

- Repetitive microtrauma from overuse of the adductor muscle–tendon unit (mostly adductor longus).
- Very common in kicking sports: soccer; Gaelic football in Ireland; and Australian rules football; and in activities with a vigorous side-to-side motion, e.g. figure skating.
- Secondary pubic symphyseal imbalance leads to laxity at the symphysis with impaction during gait producing secondary osteitis pubis (Fig. 5.33).

## History and clinical findings

- Difficult to diagnose on history and examination alone as symptoms may be difficult to precisely locate and because of long differential diagnosis.
- Pain at the pubic symphysis radiating to the groin.
- Worsening of symptoms after activity.

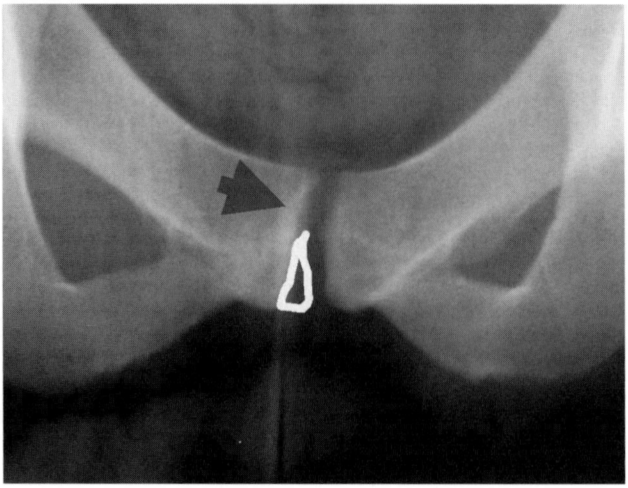

Fig. 5.34 Radiograph showing marked osteolysis on the right at the adductor attachment due to chronic repetitive distraction forces imposed by twisting and turning during fitness training in a player with right groin pain.

- Tenderness felt over the origin of the adductor longus, which is aggravated by resisted hip adduction.

## Imaging findings

### Radiography

- Look for coexistent osteitis pubis ('flamingo views') (Fig. 5.34).

### Ultrasonography

- Operator dependent; it may show anechoic fluid at the adductor insertion, and a hypoechoic focal area of linear muscle fibers indicates a tear.



### Symphysography

- Symphyseal contrast injection under fluoroscopy parallels findings at MRI with contrast leakage to the site of adductor attachment on the affected side (Figs 5.35 and 5.36).

### Magnetic resonance imaging

- The 'accessory cleft sign' is visible; high-signal fluid extending from the symphyseal cleft to the adductor attachment on the symptomatic side.
- Coronal STIR weighting most useful.
- Symphyseal irregularity and para-articular bone edema present if there is coexistent osteitis pubis (Fig. 5.37).

## Management

### Non-surgical

- This is difficult to treat as the adductor attachment is stressed each time the patient walks and healing is compromised. Tendon–bone apposition is prevented by interposed fluid arising from the fibrocartilaginous cleft to the secondary cleft identified at MRI (Fig. 5.38).
- Rest with activity modification; heat pads in the short term.
- Antiinflammatories.
- Image-guided symphyseal cleft injection of steroid and bupivacaine hydrochloride provides relief in some cases but the effects are generally temporary in the majority.
- Therapeutic ultrasound.

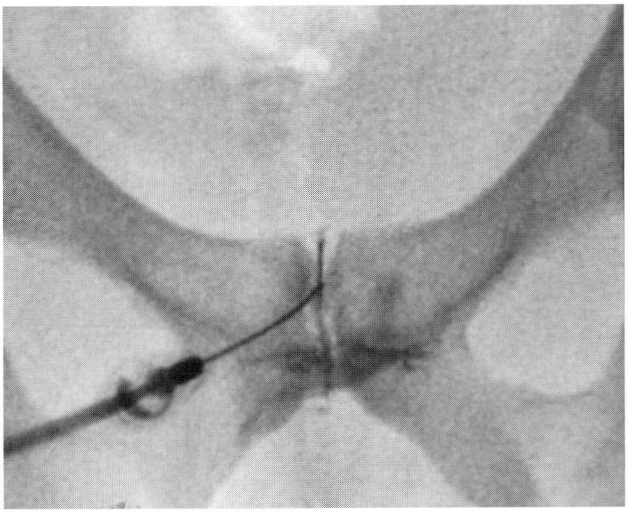

(a)

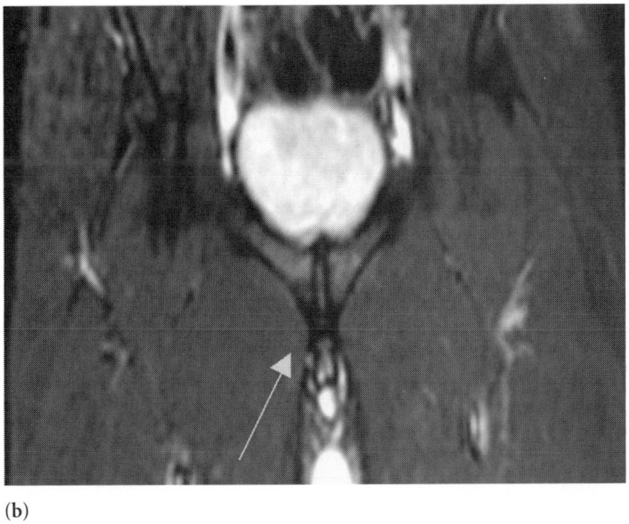

(b)

**Fig. 5.35** (**a**) (**b**) Normal contrast injection to the symphyseal cleft (left) with a normal MRI scan in the same patient showing normal adductor attachments inferiorly.

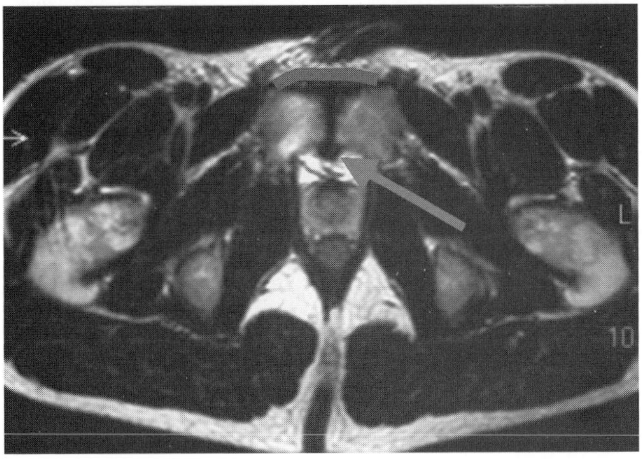

**Fig. 5.36** Axial MR image in the same patient as in Fig. 5.35 showing anterior symphyseal stabilization by an aponeurosis of the right and left adductor and gracilis tendons, with minimal subluxation of the symphyseal fibrocartilage posteriorly to the preprostatic fascia. (This is identified with increasing frequency in adulthood.)

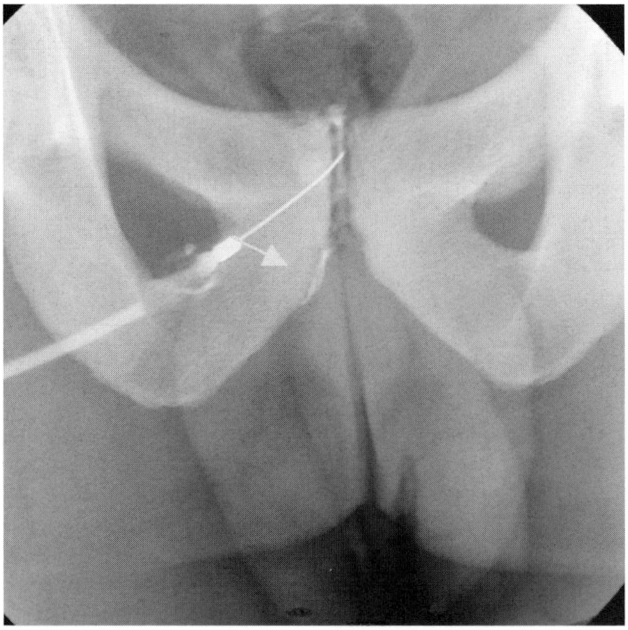

(a)

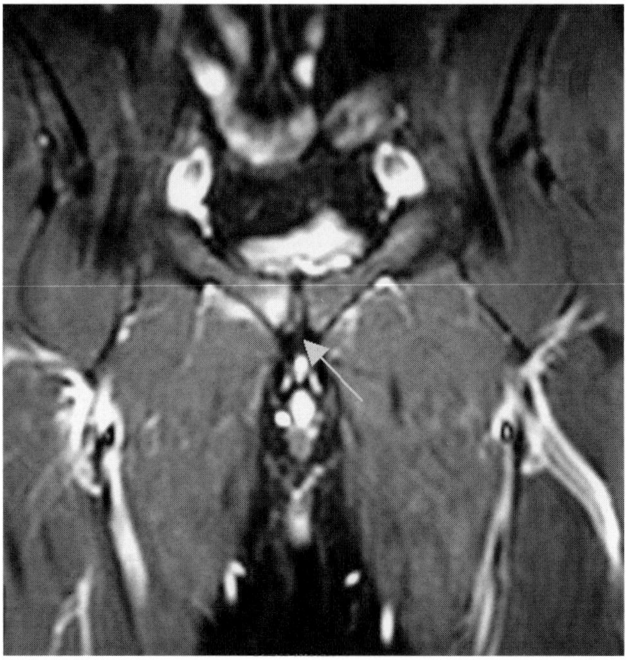

(b)

**Fig. 5.37**
(**a**) Symphysography showing contrast filling of a right-sided accessory cleft due to a microtear at the right adductor attachment, with (**b**) focal distraction-induced focal bone edema on the right at the site of tear identified at MRI.

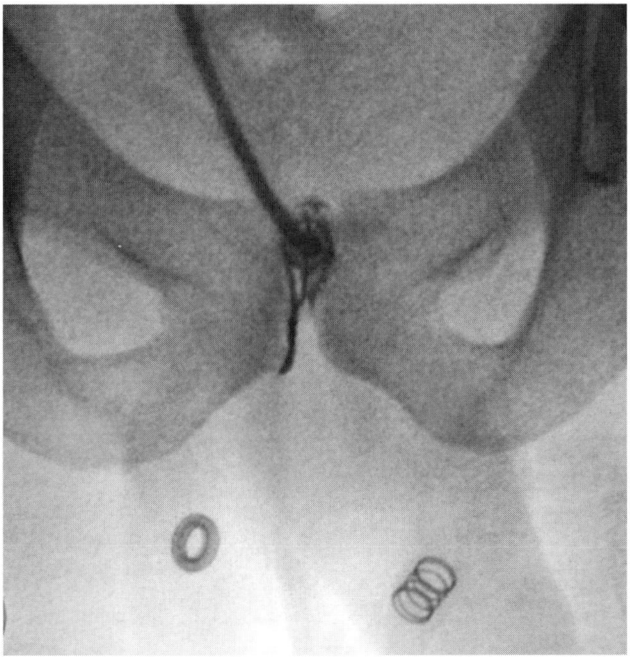
(a)

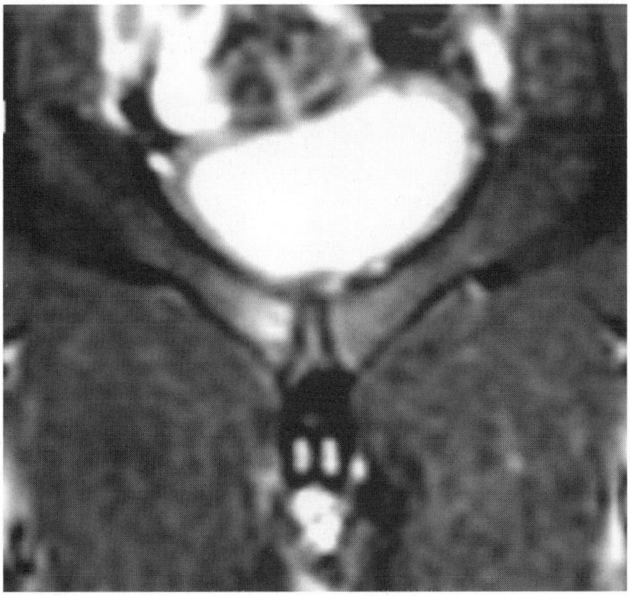
(b)

**Fig. 5.38**
(**a**) (**b**) Symphysography and MRI showing a right-sided accessory cleft due to a microtear at the right adductor attachment in a patient with right-sided groin pain.

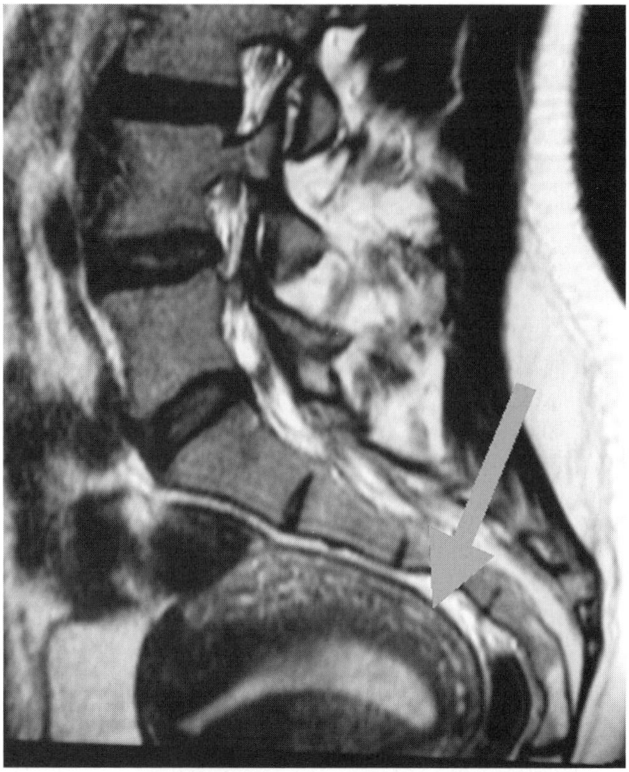

(a)

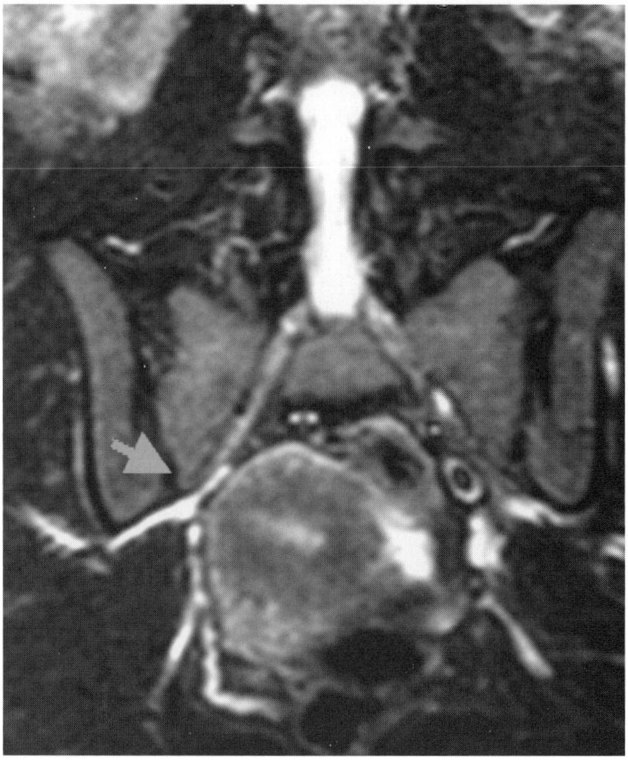

(b)

**Fig. 5.39** (**a**) (**b**) MRI showing a retroverted uterus (left) deviating to the right and displacing the associated sacral nerve plexus in an elite hockey player presenting with right-sided cyclical groin pain worse pre-menses.

- Muscle training program to strengthen the abdominal muscles and hip flexors, in addition to the hip adductors.

## Surgical

- For failed conservative management.
- Open adductor tenotomy with the excision of any granulation tissue (Figs 5.39 and 5.40).

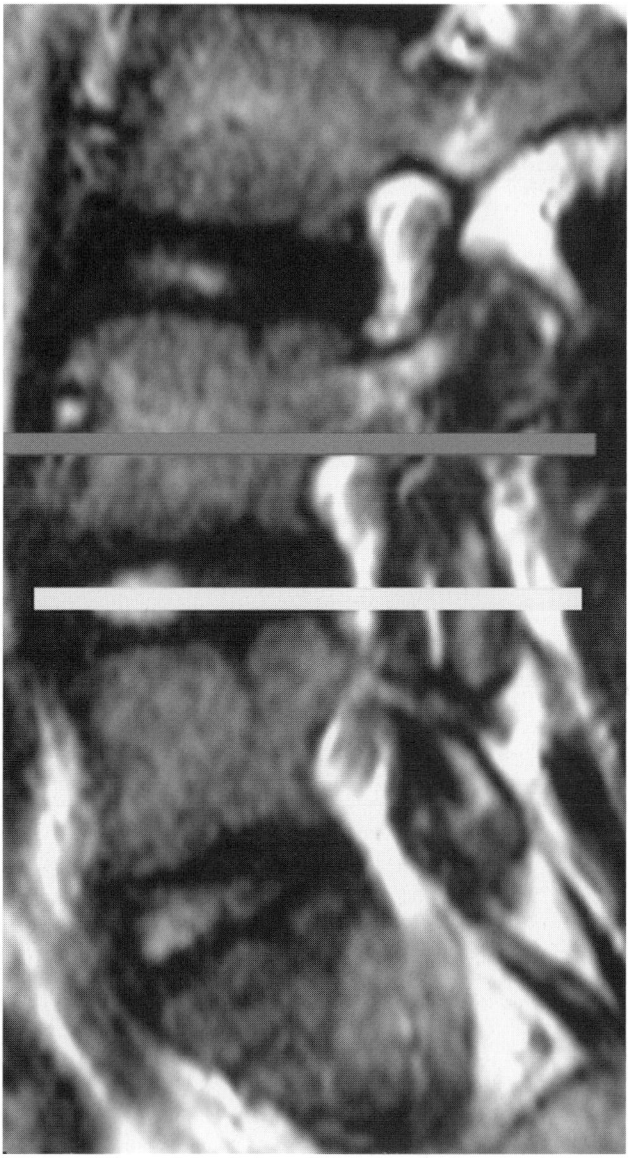

(a)

**Fig. 5.40**
(**a**) Spondylolysis presenting as groin pain in a teenage soccer player (sagittal MR image).

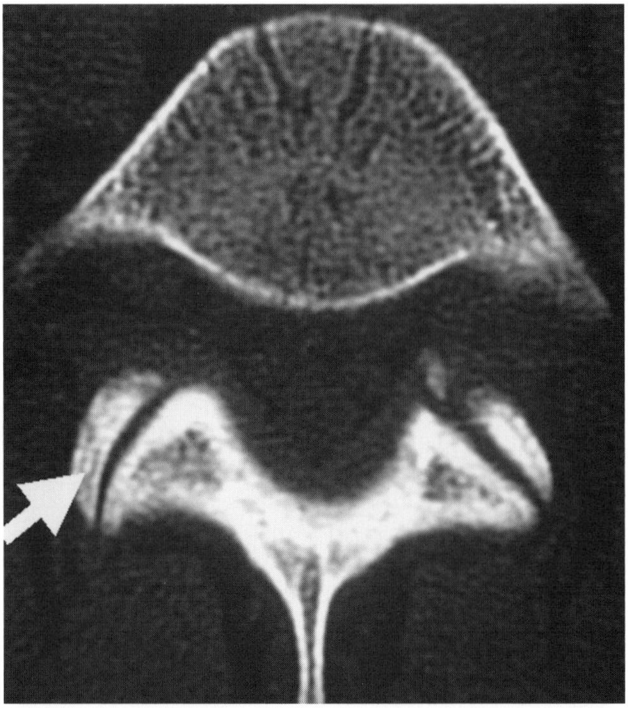

(b)

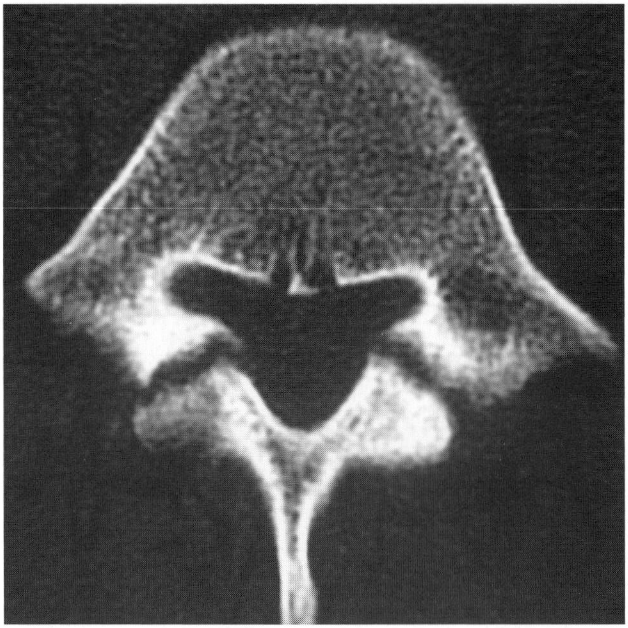

(c)

**Fig. 5.40** (**b**) Axial image through the level of the disk in this patient traversing the facet joint. (**c**) Axial image through the level of the pedicle showing a fracture through the posterior element at the site of spondylolysis.

# Iliopsoas bursitis

## Anatomy

- The iliopsoas bursa is a fluid-filled sac located between the anterior hip capsule and the posterior aspect iliopsoas muscle.

## Mechanism of injury

- Iliopsoas bursitis is inflammation of the iliopsoas bursa secondary to overuse with repetitive hip flexion and extension.
- Seen in gymnasts, dancers and runners.

## History and clinical findings

- Anterior groin mass.
- Pain in the femoral triangle with occasional radiation to the thighs and knees.
- Pain is worse on flexion, abduction and external rotation.
- Rarely, there is limitation of stride due to pain on hip extension.

## Imaging findings

### Radiography

- Usually normal.
- If large, may see soft-tissue mass at the hip joint.
- There is often coexistent hip arthritides.

### Ultrasonography

- Well-defined fluid collection anterior to the hip joint (anechoic or hypoechoic if internal debris is present).

### Computerized tomography

- Usually not required; fluid attenuation mass.

### Arthrography

- The anterior bursa may fill with injected contrast.

### Magnetic resonance imaging

- Fat-suppressed axial images show a rounded high-signal fluid collection posteromedial to the iliopsoas muscle.
- Communication with the hip joint medially is often identified (better for this than CT or ultrasound).
- Most sensitive method for bursal size (Fig. 5.41).

## Management

### Non-surgical

- Rest, heat application.
- Ultrasound therapy.
- Antiinflammatories.
- Hip strengthening exercises.
- Rarely requires steroid injection.

### Surgical

- The release of the iliopsoas tendon is very rarely performed.

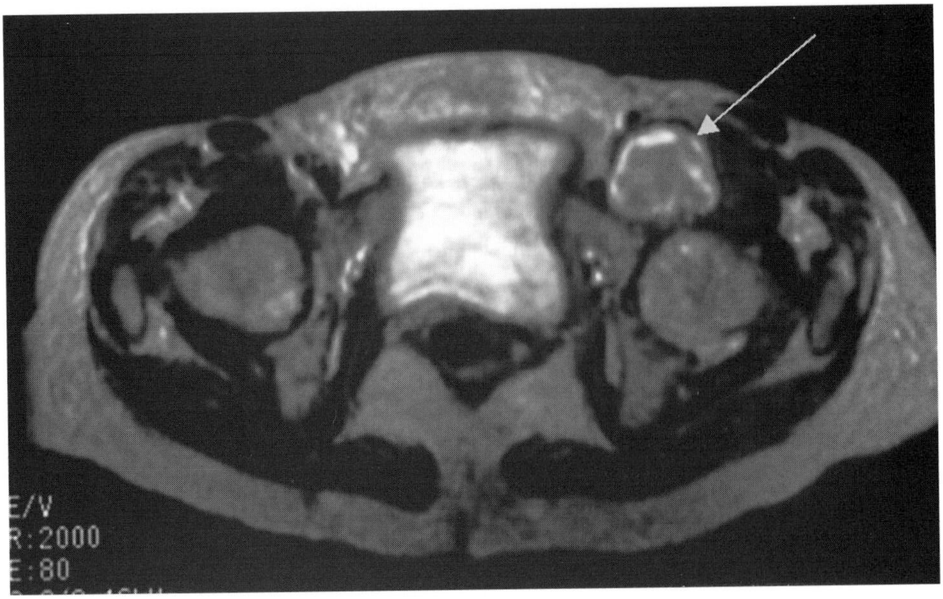


**Fig. 5.41** Axial MR image showing a distended inflamed ileopsoas bursa on the left anterior to the left hip.

# Sports hernias

## Anatomy

- The posterior wall of the inguinal canal is formed by the fascia transversalis, reinforced in its medial third by the conjoint tendon.
- The conjoint tendon is the common tendon of insertion of the internal oblique and transversus abdominus and attaches to the pubic crest and pectineal line.
- The superficial inguinal ring lies anterior to the conjoint tendon.

## Mechanism of injury

- Congenital weakness of the posterior wall of the inguinal canal, which does not result in a visible bulge and which causes chronic groin pain.
- Gilmore has described findings at surgery including dilatation of the superficial inguinal ring, tearing of the conjoint tendon and dehiscence between the torn conjoint tendon and the inguinal ligament.
- Speculated to originate from adductor dysfunction, which is also implicated in osteitis pubis and adductor microtears.

## History and clinical findings

- Insidious unilateral deep groin pain during activities such as twisting, running and straining.
- Pain may radiate to the adductors and/or the scrotum.
- Difficult to detect at clinical examination.
- Patient may have tenderness over the pubic tubercle (conjoint tendon) and at the external inguinal ring.
- Dilated superficial ring.
- Pain worse on resisted sit-up.
- No clinically recognizable hernial sac.

## Imaging findings

- Used primarily to rule out other causes of groin pain.

### Radiography

- Normal in the absence of groin pathologies.

### Ultrasound

- Maneuvers to increase intra-abdominal pressure, e.g. straining and coughing, may allow dynamic visualization of the posterior wall weakness.

### Herniography

- Generally not recommended due to associated morbidity.

## Management

### Non-surgical

- Any coexistent pathology that may contribute to groin pain should be treated.
- Poor response if there is an isolated sports hernia.

### Surgical

- Reinforcement of the posterior wall of the inguinal canal (similar to a normal hernia repair).
- A Gilmore groin repair involves modified herniorrhaphy with placation of the transversalis fascia and repair of the conjoint tendon with reattachment to the pubic tubercle and inguinal ligament.
- Return to sports is possible after 6 weeks' rehabilitation.

# Mechanical sacroiliitis

## Anatomy

- The sacral ala articulates with the ilium at the synovial SI joint, the lower two-thirds of the joint space being lined with synovium.
- The SI joints usually only move millimeters during weight-bearing and forward flexion as a 'gliding' motion. This movement comes from giving or stretching.
- The SI joint provides shock absorption for the spine by stretching in various directions.
- Sacroiliac joints are enveloped by a large amount of ligamentous and fibrous tissue (including the iliolumbar, sacrotuberous and sacrospinous ligaments) for added stability.

## Mechanism of injury

- Direct trauma versus repetitive microtrauma.
- Forceful contraction of the hamstrings or abdominal muscles producing a sudden load on the buttocks.
- Forceful straightening from a crouched position.

## History and clinical findings

- Lower lumbar ache, worse with rest, e.g. on waking.
- Radiation to the thighs, hip or groin.
- Restricted daily activities such as turning over in bed or putting shoes on.
- Absence of peripheral neurologic findings.
- Various tests for the SI joints are available:
  - *Posterior pelvic pain provocation test (thigh thrust)* – with the patient supine, the hip is flexed to 90° and the knee is bent. The posterior shearing stress is applied to the SI joint through the femur, avoiding excessive adduction of the hip.
  - *Gaenslen's test* – sitting at the edge of a table with one leg flexed to the chest, the unsupported leg dropping over the edge. In this position, SI joint problems will cause pain because of stress to the joint.
  - *Distraction test* – the SI joint is stressed by the examiner, attempting to pull the joint apart.
  - *Compression test* – the two sides of the joint are forced together. Pain may indicate that the SI joint is involved.
  - *Patrick's test* – stresses the hip and SI joint by flexion, abduction and external rotation of the hip. A positive test produces back or buttock pain, whereas groin pain is more indicative of hip joint pathology.
  - *Sacroiliac shear test* – with the patient prone, the palm of the examiner's hand is placed over the posterior iliac wing. An inferiorly directed thrust produces a shearing force across the SI joint.



## Imaging findings

### Radiography

- Generally not helpful. This may show SI joint osteophytes but there is poor correlation with symptoms (Fig. 5.42).

### Isotope bone scan

- Specific but too insensitive to be of real value.

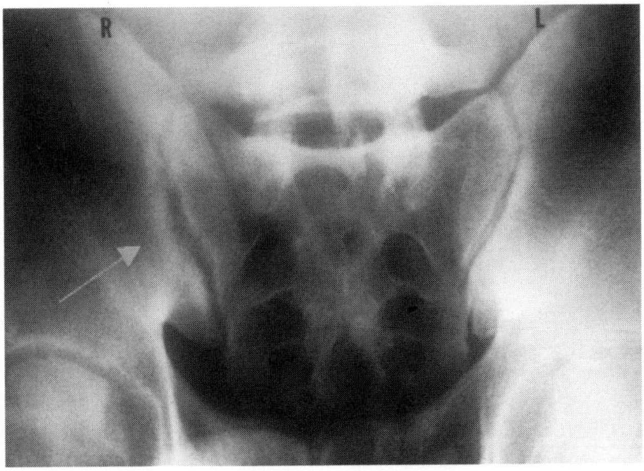


(a)

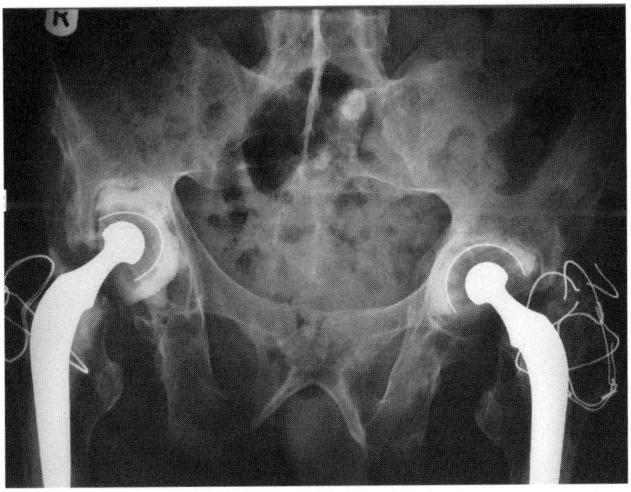


(b)

**Fig. 5.42** (**a**) PA view showing widening and erosion of the right sacroiliac joint secondary to unilateral sacroiliitis. (**b**) PA view in a patient with longstanding ankylosing spondylitis showing fused SI joints, fused bamboo spine and bilateral total hip replacements.

## Arthroscopy

- A diagnostic and therapeutic local anesthetic injection under fluoroscopy is the 'gold standard' to show SI joints as the source of pain.
- Does not assess supporting soft tissues.

## Computerized tomography

- As with plain radiography but gives improved SI joint visualization in the axial plane (Fig. 5.43).

## Magnetic resonance imaging

- Poor specificity.
- May demonstrate hyperintensity at SI joints on STIR, indicating edema.
- Sclerosis appears as low-signal intensity on $T_1$- and $T_2$-weighted images.
- Superior surrounding soft-tissue visualization (Fig. 5.44).

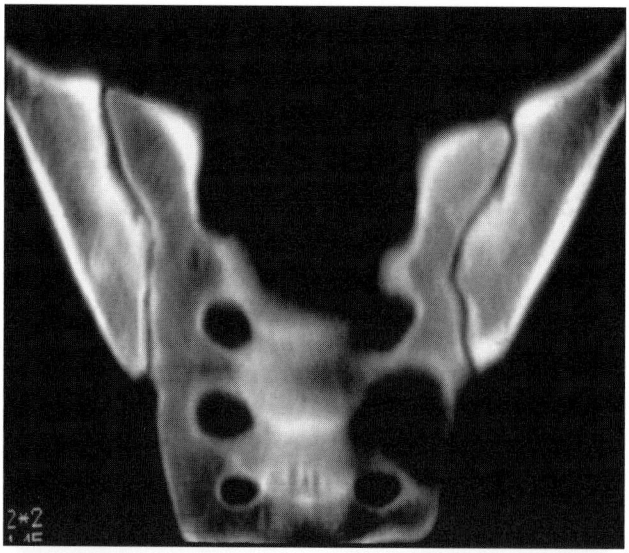

**Fig. 5.43** CT scan coronally oriented to the long axis of the SI joints showing normal corticated articular surfaces.

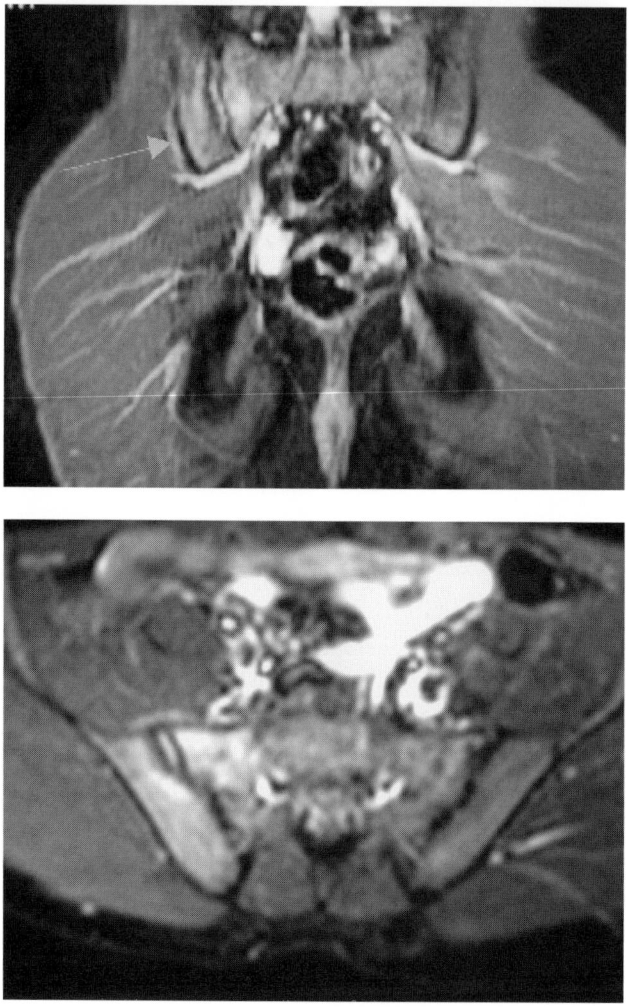

(a)

(b)

**Fig. 5.44** (**a**) (**b**) Coronal MRI showing hyperintense fluid within the right sacroiliac joint with associated para-articular bone edema secondary to active right-sided sacroiliitis.

## Management

### Non-surgical

- Antiinflammatories and rest.
- Rehabilitation program with back muscle strengthening, especially the hip abductors.
- Sacroiliac joint bracing.
- Steroid injection under fluoroscopy.
- Lumbar heat pad and massage for muscle tension.

### Surgical

- Sacroiliac joint arthrodesis is rarely required.

# Hip osteoarthritis

## Anatomy

- The hip joint is a common site of osteoarthritis (OA): 1 in 4 over the age of 60.

## Mechanism of injury

- Articular cartilage degenerative change with hip joint space narrowing.

## History and clinical findings

- Primary or secondary.
- Gradual onset of groin and thigh pain with or without radiation to the gluteal region.
- Hip joint stiffness (worse in the morning) and with weight-bearing activities.
- Pain and reduced internal rotation.

## Imaging findings

### Radiography

- Narrowing of the weight-bearing superior joint space, with relative preservation of the medial joint space.
- Subchondral cyst formation on both sides of the articulation.
- Ring osteophyte formation: lateral acetabulum and subcapital.
- Periarticular sclerosis.
- Superior migration of the femoral head (Fig. 5.45).

### Isotope bone scan

- Increased radiotracer uptake is secondary to subchondral fractures, cysts or generalized sclerosis (Fig. 5.46).

### Computerized tomography

- Similar features to plain radiography.



### Magnetic resonance imaging

- More sensitive than plain films in early OA.
- $T_1$-weighted images show cartilage loss and hypointense sclerosis at the anterosuperior femoral head.
- $T_2$-weighted images show high-signal fluid extending to the osseus surface.

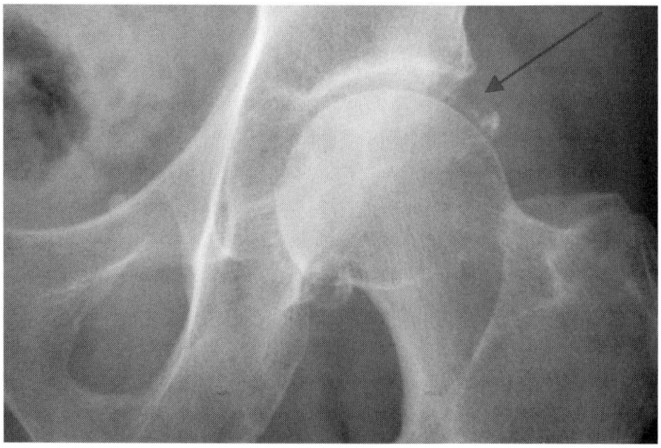

**Fig. 5.45** Radiograph showing chondrocalcinosis of hyaline articular cartilage of the left hip joint in a young athlete with hip pain. Investigation revealed background hemochromatosis.

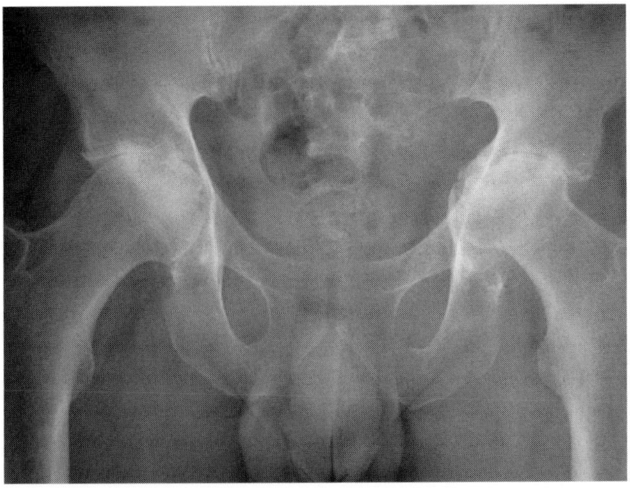

**Fig. 5.46** Radiograph showing advanced bilateral osteoarthritis which is worse on the left where there is a secondary protrusion deformity.

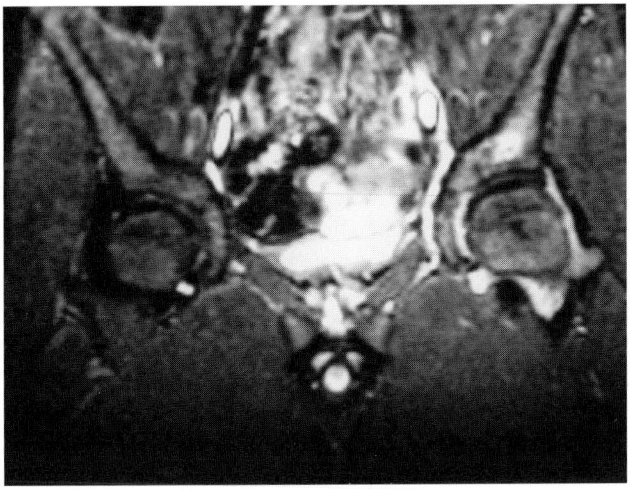

**Fig. 5.47** Coronal MRI showing inflammatory arthritis in a young athlete with left hip pain. The image shows joint effusion, synovitis and para-articular bone edema.



through cracks in denuded isointense cartilage with or without hyperintense joint effusion.

- Subchondral cysts follow fluid signal (generally high signal on $T_2$-weighted and low signal on $T_1$-weighted studies) (Fig. 5.47).

## Management

### Non-surgical

- Antiinflammatories.
- Physiotherapy.
- Intra-articular steroid injection under fluoroscopy in acute flare-ups.
- Intra-articular hyaluronate injection.

### Surgical

- Total hip arthroplasty.

# Femoroacetabular impingement

## Definition

Femoroacetabular impingement (FAI) results from abnormal morphology of the femoral head-neck junction and/or the acetabulum causing repetitive abutment between the femoral neck and the acetabular rim.

## Mechanism of injury

Two types of femoroacetabular impingement have been described (see Fig. 5.48).

Cam impingement:
- Results from abnormal morphology of the anterior femoral head–neck junction causing abutment of the femoral neck against the acetabular rim with flexion, adduction and internal rotation.
- More common in young males.

Pincer impingement:
- Results from overcoverage of the acetabulum (retroversion).
- More common in older women.

In both types repetitive impingement results in labral and chondral injuries leading to progressive osteoarthritis.

## Clinical presentation

History
- FAI often becomes symptomatic in the second or third decade of life in patients with increased sports activity or minor trauma.
- Patients present with slow onset of groin pain which is initially intermittent, particularly on sitting for a prolonged period.
- Occasionally patients have a history of SUFE as a child.
- Often diagnosed late.



Examination
- Examination of the hip often reveals limitation of motion, particularly internal rotation and adduction in flexion.
- The impingement test is almost always positive.

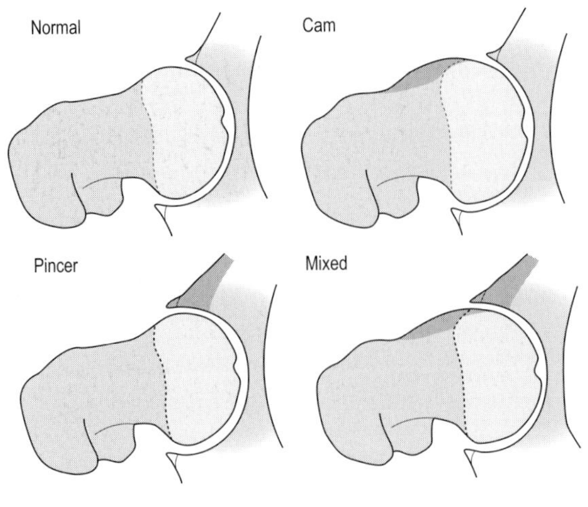


**Fig. 5.48** Cam and pincer impingement.

## Imaging findings

**Radiography**
(AP and lateral)

- Early:
  - Presence of a bony prominence in the anterolateral head and neck.
  - Reduced offset of the femoral neck and head junction (see Fig. 5.49).
  - Changes on the acetabular rim such as an os acetabuli.
  - Acetabular retroversion, relative anterior overcoverage, protrusio acetabuli.
- Late: Degenerative changes.

**Magnetic resonance imaging ± arthrography**
(see Fig. 5.50)

- Abnormal femoral head morphology.
- Low offset of the neck.
- Ossification of acetabular rim.
- Labral and chondral lesions.
- Arthrography may also aid diagnosis by alleviation of symptoms with steroid and analgesic injection.

## Management options

- NSAIDs.
- Physiotherapy.
- Intra-articular steroid injections.
- Surgery:
  - A combination of acetabular and femoral morphological aberrations often coexist.
  - Acetabular: resection osteoplasty of the excessive acetabular rim or reorientation of a retroverted acetabulum by a periacetabular osteotomy.
  - Femoral: resection osteoplasty of the prominent anterior neck or reorientation of the proximal femur with a flexion-valgus intertrochanteric osteotomy.



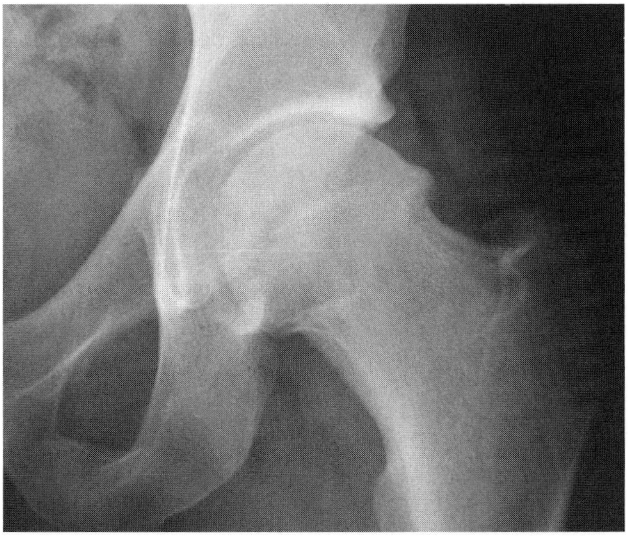

**Fig. 5.49** Radiograph of left hip showing the presence of a bony prominence in the anterolateral head and neck and reduced offset of the femoral head–neck junction. Cam impingement type.

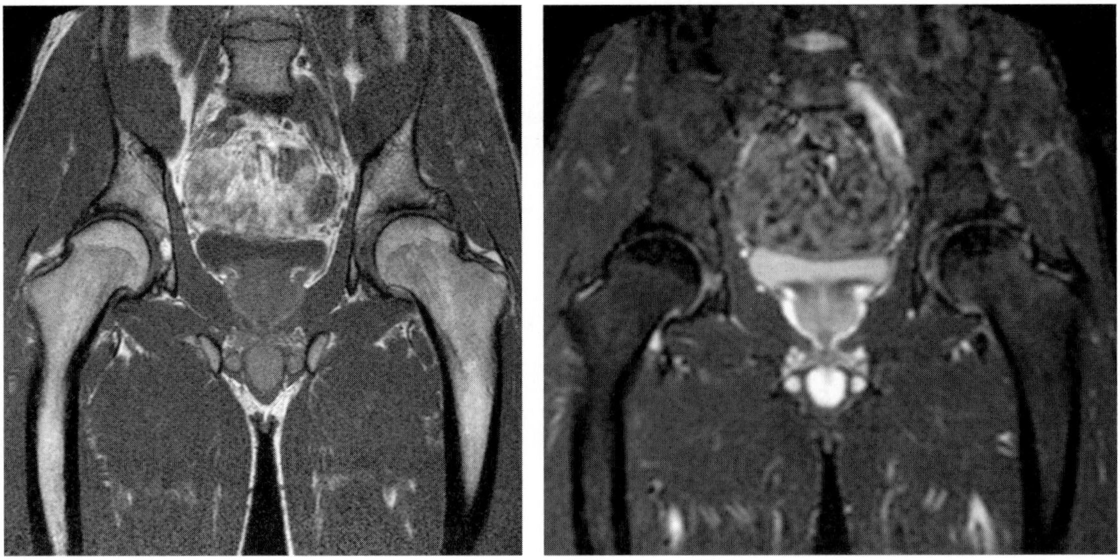

(a) (b)

**Fig. 5.50** T1 (left) and STIR (right) coronal MR images demonstrate ossification of the left acetabular rim with cartilage loss and subchondral edema.

# Further reading


Adam P, Labbe JL, Alberge Y et al. The role of computed tomography in the assessment and treatment of acetabular fractures. Clin Rad 1985; 36: 13–18.

Ben-Menachem Y, Coldwell DM, Young JWR, Burgess AR. Hemorrhage associated with pelvic fractures: causes, diagnosis, and emergent management. Am J Roengenol 1991; 157: 1005–1014.

Blickenstaff LD, Morris JM. Fatigue fracture of the femoral neck. J Bone Joint Surg 1966; 48A: 1031–1047.

Brandser EA, El-Khoury GY, Kathol MH. Adolescent hamstring avulsions that simulate tumors. Emerg Radiol 1995; 2: 273–278.

Brandser EA, El-Khoury GY, Kathol MH, Callaghan JJ. Hamstring injuries: radiographic, conventional tomographic, CT and MR imaging characteristics. Radiology 1995; 197: 257.

Davies AM. Stress fractures: current concepts. Am J Roengenol 1992; 159: 245–252.

Fernbach SK, Wilkinson RH. Avulsion injuries of the pelvis and proximal femur. AM J ROENGENOL 1981; 137: 581–584.

Fleckenstein JL, Shellock FG. Exertional muscle injuries: MRI evaluation. Topics Magn Res Imaging 1991; 3: 50–70.

Garret WE. Muscle strain injuries: clinical and basic aspects. Med Sci Sports Exerc 1990; 22: 436–443.

Hodler J, Yu JS, Goodwin D, Haghighi P et al. MR arthrography of the hip: improved imaging of the acetabular labrum with histologic correlation in cadavers. Am J Roengenol 1995; 165: 887–891.

Hofman S, Engel A, Neuhold A et al. Bone marrow edema syndrome and transient osteoporosis of the hip. J Bone Joint Surg (Br) 1993; 75B: 210–216.

Keane GS, Villa RN. Arthroscopic anatomy of the hip: an in-vivo study. Arthoscopy 1994; 10: 392.

Lecouvet FE, Vande Berg BC, Malghem J et al. MR imaging of the acetabular labrum: variations in 200 asymptomatic hips. Am J Roengenol 1996; 167: 1025–1028.

Metzmaker JN, Pappas AM. Avulsion fractures of the pelvis. Am J Sports Med 1985; 13: 349–358.

Pennal GF, Tile M, Waddell JP et al. Pelvic disruption. Assessment and classification. Clin Orthop 1980; 151: 12–21.

Schneider R, Kaye JJ, Ghelman B. Adductor avulsive injuries near the symphysis pubis. Radiology 1976; 129: 567–569.

Tile M. Fractures of the pelvis and acetabulum. Baltimore, Williams & Wilkins, 1984.

Vaccaro JP, Sauser DD, Beals RK. Iliopsoas bursa imaging : efficacy in depicting abnormal iliopsoas tendon motion in patients with internal snapping hip syndrome. Radiology 1995; 197: 853.

Zarins B, Ciullo JV. Acute muscle and tendon injuries in athletes. Clin Sports Med 1983; 2: 167–182.

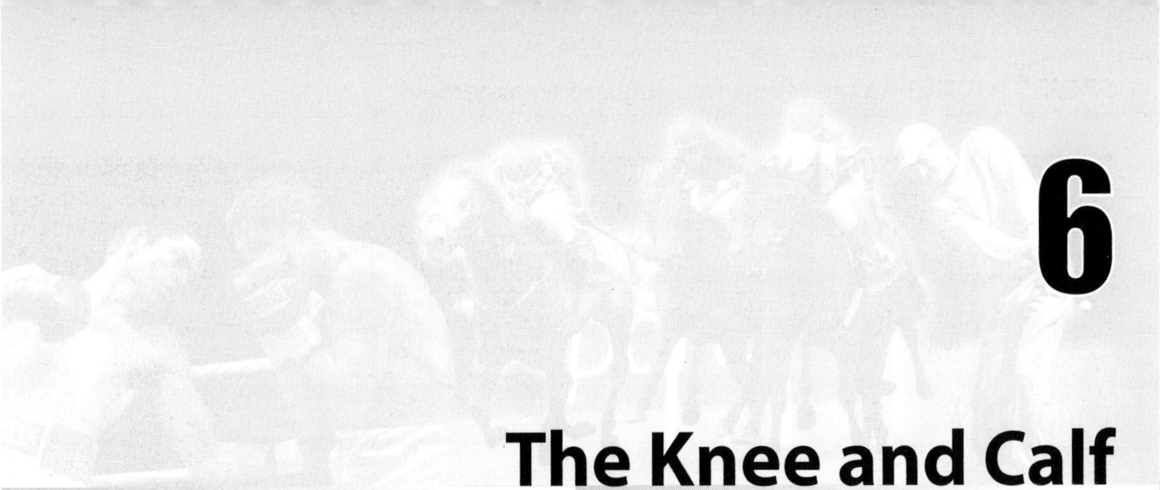

# 6

# The Knee and Calf

# CLINICAL EXAMINATION

## Clinical history

History must include sport played, mechanism of injury, onset of symptoms, aggravating and relieving factors, location and type of pain, and chronicity. This will frequently identify the likely injured structure.

## Physical examination

The physical examination should be gently initiated. Examination of the non-injured knee first can alleviate some apprehension (Figs 6.1 and 6.2).

A standard systemized examination with recording of all findings is essential. Performing and recording normal test results are just as valuable as noting abnormal findings.

Careful evaluation is essential to examine for other injury or pathology after the obvious abnormality has been identified.

The initial physical examination should include an overview of anthropometric measurements. Body height and weight, ectomorphic, endomorphic or mesomorphic somatotype (body build), and overall muscular mass and tone are recorded. The amount of injury and disability can be assessed by observing stance and gait: walking normally or with a limp, or using a walking stick. The alignment of right and left lower limbs when standing, walking and in prone positions; and the degree of genu varum and valgum in each knee and of internal or external tibial torsion of each lower leg are recorded.

### Functional tests

The patient is then asked to perform various functional tests, which are extremely important in both the disability evaluation and the determination of knee joint instability or laxity.

These tests consist of a stationary jog and, if possible, a fast stationary jog with high knee and hip flexion. Squatting, kneeling erect, kneeling backwards and 'duck waddling' are performed, if possible. The leaning hop test is an excellent test to examine for functional instability of the knee; this is performed by holding the unaffected lower limb in abduction producing a valgus stress force to the knee joint and then hopping on the affected lower limb in clockwise and anticlockwise directions. The same maneuver will place a varus stress force to the knee joint when the unaffected leg crosses in front of the affected leg.



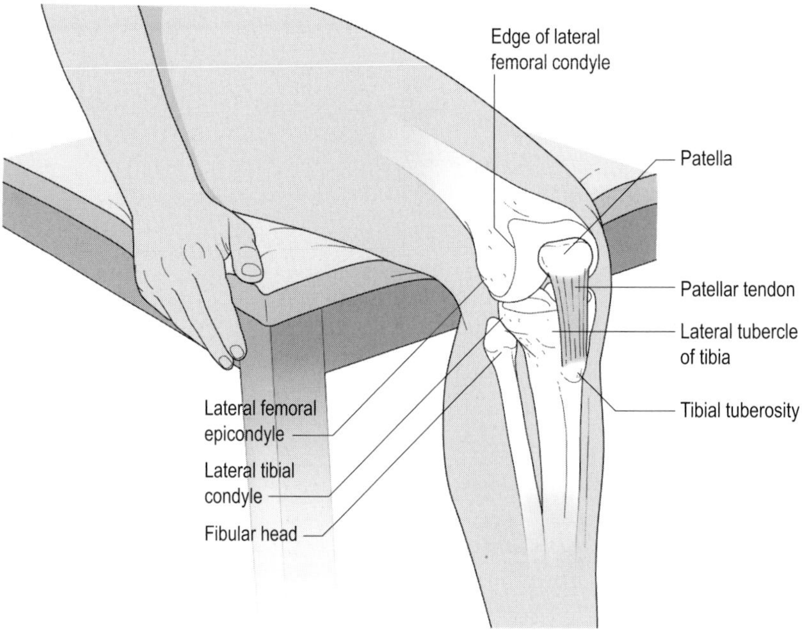


**Fig. 6.1** Anatomy of the knee joint (anterolateral aspect).

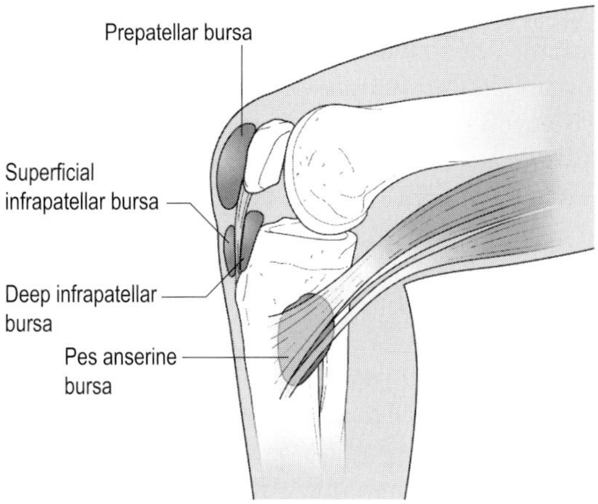


Fig. 6.2 Clinically significant bursae of the knee.

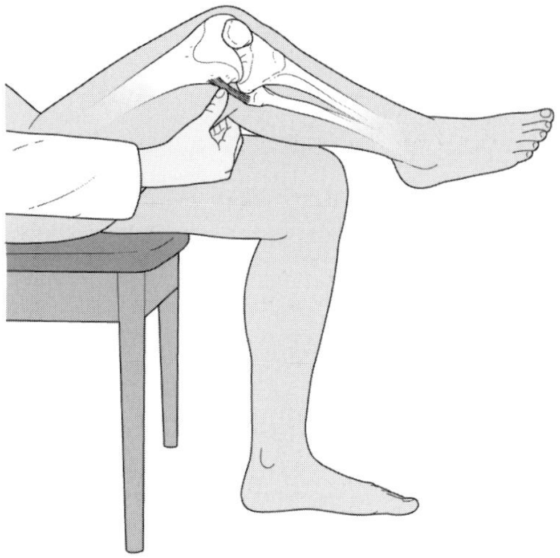

Fig. 6.3 The quadriceps muscle test (palpation of lateral collateral ligament).

## Measurements

Circumferential measurements are made of the thigh girth, vastus medialis obliquus (VMO) area, mid-patellar area and the mid-calf of both lower limbs to identify for muscle wasting.

## Motions

Active and passive ranges of knee joint motion are measured and compared with the opposite side, noting if forced extension, flexion, or varus or valgus stress or strain cause pain. The ranges of motion of the contralateral knee joint and hip and ankle joints should be examined.

Alignment of the lower limbs is assessed for malalignment such as pes planus or cavus, which may cause medial or lateral knee stress. Soft-tissue and joint swelling about the knee is palpated and balloted to determine if the swelling is intra-, extra- or periarticular.

The extensor mechanism is evaluated from a superior to inferior direction. The quadriceps tendon is palpated for integrity and tenderness. The quadriceps femoris muscles are inspected for wasting, atrophy, tenderness and tone. The vastus medialis and VMO are inspected for atrophy suggesting knee injury and disability (Fig. 6.3)

## Patellar examination

The position of the patella is identified: midline; subluxated; or dislocated. Patellar height is important in linking a high-riding patella (patella alta) to possible patellar subluxation, and a low-riding patella (patella baja or infera) to chondromalacia patellae. The mobility of the patella should be assessed and correlated with the patellar apprehension sign of prior patellar subluxation or dislocation (Fig. 6.4). Chronic or subacute patellar and patellofemoral injuries allow increased motion and possible dislocation of the patella. The individual medial and lateral patellar facets can be palpated for tenderness. Retropatellar grating or joint crepitus may be present with or without pain. This grating is reproduced easily through palpation of the patella while the patient squats and stands erect. The medial and lateral joint lines, patellar tendon, medial and lateral infrapatellar fat pads, and tibial tubercle are examined for tenderness and size.

The quadriceps angle (Q angle) is measured bilaterally, with the recognition that an angle of 20° or more may still be asymptomatic in the normal population. The dynamic Q angle representing the change in Q angle from an extended knee to a flexed knee can be measured. Increased Q angle excursion may be important in pathologic conditions such as patellar tendinitis and subluxation of the patella.

## Anatomical tenderness

All anatomical structures are palpated for tenderness and swelling. Traumatic and surgical scars are palpated for tenderness and signs of neuroma. The femoral and tibial contour is palpated with specific reference to osteochondral defects and tenderness

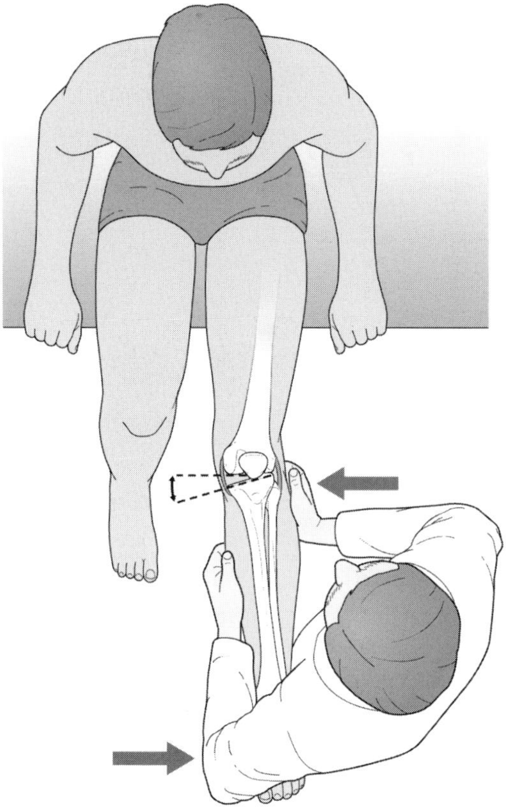

Fig. 6.4 The valgus stress testing of medial collateral ligament.



over osteophytic marginal bone spurs. The popliteal fossa is inspected and palpated for tenderness or swelling consistent with a tumor or Baker's popliteal cyst or popliteal artery aneurysm.

Neurovascular examination of the lower limb is performed.

## Meniscal injuries

The mechanism of the injury is usually a twisting force applied to the weight-bearing knee, causing entrapment of the meniscus between the tibial and femoral condyles. The resulting tear is usually longitudinal. If the tear is extensive the upper portion may displace into the joint causing the knee to lock (a 'bucket handle' tear). This locking may be intermittent as the torn portion flips in and out of the joint. A tear may extend to the inner margin of the meniscus forming a 'parrot beak' tear. The flap formed can displace into the joint causing intermittent locking; peripheral meniscal detachment may also occur. In the older age group, where the meniscus is less elastic, degenerative tears can occur. These tears are usually horizontal cleavage tears or radial tears running into the substance of the meniscus.

The history of an acute meniscal tear in a young adult is often characteristic. There is a twisting injury causing immediate severe pain. The patient is unable to bear any weight and may be unable to extend the knee fully if a bucket handle tear has lodged in the joint. The knee swells within several hours. If a cruciate ligament rupture is also present a hemarthrosis will accumulate within an hour. The patient complains of pain well localized to the joint line.

Examination reveals a painful knee with tenderness over the joint line adjacent to the tear. An effusion is virtually always present and, if the torn portion has displaced into the joint, a springy block to full extension is felt.

In a chronic tear the patient may complain of pain over the joint line and a feeling of 'catching'. Joint line tenderness is usually present. True locking occurs when the torn portion of the meniscus displaces into the joint causing loss of full extension. Locking due to a meniscal tear always occurs with the knee flexed although not necessarily when weight bearing. Examination of a knee locked due to a meniscal tear reveals a springy block to extension; forced extension is painful. Flexion is usually full or only mildly reduced due to pain.

Patients often confuse locking with stiffness and it is important to distinguish between the two. If the knee unlocks with a click or a clunk it is suggestive of a meniscal tear.

McMurray's test, which is widely used to diagnose meniscal tears (Fig. 6.11), involves flexing and extending the knee while the tibia is first internally rotated and then externally rotated, with the thumb and fingers over the joint line. Pain and an associated click are said to be diagnostic of a meniscal tear.

Apley's grinding test is performed with the patient prone and the knee flexed. Downward pressure is exerted on the tibia while it is internally and externally rotated. Pain or a clicking sensation are said to be suggestive of a meniscal tear. However, these tests are not specific.

## Ligamentous stability

Medial collateral ligament (MCL) instability is tested in the supine position (Figs 6.6 and 6.7). Valgus stress force is applied in flexion to the extension. Medial

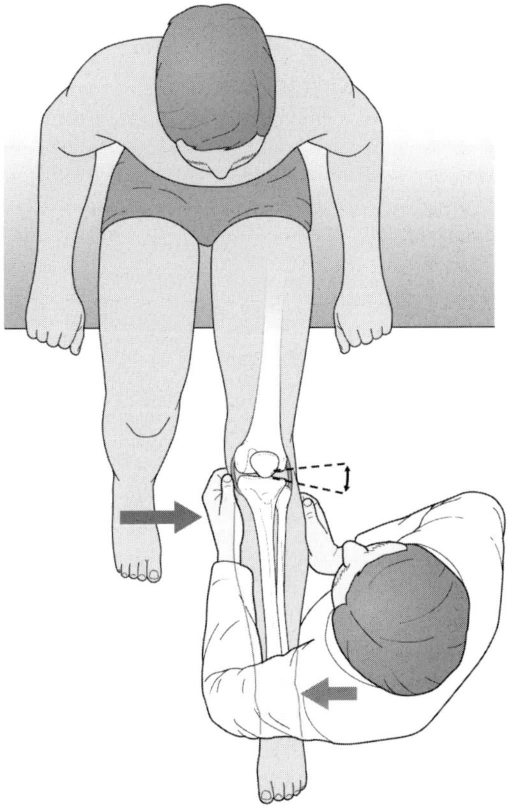

Fig. 6.5 To test the lateral knee for stability, apply varus stress to open the knee joint on the lateral side.

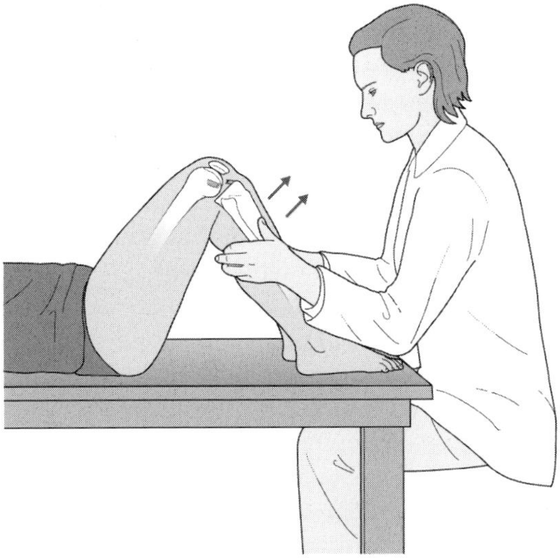

Fig. 6.6 A positive anterior drawer sign; torn anterior cruciate ligament.

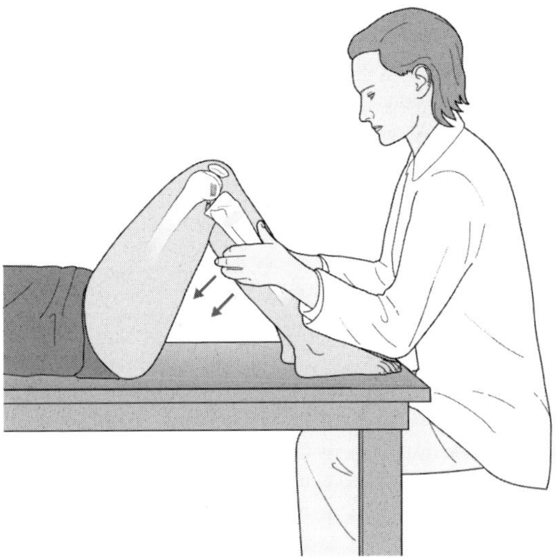

Fig. 6.7 A positive posterior drawer sign; torn posterior cruciate ligament.

instability in full extension indicates injury to the superficial or tibial collateral ligament, the middle third of the capsule or MCL, the posterior third of the capsule, the posterior oblique ligament, and possibly the anterior cruciate ligament (ACL) or posterior cruciate ligament (PCL) or both. Medial valgus stress instability at 30° involves the MCL and possibly tibial collateral ligament and/or the ACL.

Lateral collateral instability is examined in the supine position (Fig. 6.7). Varus stress is applied in flexion to the extension. Lateral instability in full extension indicates injury to the lateral collateral and ligament and the lateral capsule, and possible injury to the ACL and PCL, iliotibial tract, popliteus tendon, arcuate ligament and the biceps femoris tendon complex. Varus instability at 30° suggests injury to the lateral collateral ligament (LCL), the iliotibial tract and the lateral capsule. Integrity of the peroneal nerve must be examined with any injury to the lateral aspect of the knee joint or a varus injury.

Examination of hyperextension is performed by lifting the lower limb with straight leg raising and comparing the contralateral side. Hyperextension may be normal with generalized constitutional ligamentous laxity or abnormal due to acute injury to the ACL or PCL and the posterior capsule.

Anterior cruciate ligament instability is examined in the supine position. Lachman's and the anterior drawer tests are both performed to assess integrity of

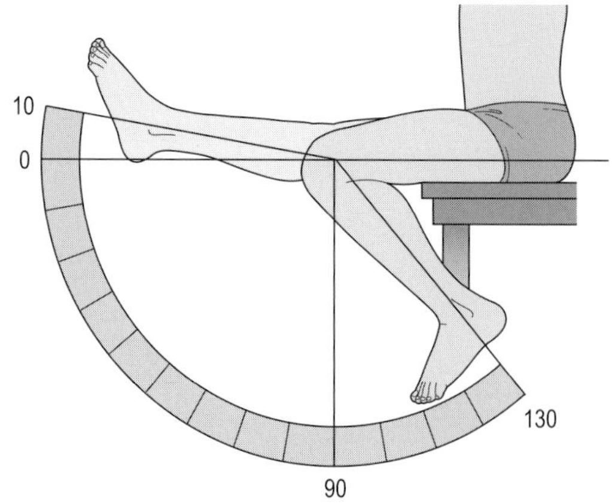


**Fig. 6.8** The range of knee motion in flexion and extension.

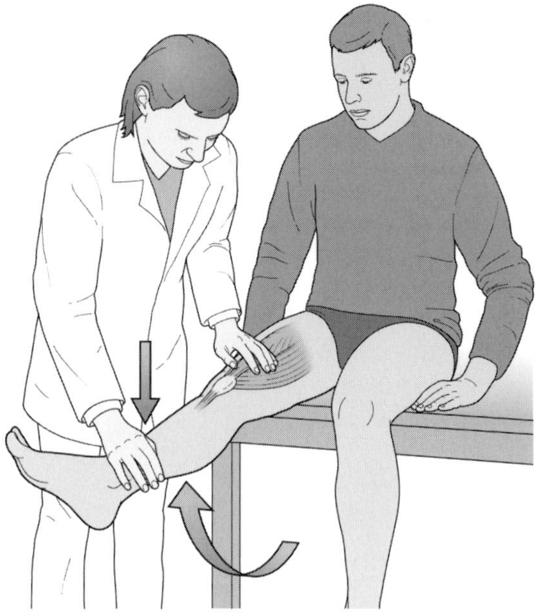

**Fig. 6.9** The quadriceps muscle test.

the ACL in the supine position with the knee flexed at 90° in neutral tibial rotation. The thumbs are placed on the anterior tibial plateau area to detect differences in anterior displacement and the index fingers palpate the hamstring muscles (Fig. 6.8). Lachman's test is performed in 20–30° of flexion with one hand holding and stabilizing the distal thigh and the other applying anterior stress to the posterior proximal tibia. The more extension one uses in Lachman's test, the more reflective the test is of posterolateral bundle injury.



Posterior cruciate ligament instability is tested by applying the posterior drawer test at 90° and in neutral rotation. Flexing the hips and knees to 90° in the supine patient may detect sagging of the tibial tubercle and proximal tibia when viewed from the side of the patient (Godfrey's test). These tests primarily evaluate the PCL and secondarily the posterior capsule and ligament complex.

Anteromedial rotatory instability is examined by the anterior drawer test at 90° in external tibial rotation. The pathologic structures involved are the ACL, the tibial collateral ligament, the MCL and/or the posterior oblique ligament (Fig. 6.6).

Posteromedial rotatory instability is rare. The posterior drawer test performed at 90° in internal rotation assesses posteromedial rotatory instability. A positive test is reflective of a partial or complete tear of the PCL and tibial collateral ligament, medial capsule, the posterior oblique ligament and/or the semimembranosus complex. Posterolateral rotatory instability is examined by the posterior drawer test at 90° in external tibial rotation or the external rotation recurvatum test. The external recurvatum test is performed by lifting the affected extremity by the hallux (big toe) and assessing any abnormal external rotation of the tibia, posterior displacement of the tibia or genu recurvatum. The posterior drawer test at 90° may be performed in the supine patient with hip flexion and the application of an active external torque to the tibia. Posterolateral rotatory instability indicates injury to the PCL and arcuate complex and possible injury to the popliteus tendon, the biceps femoris tendon, and the LCL and the lateral and/or medial head of the gastrocnemius tendon (Fig. 6.7). The 'pivot shift' maneuver performed in reverse (varus and external rotation) may also be positive in posterolateral rotatory instability.

Anterolateral rotatory instability is examined by the flexion–rotation drawer test (Noyes' test) and the anterolateral rotatory instability test with the patient in the lateral position (Slocum's test), which is more easily tolerated than the classic pivot shift jerk tests (McIntosh's or Loose tests). The latter tests may induce extreme apprehension in the patient, and many patients guard against this jerk so heavily that it is not reproducible without anesthesia. These tests are primarily reflective of injury to the ACL and, to a

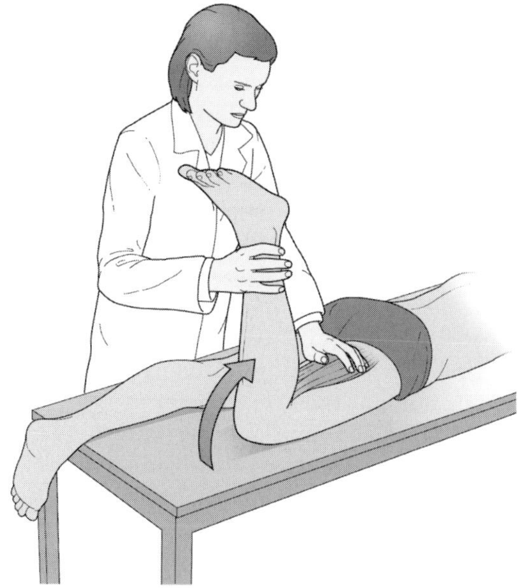

Fig. 6.10 Hamstring muscle test.

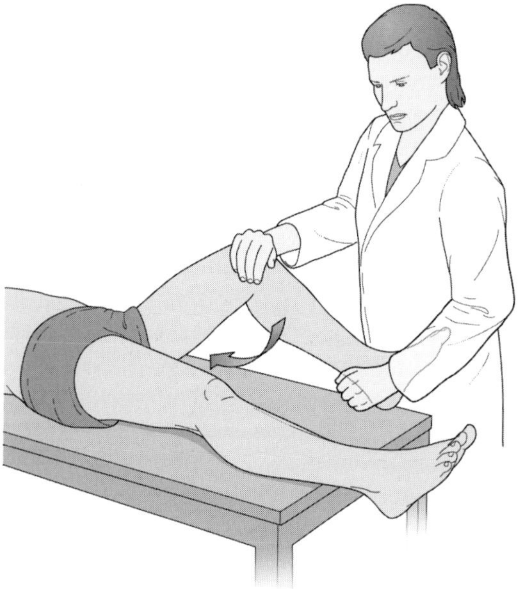

Fig. 6.11 McMurray's test for meniscal tears. Flex the knee.

lesser degree, the lateral capsule and the LCL. The intact iliotibial tract reduces the tibia back into a reduced position as the tibia proceeds from the subluxated position in extension to the reduced position in flexion. Therefore if the band is completely torn the pivot shift will be absent.

The causes of a pivot shift may be ACL injury or deficiency and anterolateral laxity, a displaced meniscal tear or an irregular tibial plateau surface.

# Patellofemoral examination

Examination of the patellofemoral joint is divided into three components: standing; sitting; and supine. Inspection and palpation are the examination techniques used in the examination. Specific tests are undertaken to complete a comprehensive examination of the patellofemoral joint and lower extremity.

## Standing examination

The standing physical examination of the patellofemoral joint begins with examination from the front with the patient directly towards the examiner, and the feet slightly apart and aligned straight ahead. The patient should wear shorts so that the lower extremity may be observed in its entirety. The overall

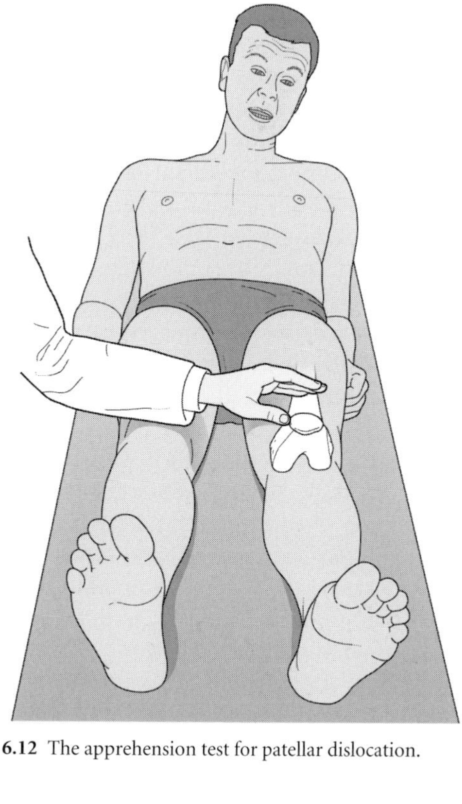

Fig. 6.12 The apprehension test for patellar dislocation.

alignment of the lower extremity is observed and attention is directed to any excessive genu valgum or varum deformities. If genu valgum is present, it effectively increases the Q angle and can be associated with patellofemoral pain. The extremity is also viewed from the side for flexion contractures or genu recurvatum, which may be an expression of a generalized ligamentous laxity or may be associated with patella alta.

Rotational malalignment may also cause patellofemoral pain and can be detected by noting the position of the patella with the feet straight ahead. 'Squinting' patellae, in which both patellae point inward in a medial fashion, can be a sign of excessive femoral anteversion or increased femoral torsion and have been associated with abnormal patellofemoral mechanics. Rotational abnormalities may also be detected by observing the angle of gait while walking or running. A deviation of the longitudinal axis of the foot greater than 10° from the line of progression is believed to be abnormal and is suggestive of excessive femoral anteversion or retroversion and excessive internal or external tibial torsion.

The lower leg and foot are next examined and the angle of the lower tibia to the floor is measured. If a lateral angulation of the tibia-to-floor angle is 10° or greater, the extremity requires an excessive amount of subtalar joint pronation to produce a plantigrade foot which can occur in both genu varum and tibia vara. The neutral position of the subtalar joint is determined to ascertain the weight-bearing status of the foot and detect any excessive pronation. This is performed by palpating the talar head between the index finger and thumb over the anterior aspect of the ankle. The patient transfers his or her weight to the lateral aspect of the foot, lifting the medial border of the heel off the floor, and the talar head can be palpated as a bulge over the lateral aspect of the ankle. Next, the patient relaxes the foot, allowing the subtalar joint to unlock and slowly pronate. As this pronation occurs, the subtalar joint is felt to be in the neutral position when the talar head can be palpated equally over the anterolateral and anteromedial aspects of the ankle. With further pronation, the talar head becomes prominent medially and the subtalar joint is now out of the neutral position. The normal weight-bearing foot should demonstrate a mild amount of pronation but should still allow for additional pronation if necessary. If the patient is weight-bearing or running with the foot out of the neutral position and near full pronation, an obligatory internal tibial rotation occurs and is actually prolonged, and there is an increased force that is absorbed by the soft tissues of the knee.



Thus it is important when examining the patient with a patellofemoral complaint to examine the entire lower extremity in the standing position and not just concentrate on the knee. Lower extremity malalignment is a common cause of anterior and peripatellar knee pain, particularly in the athletically active individual, especially the runner. The common denominator in these malalignment syndromes appears to be abnormal subtalar joint pronation, either primary or compensatory. Those entities that will produce compensatory subtalar joint pronation include genu varum, tibia vara, triceps surae contractures, hindfoot varus or forefoot supination. The excessively pronated foot is accompanied by a compensatory internal tibial rotation, and an increased amount of rotatory stress is absorbed through the peripatellar soft tissues at the knee joint.

## Sitting examination

Following the standing examination of the patellofemoral joint, the knee is examined with the patient seated on a routine examination table, the legs hanging free and the knees flexed approximately 90°. The position of the patellae over the distal aspect of the femur is first evaluated. The normal patella should sink deeply within the patellofemoral sulcus with 90° of knee flexion. If patella alta is present, the patellae are quite protuberant, do not sink into the normal sulcus, and appear to point toward the ceiling. Conversely, in patella infera, the normal smooth, rounded contour over the distal femur is lost as the patella is displaced inferiorly. The alignment of the patella and patellar tendon at its insertion into the tibial tubercle is also assessed. With the knees flexed, the tibia normally derotates and effectively reduces the quadriceps angle, with the patellar tendon orienting itself in the same longitudinal axis as the anterior crest of the tibia. Patellar tracking is next evaluated. The patella normally has 5–7 cm of longitudinal excursion with flexion and extension as it enters and exits the trochlear groove of the femur. There should be a smooth longitudinal trajectory, with only small amounts of physiologic rotation occurring. Any abrupt or sudden movements, particularly as the patella enters and exits the femoral trochlea at 10–30° of flexion, should be considered abnormal. Ficat's classification describes the following three abnormal patellar tracking trajectories:

1. A bayonet movement with abrupt lateral translation just before full extension and then further extension in a straight line.
2. An abrupt lateral movement at the end of extension.
3. A semicircular route as if the patella were pivoting around the lateral trochlear facet of the femur.

Abnormal patellar tracking is often caused by abnormalities of the patellofemoral configuration or deficiency of the supporting structures. One further sign of abnormal patellar position and tracking is the 'grasshopper eye' patella. This lateral tilting of the patella can be noted quite easily as the patient flexes the knee to 90° and is considered to be one of the most reliable diagnostic signs of patellar subluxation.

An often overlooked entity that may also interrupt patellar motion is plica syndrome. As these remnants of developmental synovial tissue become thick and fibrotic and lose their elastic properties, they may cause pain and popping within the knee. The patella will often catch momentarily during flexion and extension, which is frequently associated with a high-pitched or audible snap. In a series by Hardaker, 71% of patients with a plica syndrome had an audible or palpable snapping sensation and 90% demonstrated some tenderness over the superior pole of the patella or the medial femoral condyle. This tenderness over the medial femoral condyle is caused by direct irritation from the plica as it impinges on the femoral condyle. This area of tenderness is well above the joint line and should be distinguished from joint line tenderness associated with meniscal pathology. The symptomatic plica can often be palpated as a tender, band-like structure coursing near the medial border of the patella and will demonstrate tenderness as it rolls over the medial femoral condyle with flexion and extension.

The sitting examination of the patellofemoral joint is concluded by evaluation of the patella for crepitation as the patient actively flexes and extends the knee. The presence of crepitation does not always correlate with pain or the degree of patellar involvement, as there may be either marked pain with minimal crepitation or minimal pain with marked crepitation. Crepitation or pain may be elicited by having the patient actively extend the knee against forced resistance, holding the knee at 30° of flexion. This will often reproduce the retropatellar or anterior knee pain. Another method of testing for pain and crepitation is to have the patient perform deep knee bends while the patella is palpated.

## Supine examination

The supine examination of the patellofemoral joint and lower extremity is performed with the patient positioned on a routine examination table. In the examination of the patient with chronic complaints related to the patellofemoral joint, the supine examination is preceded by the standing and sitting examinations. However, if the patient presents with an acutely subluxated or dislocated patella, often only a supine examination may be performed.

Owing to the ease of reduction, many patients with an acutely dislocated patella are initially seen with the patella spontaneously reduced.

If the patient does present with the patella spontaneously reduced and examination of the patellofemoral joint is performed several hours, or even several days, following the acute dislocation, the physical findings are quite characteristic. There may be a considerable hemarthrosis; however, this is usually not under tension because the synovial membrane has been torn along with the retinaculum. There may be tenderness along the medial edge of the patella if the medial retinaculum has been torn from the patella, and there will be muscular tenderness more medially and proximally if the vastus medialis obliquus has been torn near the area of the adductor magnus. Although most of the tenderness in an acutely subluxated or dislocated patella is appreciated medially or superomedially, there may be mild tenderness over the anteromedial joint line. This joint line tenderness has been attributed to a tear of the insertion of the patellomeniscal ligament at the anterior horn of the medial meniscus. In the acute or subacute subluxation of the patella, it is usually hypermobile laterally and the Fairbank or apprehension sign is often present. This test is best performed with the patient's leg supported at approximately 30° of flexion to the examiner's leg. This insures the appropriate amount of flexion and muscle relaxation as well as reassures the patient.

With the patient's quadriceps mechanism relaxed. the examiner applies a firm, laterally directed force to the medial aspect of the patella, attempting to subluxate it laterally while applying a small amount of passive flexion to the knee. The test is positive if the patient experiences acute apprehension as if the patella were about to dislocate. If the patient does experience this sensation, he or she will contract the quadriceps, which re-centers the patella and prevents further flexion and further subluxation. Pain is variably associated with this maneuver; fear of dislocation is the major component of a positive test.

One is most often called upon to evaluate the patellofemoral joint in a patient with symptoms of chronic pain or instability. Abnormality of the supporting structures is one of the major causes of chronic patellofemoral disorders, and many of these abnormalities are best appreciated with the patient in the supine position. The examination begins with an inspection of the quadriceps mechanism, and the Q angle is measured. The Q angle is formed by two lines, one projecting from the anterior superior iliac spine to the mid-patella and the second from the mid-patella to the tibial tubercle. The average Q angle in men is 10° and the normal value in women is approximately 15°. The higher Q angle in women is caused by a wider pelvis. Abnormalities that may increase the Q angle are excessive femoral anteversion or femoral torsion, external tibial torsion and genu valgum. With gross subluxation of the patella, the quadriceps angle may actually be decreased because the patella rides laterally and faces outwards. The Q angle is not diagnostic of any particular patellofemoral disorder; however, an increased angle should be viewed as an indication of a potential problem that may act to subluxate or dislocate the patella.



The quadriceps musculature is next evaluated, with particular attention paid to the vastus medialis obliquus muscle. This muscle should be inspected for atrophy, hypoplasia or frank dysplasia. In addition, the level of the insertion of the vastus medialis into the medial border of the patella is ascertained. The level of patellar attachment of this muscle is directly related to its effectiveness in stabilizing the patella. The normal VMO inserts approximately one half tone third of the way down the medial aspect of the patella. The lower the insertion of the vastus medialis, the more muscle is attached to bone and the greater is its effectiveness in stabilizing the patella against lateral forces. The position of the patella is ascertained with particular attention paid to the patella that is laterally deviated or proximally located. As previously noted, in patients with patella alta, the patella fails to sink into the femoral sulcus with the knee flexed 90° and stands out facing the ceiling as the patient sits. With the patient in the supine position, the high-riding patella appears to be located more proximally and there is often a prominence of the anterior fat pad beneath the inferior aspect of the patella.

Patellar stability is also evaluated. In patients with normal extensor mechanism musculature and supporting structures, the patella can be displaced medially or laterally no more than one half the width of the patella with the knee in full extension. With the knee in 30° of flexion, the patella should be quite secure in the femoral sulcus and demonstrate little or no lateral or medial movement. Patients with recurrent subluxation of the patella will demonstrate hypermobility of the patella in a lateral direction and may have a positive apprehension sign.

The patella may also demonstrate decreased mobility, usually in the medial direction. It may also appear to be tethered or tilted by tight lateral retinacular structures. Occasionally, a thickened fascial band extending from the iliotibial tract to the lateral inferior margin of the patella may be palpated as the patella is pushed and held medially, in so doing stretching the lateral structures. Another method of palpating tight lateral structures is to displace the patella laterally, thus placing the retinacular structures under tension while they are brought away from the underlying synovium and soft-tissue structures. The final phase of the supine examination of the patella involves palpating the patellar and peripatellar soft tissues for tenderness.

There are three methods commonly used to elicit patellar discomfort:

1. One is to pull the patella distally into the superior entrance of the trochlear sulcus of the femur and have the patient contract the quadriceps.
2. A second is task the patient to extend the knee actively against forced resistance with the knee held at 30–45° of flexion.
3. The last method is direct palpation of the patellar facets.

These tests may be accompanied by a palpable or audible patellofemoral crepitus. In patients demonstrating patellofemoral abnormalities such as chondromalacia and subluxation of the patella, as well as in the lateral patellar compression syndromes, the medial facet is usually the most tender. The medial facet is best palpated by displacing the patella in a medial direction with the knee flexed approximately 30° and supported by the examiner's leg. This causes a tilting of the patella in a lateral direction as it ascends the proximal portion of the medial femoral condyle and will uncover the medial facet. The amount of dorsiflexion available at the ankle should be recorded in a patient complaining of peripatellar or patellar pain. For normal weight-bearing mechanics, the dorsiflexion required is at least 10° for walking and approximately 15° for running. Patients with less dorsiflexion than this may compensate for the tightened heel cord by compensatory pronation of the subtalar joint and, as mentioned previously, will have an obligatory internal rotation of the tibia, thus transmitting an increased energy absorption and stress at the peripatellar tissues.

The supine examination of the patellofemoral articulation is concluded with the usual tests to rule out meniscal pathology as well as straight or rotatory ligamentous instabilities.

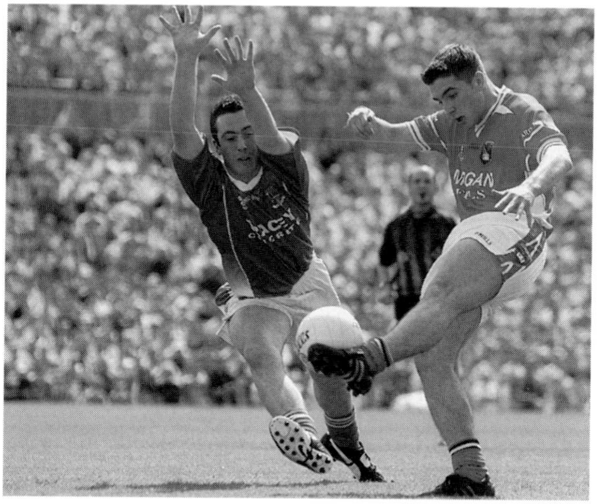

**Fig. 6.13** Sportsfield.

## PATHOLOGIES

# Anterior cruciate ligament tear

### Anatomy

- Intracapsular, extrasynovial ligament, roughly 3.5 cm long.
- Restrains anterior tibial movement in relation to the femur.
- Runs obliquely from the medial aspect lateral femoral condyle to the anterior insertion on the intercondylar notch (running lateral to medial, posterior to anterior) parallel to Blumensaat's line.
- Two components ensuring that functional tension is maintained throughout gait cycle:
  - anteromedial band (stronger): resists anterior tibial displacement in flexion
  - posterolateral band: resists posterior femoral displacement in extension.

### Mechanism of injury

- Rotational torque injury, e.g. during a pivot maneuver, especially when the foot is planted.
- A valgus stress to the joint may be described, e.g. Segond's fracture.
- Injury often occurs in combination with other soft-tissue injuries in the knee:
  - lateral knee impact (forced external rotation and valgus strain) causing ACL, MCL and medial capsular damage
  - medial knee impact (forced internal rotation and varus strain) causing ACL, LCL and posterolateral capsule
  - hyperextension or hyperflexion impacts causing combined ACL and PCL damage +/- knee dislocation.
- Avulsion of the tibial insertion site is common in younger athletes (Fig. 6.14).



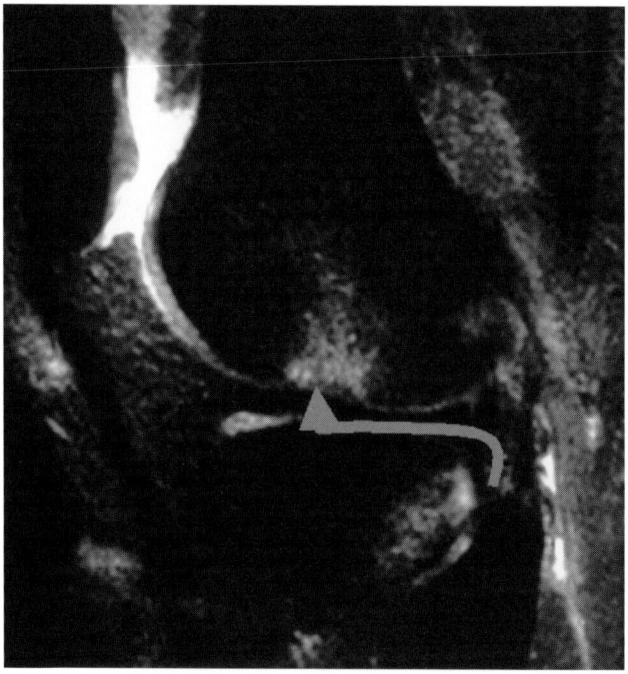

**Fig. 6.14** Following a pivot shift injury, a sagittal fat-suppressed image shows contrecoup impaction bone bruises of the posterolateral tibial plateau and of the mid-lateral femoral condyle. This indicates a gross anterior translation of the tibia only allowed by significant injury to the ACL.

## History and clinical findings

- Acute history:
  - twisting injury to the knee with a popping sensation at the time of the injury
  - patient may perceive the knee to be buckling
  - pain and immediate swelling (from traumatic hemarthrosis).
- Chronic history:
  - instability (pain and swelling subside after 2–4 weeks).
- Positive Lachman's test (main clinical examination test): (likelihood ratio of ACL tear of 42.0). At 15–30° of knee flexion, the tibia is pulled forward in relation to the femur with the tibia in neutral rotation.
- Anterior drawer test:
  - at 70–90° of knee flexion, the tibia is pulled forward in relation to the femur with the knee in neutral or internal rotation
  - false negatives are possible due to the hamstrings and the posterior horn of the medial meniscus resisting pull.
- Pivot shift test for chronic ACL injury: apply valgus force during flexion and extension to exaggerate subluxation or reduction of the tibia.
- Other findings depend on associated soft-tissue damage (e.g. valgus instability with MCL tear) and joint effusion.
- Swelling over the medial or lateral aspects of the joint may be associated with collateral ligament injury.
- There are three grades of ligamentous laxity:
  - grade I injury: no change in ligament length (intraligamentous injury)
  - grade II injury: increase in ligamentous length with intraligamentous injury
  - grade III injury: complete knee instability with ligament disruption.



## Imaging findings

### Plain radiography

- Lateral notch sign.
- Non-specific but may show knee effusion, associated fracture (e.g. Segond's fracture) or degenerative change (Fig. 6.15).

### Magnetic resonance imaging

- This is best evaluated in sagittal oblique plane (with the knee externally rotated 15°).
- ACL thinner (usually) and with a higher signal than the PCL.
- Primary findings:
  - discontinuity of low-signal ACL
  - contour abnormality: thickening; irregularity
  - high signal abnormality on $T_2$-weighted images
  - axis abnormality (Fig. 6.16).
- Secondary findings:
  - contrecoup bone bruising is present in 95% of cases, the typical pattern involving the mid-lateral femoral condyle and posterolateral tibial plateau
  - deep lateral notch
  - anterior tibial displacement by >5 mm
  - posterior horn subluxation
  - PCL buckling.

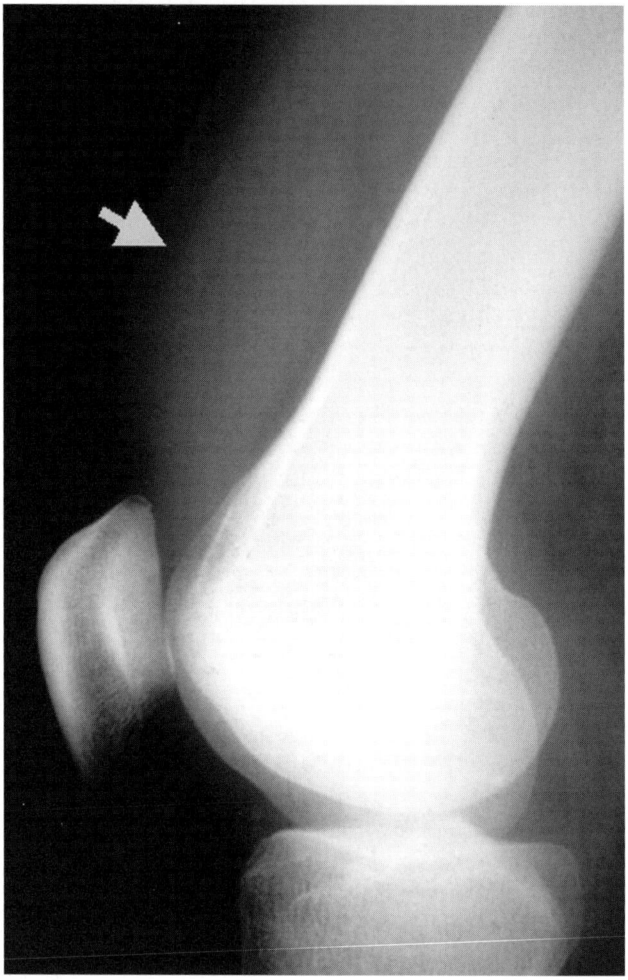

**Fig. 6.15** Lateral radiograph showing a suprapatellar swelling due to acute joint effusion in a patient with sports injury and acute disruption of the ACL.



## Management

This depends on age, desired activity level, chronicity of injury and coexistence of other injuries, and it is customized to individual needs.

### Non-surgical

- Suitable for patients with low activity levels and those who do not participate in contact sports.
- Acute management to provide symptomatic relief: ice; antiinflammatories; and analgesics.
- Early muscle rehabilitation.
- Bracing for sports involving rotational movements.
- Avoidance of 'high-risk' sporting activities (stopping or starting abruptly or pivoting) for 6–12 weeks.

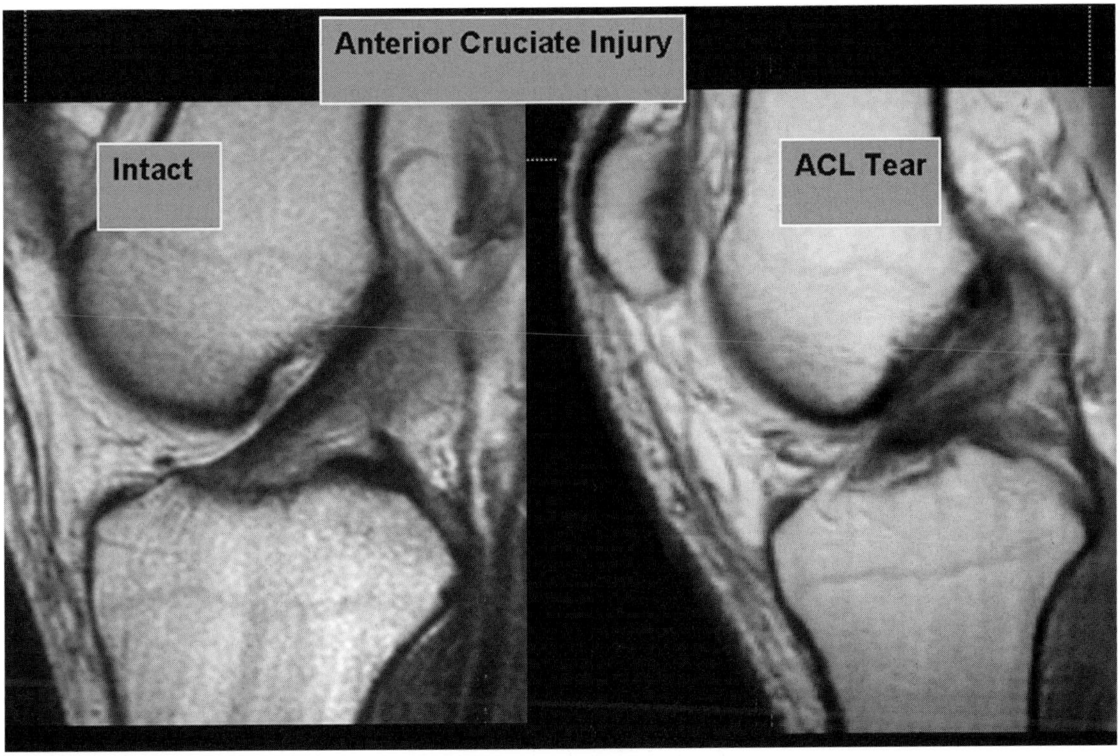


(a) (b)

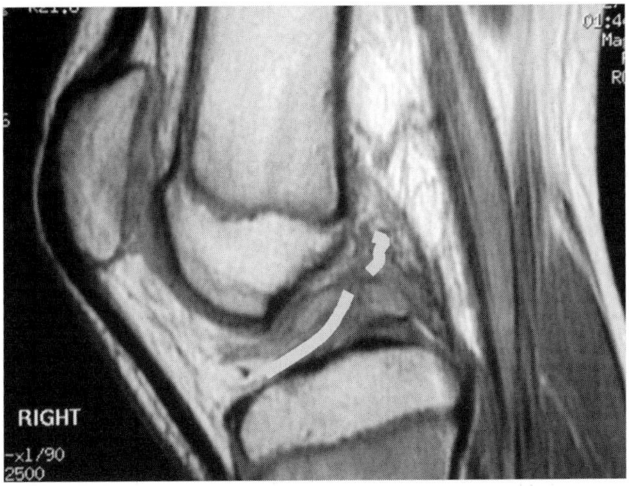


(c)

**Fig. 6.16** Anterior cruciate ligament injury. (**a**) Intact; (**b**) ACL tear; (**c**) ACL tear.

### Surgical

- For patients with recurrent marked instability or pain, high activity expectations or serious coexisting injury.
- Optimum timing of repair is at 3–8 weeks post-injury (isolated ACL tear).
- Success rate of 80–95%.
- ACL reconstruction with a graft (patellar tendon graft or semitendinosus/hamstring graft) to prevent the development of subsequent osteoarthritis in younger patients.
- Patellar tendon graft: the middle third of the patellar tendon with bone block from the tibia and femur is removed for the replacement graft of the ACL.
- Semitendinosus graft : the semitendinosus and gracilis hamstrings are removed to form a bundle graft to replace the torn ACL.
- Combined acute ACL and grade 3 MCL requires initial MCL repair with interval ACL reconstruction at 6 weeks.

### Rehabilitation

- Treat pain and swelling, which can limit movement at the joint.
- Early exercises for quadriceps and hamstrings.
- Initial range of motion limited to up to 70° flexion post-operatively, increasing to full motion.
- Graded reintroduction of sporting activities but avoidance of sports involving rotational or cutting movements for at least 4–6 months.

# Anterior cruciate ligament graft tear

## Anatomy

- The ACL is replaced by a graft composed of three components:
  - femoral tunnel (intersection of the posterior femoral cortex and physeal scar)
  - tibial tunnel (posterior to midpoint of tibial ACL footprint)
  - interposed graft runs parallel to the roof of the intercondylar notch (Blumensaat's line).
- Types of graft: patellar tendon; hamstring; or synthetic.
- The goal of reconstruction is to maintain isometric tension in the graft, i.e. a taut graft in both flexion and extension as occurs in native ACL.

## Mechanism of injury

- Post-trauma.
- Chronic impingement from the intercondylar notch roof.

## History and clinical findings

- Pain and instability after ACL reconstruction.
- Impingement leads to pain, reduced extension, recurrent instability and joint effusions.

## Imaging findings

### Plain radiography

- Non-specific but may show osteophyte development in the intercondylar notch causing impingement.

### Magnetic resonance imaging

- Best evaluated in the sagittal oblique plane.
- Intact grafts seen as a continuous low-signal band (patellar graft) or as two low-signal bands inside a high-signal fluid/synovial compartment on $T_2$-weighted sequences (hamstring grafts) (Fig. 6.17).
- A slight increase in graft signal intensity is seen on both $T_1$- and $T_2$-weighted sequences 6 weeks to 8 months after grafting due to revascularization.
- Primary findings in graft tear:
  - increased graft signal intensity on $T_2$-weighted sequences
  - thickening and laxity of graft
  - discontinuity of graft.
- Secondary findings in graft tear:
  - other injuries: meniscal injury; collateral ligament tear; or bone bruising
  - a tibial tunnel that is placed too anteriorly
  - cyclops lesion: fibrotic mass anterior to graft.
- Graft impingement findings:
  - tibial tunnel anteriorly placed with intercondylar roof causing graft impingement
  - increased signal intensity on all sequences.

## Management

### Non-surgical

- As for native ACL tear.

### Surgical

- Resection of osteophytes for impingement.
- Graft replacement if torn.
- Arthroscopic resection of cyclops lesion.

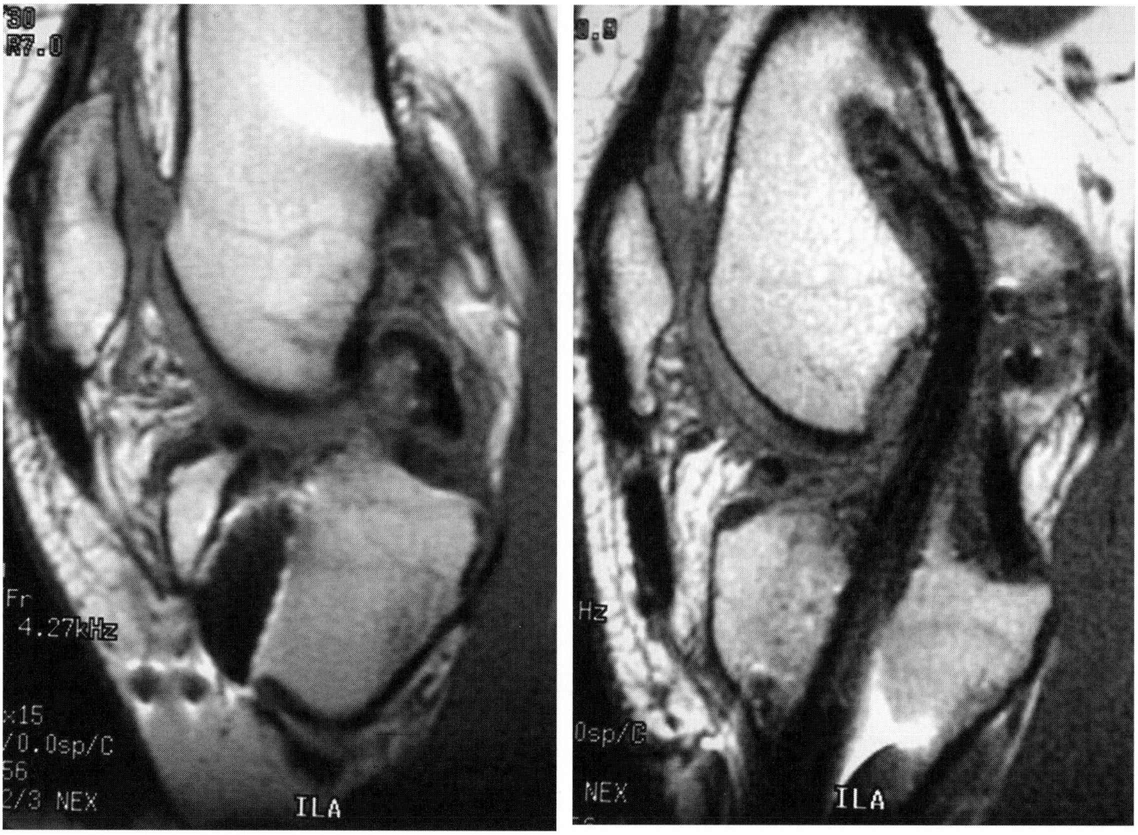


(a) (b)



**Fig. 6.17** (**a**) Sagittal MR image showing a disrupted ACL graft, with (**b**) subsequent second reconstruction using a gracilis, semitendinosis tendon graft.

# Anterior cruciate ligament ganglion cysts

## Anatomy

The ACL is an intrasynovial extracapsular ligament responsible for restraining anterior displacement or translation of the tibia on flexion or extension.

## Mechanism of injury

Occasionally, complicating a pivot shift injury, some of the intrasynovial ACL fibers are torn but in the presence of predominantly intact ligament fibers their presence is not immediately appreciated. Leakage of serum and interstitial fluid at the site of the fiber tear results in the development of a localized fluid collection which ultimately becomes encapsulated: an ACL ganglion cyst.

## History and clinical findings

- Patients typically complain of pain deep within the knee on flexion (as flexion results in compression of the cyst within the notch).
- There are no definite clinical findings beyond the demonstration of pain on knee flexion.

## Imaging findings

### Ultrasound

- This may allow the identification of large cysts extending out of the intercondylar notch.

### Magnetic resonance imaging

- This demonstrates a well-circumscribed loculated hyperintense fluid collection intimately related to the ACL, often hugging the inner aspect of the lateral femoral condyle 1–3 cm in diameter (Figs 6.18 and 6.19).



## Management

### Non-surgical

- NSAIDs, intra-articular steroid injection and CT-guided percutaneous drainage (favored over surgery).

### Surgical

- Arthroscopic localization with associated incision and drainage.

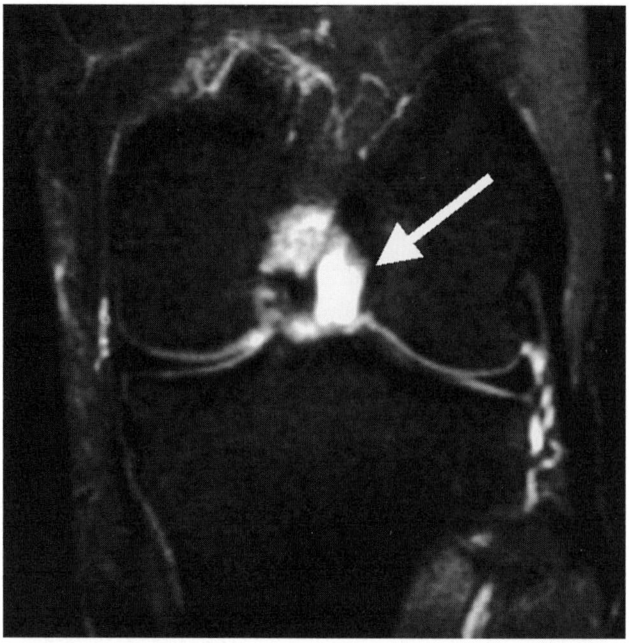

(a)

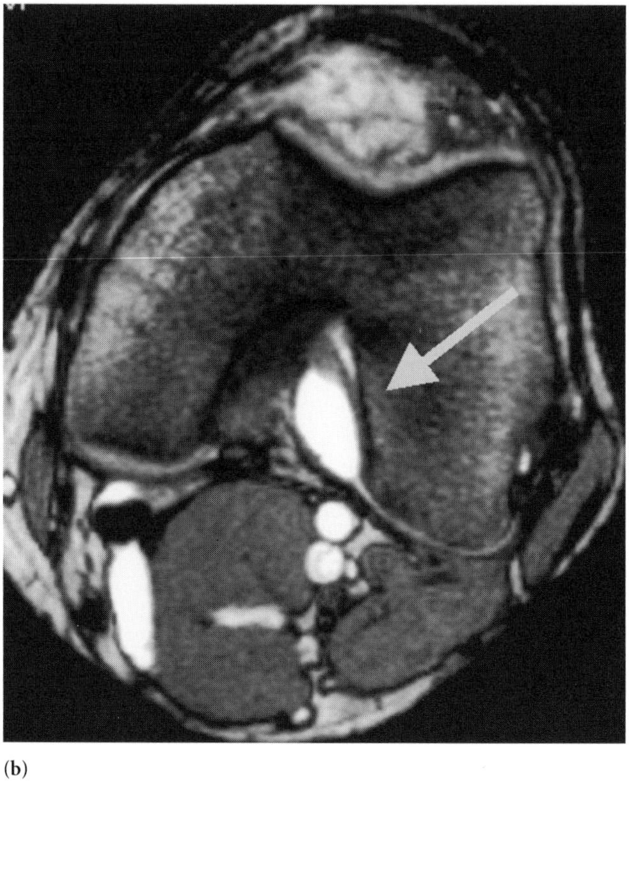

(b)

**Fig. 6.18** (**a**) Coronal, fat-suppressed image showing a cruciate ganglion cyst within the intercondylar notch, (**b**) identified hugging the inner aspect of the lateral femoral condyle on the axial image.

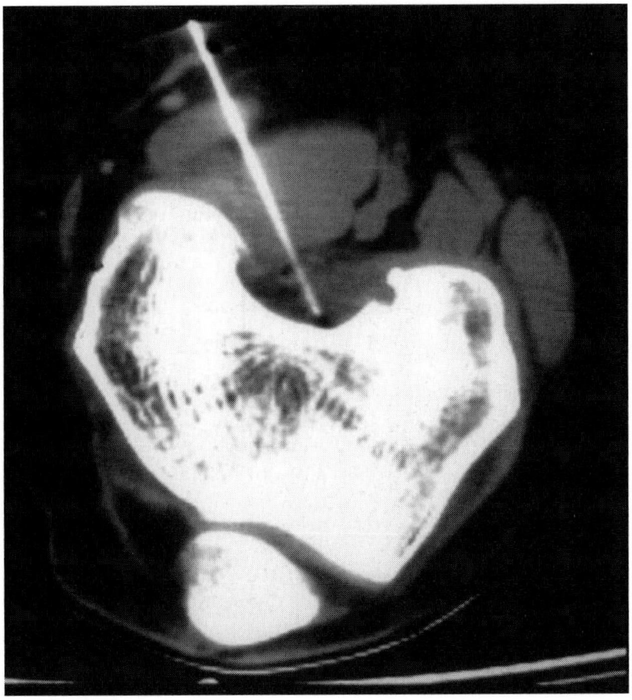

**Fig. 6.19** CT scan showing needle drainage of an ACL ganglion cyst approached via the posteromedial soft tissues.

# Posterior cruciate ligament injury

## Anatomy

- Intrasynovial extracapsular ligament.
- Resists posterior translation of the tibia and limits hyperextension.
- Primarily responsible for resisting posterior translation of the tibia during maximal flexion.
- It is 13 mm long and is comprised of a dominant anterolateral bundle (taut in flexion) and a smaller posteromedial band (taut in extension).
- Arises from the inner aspect of the medial femoral condyle running posteriorly in a C-shaped configuration to attach in a midline depression in the posterior margin of the tibial plateau.

## Mechanism of injury

- This is a direct blow to the patella or anterior tibia in the planted foot position forcing posterior tibial translation. This injury most frequently follows dashboard impaction in a motor vehicle accident but also occurs in sport-related impaction injuries.
- A fall on a flexed knee with rapid deceleration when the foot is in plantar flexion.
- Rarely during unexpected hyperextension of the knee.
- Rarely as a part of total knee dislocation.

## History and clinical findings

- A history of an acute blow to the anterior knee.
- The patient often describes a sensation of 'something snapping'.
- Pain on flexion beyond 90°.
- Swelling less than in an ACL tear.
- Posterior drawer test performed at 90° knee flexion with the tibia in neutral rotation:
  - *partial PCL tear* – <10 mm posterior tibial translation
  - *complete PCL tear* – >10 mm posterior tibial drawer.
- False negative results if posterolateral corner structures limit posterior tibial movement.
- Posterior sag test (Godfrey's test): patient supine with knee flexed to right angles; tibia sags into posterior subluxation relative to the femur.
- Quadriceps active test: tibia moves anteriorly on contraction of the quadriceps.
- Pathological hyperextension.



## Imaging findings

### Radiography

- Avulsion fractures of the posterior tibia (Fig. 6.20).

### Magnetic resonance imaging

- The normal PCL is uniformly hypointense.
- The majority of tears are mid-substance and characterized by apparent ligamentous swelling and signal change.
- Rarely, the PCL is avulsed from its posterior tibial plateau attachment.
- Secondary bone contusion in the anterior tibia and femur in hyperextension injuries.

## Management

### Non-surgical

- The majority of PCL injuries are treated non-surgically: NSAIDs; bracing.
- Early mobilization physiotherapy, especially quadriceps conditioning.

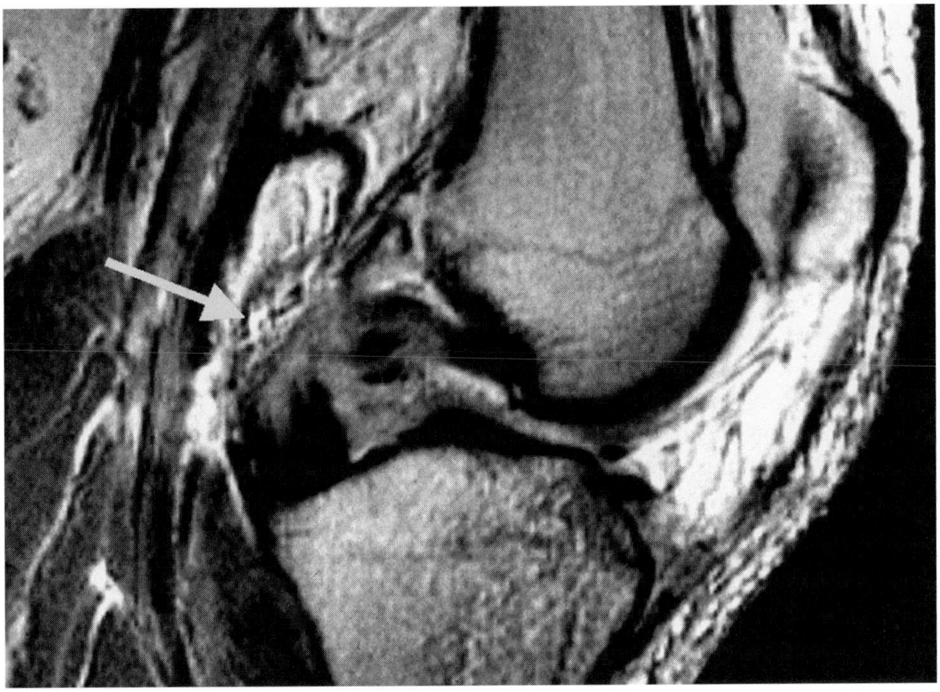

**Fig. 6.20** Sagittal image showing intrasubstance rupture of the mid-posterior cruciate ligament.

- Return to sports normally by 8 weeks in an isolated tear.
- Increased patellofemoral osteoarthritis after many years (contact between the tibia and femur shifts anteriorly).



## Surgical

- Recommended if there is more than 10 mm of posterior translation on a drawer test or if combined with other injuries.
- Employs a patellar or quadriceps tendon graft, Achilles allograft or hamstring augmentation.
- Open reduction with fixation in dislocated PCL bone avulsions.

# Medial meniscus tear

## Anatomy

- The medial meniscus is an open C-shaped fibrocartilage ring between the medial femoral condyle and the medial tibial plateau (Fig. 6.21).
- Attachments:
  - intercondylar notch of the tibia anteriorly and posteriorly
  - anterior horn of the lateral meniscus in 40% of the population (via the transverse meniscal ligament)
  - posterior capsule of the knee joint
  - MCL.
- Organized into an outer circumferential zone and an inner transverse zone.
- Poorly vascularized in adulthood (only the outer third receives a supply via the geniculate branches); poorer healing post-injury.
- Buffering function to protect articular cartilage.
- Important also in joint stability and lubrication.
- Subject to rotational forces on flexion and extension to distribute the strain of weight-bearing.

## Mechanism of injury

- About five times as common as lateral meniscal injury.
- Acute:
  - twisting impact on the joint, e.g. a soccer tackle to the lateral knee
  - forced external rotation of the foot
  - hyperflexion or hyperextension injury.
- Chronic:
  - minor trauma (e.g. squatting or climbing stairs) superimposed on meniscal degeneration; this is usually in older patients.



## History and clinical findings

- Acute history:
  - twisting injury to the knee with a popping sensation at the time of injury
  - patient may perceive the knee to be buckling
  - pain and immediate swelling
  - 'locking' sensation if there is a bucket handle tear.
- Chronic history:
  - instability (pain and swelling subside after 2–4 weeks).
- Point tenderness over the medial knee joint.
- Pain on either hyperflexion or hyperextension of the knee.
- Pain when the lower leg and foot are externally rotated with the knee in 90° flexion.
- Weakening of the quadriceps muscle.

## Imaging findings

### Magnetic resonance maging

- Best evaluated in sagittal oblique plane (Fig. 6.22).
- Hypointense normally on all sequences.
- The posterior horn of the medial meniscus is twice the size of the anterior horn and most commonly torn in cases of trauma.
- Body of meniscus seen only on the outer two slices.

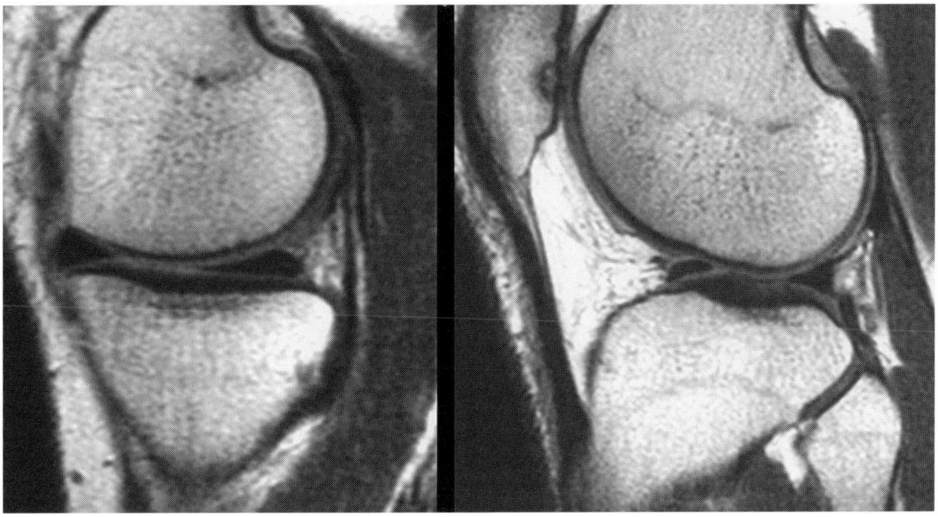

(a) (b)

**Fig. 6.21** (**a**) Normal medial meniscus and (**b**) normal lateral meniscus with bow-tie configuration. Note the proximity of the popliteus tendon to the posterior horn of the lateral meniscus.

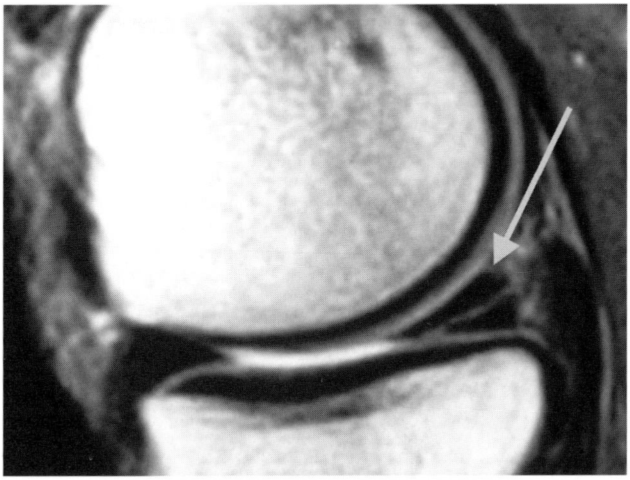

**Fig. 6.22** Sagittal image showing an oblique tear of the posterior horn of the medial meniscus.



- Grading system for meniscal tears:
  - grade I: focal signal abnormality (slight $T_1$ and $T_2$ hyperintensity)
  - grade II: linear or diffuse globular signal abnormality not extending to a meniscal surface
  - grade III: signal abnormality, either linear or globular, with definite extension to a meniscal surface.
- A grade II-type signal abnormality is occasionally seen in the periphery of normal menisci in children (perforating vessels).

- Signal orientation provides a clue to etiology
  - vertical tear: traumatic
  - horizontal tear: degenerative.
- Vertical tears may be parallel to the long axis of the meniscus, radial ('parrot beak') versus perpendicular to the long axis, a longitudinal (bucket handle) tear.
- Pitfalls: a grade II signal change in the posterior horn is secondary to the magic angle phenomenon.
- Arthroscopy may miss inferior surface tears.

## Management

### Non-surgical

- No operation is required if the tear comprises small stable vertical tears, especially if peripherally located.

### Surgical

- Arthroscopy and meniscal repair (in younger patients) or partial meniscectomy (in older patients).
- Meniscal repair is performed with T-fixes, resorbable staples or screws.
- The aim is to preserve as much meniscus as possible.
- Degenerative changes are commonly seen after total meniscectomy.
- Early quadriceps muscle strengthening is paramount post-surgery.
- A return to training is possible in 3–6 weeks (large posterior horn tears take longer).

# Lateral meniscus tear

## Anatomy

- The lateral meniscus is a circular fibrocartilage ring between the lateral femoral condyle and the lateral tibial plateau.
- Attachments:
  - intercondylar notch of the tibia anteriorly and posteriorly
  - anterior horn of the medial meniscus via the transverse meniscal ligament
  - meniscofemoral ligament attachments to the inner aspect of the medial femoral condyle (Humphry's anteriorly, Wrisberg's posteriorly)
  - loosely attached to the capsule of the knee joint.
- Not attached to the LCL.
- It is attached less firmly to the tibia via capsular attachments than the medial meniscus (more mobility in an AP direction).

## Mechanism of injury

- Lateral meniscal injury is less common (more mobile and fewer capsular attachments).
- Forced internal rotation of the foot in relation to the femur.
- Hyperflexion or hyperextension injury.
- Free edge tears of the lateral meniscus often accompany rotational torque injuries, with frequent coexistent ACL damage.

## History and clinical findings

- Acute history
  - twisting injury to the knee with popping sensation at the time of injury
  - pain and immediate swelling
  - locking sensation if bucket handle tear.
- Chronic history
  - instability.
- Point tenderness over the lateral knee joint.
- Pain on either hyperflexion or hyperextension of the knee.
- Pain when lower leg and foot are internally rotated with the knee in 90° flexion.
- Weakening of the quadriceps muscle.

## Imaging findings

### Magnetic resonance imaging

- Best evaluated in sagittal oblique plane.
- The posterior horn is the same size as the anterior horn (cf. medial meniscus).
- Grading system as for medial meniscus.
- Vertical radial tears extending from the free edge to the periphery of the meniscus are more common than in medial meniscus ('parrot beak' tear).
- Pitfalls: the popliteus tendon may mimic a tear in the posterior horn of the lateral meniscus.

## Management

- As for medial meniscus tear (Figs 6.23 and 6.24).

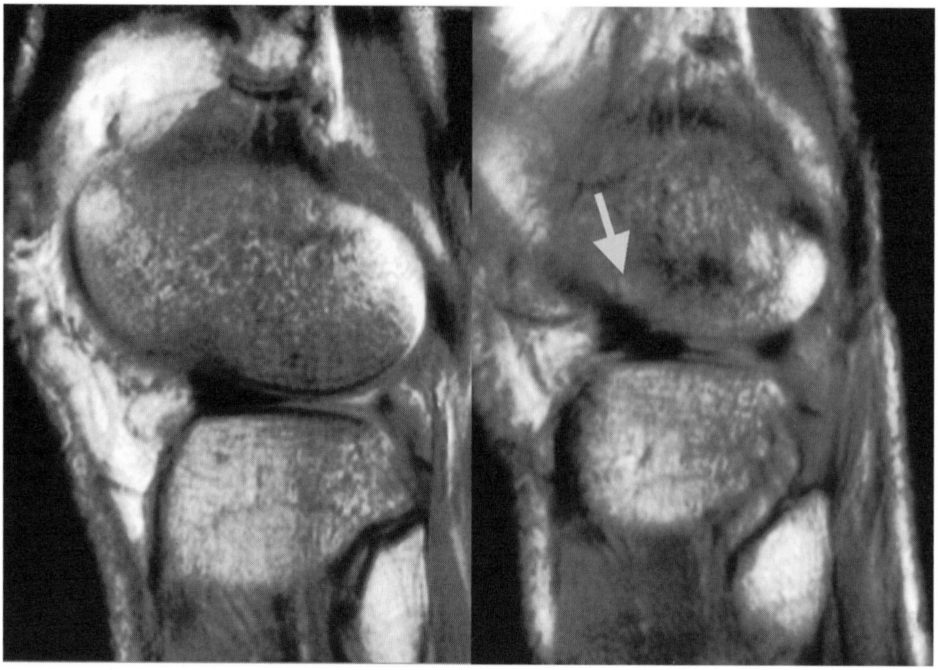

Fig. 6.23 A double anterior horn sign due to a bucket handle tear of the lateral meniscus in a patient following pivot shift injury.



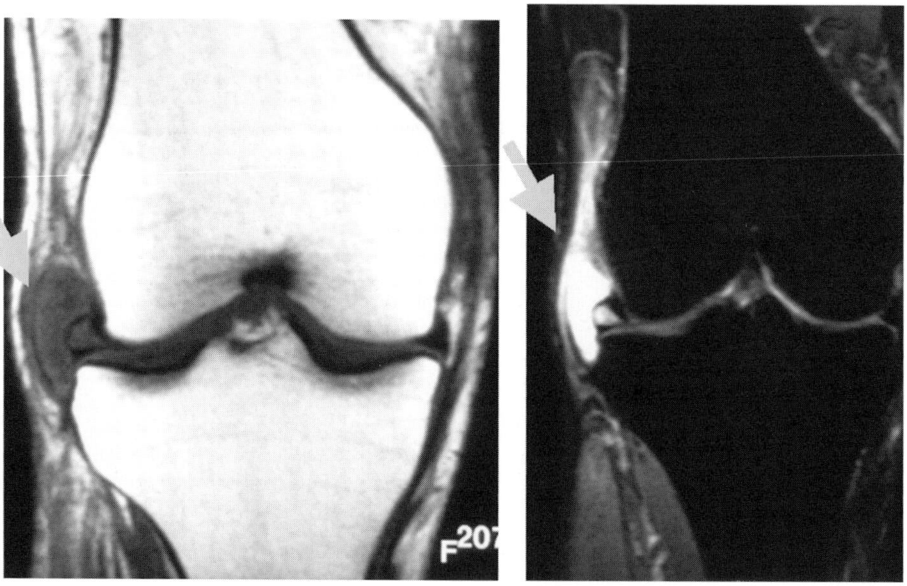


(a) (b)

Fig. 6.24 (a) (b) MR images showing a chronic tear of the lateral meniscus complicated by the formation of a lateral meniscal cyst.

# Bucket handle tear

## Anatomy

- Vertical peripheral tear (2–5 mm long) with a displaced inner fragment into the intercondylar notch of the knee.
- This occurs more frequently in the medial than the lateral meniscus.

## Mechanism of injury

- Usually an acute meniscal tear but relatively uncommon.
- A sudden impact splits the meniscus.

## History and clinical findings

- Pain and locking post-trauma.
- Locking preventing full extension and weight-bearing.
- Sensation of giving way.
- Joint line tenderness.

## Imaging findings

### Magnetic resonance imaging

- 'Double PCL sign': displaced fragment beneath the PCL at the notch, appearing like two PCL ligaments (Fig. 6.25).
- Two meniscal fragments seen on coronal images at the notch (body of meniscus plus meniscal fragment).
- 'Double delta sign': two triangular fragments of meniscus adjacent teach other anteriorly in the notch (anterior horn of donor meniscus and flipped torn segment).
- Smaller than normal remaining meniscus (blunting of donor).
- Can be confirmed by MR arthrography (contrast surrounds bucket handle tear).

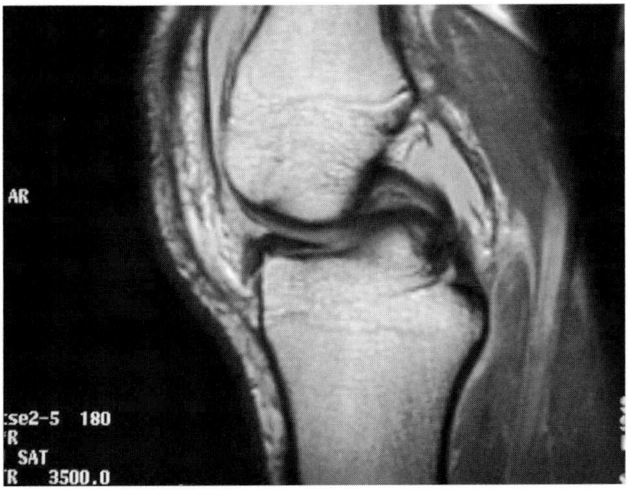


**Fig. 6.25** Sagittal MR image showing a double posterior cruciate ligament sign due to reflected meniscal fragment to the intercondylar notch, the so-called double PCL sign due to bucket handle tear of the medial meniscus.

### Management

**Non-surgical**

- As for other meniscal tears.

**Surgical**

- The aim is to preserve as much remaining meniscus as possible.
- Surgical removal of any free fragments if separated from the parent meniscus or if they affect the free edge of the meniscus (non-vascularized).
- Surgical repair if the fragment is not displaced or affects the peripheral vascularized zone.

## Discoid meniscal injury

### Anatomy

- This is an anatomical variant occurring in 2–15% of the world's population.
- More common on the lateral side.
- The normal open configuration of the meniscus is replaced by a solid appearance, which totally or partially covers the surface of the tibial condyle.
- Configuration lacks normal biomechanical integrity: a predisposition to tear.
- Posterior segment may become hypermobile.

### Mechanism of injury

- As for meniscal injury.

### History and clinical findings

- Occasional 'slapping knee syndrome'.
- 'Snapping' sound heard on knee motion.
- Sensation of giving way.



### Imaging findings

**Magnetic resonance imaging**

- Identification of the body of the meniscus on more than three contiguous 4 mm slices.
- Lack of rapid tapering from the periphery to the free edge of meniscus.
- Abnormally wide meniscal body on coronal images (loss of normal triangular configuration) with encroachment into the intercondylar notch.

### Management

**Non-surgical**

- No treatment required for incidentally discovered asymptomatic discoid meniscus.

**Surgical**

- Subtotal arthroscopic meniscectomy if torn or unstable.

# Medial collateral ligament injury

## Anatomy

- Originates from the medial femoral condyle and inserts distally on the anteromedial tibia below the insertion for the pes anserinus.
- Resists valgus strain and external rotation of the tibia.
- Deep and superficial parts separated by the medial collateral ligament bursa.
- Deep fibers (medial capsular ligament): meniscofemoral and meniscotibial ligamentous attachments.
- Superficial fibers (MCL proper): meniscotibial ligament.
- Medial knee stability posteriorly, also from the posterior oblique ligament (condensation of the capsular fascia), which inserts into the posterior horn of medial meniscus.

## Mechanism of injury

- This is the most commonly injured knee ligament.
- Acute valgus injury: forceful lateral blow to lower thigh/upper leg.
- External rotation injury (MCL is taut in external rotation).
- Frequent (95%) coexistent ACL rupture in grade III tears of the MCL.

## History and clinical findings

- Pain at time of injury.
- Swelling is unusual unless the MCL injury is complicated by other ligamentous damage (ACL, etc.).
- Tenderness over the medial femoral condyle.
- Valgus stress test the laxity of the MCL at 30° knee flexion (false negatives are possible at full knee extension if the PCL and posterior capsule are intact).
- There are three grades of ligamentous laxity:
  - grade I sprain: minimal joint opening (4 mm or less)
  - grade II sprain: moderate joint opening (5–10 mm)
  - grade III sprain: marked joint laxity (opening >10 mm); there is no firm endpoint to abduction stress.
- Swelling over the medial or lateral aspects of the joint may be associated with collateral ligament injury.

## Imaging findings

### Plain radiography

- Non-specific but may show associated fracture, e.g. Pellegrini–Stieda lesion (Fig. 6.26).

### Magnetic resonance imaging

- Best evaluated in the coronal plane.
- Grades of injury:
  - grade I: fluid on either side of the superficial fibers of the MCL
  - grade II: fluid on both sides of the ligament without discontinuity
  - grade III: tendon disruption and complete discontinuity.
- Contrecoup bone bruising ('kissing contusion') in the mid-lateral femoral condyle and mid-lateral tibial plateau due to valgus strain.

## Management

### Non-surgical

- Isolated grades I and II MCL tears are treated conservatively (e.g. pain relief, antiinflammatories and bracing) with early rehabilitation.

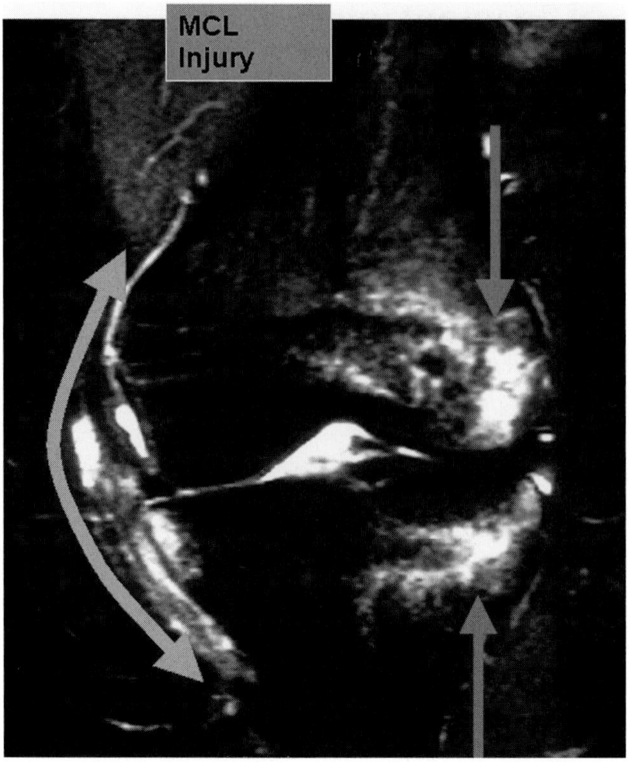


**Fig. 6.26** Coronal, fat-suppressed image showing disruption of the medial collateral ligament incurred by acute valgus injury with contrecoup impaction bruises of the mid-lateral femoral condyle and mid-lateral tibial plateau.

- Early mobilization, weight-bearing and physiotherapy reduce stiffness.
- A return to sports following an uneventful recovery is anticipated by 2–4 weeks in grade I and II tears.
- Isolated grade III tears usually heal as long as other serious injury to the knee structures is not present.



## Surgical

- For isolated grade III injuries, if there is severe capsular disruption and the two ends are widely spaced early surgical repair (<2 weeks) is recommended.
- Surgical repair if combined with ACL tear.
- Delayed return to sporting activities (6 to 9 months at least).

# Lateral collateral ligament complex injury

## Anatomy

- Resists varus stress on the knee.
- Runs from the lateral femoral condyle to the fibular head (inserts with the biceps femoris tendon).
- The primary restraint to external rotation in the posterolateral complex (PLC).
- Extracapsular and not attached to the lateral meniscus.
- There are three components:
  - superficial layer composed of an iliotibial band (ITB) anteriorly and continuous with the biceps femoris tendon posteriorly
  - middle layer composed of a posterior fibular collateral ligament
  - deep layer composed of a popliteus tendon, an arcuate ligament and the knee capsule.

## Mechanism of injury

- Uncommonly injured knee ligament and rarely torn in isolation.
- Acute varus injury, especially in hyperextension; forceful medial blow to the lower thigh or upper leg, e.g. motorcycle accident with the bike falling on the knee.
- Injury normally occurs at the proximal origin.
- Frequent coexistent posterolateral corner and/or cruciate ligament injury.

## History and clinical findings

- Posterolateral pain at the time of injury.
- Varus instability.
- Buckling to hyperextension when weight-bearing.
- Swelling is unusual unless the injury is complicated by other ligamentous damage.
- Lateral joint line tenderness.
- Varus instability test (with the knee in 30° flexion).
- There are three grades of ligamentous laxity:
  - 5 mm laxity: LCL insufficiency
  - 5–10 mm laxity: combined LCL and popliteus injury

  >10 mm laxity: LCL, popliteus and cruciate ligament injury.

## Imaging findings

### Plain radiography

- Non-specific but may show associated fracture or effusion (Fig. 6.27).

### Magnetic resonance imaging

- Best evaluated in the coronal plane.
- Discontinuity of LCL fibers in a complete tear.
- Thickening and high-signal abnormality on $T_2$-weighted images in partial tears.
- Contrecoup bone bruising in the medial femoral condyle and medial tibial plateau.
- Important to check for associated damage to other posterolateral structures.

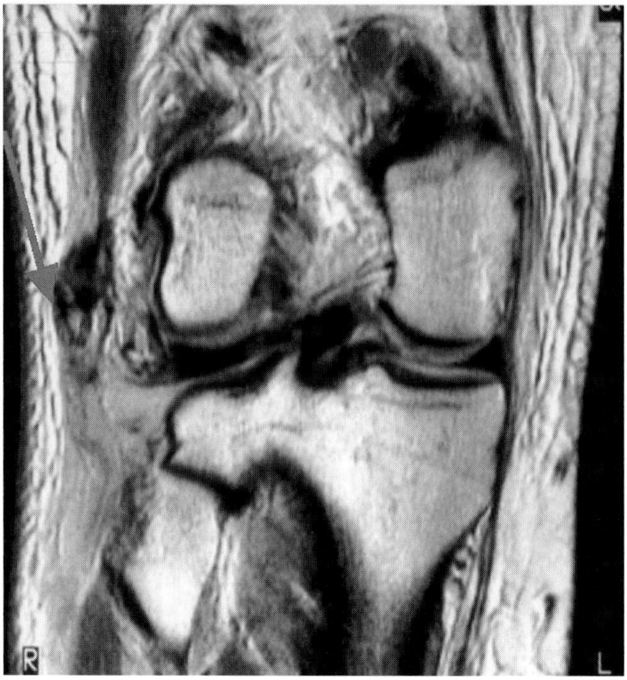


**Fig. 6.27** Coronal MR image showing a biceps tendon avulsion from the fibula head complicating an acute varus injury in a young football player.

## Management

### Non-surgical

- Isolated minor LCL tears treated conservatively (similar to MCL tears).
- Splint in full extension for 2 weeks.
- Subsequent mobilization, weight-bearing and physiotherapy reduce stiffness.



### Surgical

- Advanced LCL tears only, especially when associated with posterolateral corner injuries or cruciate ligament tears.

# Posterolateral corner injury

## Anatomy

- Components of the PLC:
  - lateral head of the gastrocnemius tendon
  - arcuate ligament
  - LCL
  - popliteus muscle and tendon
  - popliteofibular ligament
  - posterolateral joint capsule.
- Resists varus stress and external rotation.
- Adjacent to the tibiofibular joint.
- The biceps femoris tendon and ITB also provide posterolateral stability.

## Mechanism of injury

- Acute varus injury with rotation, e.g. in skiing or football/soccer.
- Direct blow to the anteromedial tibia with the knee extended.
- Commonly injured with the LCL and cruciate ligaments.
- Severe disability can result.

## History and clinical findings

- Posterolateral pain.
- Buckling in hyperextension and posterolateral instability.
- Reverse pivot shift test to detect posterolateral instability: place the knee in flexion and the foot in external rotation to posteriorly sublux the lateral tibial plateau.
- Extend the knee with pressure in the lateral tibial plateau.
- Joint relocates at about 30° of flexion (the 'shift').
- Reverse pivot shift test findings occur in up to a third of normal individuals.
- Posterolateral drawer test.
- Increased external rotation of the foot on walking.
- Painful heel strike.
- Varus instability on weight-bearing.



## Imaging findings

### Plain radiography

- Fractures of the fibular head, posterolateral tibia and lateral femoral condyle are common.
- Effusion and posterolateral soft-tissue swelling.

### Magnetic resonance imaging

- Discontinuous ligament or tendon fibers.
- Increased signal in structures of the PLC on $T_2$-weighted or short tau inversion recovery (STIR) sequences.
- Bone bruising in the posterolateral aspect of the knee.
- With or without a fibular head avulsion fracture or other fractures of the posterolateral corner.

## Management

### Non-surgical

- Significant injuries to the PLC usually require surgery.

### Surgical

- For acute posterolateral instability.
- Early repair (<2 weeks) is essential to avoid disability later.
- Restricted weight-bearing and motion with bracing post-operatively.

# Iliotibial band syndrome

## Anatomy

- Origin is the tensor fascia latae and inserts into the lateral tibial condyle.
- Part of the LCL complex.

## Mechanism of injury

- The ITB passes over the lateral epicondyle of the femur as the knee flexes.
- Inflammation with or without bursitis occurs with repeated microtrauma.
- Chronic frictional trauma when the ITB rubs on the outer aspect of the lateral femoral condyle.
- This syndrome especially affects downhill runners.
- Associated factors include excessive foot pronation, genu varum, tibial rotation and excessive tightness of the ITB.

## History and clinical findings

- Anterolateral knee pain (at the site of the ITB).
- Pain is worse on exercise and relieved with rest.
- Running downhill or climbing stairs are typical aggravating activities.
- Tenderness just proximal to the lateral joint line.
- Noble's test: pain is worst at 30° knee flexion (when the ITB crosses the lateral tibial condyle) when the lateral condyle is compressed.
- Ober's test: to evaluate ITB tightness.

## Imaging findings

### Magnetic resonance imaging

- $T_2$-weighted and STIR sequences may show partial or complete tear with or without early peritendon edema.
- Chronic change: thickened tendon with areas of focal high-signal intensity on $T_2$-weighted sequences (collagen degeneration) (Fig. 6.28).



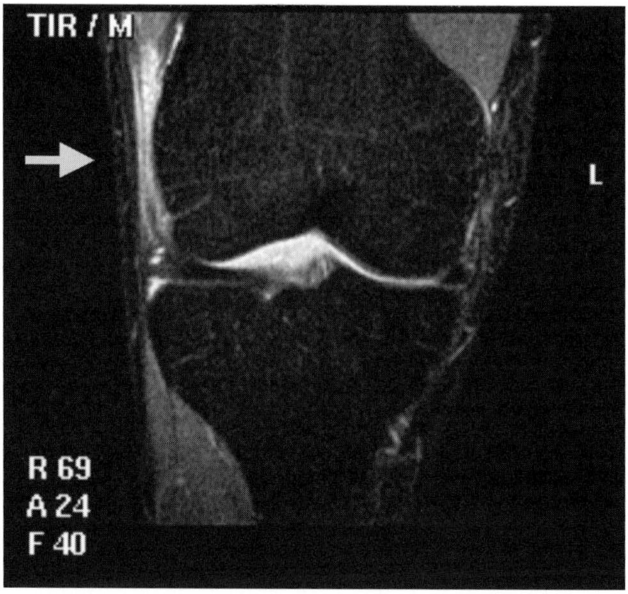


**Fig. 6.28** Coronal, fat-suppressed image showing an inflammatory reaction inside and outside the anterior margin of the iliotibial band in an elite athlete.

## Management

### Non-surgical

- Modification of sporting activity to reduce aggravating factors and allow healing.
- Conservative (heat pack application before activity with ice application afterwards; antiinflammatories and steroids injected locally).
- Static stretching of the lateral thigh.
- Wedge orthosis for a tight ITB.

### Surgical

- Incision posterior to the ITB over the lateral condyle with the knee in 30° flexion.

# Quadriceps tendon injuries

## Anatomy

- The quadriceps tendon links the quadriceps muscle to the patella and patellar retinaculum.

## Mechanism of injury

- Rupture of the quadriceps tendon at the patellar insertion site.
- Mostly found in older patients with repeated inflammation and pre-existing tendinosis, often with an exacerbating incident (a fall or slip on a slope).
- Rupture is rare in younger athletes, e.g. when lifting excessive loads.
- Overuse injury occurs in athletes repeatedly extending their knees under excessive force, e.g. weightlifters, or frequent jumpers, e.g. in basketball.

## History and clinical findings

- Rupture:
  - a sudden 'pop' when the extensor mechanism is put under strain
  - complete disruption is usually clinically evident with an inability to bear weight, and distal patellar displacement
  - pain not prominent in a complete tear.
- Overuse injuries: pain when pushing off or rising from a squatting position.
- Rupture:
  - hemarthrosis and mobile patella
  - impaired knee extension
  - inferior patellar displacement in complete rupture.
- Overuse:
  - tenderness over the proximal patella where the quadriceps tendon inserts
  - discomfort when contracting quadriceps muscle, especially against a force.

## Imaging findings



### Plain radiography

- May show an inferiorly displaced patella (patella baja) with knee effusion (Fig. 6.29).

### Magnetic resonance imaging

- Discontinuity of the low-signal quadriceps tendon in complete rupture.
- Incomplete tears show a thickened tendon with high-signal abnormality with continuity of fibers.
- Hyperintense fluid or blood at the tear site on $T_2$-weighted sequences or STIR.

## Management

### Non-surgical

- Partial ruptures do not normally require surgery.
- Bandaging and support.
- Early mobilization with strength and mobility training.
- Refrain from sports for 4–6 months.
- Overuse injuries require strengthening and stretching exercises.

### Surgical

- For complete ruptures or high-performance athletes: best results when repaired within 48 hours.

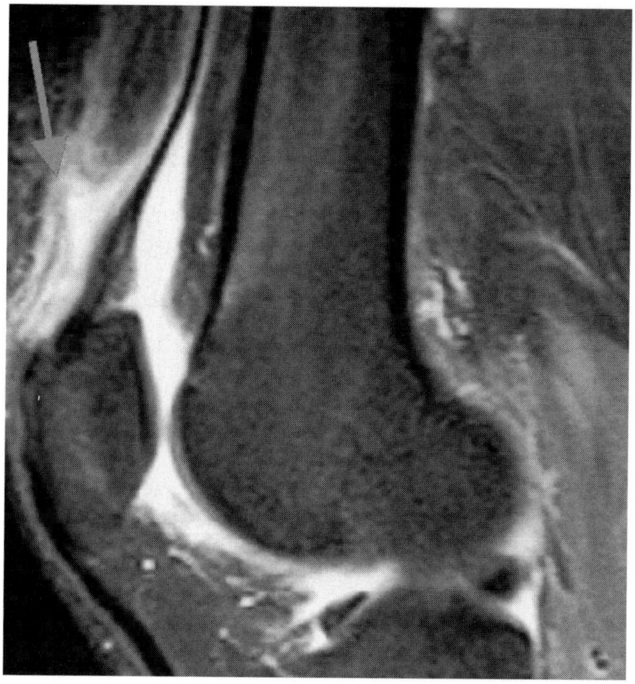

**Fig. 6.29** Sagittal fat-suppressed image showing an incomplete tear with local hemorrhage of the distal quadriceps tendon immediately above the patella.

# Patellar tendon injuries

## Anatomy

- Links the patella and patellar retinaculum to the tibial tuberosity.

## Mechanism of injury

- Rupture of the patellar tendon (usually the proximal third).
- Less common than quadriceps rupture.
- Mostly found in older patients with repeated inflammation and pre-existing degenerative tendinosis, often with an exacerbating incident (a fall or slip on a slope).
- Rupture is rare in younger athletes, e.g. when lifting excessive loads (Fig. 6.30).

## History and clinical findings

- Complete disruption is usually clinically evident with an inability to bear weight, and proximal patellar displacement.
- Pain when pushing off or rising from a squatting position.
- Hemarthrosis and mobile patella.
- Impaired knee extension.
- Superior patellar displacement and palpable defect in complete rupture.

## Imaging findings

### Plain radiography

- May show a superiorly displaced patella (patella alta) with knee effusion or small avulsion at the inferior patellar pole (Fig. 6.31).

### Magnetic resonance imaging

- Discontinuity of the low-signal patellar tendon in complete rupture on sagittal images.
- Incomplete tears show a thickened tendon with high-signal abnormality with continuity of fibers.
- Hyperintense fluid or blood at the tear site on $T_2$-weighted sequences or STIR.



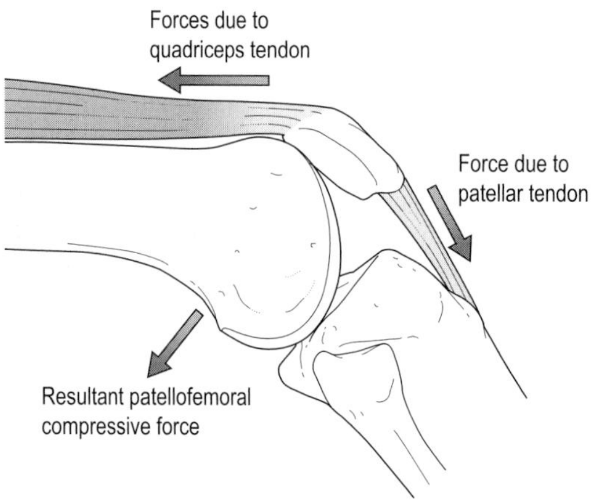


**Fig. 6.30** Rupture of the patellar tendon.

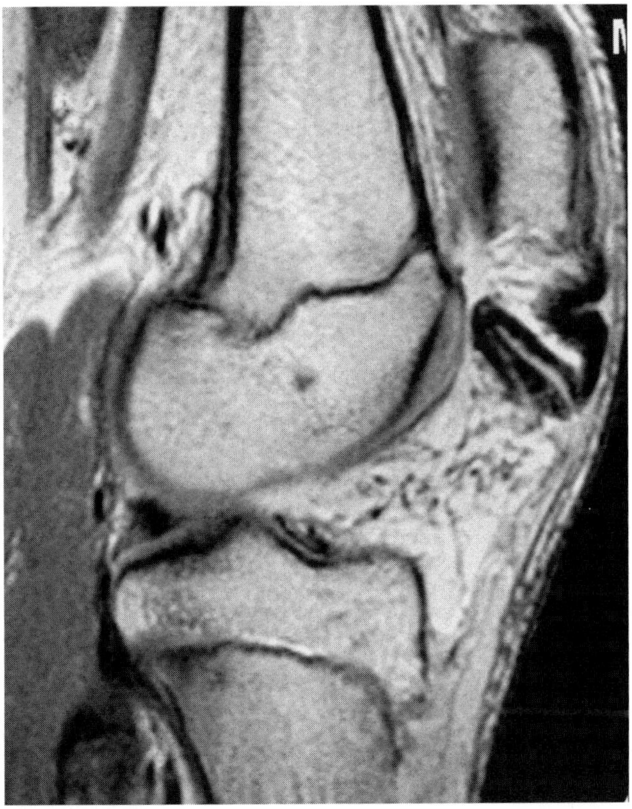

**Fig. 6.31** Sagittal MR image showing a complete avulsion of the patellar tendon from the tibial tuberosity in an adolescent basketball player, incurred during forced knee extension during an attempted scoring lay-up.



## Management

### Non-surgical

- Partial ruptures do not normally require surgery.
- Immobilization for 3–6 weeks.
- Early mobilization with strength and mobility training.

### Surgical

- For complete ruptures or high-performance athletes: best results when repaired within 48 hours.
- End-to-end suturing.

# Patellar tendinitis ('jumper's knee')

## Anatomy

- Links the lower pole of the patella with the anterior tibial tuberosity.

## Mechanism of injury

- Inflammation of the patellar tendon secondary to repetitive trauma, e.g. as seen in jumping sports (basketball, tennis).
- Usually etiology is chronic overuse.
- Especially posterior proximal third of the tendon (Fig. 6.32).

## History and clinical findings

- Pain during or after activity:
  - phase I: pain after activity
  - phase II: pain during activity but which does not limit participation
  - phase III: pain during and after participation, which interferes with activity
  - phase IV: complete tendon disruption.
- Excessive foot pronation.
- Tenderness over the patellar tendon and inferior patellar pole.

## Imaging findings

### Radiography

- Limited utility but may show patellar tendon thickening or secondary fragmentation of the tibial attachment (Osgood–Schlatter disease).

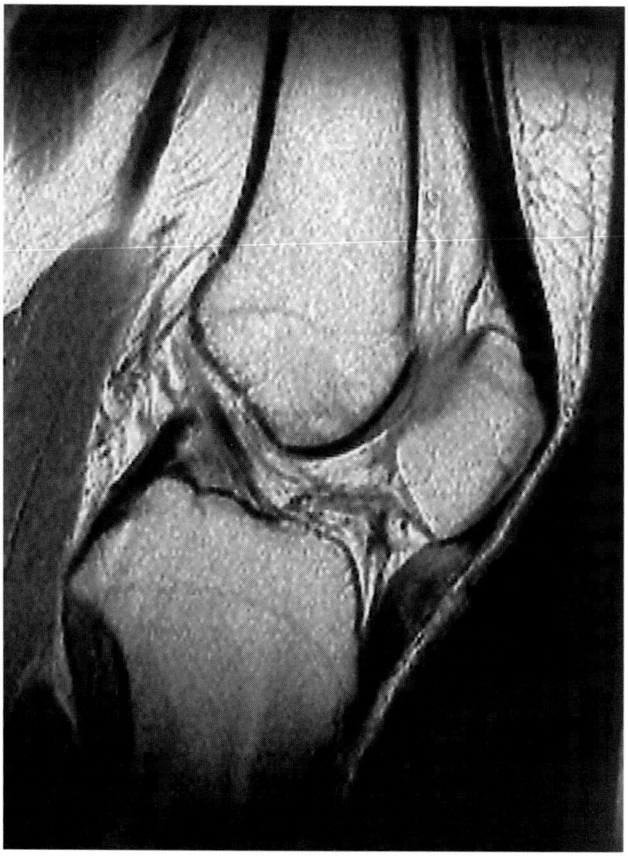

**Fig. 6.32** Sagittal MR image showing thickening and shortening of the patellar tendon due to chronic tendinitis in a basketball player: 'jumper's knee'.

Ultrasound

- Thickened hypoechoic tendon.

Magnetic resonance imaging

- Patellar tendon thickening (including increase AP dimensions and convex posterior margin).
- $T_2$-weighted and STIR sequences may show partial or complete tear with or without peritendon edema early.
- Chronic change: thickened tendon with areas of focal high-signal intensity on $T_2$-weighted (collagen degeneration).
- Lower pole patella bone edema (reactive).
- Beware magic angle effect (mimics tendinosis).

## Management

Non-surgical

- Cessation of jumping sports to prevent progression to tear and allow healing.
- Conservative (rest, ice, NSAIDs and steroids).

Surgical

- Maquet's procedure: decreases the force on the patellar tendon by elevating the anterior tibial tubercle.

# Sinding–Larsen–Johansson disease: patellar tendon apicitis

## Mechanism of injury

- Traction tendinitis of the distal pole of the patella.
- Repetitive microtrauma during running and jumping.
- Growing active patients.

## History and clinical findings

- Low-grade ache, worse with activity and localized to the lower pole of the patella.
- Swelling and limitation of movement.
- Symptoms during rapid growth period (during formation of the secondary ossification center) in younger patients (10–15 years old).
- Tenderness around the inferior pole of the patella.

## Imaging findings

### Radiography

- Fragmentation of the distal patellar pole at the insertion of the tendon.

### Isotope bone scan

- Positive in cases of inferior pole patella apophysitis.

### Magnetic resonance imaging

- Increased signal intensity in the patellar tendon at the insertion on the inferior pole patella, with tendon thickening.
- Fragmentation of the inferior patellar pole.
- Rarely, fluid in the infrapatellar bursa (Fig. 6.33).



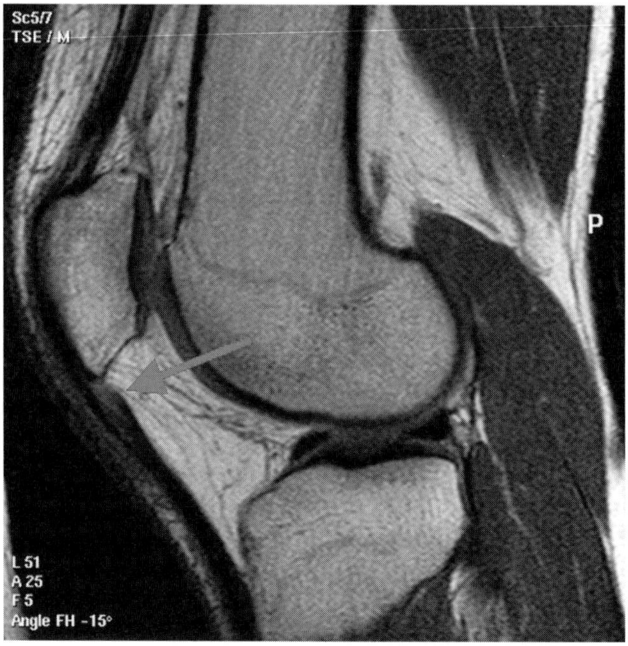


**Fig. 6.33** Sagittal MR image in a soccer player with chronic infrapatellar discomfort secondary to patellar tendon apicitis (Sinding–Larsen–Johansson disease). The image shows a microtear of the deep fibers of the patellar tendon at their attachment to the inferior pole of the patella where there is signal change and thickening.

## Management

Non-surgical

- Usually self-limited (<12 months) and prognosis is excellent.
- Restriction of activities during symptomatic periods.
- Muscle strengthening.

Surgical

- Not normally required.
- Arthroscopic debridement of the deep fiber attachment to the inferior pole of patella in refractory cases.

# Osgood–Schlatter disease

## Mechanism of injury

- Traction apophysitis of the patellar tendon insertion on the tibial tubercle (repetitive microtrauma); common in jumping sports.
- Young active patients (occurs during contraction of strong extensor mechanism).

## History and clinical findings

- Low-grade ache, worse with activity and localized to the tibial tuberosity.
- Symptoms during rapid growth period (during formation of the secondary ossification centre) in younger patients (10–15 years old).
- Aggravated by acceleration or deceleration.
- Bilateral frequently (15–30%).
- Tenderness around the patella and patellar tendon.
- Pain on resisted knee extension.
- Muscle tightness of the quadriceps, hamstrings and ITB.

## Imaging findings

### Radiography

- Hypertrophy and possible fragmentation of the tibial tuberosity.
- Soft-tissue swelling >4 mm over the anterior proximal tibia.

### Isotope bone scan

- Positive in cases of tubercle apophysitis.

### Magnetic resonance imaging

- Increased signal intensity in patellar tendon at insertion on tibial tubercle, with tendon thickening.
- Fluid in the infrapatellar bursa.
- Fragmentation and hypertrophy of the tibial tuberosity.



## Management

### Non-surgical

- Usually self-limited and prognosis is excellent.
- Rehabilitation and conditioning of the extensor mechanism.
- Bracing or infrapatellar strapping.

### Surgical

- For refractory cases.
- Operative bone plug placement or, less commonly, tuberosity drilling.
- Tuberosity debulking or osteotomy.
- Surgical removal of loose bodies formed at the site of patellar tendon attachment.

# Popliteus tendon injury

## Anatomy

- Inserted inferomedially into the Achilles tendon.
- Extends superolaterally through the calf to buttress the posterolateral aspect of the knee joint.
- Inserts into the popliteus recess of the lateral femoral condyle.

## Mechanism of injury

- Gross rotational torque injury with varus, e.g. running downhill.
- Commonly accompanies other soft-tissue derangement of the knee caused by varus injury, e.g. ACL or LCL tears.
- Rarely occurs as an isolated entity.
- Tendinosis is much more common than complete rupture.

## History and clinical findings

- Pain at the lateral femoral condyle.
- Worse with weight-bearing with the knee flexed, e.g. walking or running downhill.
- Pain on internal rotation of the tibia.
- Local tenderness over the site of tendon attachment on the lateral femoral condyle.
- Posterolateral instability with a varus opening of more than 5 mm.
- Increased external rotation of the lower leg with the knee flexed.
- Other injuries (e.g. ACL tear, lateral meniscal injury) should be assessed.

## Imaging findings

### Magnetic resonance imaging

- Type 1 injury: rupture of tendon at its insertion in the popliteal recess.
- Type 2 injury: rupture in the mid substance of the tendon.
- Type 3 injury: rupture at the junction of the proximal tendon and muscle belly.



## Management

### Non-surgical

- Avoid running on downhill inclines.
- Heat packs before exercise and ice packs afterwards.
- Antiinflammatories, steroids and physiotherapy.

### Surgical

- Rarely required; only for persistent refractory cases.

# Gastrocnemius tear

## Anatomy

- This muscle tears most commonly during vigorous exercise. The gastrocnemius crosses two joints, has abundant fast-twitch fibers and has an eccentric contraction (it lengthens during contraction); all these features are known to predispose to tearing.
- The muscle belly has two components: the medial and lateral heads. In most people the medial head is considerably larger and stronger than the lateral head, and therefore more vulnerable to tear as a result of the vast forces generated during contraction.
- The gastrocnemius merges with the muscle belly of the soleus, which together pass inferiorly to form the Achilles tendon attaching to the calcaneum.
- The medial and lateral heads of the gastrocnemius merge with the soleus over a larger footplate of up to 5 cm. The lower part of the aponeurosis is exposed to the greatest force during contraction and so this is the site that usually tears.
- Extension of the tear more proximally to completely detach from the soleus allows retraction and occasionally the development of a large interposed hematoma at the site of injury.

## Mechanism of injury

- Muscle tear most frequently occurs in poorly conditioned athletes engaging in unaccustomed exercise, tennis and cricket.
- With increasing frequency, muscle tears are being identified in sportsmen who have built up muscle bulk to such a level that contraction and generated force overcomes the bond at the level of the aponeurosis.
- Front row forwards in rugby place dramatic pressure on the contracting gastrocnemius during scrummaging, accounting for the frequency of this injury in this subgroup.
- The lateral head of gastrocnemius, being less bulky, generates less force during contraction and therefore less frequently tears.
- Occasionally, lateral head of gastrocnemius tears are identified in soccer players who have built up this muscle group by repeatedly kicking with the outside of the foot.



## Imaging findings

### Ultrasound

- Allows clear visualization of the aponeurosis between the gastrocnemius and the soleus muscle belly. Ultrasound allows the identification of disrupted muscle bundles usually manifest as a hypoechoic fluid-filled defect.

### Magnetic resonance imaging

- Fat-suppressed imaging sequences allow the identification of muscle tears as a result of sensitivity to the detection of fluid, hemorrhage and edema at the site of the injury. $T_1$- and proton density-weighted sequences allow detailed anatomic evaluation of the extent of the injury (Fig. 6.34).
- Gastrocnemius tears are best identified on sagittal and axial scans. Sagittal images allow the assessment of the amount of retraction at the site of the tear. Axial images show the extent of local hemorrhage and edema within the muscle belly, which is typically most marked in the deeper fibers abutting the aponeurosis.

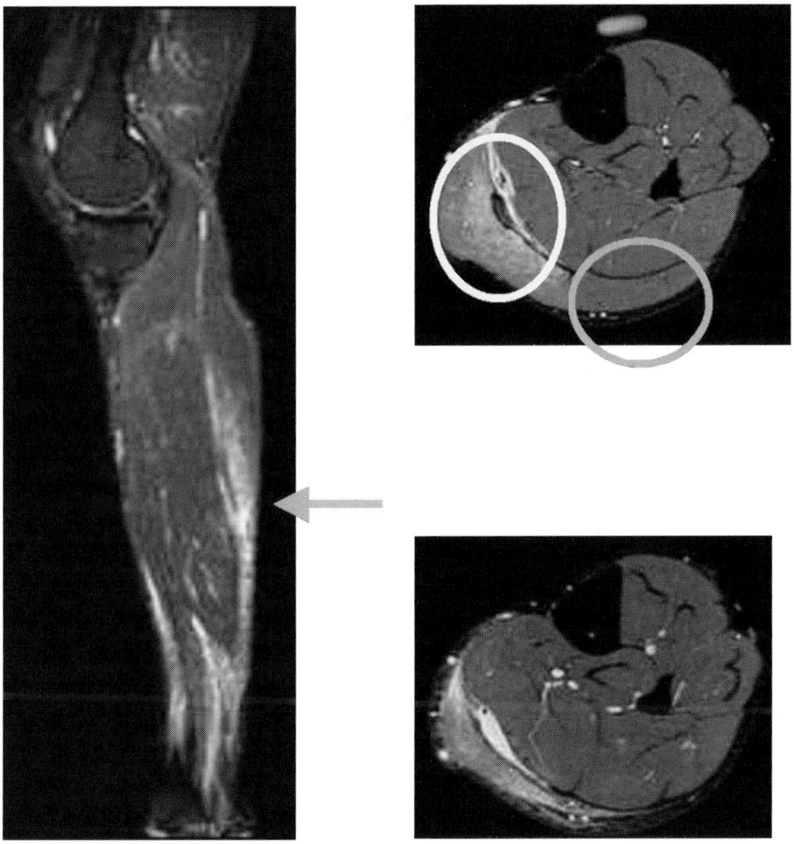

**Fig. 6.34** **(a, b, c)** Sagittal image (above) showing focal hemorrhage and edema at the aponeurosis of the medial head of the gastrocnemius muscle, with a normal signal identified in the lateral head on axial images acquired at the level of the tear in a poorly conditioned athlete stretching at tennis.



## Management

### Non-surgical

- Muscle healing requires apposition at the margins of the tear and immobilization. Apposition of the gastrocnemius is maximized in the plantar flexed position, while immobilization is maximized in a cast, the logic behind a growing use of short-term cast fixation in the early treatment of this injury (2–4 weeks).
- Local inflammation and pain are usually addressed with conventional oral antiinflammatories; there is little evidence to support the use of steroids.
- Reflecting the requirement for oxygen to promote cellular metabolism and healing, many advocate the use of hyperbaric oxygen although in controlled study this approach has not been proven (see Chapter 2). These authors have, however, had significant success with this approach.
- Healing is delayed if muscle surfaces at the site of the tear are displaced and held apart by hematoma. Healing in this setting may be accelerated by hematoma aspiration, often performed with ultrasound guidance.

- Physiotherapy employing heat treatment may enhance healing but is primarily employed in the slowly controlled reintroduction of exercise and muscle contractions.

### Surgical

- Primary suture repair is uncommon but effective in generating immediate apposition at the site of the tear and when undertaken can effect more rapid recovery. Such an approach is more commonly adopted with larger grade II tears and should be undertaken in grade III injuries with complete detachment of the muscle head.

# Soleus muscle tear

## Anatomy

- The soleus muscle lies deep to the gastrocnemius in the calf.
- Crossing a single joint and lacking fast-twitch fibers, the muscle tears less frequently than the gastrocnemius.

## Mechanism of injury

- The soleus functions in a similar way to the gastrocnemius in executing plantar flexion and push-off in the toe phase of the gait cycle. It therefore tears in those undertaking unaccustomed exercise. Similarly to gastrocnemius tears, soleus belly tears are now also encountered in rugby players during scrummaging, particularly players in the front and second rows.

## Imaging findings

### Ultrasound

- Ultrasound employing linear-array high-frequency probes above 6 MHz readily allows identification of muscle belly tears. Subtle tears often become conspicuous as a result of local hyperemia demonstrated on flow-sensitive color or power Doppler images.

### Magnetic resonance imaging

- MRI employing fat-suppressed sequences readily allows the identification of soleus tears; these are usually better identified in the axial plane. There are no data to support the use of contrast media to improve the conspicuity of tears (Fig. 6.35).

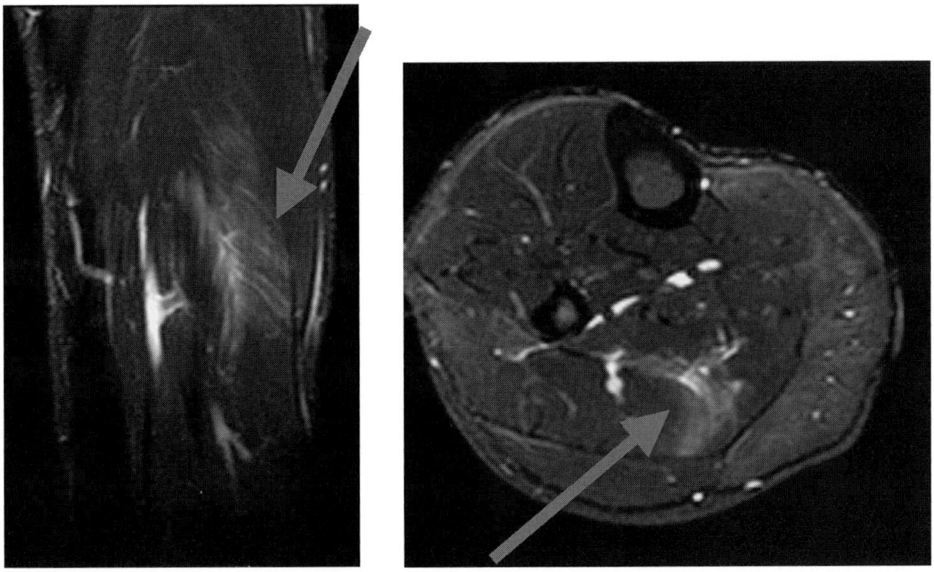

(a) (b)

**Fig. 6.35** In a professional rugby player (**a**) sagittal and (**b**) axial MRI images show hemorrhage in the mid belly of the soleus incurred during attempted calf contraction while scrummaging.

## Management

### Non-surgical

- The majority of soleus tears resolve with conservative approaches, combining rest, antiinflammatories and deep massage. Physiotherapy is employed to monitor scientifically the reintroduction of muscle contractions.

### Surgical

- The surgical repair of grade III muscle tears may be undertaken although this is an approach not encountered by the authors of this book.

# Interosseous membrane rupture

## Anatomy

- The interosseous membrane bridges the tibia and fibula and runs from a point just above the inferior tibiofibular articulation to a point proximal to the superior tibiofibular articulation below the knee.

## Mechanism of injury

- The membrane is most commonly ruptured and torn as part of a severe ankle sprain, usually with eversion strain. In this setting the ligament occasionally tears superiorly to the level of the proximal neck of the fibula where it may be associated with a spiral fracture of the fibula. In this setting eversion produces a transverse fracture of the medial malleolus with associated torque decompressed by rupture of the interosseous membrane and fracture of the proximal neck of fibula (Maisonneuve's fracture).
- Occasionally isolated membrane rupture occurs as a result of direct trauma such as from a kick to the shin in soccer and presents with severe localized pain and swelling (Figs 6.36 and 6.37).

## Imaging findings

- Membrane rupture may be identified on both ultrasound and MRI.

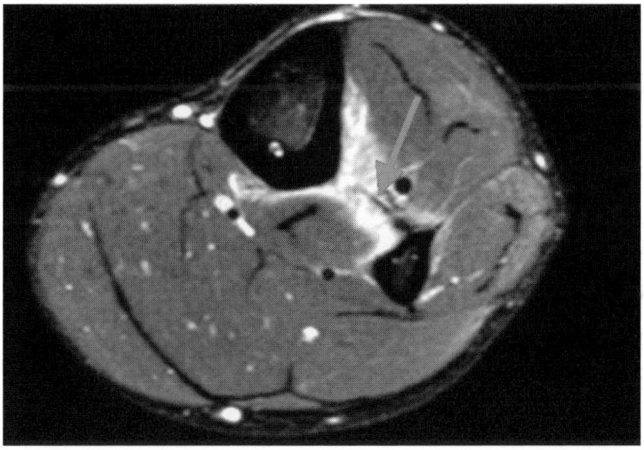

**Fig. 6.36** Axial image showing an intact interosseous ligament.

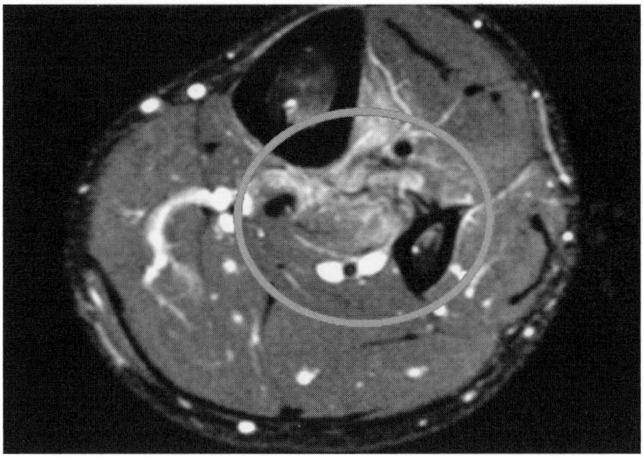

**Fig. 6.37** Axial image showing a disrupted interosseous ligament in a professional soccer player following a blunt kick to the shin.

## Management

### Non-surgical

- Membrane rupture (particularly isolated) produces marked local pain and swelling which is best treated by a combination of oral antiinflammatories, ice and rest. Deep massage may be employed to promote hematoma resorption and prevent scar and heterotopic ossification.

### Surgical

- Primary surgical repair is rarely undertaken. When membrane tear is accompanied by fractures of proximal neck of the fibula, cast fixation minimizes motion between the fibula and tibia and allows membrane healing without direct intervention.

# Compartment syndromes

## Anatomy

- The calf muscles are divided into four recognizable compartments.
- Each compartment is composed of muscles invested by a fascial sheath.
- The anterior compartment contains the extensors of the ankle, the extensor hallucis longus, the extensor digitorum longus and the tibialis anterior muscles.
- The peroneal compartment contains the peroneus longus and brevis muscles.
- The deep posterior compartment contains the tibialis posterior, the flexor hallucis longus and the flexor digitorum longus muscles.
- The superficial posterior compartment contains the soleus and the medial and lateral heads of the gastrocnemius muscles.
- Compartment syndrome describes acquired elevation of pressure to over 35 mmHg either occurring acutely following trauma and intracompartmental hemorrhage or chronically following chronic exertion with muscular overuse and swelling.
- In all types, raised pressure impairs blood supply to muscles with accumulation of lactic acid and pain.
- Acquired acidosis results in further capillary leakage with accumulation of fluid, and further elevation of pressure with associated sequelae.

## Mechanism of injury

- Acute:
  - direct blow with secondary hemorrhage
  - fracture with secondary hemorrhage
  - acute overuse with acute muscle swelling.
- Chronic:
  - overtraining with muscle hypertrophy and swelling during chronic exercise; this is the most frequently encountered form in sportsmen
  - compartment syndrome involving the superficial posterior muscles is extremely uncommon. More frequently, muscle discomfort develops secondary to overuse as a result of gait abnormality. Persistent running off the toes (either idiopathic or secondary to impaired dorsiflexion at the tibiotalar joint as a result of footballer's ankle-type impingement) results in overuse of the soleus and gastrocnemius musculature to maintain ankle extension, and presents as pain.



## Clinical findings

### Anterior compartment syndrome

- Acute: pain, numbness and occasionally acute arterial occlusion resulting in dramatic temperature change and numbness over the dorsum of the foot.
- Chronic: pain induced by exercise and resolving progressively with rest, weakness, numbness extending to the dorsum of the foot. Symptoms aggravated by dorsiflexion at the ankle (Figs 6.38–6.40).

### Peroneal compartment syndrome

- Acute: pain and numbness over the lateral calf aggravated by eversion at the ankle.
- Chronic: pain, numbness and parasthesia extending from the lateral calf to the lateral foot aggravated by ankle eversion.

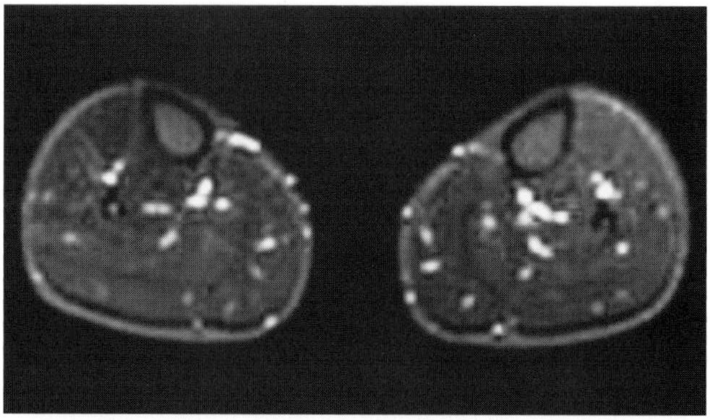

**Fig. 6.38** Axial images showing uniform signal changes within the muscles of the calf pre-exercise.

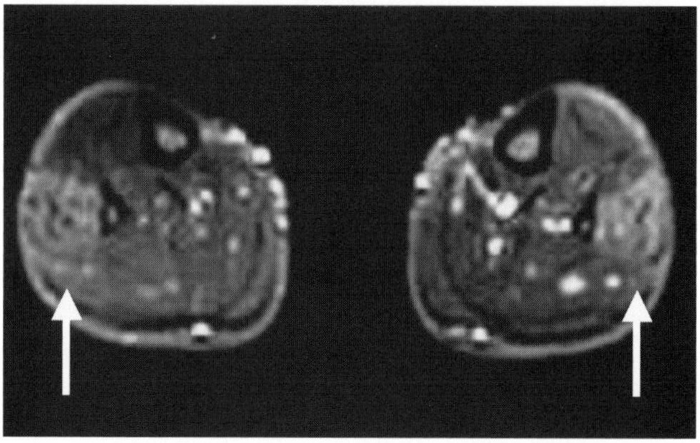

**Fig. 6.39** Axial image post-exercise showing signal hyperintensity within the lateral peroneal compartment secondary to peroneal compartment syndrome.



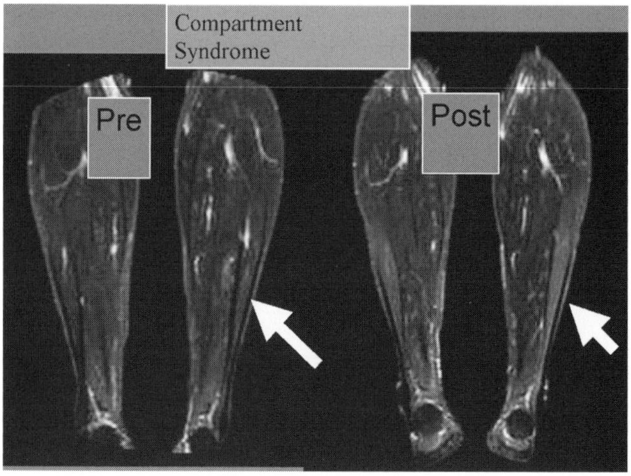


(a) (b)

**Fig. 6.40** (**a**) Coronal MR images pre-exercise showing uniform signal with (**b**) peroneal signal hyperintensity identified post-exercise secondary to compartment syndrome.

| | |
|---|---|
| Deep posterior compartment syndrome | • Acute: pain in the posterior mid calf.<br>• Chronic: pain in the mid calf aggravated by plantar flexion. |
| Superficial posterior compartment syndrome | • Calf pain induced by exercise and relieved by rest referable to the superficial musculature of the posterior calf. No discrete clinical abnormality is detected at examination. |

## Imaging findings

- Compartmental pressure studies greater than 35 mmHg following exercise. (Measurements in the deep posterior compartment are variable as catheter localization for pressure measurement in this compartment is difficult in the absence of ultrasound guidance.)
- Pre- and post-exercise MRI showing muscle swelling and accumulation of fluid post-exercise manifest as the development of muscle hyperintensity throughout the involved muscle group. Signal changes are best identified on fat suppressed scans (STIR). It is critical that exercise reproduces symptoms before imaging and that when undertaken images are acquired immediately following cessation of activity.

## Management

- Acute: treated acutely with diuretics and antiinflammatories including steroids. Surgical decompression with fasciotomy is undertaken as definitive therapy.
- Chronic: surgical fasciotomy is the definitive treatment. This is readily performed for the anterior compartment and in proven cases often results in dramatic resolution of symptoms. Fasciotomy of the deep posterior compartment is technically more involved and although reported successful outcome rates are more variable; in proven cases this occurs in up to 80% of cases.
- Superficial posterior compartment syndrome can be treated by addressing primary abnormality, such as 'toe gait'.

# Bone injury: supracondylar and condylar fractures of the femur

| | |
|---|---|
| **Anatomy** | • The supracondylar femur is that portion between the femoral condyles and the metaphysis of the distal femur (approx. 9 cm long). |
| **Mechanism of injury** | • In younger patients distal femoral fractures are usually secondary to complex injuries.<br>• In older patients minor trauma is imposed on osteoparotic bones. |
| **History and clinical findings** | • Deformities following fractures reflect the initial direction of displacement and the pull of the thigh muscles, e.g. the gastrocnemius pulls the distal fragment medially, hamstrings and quadriceps result in shortening and overlap. |
| **Imaging findings** | • Fractures are divided into intra- and extra-articular (extra-articular fractures are divided into supracondylar and condylar). |
| Radiography | • Lucent fracture line with or without comminuted fragments.<br>• Lipohemarthrosis if there is intra-articular extension. |
| Isotope bone scan | • If normal, an initial radiograph (and high clinical suspicion) may show increased uptake after 24–72 hours in insufficiency fractures. |
| Computerized tomography | • As above.<br>• For fragment localization in cases of intra-articular extension and planned surgery. |
| Magnetic resonance imaging | • Used with soft-tissue injuries associated with intra-articular fractures.<br>• Used for the assessment of associated fractures of the tibial plateau, fibular head or patellar subluxation.<br>• Concern about integrity of underlying bone (suspected metastatic disease). |
| **Management** | • Factors influencing management and outcome include the amount of displacement, the degree of comminution, the extent of soft-tissue injury, the amount of osteoporosis and the presence of intra-articular extension. |
| Non-surgical | • For supracondylar fractures with no intra-articular extension: closed reduction, skeletal traction and immobilization.<br>• The goal is to restore length and axial alignment. |
| Surgical | • Open reduction and internal fixation, e.g. blade and screw fixation.<br>• Solitary lag screws are occasionally used in the fixation of condylar fractures. |

# Bone injury: tibial plateau fractures

**Mechanism of injury**

- Classically 'bumper'/'fender' fractures.
- Can follow acute valgus or varus impact, axial loading or combination of these, e.g. motor vehicle accident.
- Shearing and compression forces also lead to a high incidence of accompanying soft-tissue injuries.
- Up to 70% involve the lateral tibial plateau (valgus force) and 20% the medial plateau; in 10% the fractures are combined.

**History and clinical findings**

- Knee effusion and pain after trauma.
- History of motor vehicle accident or fall.
- Apply varus and valgus stress to the knee to assess for stability: >10° of laxity indicates articular depression or ligamentous laxity.

**Imaging findings**

Schatzker described six types of tibial plateau fractures based on anatomic location:

1. Vertical split of the lateral tibial plateau.
2. Vertical split plus depression of the lateral tibial plateau.
3. Depressed fracture of the lateral tibial plateau without the vertical component.
4. Medial plateau fracture (wedge, split, depressed, comminuted) (Fig. 6.41).
5. Bicondylar fractures.
6. Tibial fracture, which separates the tibial metaphysis and diaphysis in combination with a tibial plateau fracture.

- Type 1 fractures are common in young adults and are often associated with lateral meniscal tears and, after a valgus stress, also with ACL or medial collateral ligament damage.
- Type 2 fractures occur in patients older than 40 years and tibial plateau depression has a protective effect of decreasing the valgus strain on the collateral ligaments.
- Type 3 fractures have frequent coexistent meniscal damage; posterior depressions are more unstable and likely to require surgical repair.
- Complex type 6 fractures may be accompanied by popliteal artery injury and compartment syndromes (Figs 6.42 and 6.43).

Radiography

- Most depressed fractures are visible: fracture line or comminuted fragment.
- Lipohemarthrosis on lateral shoot-through films.

Computerized tomography

- For pre-operative planning (multiplanar visualization with multislice CT and 3D reconstruction).
- Degree of displacement, fragment distraction and articular margin step-off.

Magnetic resonance imaging

- As for CT.
- Decreased signal intensity fracture line on all sequences.
- Also allows superior visualization of adjacent soft tissues.
- Addition of MR angiography if a compartment syndrome is suspected.

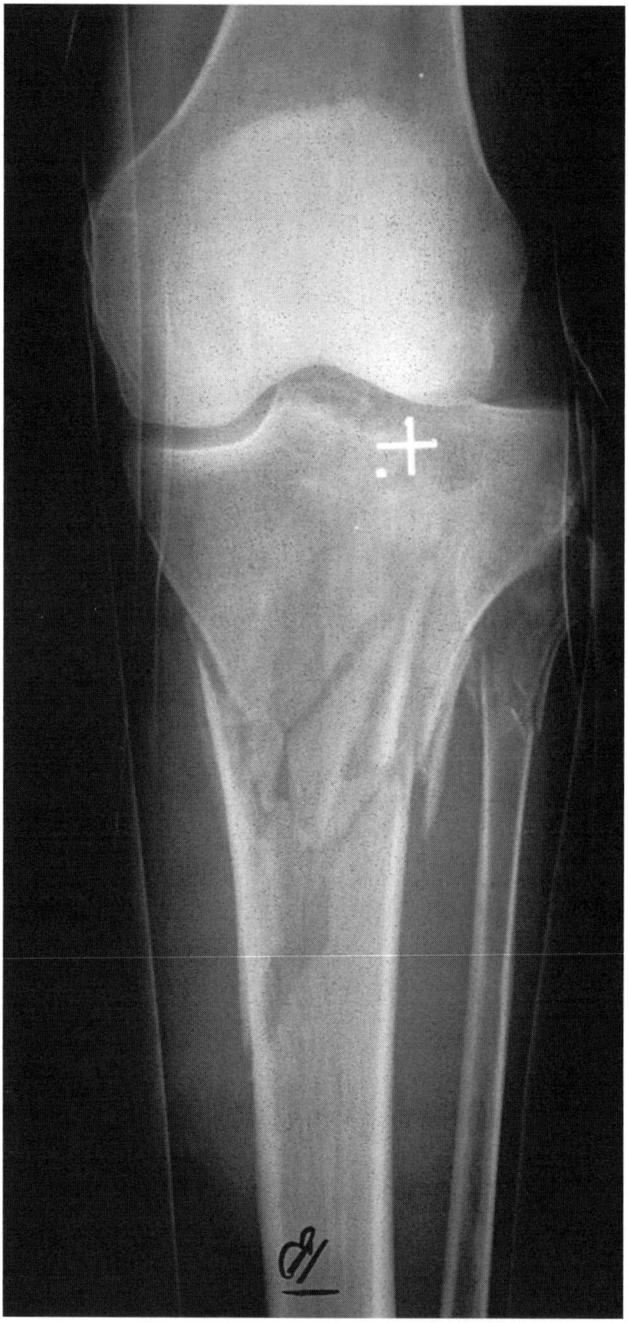

**Fig. 6.41** Radiograph showing a comminuted lateral tibial plateau fracture complicating valgus injury.

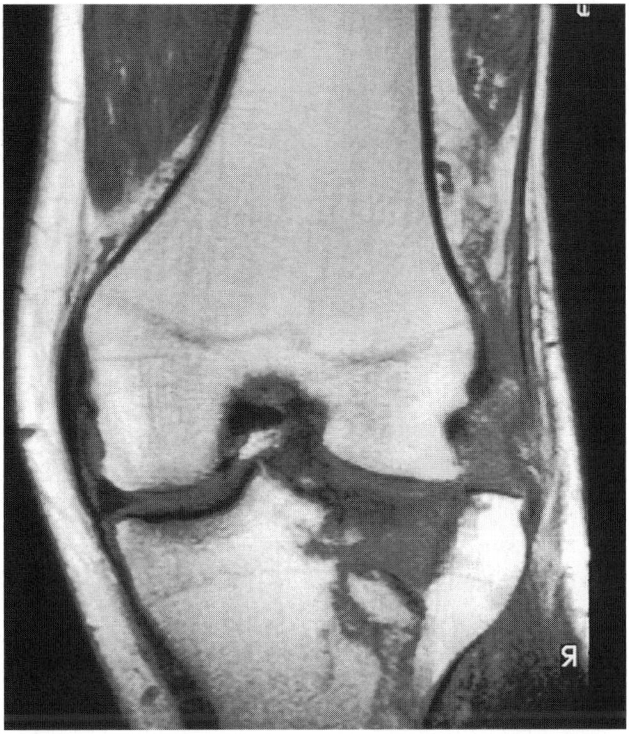


(a)

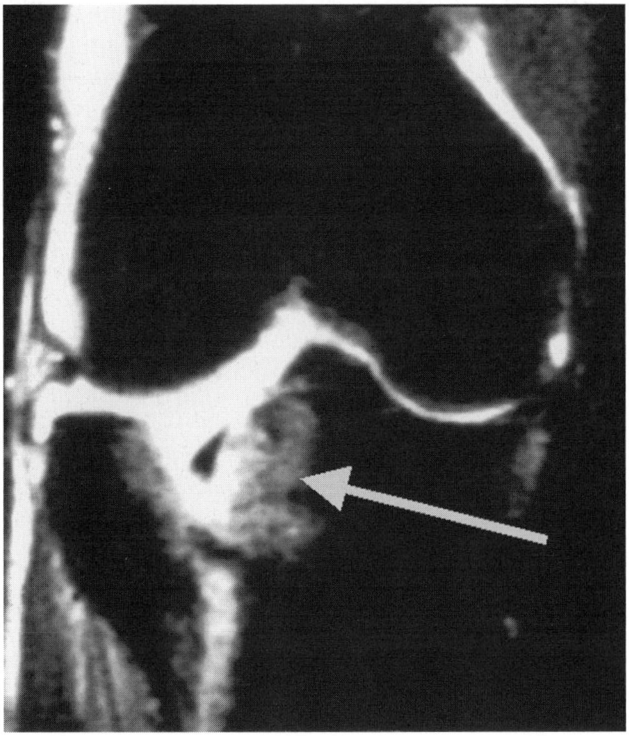

(b)

**Fig. 6.42** Coronal MR images showing (**a**) a lateral tibial plateau fracture with associated lateral meniscal disruption. (**b**) Coronal fat-suppressed image showing a lateral tibial plateau split fracture with the lateral meniscus displaced into the fracture cleft.

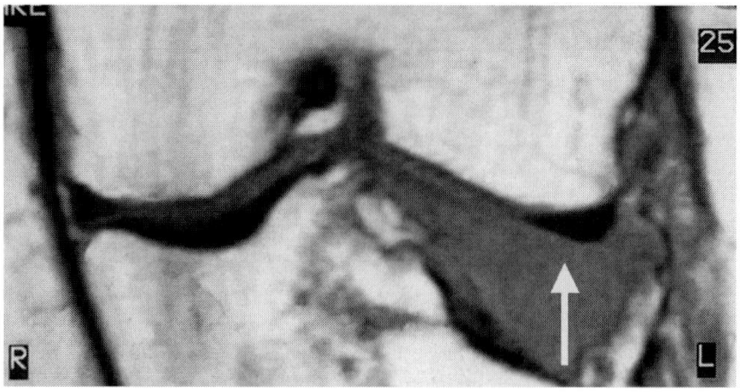


**Fig. 6.43** MR image showing a lateral tibial plateau fracture with an intact lateral meniscus.

## Management

### Non-surgical

- Cast immobilization in undisplaced fractures with no internal knee derangement.

### Surgical

- For fractures with a significant articular margin step-off (>5 mm) or displacement or distraction (>4 mm).
- For coexistent tendon or ligamentous damage; this requires combined intra-articular repair of soft-tissue injury in conjunction with extra-articular buttressing.
- Failure to repair ligaments or menisci leads to poorer postoperative stability.
- Inadequately corrected depression leads to accelerated osteoarthritis.
- Early mobilization postoperatively (<3 weeks) is important.

# Bone injury: Segond's fracture

## Anatomy

- Cortical avulsion of the meniscotibial portion of the lateral capsular ligament resulting in a small avulsion of the lateral tibial plateau margin.
- Described by Paul F Segond (1851–1912) in 1879.
- The lateral capsular ligament runs from the patella and patellar tendon to the PCL.
- The ligament is divided into three segments.
- The site of the injury is the middle section (ITB anteriorly to the fibular collateral ligament).

## Mechanism of injury

- Acute varus strain with rotation avulses the ligament from its meniscotibial insertion.
- Accompanied by ACL rupture in 90% of patients and meniscal tear in up to 70% (similar forces causing injury).

## Imaging findings

### Radiography

- Avulsed fragments originating below the lateral tibial plateau, posterior and superior to Gerdy's tubercle.
- May be accompanied by other avulsions, e.g. of the fibular head.

### Computerized tomography

- As above.
- Used for fragment localization.

### Magnetic resonance imaging

- As above (Fig. 6.44).



## Management

- Immobilization and a support bandage.
- Arthroscopic repair of associated ACL injury.

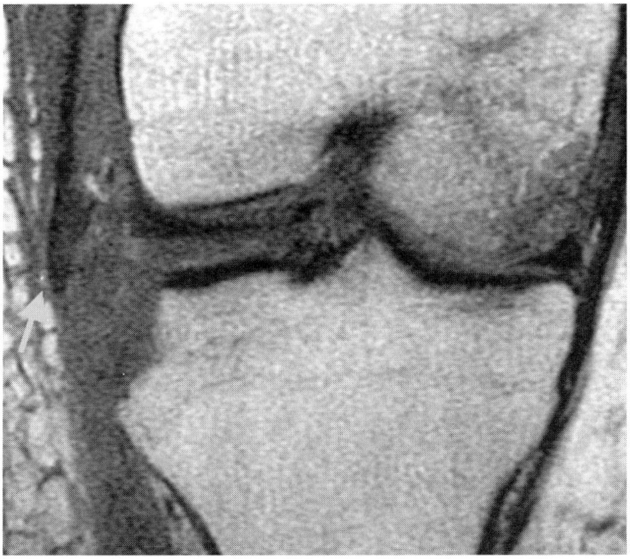

**Fig. 6.44** MR image showing a lateral capsular avulsion fracture (Segond type) in a patient with concomitant disruption of the ACL.

# Bone injury: Pellegrini–Stieda fracture

**Mechanism of injury**

- Medial collateral ligament avulsion of its femoral attachment.
- Follows acute valgus strain with torque.
- Intrasubstance ligamentous rupture is more common.

## Imaging findings

Radiography

- Heterotopic ossification at the medial femoral epicondyle.
- Effusion if accompanying internal knee derangement is present.

Magnetic resonance imaging

- $T_2$ gradient echo sequences are useful.
- Soft-tissue assessment for coexistent injuries.

**Management**

- Normally non-operative conservative methods are enough.

# Bone injury: patellar tracking disorders

## Anatomy

- Passive stability of the patellofemoral joint is maintained by the joint articulation between the patella and trochlea of femur, lateral and medial retinacular fibers and patellar ligament.
- Active stability of the joint is mainly achieved by the quadriceps muscles.
- Instability of the joint is caused by developmental anomalies of the patella and trochlea, and exacerbated by muscle imbalance.

## Mechanism of injury

- *Grade I* – lateral patellar tracking:
  - in which the patella moves laterally first before moving superiorly when the quadriceps is contracted
  - causes a lateral patellar compression syndrome
  - in which the patella does not dislocate but tracks laterally on quadriceps extension
  - requires the negative apprehension test.
- *Grade II* – patellar subluxation due to:

i. Patellar lateral tilt:
  - lateral retinaculum and capsule thickening occur
  - during flexion, the lateral patellar facet impinges on the trochlea
  - chronic lateral compression and tilt lead to cartilage damage.

ii. Patellar lateral subluxation:
  - straight subluxation of the patella during quadriceps contraction
  - recurrent subluxation causes cartilage damage.

- *Grade III* – patellar dislocation:
  - recurrent instability and progressive cartilage damage occurs secondary to recurrent dislocations
  - subluxation or dislocation on quadriceps contraction
  - requires the positive apprehension test.

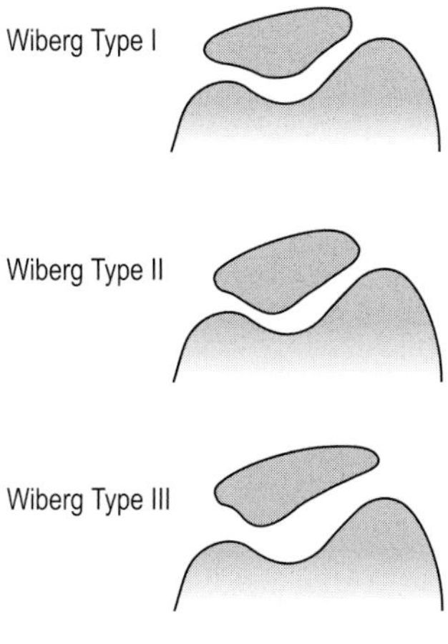


**Fig. 6.45** Wiberg's variations in patellar shape: types I–III.

## History and clinical findings

- Anterior knee pain, worse with exertion and downhill inclines.
- Pain worse on standing up or squatting.
- Local tenderness around the patella.
- Crepitus on knee movement due to chondromalacia.
- Q angle increases. This is the angle between the line through the long axes of the rectus femoris and the patellar tendons; normally $<10°$ in men and $<15°$ in women when the knee is at 30° of flexion.
- Observe for femoral anteversion, genu valgum and tightness of the lateral retinaculum, which can exacerbate lateral patellar instability.
- Apprehension test: the patella is held laterally with the knee in the neutral position. A positive test results if the patella tries to sublux on flexing the knee.
- Passive patellar tilt test.

## Imaging findings

### Radiography

- Lateral views show patellar location in relation to the knee joint.
- Skyline view (knee flexed to 40°) (Fig. 6.46).

### Isotope bone scan

- Increased uptake in the patella and femur in chronic cases.

### Computerized tomography

- Bony relationships are characterized.

### Magnetic resonance imaging

- For articular cartilage evaluation as well as alignment (Figs 6.47 and 6.48).



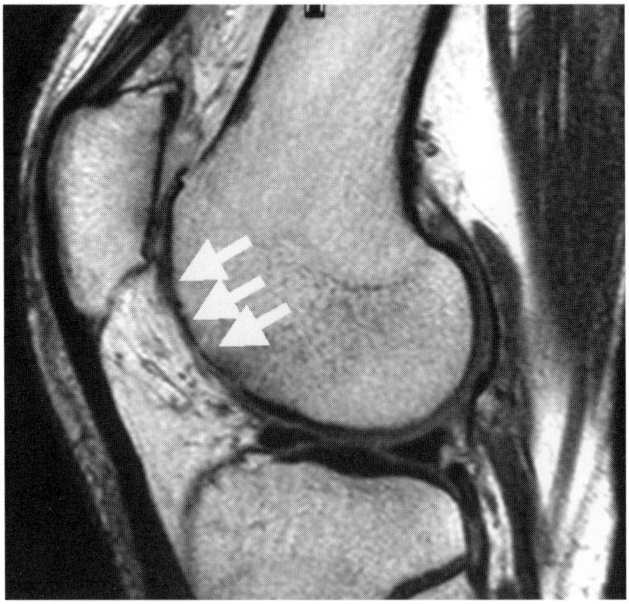

**Fig. 6.46** Sagittal image showing chondromalacia along the anterior margin of the lateral femoral condyle secondary to patellofemoral disease.

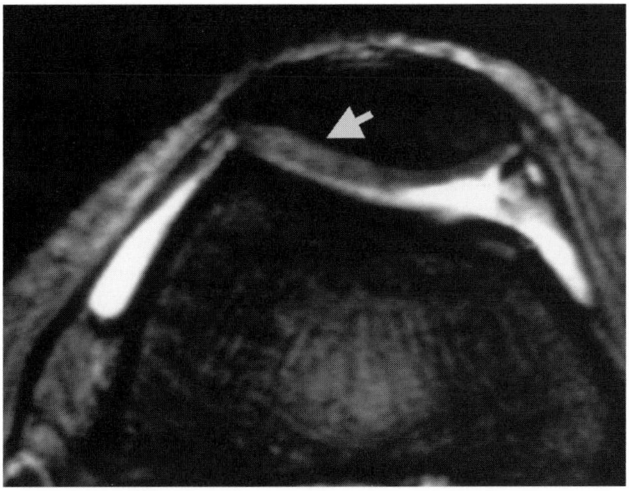

**Fig. 6.47** Axial MR image showing a heterogeneous signal within the lateral patella cartilage secondary to grade I chondromalacia and cartilage fibrillation.

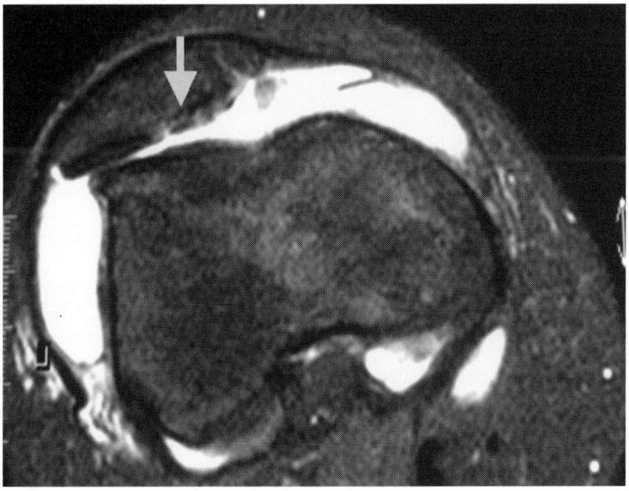

**Fig. 6.48** Axial MR image showing lateral patella tilt with impaction (chondromalacia) rent at the junction of the medial and lateral patella facets and joint effusion.

## Management

### Non-surgical

- Rest, bracing and taping.
- Strengthen the vastus medialis muscle, especially to counteract lateral forces.
- Antiinflammatories in the acute phase.

### Surgical

- Lateral retinaculum release in chronic cases.

# Bone injury: transient patellar dislocation

## Anatomy

- Predisposing factors include a shallow trochlear groove and laxity of the patellar ligaments and patella alta (loss of protective containment of the lateral femoral condyle).
- An abnormal vastus lateralis and ITB produce a lateral patellar pull.
- Wiberg's variations in patellar shapes:
  - type 1: concave facets, symmetrical and equal in size (10%)
  - type 2: smaller medial facet, concave lateral facet (65%)
  - type 3: small, convex medial patellar facet with lateral predominance (25%).

## Mechanism of injury

- Non-contact indirect injury: lateral patellar dislocation due to twisting injury with a valgus stress applied to the lateral femoral condyle.
- Rarely, direct trauma.

## History and clinical findings

- Anterolateral knee pain after twisting injury.
- Frequent relocation of the patella into the trochlear groove by extending the knee.
- Falkerson's classification:
  I. Subluxation
  II. Subluxation and tilt
  III. Tilt
  IV. No malalignment.

## Imaging findings

### Radiography

- May show patellar or anterior lateral femoral condyle fracture.



### Magnetic resonance imaging

- Bone bruise pattern characteristic: anterior aspect of the lateral femoral condyle and the medial patella (Fig. 6.49).
- Osteochondral defect in the anterior lateral femur, or a fracture.
- Medial retinacular tear: high $T_2$-weighted signal.
- hemarthrosis (fat/fluid level) with or without osteochondral free fragments.
- There may also be a tear of the vastus medialis muscle.

## Management

### Non-surgical

- Cast immobilization.
- Early physiotherapy.

### Surgical

- A torn medial patellofemoral ligament is usually surgically repaired to prevent recurrent dislocations (reinforcement with adductor magnus tendons is sometimes employed).
- Arthroscopic removal of osteochondral fragments.
- Occasional lateral retinacular release to reduce lateral pull on the patella.

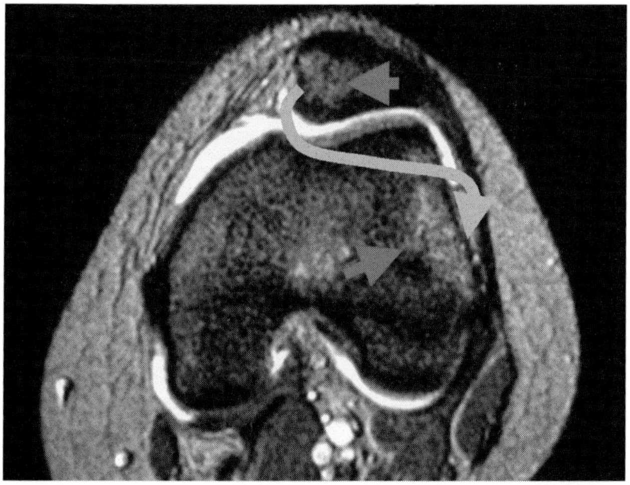

(a)

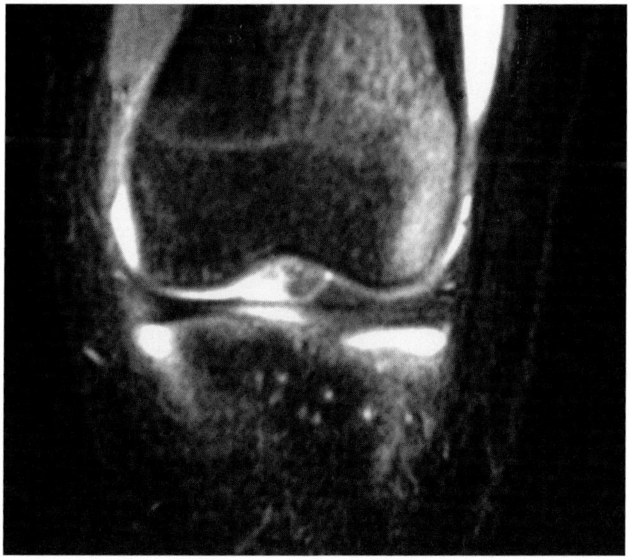

(b)

**Fig. 6.49** (**a**) Axial MR image showing a bone bruise of the medial patellar facet and of the lateral femoral condyle secondary to impaction during transient subluxation. (**b**) Coronal fat-suppressed image showing an isolated high lateral femoral condylar bone bruise typical of transient patellar dislocation.

# Bone injury: patellar fracture

## Mechanism of injury

- Transverse (common), vertical, marginal or osteochondral.
- Direct injury results in greater comminution and more articular cartilage damage, e.g. in a fall.
- Indirect injury results in less comminution and articular cartilage damage but more displacement, e.g. forced flexion on tight quadriceps.
- Transverse fractures are the most common, usually indirect trauma to the middle or distal third of the patella.
- Osteochondral defects are usually medial or inferior and often accompany patellar dislocation.
- Occasionally at donor site of a patellar graft for ACL reconstruction.

## History and clinical findings

- Found in children and adolescents more than in adults.
- Persistent pain after patellar trauma.
- Effusion (hemarthrosis).
- Proximal displacement of the patella.
- Difficulty extending the knee.

## Imaging findings

### Radiography

- Lucent fracture line with or without comminuted fragments (Fig. 6.50).
- Lipohemarthrosis.

### Isotope bone scan

- Increased uptake after 24–72 hours.



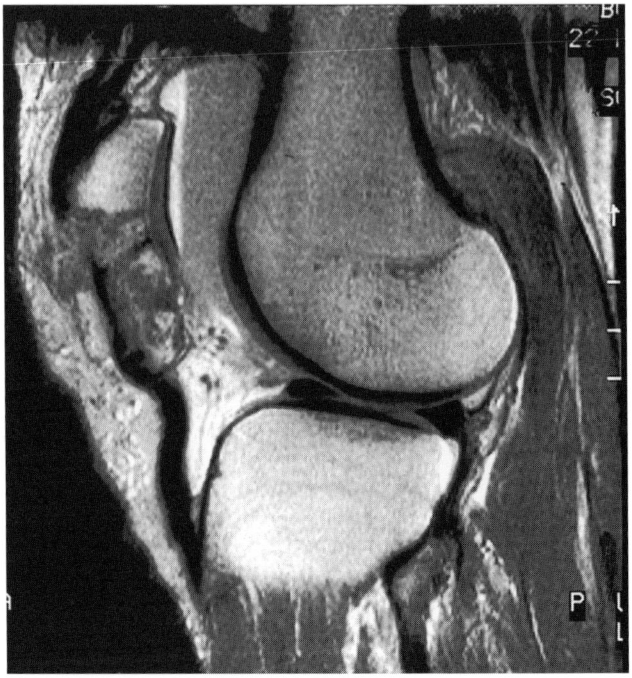

**Fig. 6.50** Sagittal image showing a comminuted patellar fracture without disruption of the articular cartilage.

Computerized tomography
- As above.
- For fragment localization in cases of reconstruction.

Magnetic resonance imaging
- As above.
- Patella alta on sagittal images.
- STIR sequences show hypointense fracture line and edema.
- Coexistent tendon/ligament disruption or joint effusion.

## Management

Non-surgical
- Non-displaced vertical, peripheral, comminuted and transverse fractures with a step-off of less than 2 mm.
- Above knee casting or immobilization cylinders for 4–6 weeks.

Surgical
- Repair if displaced to prevent subsequent fibrosis.
- Indications: step-off of over 2 mm or separation of over 3 mm.
- Patella fixed with modified tension band wiring (circular or figure of eight), lag screws or both.
- Patellectomy.

# Hyaline cartilage injury

## Anatomy

- The histology of cartilage shows five organized layers, predominantly composed of water.
- Chondrocyte size and mineralization increase in deeper layers in contrast to water content.
- Such a structure facilitates its function in cushioning impaction forces at weight-bearing articular surfaces and its role in allowing free motion supplemented by synovial joint fluid.
- In the knee, hyaline articular cartilage lines the articular surfaces of the tibia, femur and the articular surface of the patella.

## Mechanism of injury

- Damage to hyaline articular cartilage most frequently follows impaction trauma either occurring acutely following impaction such as occurs to the mid lateral femoral condyle following pivot shift injury and ACL tear, or following chronic trauma as occurs secondary to impaction in osteoarthritis.
- Less frequently, hyaline articular cartilage becomes devitalized by inflammatory proteins released in synovial fluid by inflamed synovium.

## History and clinical findings

- Cartilage itself is both poorly vascularized and innervated, accounting for relatively little pain following injury.
- Significant pain only occurs when cartilage becomes deficient or absent, allowing the insudation of synovial fluid into well-innervated subchondral bone.
- The accumulation of subchondral synovial fluid under pressure compresses trabeculae and associated nerve bundles to produce pain. In effect, the fibrillation of cartilage in early chondromalacia patellae is usually relatively asymptomatic.
- In general, knee pain in chondromalacia patellae is only encountered when discrete defects occur in cartilage.
- Similarly, stellate cracks in cartilage overlying the lateral femoral condyle following ACL impaction injuries are generally not a direct cause of pain until a discrete chondral defect appears allowing the insudation of synovial fluid.



## Imaging findings

### Radiography

- The indirect assessment of cartilage is yielded by an evaluation of joint space on weight-bearing conventional radiography.

### Ultrasound

- Ultrasound allows the visualization of superficial cartilage, which appears hypoechoic overlying hyperechoic bone cortex.

### Magnetic resonance imaging

- Because of the predominant water content, cartilage is readily visualized directly at MRI, which is the optimum imaging tool. Cartilage may appear hyperintense or bright on fat-suppressed $T_1$-weighted sequences or relatively hypoechoic against hyperintense $T_2$-weighted sequences.

## Management

### Non-surgical

- Chondroitin supplements may be injected into the joint.
- NSAIDs are used to minimize pain and inflammation.
- Non-weight-bearing regimen should theoretically decrease pain and promote healing but this approach has not been validated to date in scientific study.

### Surgical

- Osteotomy may be employed to rotate cartilage defects out of the weight-bearing plane.
- Cartilage repair may be accelerated by drilling at the site of defects through to subchondral bone to promote local hemorrhage and the delivery of mesenchymal cells to generate a local fibrous scar.
- Grafting techniques use cartilage and subchondral bone harvested from non-weight-bearing surfaces (usually the posterior femoral condyle) and transferred to the site of the defect.
- Cartilage transplantation techniques are currently undergoing scientific evaluation.

# Calf pain: medial tibial stress syndrome (shin splints)

## Mechanism of injury

- In contrast to a stress fracture induced by direct force applied to bone, repeated impaction on the fibula in long-distance runners or abnormal angular stresses imposed on trabeculae of the distal tibia in ballet dancers, medial tibial stress syndrome describes a syndrome of calf pain induced by abnormal traction effects imposed on the tibia at muscular attachments; in effect it describes a spectrum of changes primarily due to muscular overuse ultimately leading to osseous changes.
- In most cases, abnormal traction is imposed by the flexor muscles leading to changes at the flexor digitorum longus and deep crural fascial attachments along the anteromedial cortex.
- Such overuse of the flexor digitorum occurs in all running sports and may be identified in specific subgroups such as line-out jumpers in rugby, competitive long-distance and high jumpers and basketball players at all levels.

## History and clinical findings

- Patients complain of anterior calf pain usually localized to the mid and distal anteromedial cortex of the tibia. Typically, pain is induced by exercise and persists following its cessation. Initially pain resolves soon after stopping activity but as the syndrome progresses so does the time taken for symptoms to resolve.
- On examination, patients are often tender over the affected anteromedial cortex and in contrast to stress fracture tenderness is diffuse.

## Imaging findings

### Radiography

- Radiographs show a diffuse periosteal reaction along the anteromedial cortex of the distal tibia in established cases. In contrast to stress fractures, the periosteal reaction is not associated with a discrete transverse band of sclerosis unless the syndrome is complicated and advanced (Fig. 6.51).



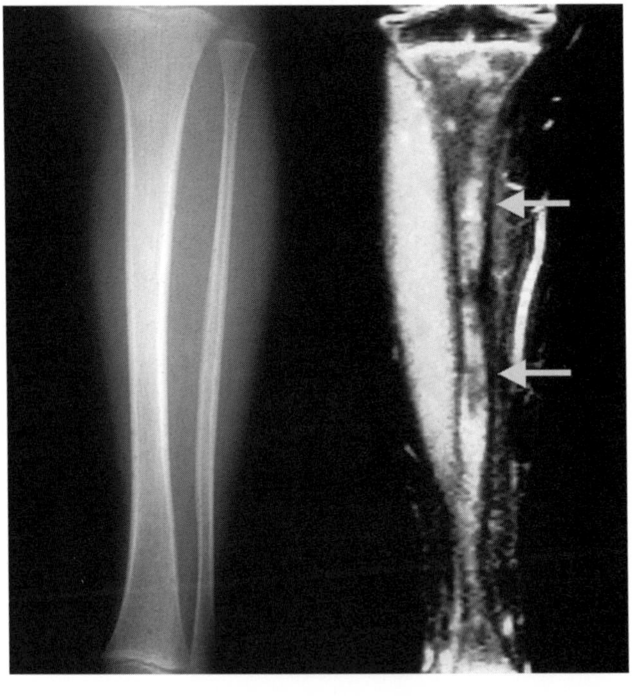

**Fig. 6.51** (**a**) Radiograph showing normal bone outlines. (**b**) In the same patient as in (a) an MR image showing multiple foci of bone edema secondary to microtrauma of shin splints.

## Magnetic resonance imaging

- MRI is favored over isotope bone scan for diagnosis as the earliest changes of the syndrome are muscular occurring at bone attachments, and manifest by local inflammation at these sites. As the syndrome progresses, MRI allows the identification of periostitis and evidence of traction-induced trabecular damage manifest as bone edema. Ultimately MRI reveals the presence of microfractures or transverse bands through the tibia perpendicular to the axis of its shaft. The progression of changes allows systematic grading on the basis of MRI grades 1–4:
  1. Soft-tissue edema and inflammation along the anteromedial cortex
  2. Soft-tissue edema with periostitis and subtle marrow edema
  3. Soft-tissue edema with periostitis and significant marrow edema (Fig. 6.52)
  4. All of the above with associated transverse bands at sites of microfractures.

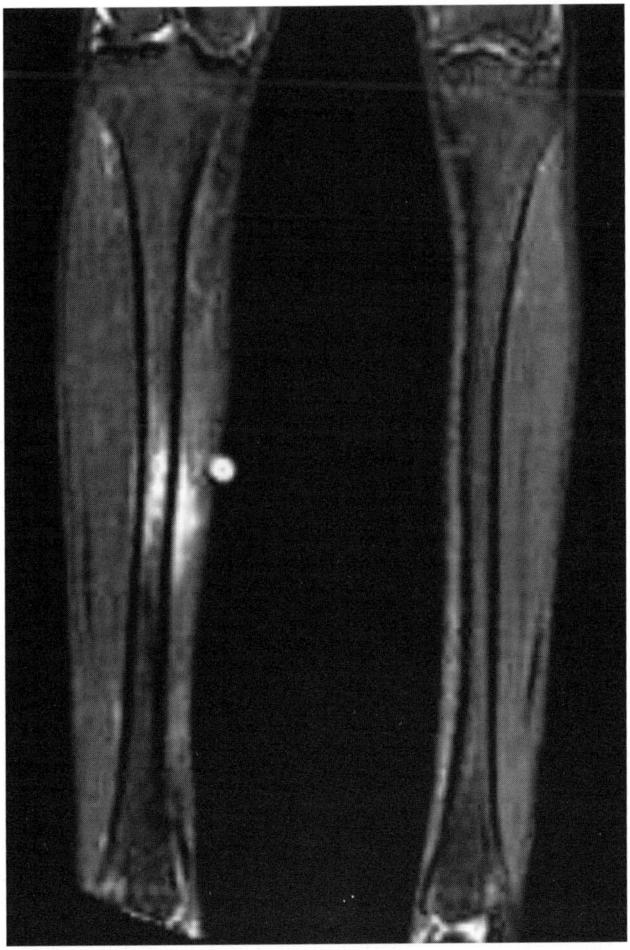

**Fig. 6.52** Coronal fat-suppressed image showing grade 3 medial tibial stress syndrome.

## Management

### Non-surgical

- Rest usually results in the resolution of symptoms over about 6 weeks.

### Surgical

- Refractory cases may require surgical intervention. Similar to tenotomy in groin pain, muscular attachments may be incised to decompress abnormal traction forces on bone. When undertaken, resolution of symptoms occurs in the majority.
- Occasionally, microfractures become complicated and lead to the development of a displaced fracture requiring realignment and immobilization.

# Calf pain: stress fracture

## Mechanism of injury

- The term 'stress fracture' is applied to a fracture through normal bone occurring due to progressive disruption of internal trabeculae secondary to repeatedly applied forces eventually leading to cortical disruption.
- 'Stress' fracture should be contrasted with 'fatigue' fracture, where fracture occurs through pathologically weakened bone as occurs in osteomalacia and osteoporosis.

## History and clinical findings

- Stress fractures present with pain exacerbated by exercise and often becoming more marked and persistent for days following activity.
- In long-distance runners stress fractures typically involve the distal fibula and pain is referable to this site.
- In ballet dancers stress fractures typically involve the mid tibia.
- In young sportsmen or women these fractures most often involve the anteromedial cortex of the tibia at the junction of the middle and lower third. In this setting, the fractures are often multiple and are preceded by predictable soft-tissue, periosteal and marrow changes termed medial tibial stress syndrome (see above, p. 208). In contrast, in long-distance walkers (typically military recruits) similar fractures more frequently involve the posteromedial cortex.
- On examination, patients with stress fractures are extremely tender at the site of injury in contrast to the more diffuse tenderness in medial tibial stress syndrome (see below).

## Imaging findings

### Radiography

- Stress fractures are characterized by the development of a sclerotic linear band perpendicular to the long axis of the affected bone. Prior to cortical disruption with associated dramatic loss of structural integrity and hence risk of displacement, stress fractures develop periosteal reaction.

### Isotope bone scan

- In patients with suspected stress fractures but without radiographic abnormality, an isotope bone scan or MRI may allow detection of occult changes. An isotope bone scan detects osteoblastic activity and therefore, although sensitive, is non-specific.

### Magnetic resonance imaging

- MRI, particularly with fat-suppressed sequences, allows the identification of marrow edema occurring at the site of stress fracture due to disruption of capillaries accompanying disrupted internal trabeculae. Concomitant identification of a fracture line increases the specificity of this technique. (Because MRI allows the exclusion of differential diagnoses, its use is preferred over an isotope bone scan when available) (Fig. 6.53).

## Management

### Non-surgical

- Undisplaced fractures are treated with rest. If medullary sclerosis is associated with periosteal reaction, rest should be combined with non-weight-bearing, short-cast immobilization and crutch support for 4–6 weeks.

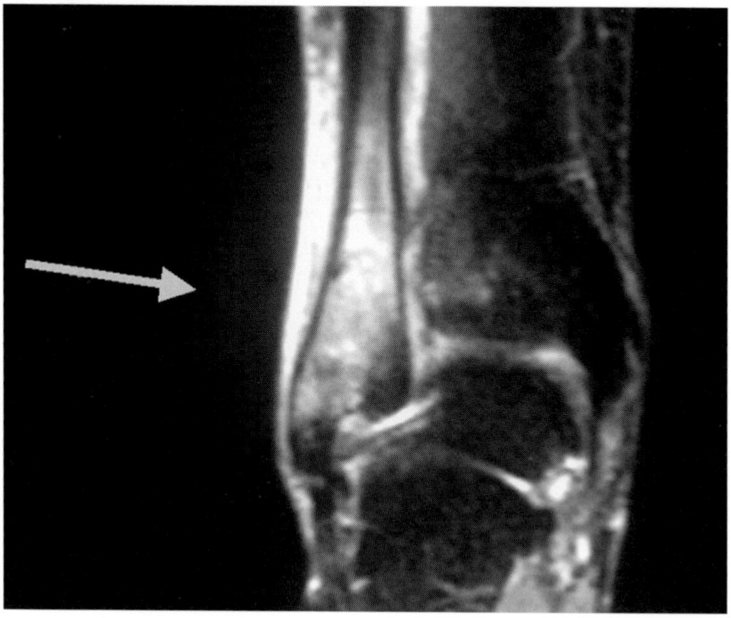

Fig. 6.53 Fat-suppressed image showing bone edema in the distal fibula at a site of undisplaced stress fracture.

## Surgical

- Displaced fractures require realignment, restoration of anatomic alignment and immobilization either by cast or surgical fixation ranging from plate and screw fixation through intramedullary rod fixation.

# Calf pain: vasculopathy

## Anatomy

- The calf is supplied directly by the popliteal artery, which trifurcates to form the posterior tibial artery, the peroneal artery and the anterior tibial artery.

## Mechanism of injury

- Injury at sport may result in acute arterial laceration requiring acute surgical intervention and repair.
- Less commonly, repeated trauma as part of sport leads to local arterial wall damage gradually decreasing flow through the central lumen.
- Two forms of arterial wall damage are recognized:
  1. Cystic adventitial necrosis is manifest as small cysts that develop within a small segment of the arterial wall, usually at the knee. Enlargement of the cysts results in gradual compression of the central lumen.
  2. Intimal fibrosis is the result of repeated intimal damage due to contusion or the trauma of repeated flexion with the development of wall scar and focal luminal narrowing. Intimal fibrosis most frequently occurs at the level of the knee although it has been reported (in cyclists) within the iliac arteries damaged by long periods of hip flexion.
- Even less commonly, aberrant muscle insertion and hypertrophy may gradually compress the main arteries with a similar outcome. In each setting, impaired flow usually only becomes manifest during exercise when the demands for oxygenated blood are maximal.

## History and clinical findings

- Affected patients complain of 'crampy' calf pain, which progressively deteriorates with exercise but gradually resolves following rest. In contrast to muscle injury the pain resolves soon after stopping activity.
- At clinical examination popliteal and dorsalis pedis pulses may be poorly detected.



## Imaging findings

### Ultrasound

- Doppler and gray-scale ultrasound readily identify the popliteal artery. Using ultrasound, the multiple cysts within the adventitial wall may be identified in patients with cystic adventitial necrosis. Similarly, acute-flow cut-off may be demonstrated in patients with intimal fibrosis.

### Magnetic resonance imaging

- MRI using tissue-specific and angiographic sequences readily allows the identification of extrinsic luminal compression in cystic adventitial necrosis and of acute vascular cut-off and collateralization in patients with intimal fibrosis.

## Management

- Cystic adventitial necrosis: cyst de-roofing results in luminal decompression. Occasionally, in extensive cases, bypass grafting is required.
- Intimal fibrosis, if localized, may be treated by image-guided stenting or, in severe cases, by bypass grafting.
- Aberrant muscle heads producing vascular compression are treated by incision or detachment and surgical reattachment.

# Calf pain: muscle hernia

## Mechanism of injury

- Muscle hernia is an unusual cause of calf pain. It describes herniation of muscle through a rent or tear in compartmental fascia in the calf. It can occur in any compartment but is most frequently encountered in the superficial posterior compartment.

## History and clinical findings

- Patients complain of a lump in the calf appearing on exercise. In the majority of cases the hernia is asymptomatic. Occasionally, patients complain of vague discomfort associated with the hernia without loss of power or impact on performance. Rarely, the neck may impair blood supply to hernia, induce ischemia during exercise and produce a cramp-like pain at the site of the hernia. Affected individuals may express concern about the cosmetic impact of the lump.
- On examination a lump can be palpated at the site of the hernia, usually becoming more pronounced on muscle contraction. Occasionally, hernia is misinterpreted as being due to soft-tissue tumor.

## Imaging findings

### Ultrasound

- Ultrasound allows the dynamic assessment of muscle with and without contraction and is the test of choice when this diagnosis is suspected.

### Magnetic resonance imaging

- MRI may be performed with and without muscle contraction and may supplement ultrasound. It may be valuable when ultrasound fails to demonstrate a hernia despite strong clinical suspicion.



## Management

### Non-surgical

- Reassurance, antiinflammatories for patients complaining of mild discomfort.

### Surgical

- Primary repair of the fascial defect should be undertaken when a discrete defect can be identified.

# Maisonneuve's fracture

## Anatomy

- The combination of a distal syndesmosis tear and a proximal fibular fracture is called a Maisonneuve's fracture.
- Implies significant medial injury to the ankle joint.

## Mechanism of injury

- Foot pronation accompanied by external rotation following medial malleolar or ligamentous injury; the anterior syndesmosis tears, and the fibula fractures in a spiral or oblique manner.
- If the torque forces are transmitted to the neck of the fibula, a Maisonneuve's fracture results.

## History and clinical findings

- Intense pain and swelling immediately after trauma.
- Inability to bear weight.
- The ankle joint should also be assessed.

## Imaging findings

### Radiography

- AP view of the ankle: widening of the mortise medially.
- Lateral view of the leg reveals a spiral or oblique fracture of the fibular neck.
- Note that a lateral view of the ankle is normal.
- A mortise view shows a widening of the mortise (normal overlap of the tibia and fibula is absent); a widening of the mortise implies injury to the syndesmosis.

### Computerized tomography

- Rarely required except in complex cases.

### Magnetic resonance imaging

- This is usually not required unless a compartment syndrome or vascular compromise is suspected.



## Management

### Surgical

- Treated operatively as Weber C or pronation–abduction/external rotation fractures.

# Knee osteoarthritis

## Anatomy

- The knee joint is the commonest site of osteoarthritis (OA); this occurs in 90% of the population over 40 years old.

## Mechanism of injury

- Primary (chronic microtrauma) or secondary (e.g. longstanding meniscal tear/postpartial meniscectomy or other predisposing factor).
- Chondromalacia and articular cartilage loss with eventual osteophyte formation and fibrosis of the capsule.

## History and clinical findings

- Gradual onset of knee pain with or without radiation to the gluteal region.
- Knee joint stiffness, which is worse in the morning and with weight-bearing activities.
- Locking if coexistent loose body.
- Pain and reduced range of motion.
- Effusion, crepitus, muscle atrophy, ligamentous laxity may be present.
- The knee joint may appear deformed or subluxed.

## Imaging findings

### Radiography

- Standing AP views.
- Narrowing of joint space: uni- or bicompartmental (Fig. 6.54).
- Subchondral cyst formation on both sides of the articulation.
- Osteophyte formation.
- Periarticular sclerosis.

### Isotope bone scan

- Increased radiotracer uptake secondary to subchondral fractures, cysts or generalized sclerosis.



### Computerized tomography

- Similar features to plain radiography.

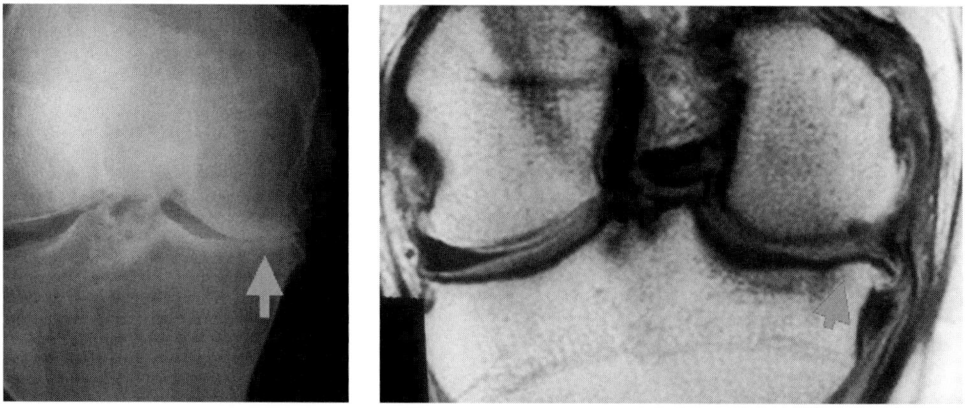

(a) (b)

**Fig. 6.54** **(a)** Radiograph showing advanced medial compartment osteoarthritis characterized by loss of joint space. **(b)** MR image in the same patient as in (a) showing meniscal extrusion, osteophytes and loss of hyaline articular cartilage.

Magnetic resonance imaging

- More sensitive than plain films in early OA.
- $T_1$-weighted images show cartilage loss and hypointense subchondral sclerosis; sagittal images are best for the patellofemoral joint, coronal images for the knee joint.
- $T_2$-weighted images show high-signal fluid extending to the osseous surface through cracks in denuded isointense cartilage with or without hyperintense joint effusion and high-signal subchondral bone edema.
- Subchondral cysts follow the fluid signal (generally a high signal on $T_2$-weighted and low on $T_1$-weighted studies).
- Gradient echosequences may be used to detect and locate loose bodies.

## Management

Non-surgical

- The aim is pain relief with improved functional mobility.
- Non-pharmacological therapy: reduced activity, weight reduction, strengthening of muscles around the joint (especially the quadriceps) and bracing/supports.
- Topical therapy: NSAIDs and capsaicin, reducing the effects of substance P, which is involved in pain transmission.
- Systemic therapy: antiinflammatories, other analgesics, glucosamine and chondroitin supplements (components of the cartilage matrix).
- Intra-articular therapy: steroid injection and hyaluronate injection (for its viscoelastic, antinociceptive, antiinflammatory, and autoregulatory functions).

Surgical

- For ongoing symptoms.
- Arthroscopy and debridement have been shown to have no better outcomes than placebo procedures.
- Knee arthroplasty.
- Realignment osteotomy in younger patients (redistributes weight-bearing to try to prevent progression of the condition).
- Newer disease modifying therapies such as autologous chondrocyte transplantation for isolated cartilage defects.

# Tibial and fibular fractures

## Anatomy

- The tibia and fibula are linked by a tight band of connective tissue (the interosseous membrane).

## Mechanism of injury

- Usually direct trauma.
- More serious injury occurs if there is a compound fracture and both lower leg bones are involved.

## History and clinical findings

- Intense pain and swelling immediately after trauma.
- Malalignment and inability to bear weight.
- Distal vessel and nerve injury may occur.
- The ankle joint should also be assessed.

## Imaging findings

### Radiography

- Lucent fracture line with or without comminuted fragments.

### Isotope bone scan

- If there is a normal initial radiograph and high clinical suspicion, the scan may show increased uptake after 24–72 hours in fibular stress fractures.

### Computerized tomography

- Rarely required except in complex cases.
- For fragment localization in cases of intra-articular extension and planned surgery.

### Magnetic resonance imaging

- Usually not required unless a compartment syndrome or vascular compromise is suspected.



## Management

Factors influencing management and outcome include the amount of displacement, degree of comminution, extent of soft-tissue injury and amount of osteoporosis.

### Non-surgical

- Plaster cast for 8–12 weeks (above-knee cast required in high tibial or fibular fractures).
- Goal is to restore length and alignment.
- Isolated simple fibular fractures only require rest with no immobilization.

### Surgical

- Open reduction and internal fixation with early postoperative mobilization.
- External fixators.

# Further reading

De Lee JC, Drez, Jr D, Miller MD. Orthopaedic sports medicine, 2nd edn. Philadelphia, WB Saunders, 2003.

Eustace S. MRI of orthopaedic trauma. Lippincott Williams & Wilkins, 1999.

Finnegan MA, Uhtoff HK. Healing of trabecular bone. In: Lang JM ed. Fracture healing, Churchill Livingstone, 1987; 33–38.

Fitzgerald RH, Kaufer H, Malkani AL. Orthopaedics. Oxford, Mosby/Elsevier, 2001.

# 7

# The Foot and Ankle



## CLINICAL EXAMINATION

### Clinical history

Elucidation of the mechanism of injury assists in making the proper diagnosis of ankle injuries. Inversion and eversion injuries of the ankle should

**Fig. 7.1** Sportsfile.

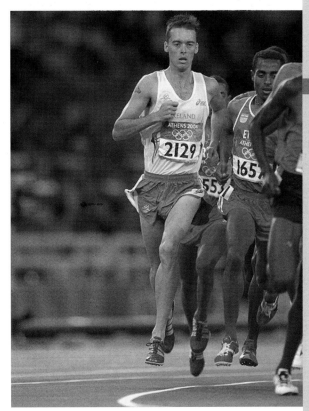

be differentiated. Eversion injuries can cause injuries to the deltoid ligament, the posterior tibial tendon and the inferior tibiofibular syndesmosis injury, and oblique fractures of the distal fibula. Acute supination, in effect plantar flexion with inversion injury, accompanied by the sudden onset of pain after an audible 'crack', suggests a serious lateral ankle ligament and capsule injury. An inability to bear weight initially followed by marked ecchymosis and subsequent feeling of giving way during ambulation is also suggestive of significant ligamentous pathology. Osteochondral fractures and peroneal tendon subluxation are associated with a 'clicking' sensation around the ankle joint and region.

## Physical examination

Without an adequate physical examination, subtle but significant pathology may go undiagnosed. Imprecise diagnosis leads to inadequate or inappropriate treatment, which may cause residual morbidity.

Determining the location of maximum tenderness and swelling is the key to predicting the nature of the injury. Within hours of injury, hemorrhage and edema into the ankle joint and soft tissues cause capsular distension, swelling and tenderness, which ultimately reduces the possibility of a precise diagnosis.



A complete examination includes palpation of the anterior talofibular ligament (ATFL), calcaneofibular ligament (CFL), posterior talofibular ligament (PTFL), syndesmosis, calcaneocuboid joint, posterior tibial and peroneal tendons, fifth metatarsal base and shaft, and the medial and lateral malleoli. Tenderness over the bony structures indicate the possibility of fracture or severe bony injury. The presence of marked ecchymosis and swelling indicates possible complete ligament tear and/or fracture. Special tests complete the routine examination.

The **anterior drawer** and **talar tilt tests** are manual stress tests to evaluate the competence of the ATFL and CFL, respectively. The anterior drawer test is performed with the patient sitting with the knee flexed at 90°. Patients have a tendency to extend the knee, which alters the resistance for translation of the talus on the tibia; therefore the examiner should make sure the patient is relaxed. With the heel grasped and pulled forward, a posterior force is placed on the tibia. Visible dimpling over the anterolateral aspect of the ankle, the **sulcus sign**, signifies incompetence of the ATFL. When examining the patient with an acute injury, there may be a joint effusion and so much soft-tissue swelling that the sulcus sign is not readily apparent. The examiner also relies on the quality of the end-point felt when performing the anterior drawer test as a clue to the extent of ligament damage. A soft end-point accompanied by increased anterior translation of the talus suggests a complete rupture of the ligament. A partial ligament tear is suggested if **anterior talar translation** of the talus is slightly increased and there is a moderate to firm end-point.

The second manual stress test of the ankle ligaments is the **talar tilt test**. To perform this, the examiner supports the medial aspect of the tibia in one hand, and the opposite hand is placed on the lateral aspect of the heel. The ankle is positioned at 0° dorsiflexion and the examiner inverts the heel forcibly. In health, excursion of the talus is limited and a firm end-point is felt. An increase in talar tilt accompanied by lateral dimpling indicates damage to the CFL.

A soft end-point indicates a complete rupture. In acute cases, anesthesia may be used to decrease involuntary guarding by the patient and improve the validity of the anterior drawer and talar tilt tests.

Syndesmosis injuries are diagnosed by the presence of tenderness over the syndesmosis and the '**squeeze test**.' This test is performed by squeezing the tibia and fibula together at the midcalf level. Pain distally at the syndesmosis or ankle joint is indicative of a syndesmosis sprain. Pain proximally at the fibula indicates Maisonneuve's fracture of the neck of the fibula. If such a fracture is suspected, a radiograph of the entire length of the lower leg is indicated. The squeeze test may be supplemented by the external rotation stress test to diagnose a syndesmosis injury. The test is performed with the patient in the sitting position with the knee flexed at 90°. The foot is externally rotated on the fixed tibia by the examiner. Pain at the syndesmosis indicates trauma to the syndesmosis ligaments and is an indication for an external rotation stress radiograph. Syndesmosis sprains are reported to occur in 1–11% of sprained ankles and may lead to a diastasis of the ankle joint, depending on the extent of the damage.

The examiner may find it difficult if not impossible to hold the leg of a large and heavy individual when performing the external rotation stress test. In this situation, a modified external rotation stress test can be performed by having the patient stand on the involved planted foot and internally rotate the ipsilateral leg and body, when comparison is made to the contralateral side. Again, the test is positive for high ankle sprain in the presence of tenderness over the syndesmosis. In general, the external rotation stress test is more specific in isolating a syndesmosis injury than the squeeze test. The **Cotton test** is used to assess syndesmosis instability with diastasis. It is performed by stabilizing the distal tibia and applying a lateral force to the foot, looking for any lateral translation of the foot, which would indicate syndesmotic instability.

Disruption of the syndesmosis can be confirmed by grasping the tibia and fibula separately and an attempt made to translate the fibula on the tibia in the sagittal plane anterior posteriorly (anterior posterior translation test). The test is positive when pain is elicited at the syndesmotic joint. Stability of the syndesmosis can also be assessed arthroscopically, where a 2 mm or greater movement between the tibia and the fibula establishes the diagnosis of instability. Under normal circumstances, there is approximately 1 mm of movement between these two bones.

The peroneal tendons are examined for subluxation or dislocation. Test for subluxation by placing the foot in a dorsiflexed and everted position; then have the patient resist inversion. With damage to the peroneal retinaculum, subluxation or dislocation of the tendons is observed. This may be treated by immobilization in a short leg cast in 30° of ankle plantarflexion for 6 weeks.

The **Thompson test** is used to diagnose Achilles tendon rupture. The test is performed by squeezing the gastrocnemius–soleus muscle complex having positioned the patient prone with the foot off the examination table. The normal finding is passive plantar flexion when the gastrocnemius–soleus muscle belly is squeezed. Absence of plantarflexion of the foot is indicative of a ruptured Achilles tendon. It is important to recognize that patients often present to the physician with a misleading history of presumed inversion ankle sprain when, in reality, the Achilles tendon has been ruptured.

If the patient is most tender over the extensor digitorum brevis muscle, one must be suspicious of injury to the calcaneocuboid joint. Injury of the calcaneocuboid joint includes fracture of the anterior process of the calcaneus or damage to the bifurcate ligament (lateral calcaneal navicular ligament and medial calcaneal cuboid ligament). The calcaneocuboid joint is tested by stabilizing the hindfoot and stressing the forefoot in adduction and abduction.

Less commonly, traction injuries occur to the superficial peroneal and sural nerves. If these nerves have been injured, they are very tender on palpation. Traction injuries of these nerves can require a prolonged recovery period. The occasional patient may develop severe **reflex sympathetic dystrophy** or **chronic pain disorder**, which markedly impact on recovery from the injury.

There are distinct differences between high-ankle and anterolateral ankle sprains in terms of the mechanism of injuries and physical findings so that the diagnosis of syndesmosis injury is usually readily apparent if the clinician takes a detailed history and performs a thorough physical examination. The swelling and ecchymosis in high-ankle sprain is usually at the syndesmosis and more proximally in the leg. Tenderness is usually localized directly over the syndesmosis region instead of the ATFL and CFL. There is the negative anterior drawer test and lateral talar tilt test, unless significant concomitant lateral ankle ligament tears are also present. The interosseous membrane is also tender when there is more proximal propagation of the soft-tissue injury. Tenderness over the fibula shaft or neck is present when there is a Maisonneuve fracture. Dorsiflexion of the ankle is painful.



## Sustentaculum tali: medial extension of the calcaneum

The sustentaculum tali (medial extension of the calcaneum) is palpable about one finger's breadth from the distal end of the medial malleolus. The sustentaculum tali may be small and may not be palpable at all but it has anatomical significance in that it supports the talus and serves as an attachment for the spring ligament. Problems within this anatomical alignment may well lead to pes planus (Fig. 7.2).

## Medial tubercle of the talus

The medial tubercle of the talus – the small and barely palpable bony prominence lying immediately

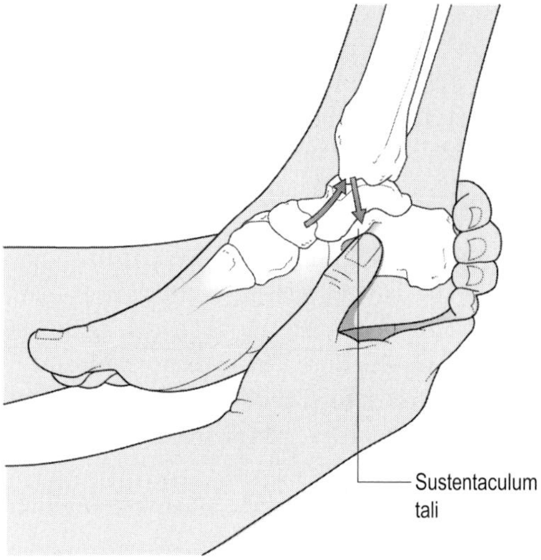


Fig. 7.2 Sustentaculum tali.

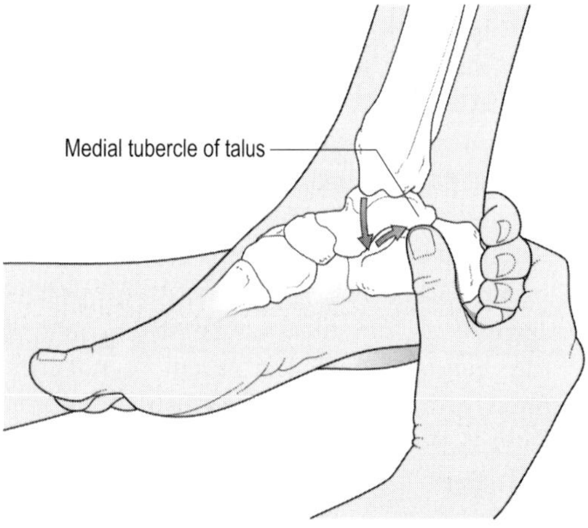


Fig. 7.3 Medial tubercle of the talus.

posterior to the distal end of the medial malleolus – is the insertion for the posterior aspect of the medial ankle collateral ligament (Fig. 7.3).

## Sinus tarsi

The sinus tarsi is an area of soft-tissue depression just anterior to and partly overlain by the lateral malleolus. It is filled by the extensor digitorum brevis muscle and an overlying fat pad. The superior dorsal aspect of the calcaneum can be palpated near its articulation with the cuboid bone through the soft tissues, and the lateral side of the neck of the talus

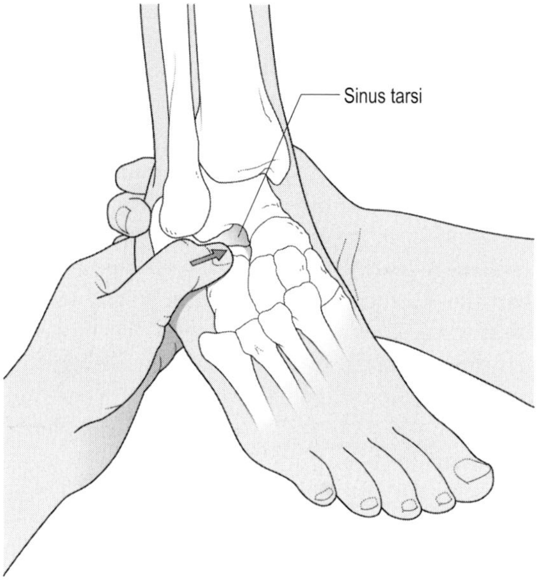


Fig. 7.4 Sinus tarsi.

may be palpated in inversion by pushing your finger deeper into the sinus tarsi (Fig. 7.4).

## Dome of the talus

A small portion of the dome of the talus becomes palpable in inversion and plantar flexion with a greater portion of its articular surface palpable on its lateral side than on the medial side. An osteochondral defect may be palpable on the articular surface of the dome of the talus in this position (Fig. 7.5).

## Inferior tibiofibular syndesmosis

This syndesmotic joint lies immediately proximal to the talus between the tibia and fibula distally. The anteroinferior tibiofibular (AITF) ligament overlies this joint and a slight depression is usually palpable. The bones of the joint may separate (diastasis) during injury to the ankle joint and region (Fig. 7.6)

## Tubercle of the navicular bone and head of the talus

The plantar portion of the head of the talus articulates with the sustentaculum tali and the anterior portion with the posterior aspect of the navicular bone is supported by the tibialis posterior tendon and the spring ligament, which runs from the sus-

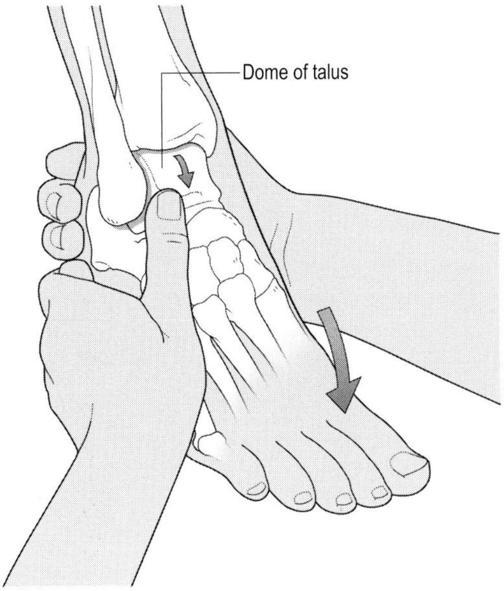


Fig. 7.5 Dome of the talus.

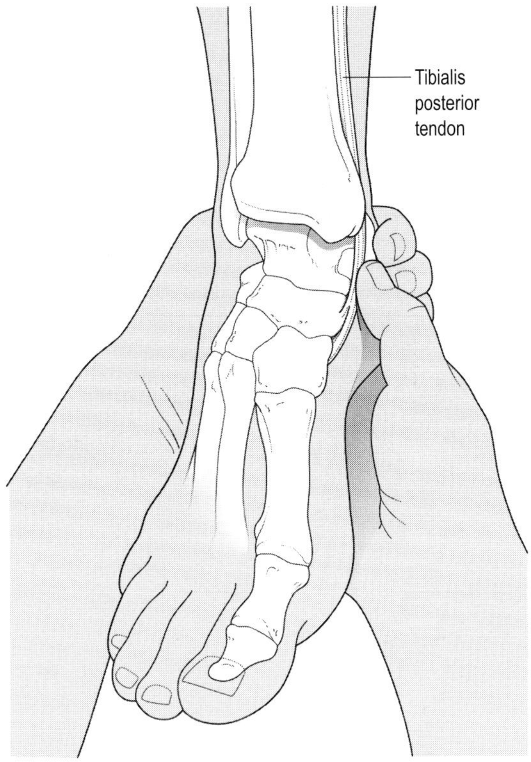


Fig. 7.7 Tibialis posterior tendon.

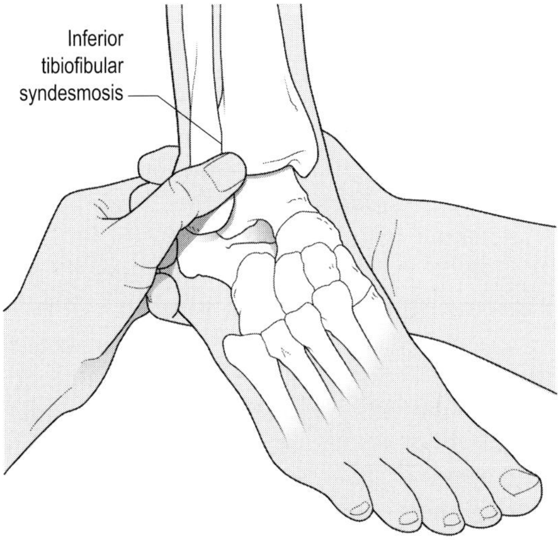


Fig. 7.6 Inferior tibiofibular syndesmosis.

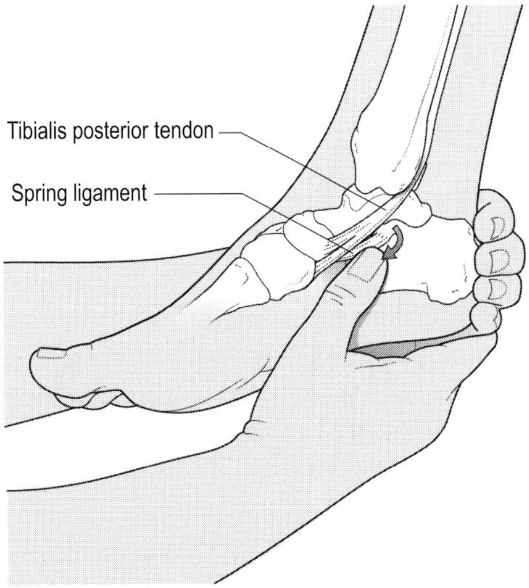


Fig. 7.8 Tubercle of the navicular bone.

tentaculum tali to the navicular bone because the head of the talus lacks bony support between these two articulations (Fig. 7.7 and Fig. 7.8).

## Deltoid ligament

Pain elicited upon eversion may be due to a sprain of the deltoid ligament (Fig. 7.9).

## Posterior tibial arterial pulse

See Figure 7.10.

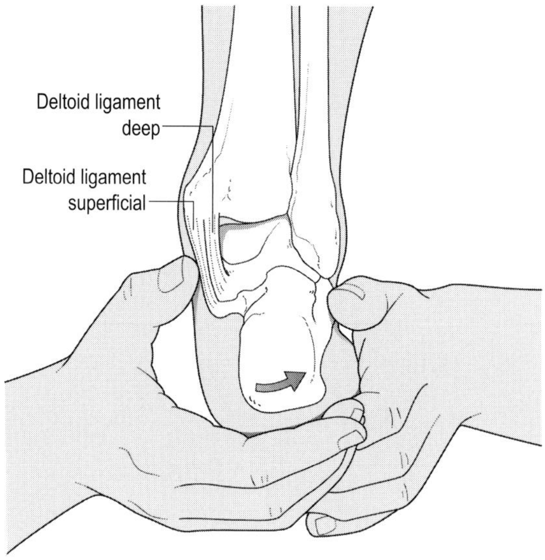


**Fig. 7.9** Deltoid ligament.

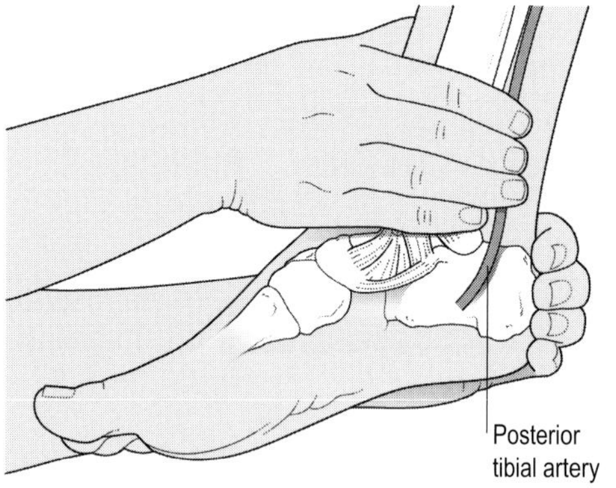


**Fig. 7.10** Posterior tibial arterial pulse.

## Dorsal pedis arterial pulse

The dorsal pedis artery lies subcutaneously between the extensor hallucis longus and the extensor digitorum longus tendons on the dorsum of the foot. It is absent in approximately 10–15% of the normal population (Fig. 7.11).

## Tibialis anterior tendon

The tibialis anterior tendon is the most prominent and most medial tendon on the dorsum of the ankle and foot. The tendon becomes prominent on dorsiflexion of the ankle and is palpable distally to its insertion onto the medial aspect of the base of the

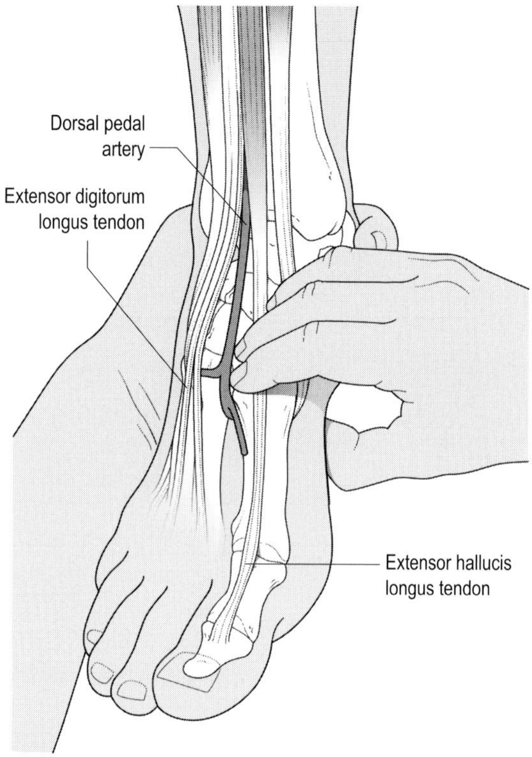


**Fig. 7.11** Dorsal pedis arterial pulse.

first metatarsal and the first cuneiform bone, and proximally along the tendon to the muscle belly on the lateral side of the shaft of the tibia (Fig. 7.12).

## Extensor hallucis longus tendon

The extensor hallucis longus tendon is situated immediately lateral to the tibialis anterior tendon and, when the hallux is actively extended, it becomes prominent and stands out immediately lateral to the tibialis anterior tendon at the level of the ankle joint. It is palpable on the dorsum of the foot to its insertion into the base of the distal phalanx of the hallux (see Fig. 7.11).

## Extensor digitorum longus tendon

The extensor digitorum longus tendon is located and palpable lateral to the extensor hallucis longus. It crosses the ankle joint and divides into four separate tendon slips, which insert into the dorsal base of the distal phalanx of the four lesser toes and become prominent for palpation on extension of the lesser toes (see Fig. 7.11).

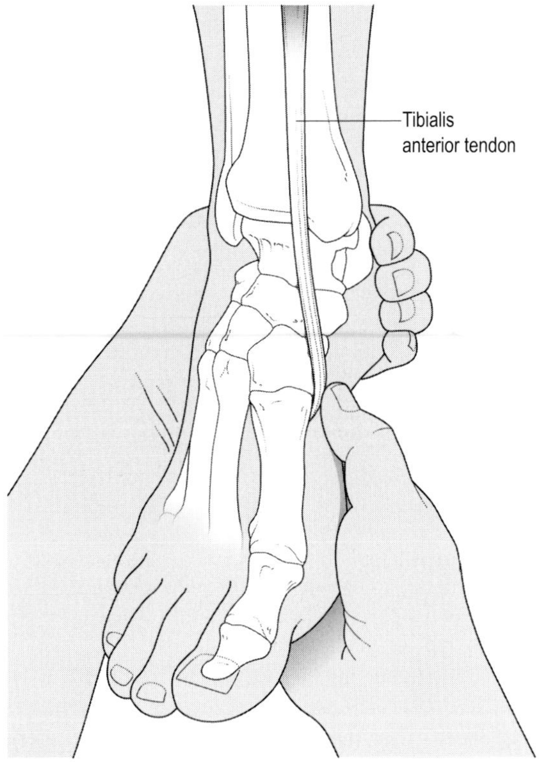


Fig. 7.12 Tibialis anterior tendon.

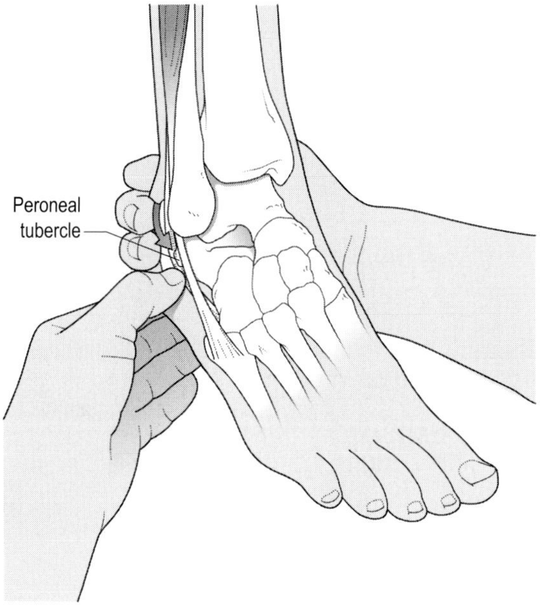


Fig. 7.13 Peroneus longus.



## Peroneus longus and brevis tendons

The peroneus longus and brevis tendons pass immediately behind the lateral malleolus as they cross the ankle joint. The peroneus brevis is closer to the bone in the peroneal groove of the lateral malleolus, and the peroneus longus lies just posterior to the brevis. The peroneal retinaculum (fascial band) holds the tendons to the lateral malleolus (Fig. 7.13).

The peroneal tendons are separated by the peroneal tubercle by a retinaculum and are surrounded by a synovial sheath. The peroneus brevis tendon is palpable down to its insertion into the styloid process of the base of the fifth metatarsal bone (Fig. 7.14).

## Lateral ligament complex

The ATFL extends from the anterior aspect of the lateral malleolus to the lateral aspect of the neck of the talus.

The CFL extends from its origin to its insertion to a small tubercle on the lateral wall of the calcaneus slightly posterior to the peroneal tubercle.

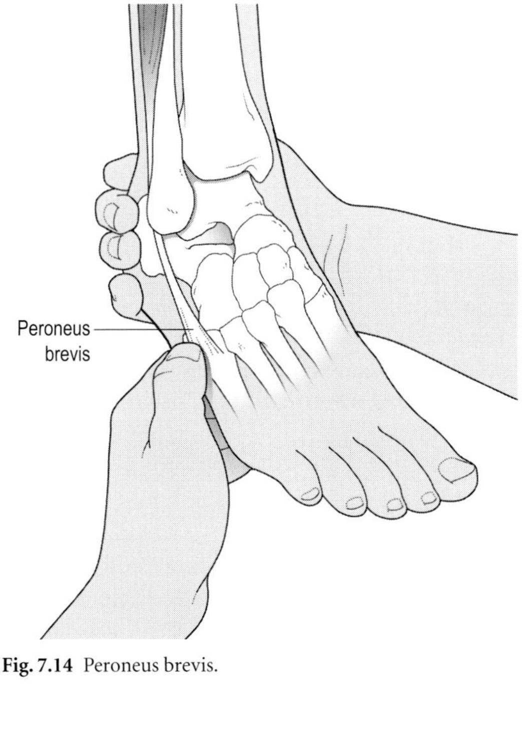


Fig. 7.14 Peroneus brevis.

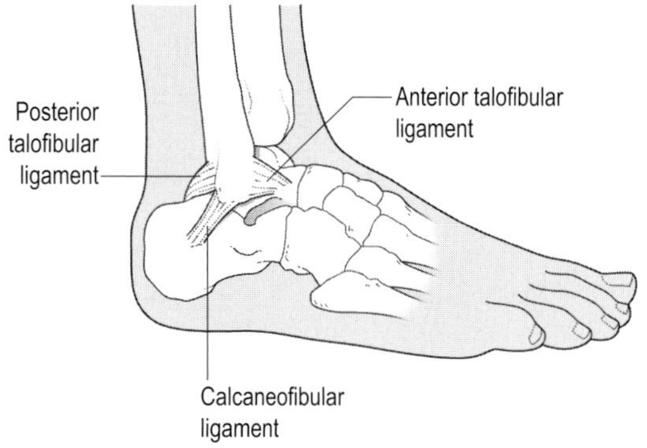


**Fig. 7.15** Lateral ligament complex.

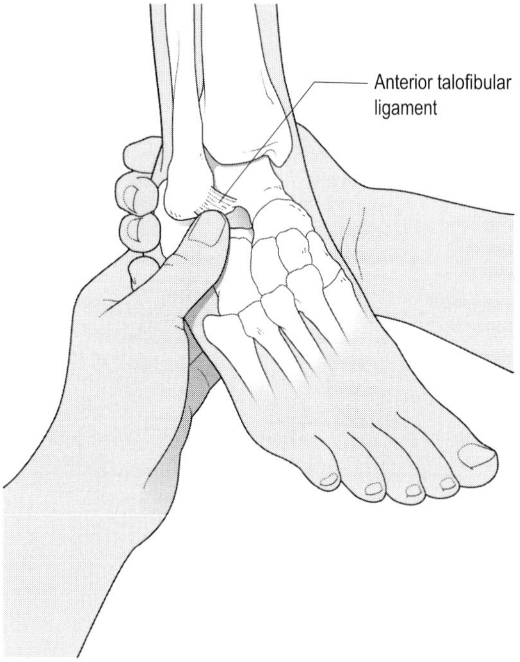


**Fig. 7.16** Lateral ankle ligament palpation.

The PTFL extends from its origin on the posterior aspect of the lateral malleolus passing posteriorly to the small lateral tubercle on the posterior aspect of the talus (Fig. 7.15).

For lateral ankle ligament palpation see Figure 7.16.

## Talar tilt test

Inversion of the calcaneum resulting in tilting of the talus out of the ankle joint mortise indicates laxity of the ATFL and CFL with resultant lateral ankle instability. The PTFL can be injured only in conjunction

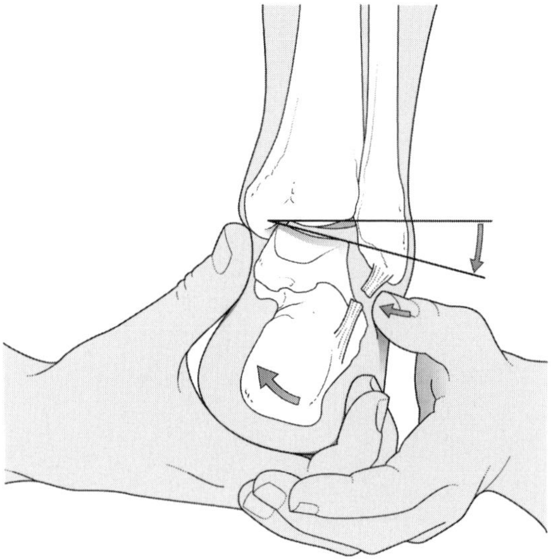

**Fig. 7.17** Talar tilt test.

with the other two components of the lateral ligament; it takes a massive trauma to the ankle joint, such as dislocation, to damage the talofibular ligament. Eversion of the calcaneum tests the stability of the deltoid ligament on the medial side There may be a palpable defect in the deltoid ligament and opening of the ankle joint space and mortise. The ankle is unstable if the ATFL and CFL are torn (Fig. 7.17).

## Anterior drawer test

This is used to evaluate the stability of the ATFL and CFL (Figs 7.18–7.20).

## Ranges of motion

Movements of the foot and ankle almost invariably involve more than a single joint. The basic ankle and foot motions are:

- Ankle joint motion:
  - dorsiflexion
  - plantar flexion.
- Subtalar joint motion:
  - inversion
  - eversion.
- Mid-tarsal joint motion (Figs 7.21–7.23):
  - forefoot adduction
  - forefoot abduction.

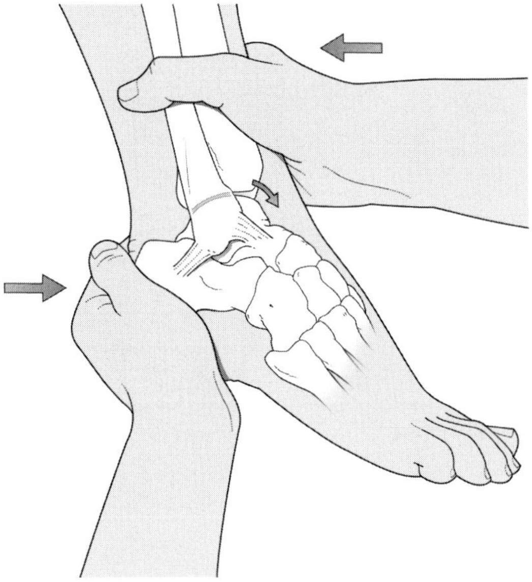

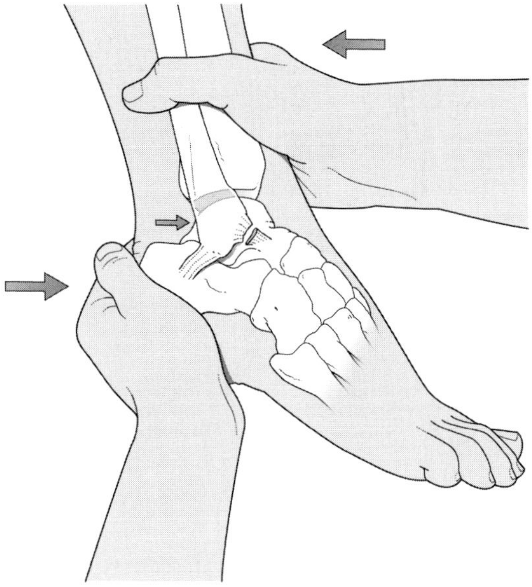

(a) (b)

Fig. 7.18 Anterior drawer test.

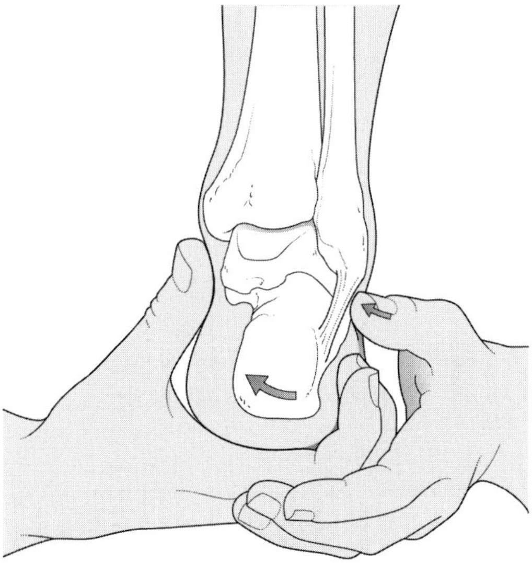

Fig. 7.19 Anterior drawer test.

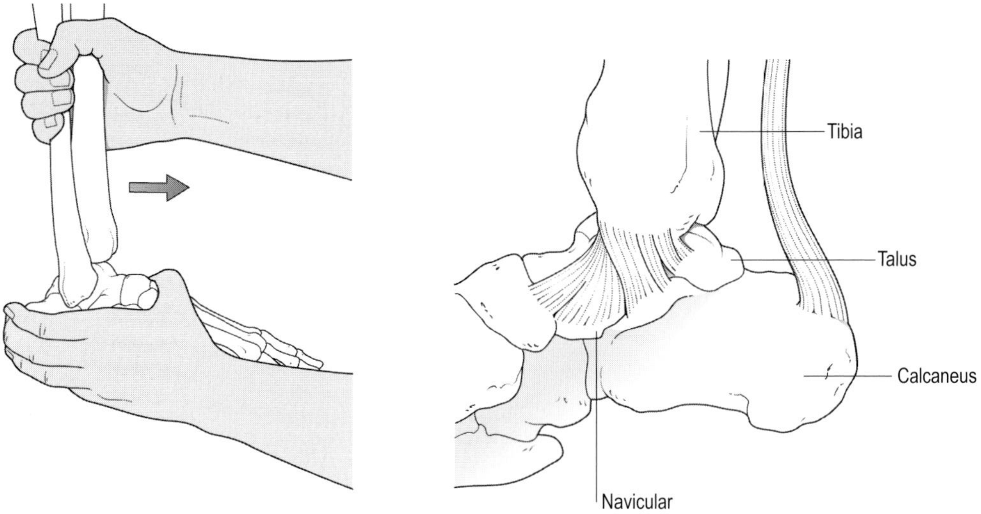


**Fig. 7.20** Anterior drawer test.

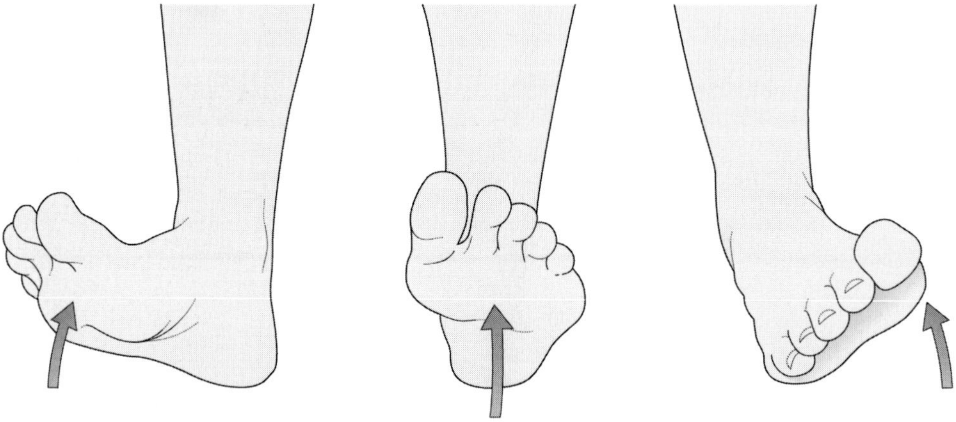

(a)

**Fig. 7.21** Mid-tarsal joint motion.

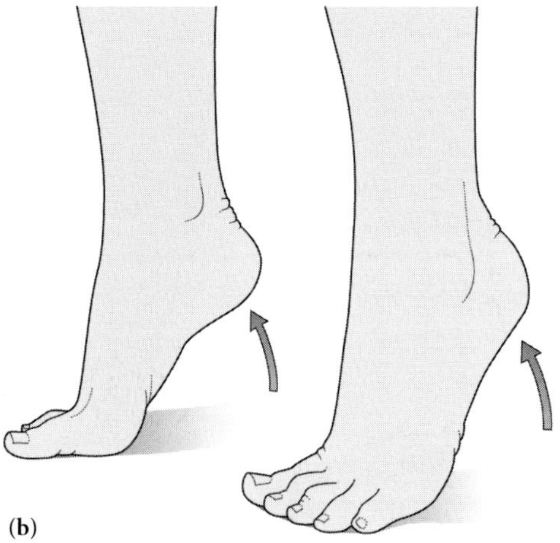
(b)

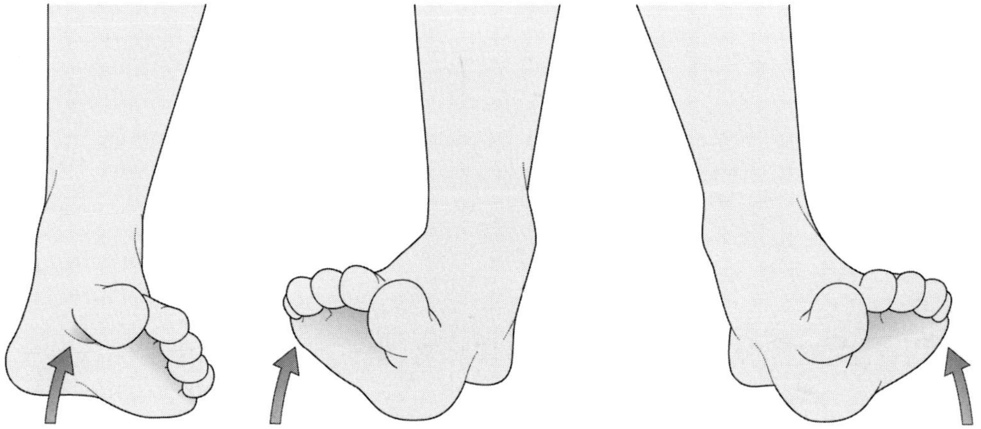
(c)

**Fig. 7.21** Mid-tarsal joint motion – *Cont'd.*

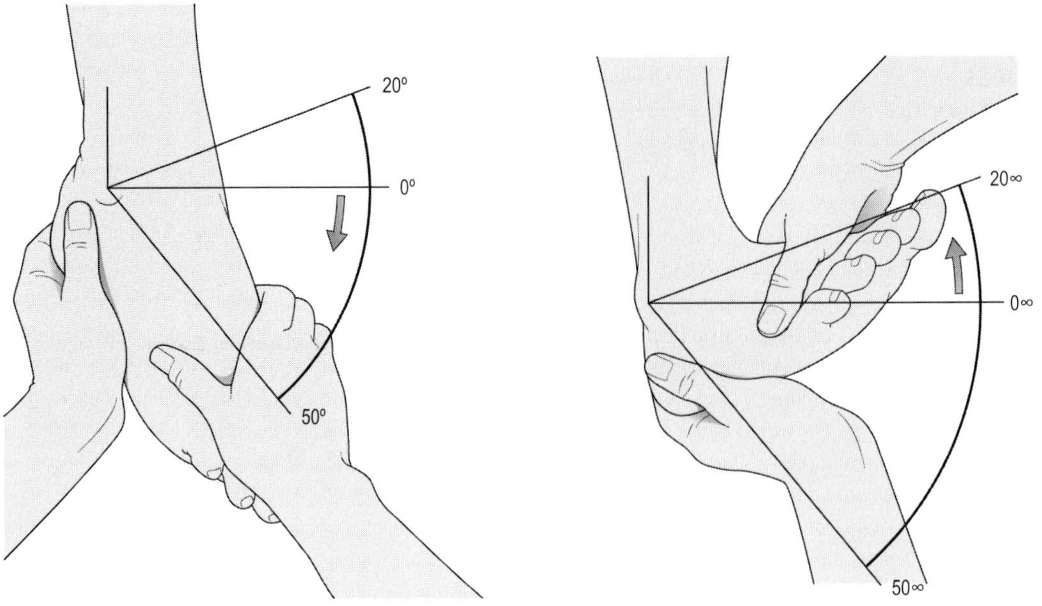


(a) (b)

**Fig. 7.22** Mid-tarsal joint motion.

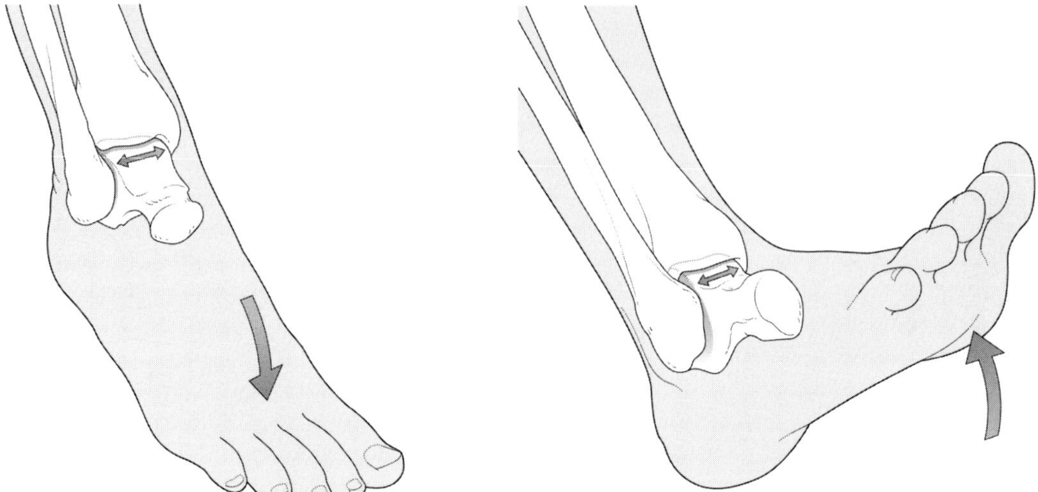

(a) (b)

**Fig. 7.23** Mid-tarsal joint motion.

## Test to distinguish between gastrocnemius and soleus muscle tightness

**The ankle dorsiflexion test**. When the ankle cannot be dorsiflexed or brought to the plantagrade position with the knee extended, and when you know the limitation of motion to be caused by either the gastrocnemius or the soleus muscles, the determination of which muscle is causing the limitation is by means of the following test. First, flex the knee joint. If you are able to achieve ankle dorsiflexion when the knee is flexed, the gastrocnemius muscle is the cause of the limitation, since flexion of the knee slackens the gastrocnemius (a two-joint muscle) by bringing its origin closer to its insertion Since the soleus is a one-joint muscle, it is not affected by flexion of the knee. If the soleus is responsible for the limited motion, the limitation will be the same whether or not the knee is flexed (Fig. 7.24).

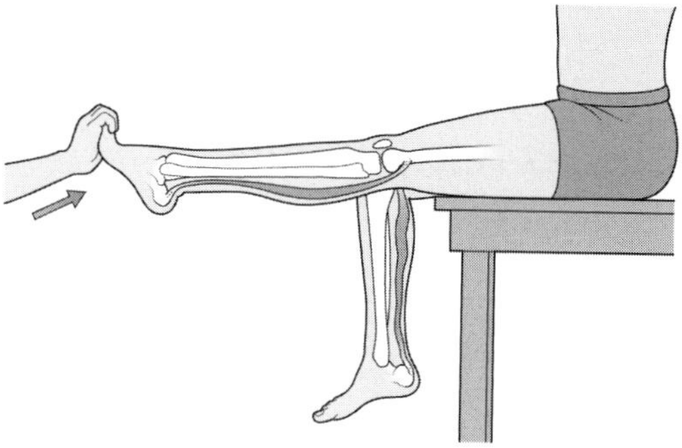

**Fig. 7.24** Test to distinguish between gastrocnemius and soleus muscle tightness.

# INJURIES AND PATHOLOGIES

## Achilles tendinitis

### Anatomy

- The Achilles tendon, formed by the merging of the gastronemius and soleus tendons, is the most commonly injured tendon in the foot.
- No synovial sheath.

### Mechanism of injury

- Insertional and non-insertional forms.
- Insertional (tendinitis at distal calcaneal insertion): found in the older population and in less active people, and usually follows chronic trauma, impingement by a bony spur (Haglund's disease) or chronic local synovitis.
- Non-insertional (more proximal; occurs at the hypovascular myotendinous junction 3–6 cm proximal to the tendon insertion): found in elite athletes usually following acute trauma.
- Secondary to eccentric loading (e.g. sprinters decelerating) or hyperpronation.
- Associated with altered foot biomechanics: forefoot varus, pes cavus and equinus deformity.
- Common in sprinters and dancers.

### History and clinical findings

- Pain on weight-bearing.
- Symptoms and pain on deep palpation: more proximal in non-insertional than insertional tendinitis (tenderness felt proximal to the retrocalcaneal bursa versus the os calcis).
- Palpable tendon nodularity.



### Imaging findings

#### Radiography

- Thickened Achilles tendon and blurring of fat planes anterior to Achilles tendon on lateral ankle view.

#### Ultrasound

- Increased tendon thickness and disruption of linear fibrillary bundles.
- Decreased tendon echogenicity, focal nodularity or diffuse hypoechogenicity.

#### Magnetic resonance imaging

- Thickened tendon with anterior convexity.
- Tendinosis (mucoid degeneration) appears as a high signal on short tau inversion recovery (STIR) images.
- If paratendinitis is present there is a generalized inflammatory change in surrounding soft tissues.
- Insertional tendinitis is associated with reactive marrow edema in calcaneus with or without a bony calcaneal prominence (Haglund's deformity) and with or without retrocalcaneal or Achilles tendon bursitis (Figs 7.25 and 7.26).

### Management

#### Non-surgical

- Icing, gentle stretching.
- Avoidance of precipitating exercise.
- Antiinflammatory medication.

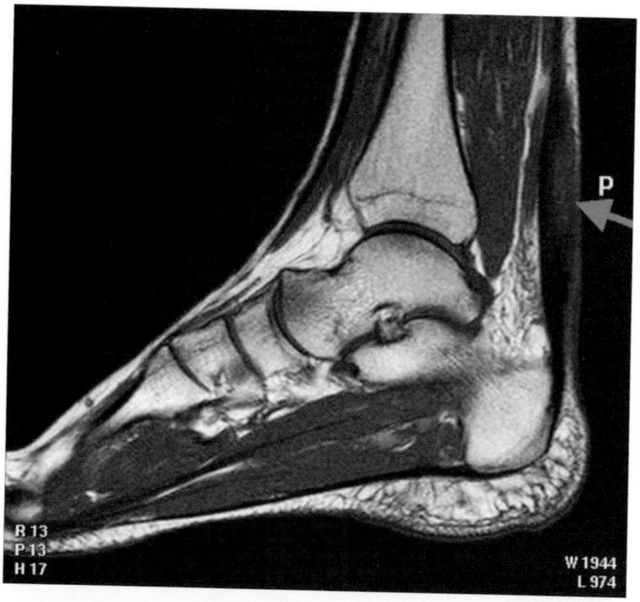


(a)

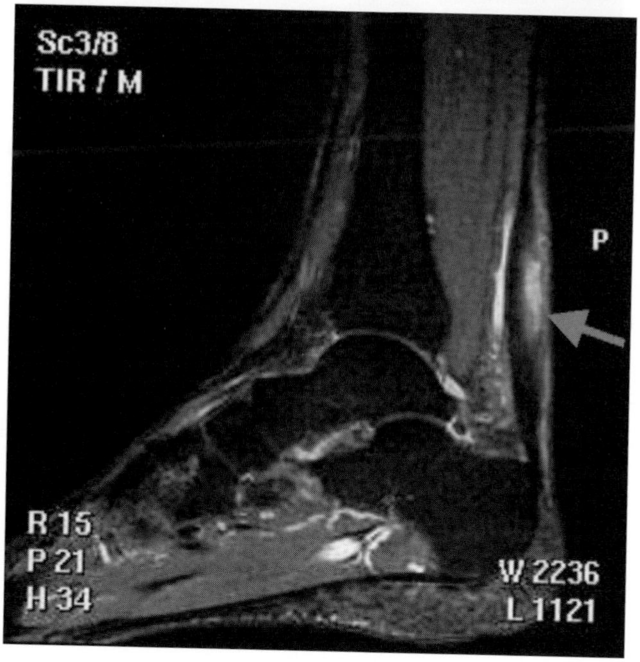


(b)

**Fig. 7.25** (**a**) Sagittal $T_1$-weighted and (**b**) fat-suppressed image showing focal signal abnormality at the musculoskeletal junction secondary to tendinitis/partial Achilles tendon tear.



- Orthotics to correct hyperpronation.
- For people with low levels of activity, casting for several weeks can be used in severe cases.

Surgical

- For chronic cases where tendinosis is evident and other methods of treatment have failed.
- Surgery is usually recommended for treatment of Achilles tendon ruptures in active, healthy patients.

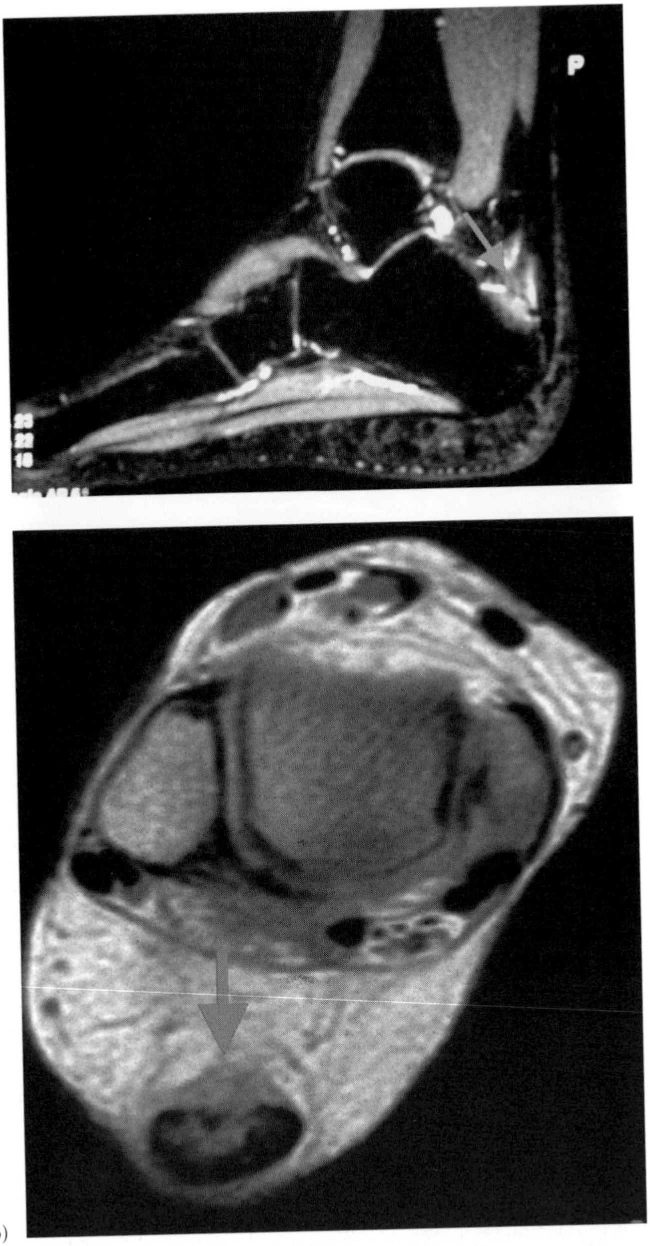


(a)

(b)

**Fig. 7.26** (**a**) Sagittal fat-suppressed and (**b**) axial $T_1$-weighted images showing focal signal abnormality and thickening of the Achilles tendon with pre-Achilles bursitis secondary to insertional Achilles tendinitis.



- Insertional tendinopathy: debridement of the retrocalcaneal bursa, calcaneal osteophyte excision and removal of the diseased tendon.
- Suture anchors, tendon transfers or allograft may be necessary when more than 50% of the tendon is excised.

## Repair of partial tears

- Release and excise the paratenon in cases of paratenonitis.
- The resumption of full athletic activity usually takes 4–6 months or longer after injury in the surgically treated patient. Surgically repaired tendons heal stronger with less chance of re-rupture.

# Achilles tendon tear

## Anatomy

- This is the third most frequent tendon rupture.
- Tears at the hypovascular area 2–3 cm above calcaneal insertion.
- Posterior fibers tear first in partial tear.

## Mechanism of injury

- Direct (less common) or indirect trauma (especially in unconditioned middle-aged athletes).
- Forced dorsiflexion of the foot.
- Overpronation of the heel causes repetitive microtears.
- Chronic tendinosis and partial tears may predispose to complete tears.

## History and clinical findings

- Pain and swelling.
- Palpable tendon defect.
- Impaired plantar flexion.
- Positive Thompson test.
- O'Brien's needle test.
- Grading of tears (Fig. 7.27):
  - type 1: <50% partial rupture
  - type 2: complete rupture with gap <3 cm
  - type 3: complete rupture with gap 3–6 cm
  - type 4: complete rupture with gap >6 cm.

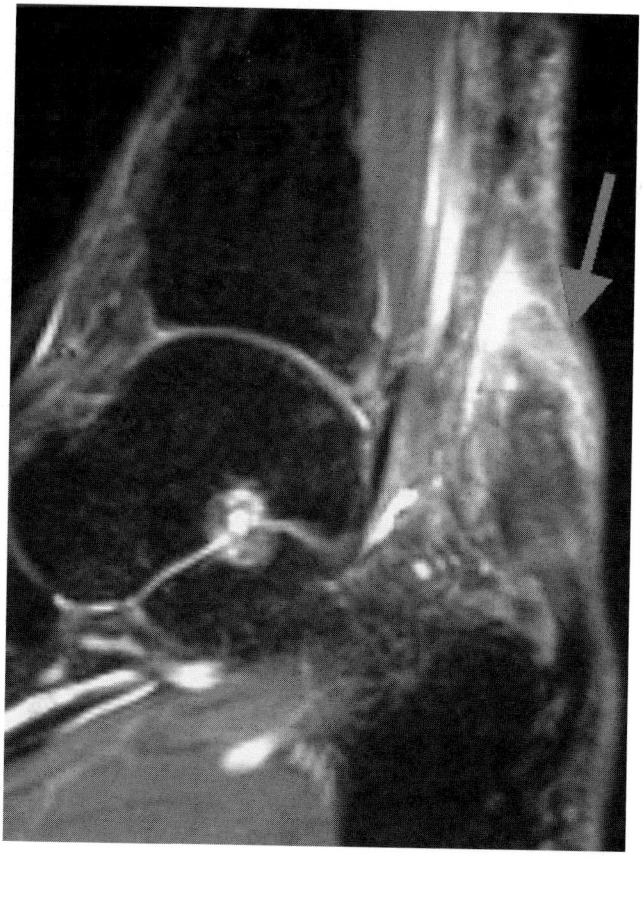

**Fig. 7.27** Sagittal fat-suppressed image of a gymnast showing a complete rupture of the Achilles tendon at the musculoskeletal junction.

## Imaging findings

### Magnetic resonance imaging

- Best evaluated on sagittal images.
- Discontinuity of uniform low signal of the tendon.
- Retraction of tendon with irregularity and enlargement of split tendon ends.
- High signal in torn tendon and adjacent soft tissues representing edema or hemorrhage.
- Useful in preoperative planning.
- Signal abnormalities may persist for at least a year following conservative management.

## Management

### Non-surgical

- Especially necessary in patients with low activity levels.
- Cast immobilization for 6–10 weeks with an above-knee cast with equinus or a below-knee cast with decreased equines.

### Surgical

- Reduced rate of recurrent rupture.
- Depends on grade of tear:
  - suturing to approximate ends for types 1 and 2
  - autogenous tendon graft flap for type 3
  - free tendon graft or synthetic tendon for type 4.
- Percutaneous repair possible.
- Alternative function bracing.
- Plantaris reinforcement.
- Casting after surgery for 4 weeks.
- Resumption of full athletic activity usually takes 4–6 months or longer after injury in the surgically treated patient.

# Tibialis posterior tendon tear

## Anatomy

- Tendinous continuation of the muscle belly within the deep posterior compartment of the calf attaches to the navicular tuberosity and six further lesser insertions in the forefoot, at the bases of the cuneiforms and the bases of metatarsals 2–4.
- Provides major support to the medial longitudinal arch during the planted foot phase of the gait cycle, and is responsible for both plantar flexion and inversion.
- Synergistic relationship with deltoid ligament.

## Mechanism of injury

- The mid-portion of the tendon is most vulnerable at the hypovascular area as it lies behind the medial malleolus and angles anteriorly.
- Compressive force of flexor retinaculum may contribute to injury.
- Chronic overuse or trauma in middle-aged females is the most frequent cause associated with arthropathies, obesity, hypertension, diabetes and steroids.
- Traumatic etiology is much less common (forced dorsiflexion with eversion, usually in young athletes).

## History and clinical findings

- Medial ankle pain and swelling.
- Weakness of supination/inversion.
- Flattening of longitudinal arch with pes planus with progressive hindfoot valgus, posterior subtalar joint subluxation and arthritis.

## Imaging findings

### Magnetic resonance imaging

- The tibialis posterior tendon is twice the transverse diameter of the other flexor tendons on images acquired perpendicular to the long axis of the tendon.
- Following injury, intrasubstance hemorrhage and edema results in tendon swelling to up to four times the transverse diameter of the other flexors (a type 1 tear or intrasubstance vertical split), often accompanied by tendon sheath inflammation, peritendinous fluid or tenosynovitis (Fig. 7.28).
- In chronicity, disrupted fibers become stretched and attenuated and the transverse diameter decreases to less than that of other flexors (a type 2 tear), finally progressing to complete disruption with discontinuity and tendon diastasis (a type 3 tear).
- May be associated with a bony spur on the posterior medial malleolus.
- Other secondary signs include loss of longitudinal arch, navicular–talus misalignment, hypertrophy of the medial tubercle of the navicular and thickening of the flexor retinaculum.
- Medial arch collapse may result in impaction bone bruising between the anterior talar process and the navicular, or between the calcaneus and the cuboid.

## Management

### Non-surgical

- Non-steroidal antiinflammatories.
- Taping to reduce the tension on the tibialis posterior.
- Tenography with ultrasound guidance and tendon sheath steroid injection.
- Orthotics with inversion with a medial heel implant to increase subtalar joint control and a lateral implant to control forefoot abduction.

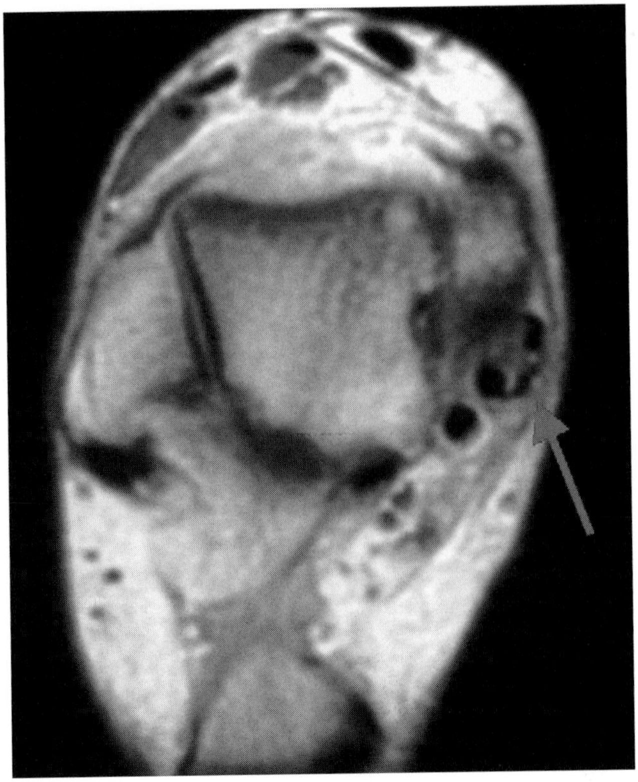

**Fig. 7.28** Axial $T_1$-weighted image showing intrasubstance signal change and swelling of the tibialis posterior tendon secondary to a type 1 tibialis posterior tendon rupture.

- Muscle strengthening exercises.
- Immobilization: lower leg cast immobilization with the foot in inversion for several weeks to months.
- If the patient is unresponsive after approximately 8 weeks of conservative treatment they are then considered surgical candidates.



## Surgical

- In type 1 injuries, peritendinous release, synovectomy and tendon debridement may be performed.
- In type 2 injuries, synovectomy, insertion reattachment or a transfer of flexor digitorum longus may be attempted.
- In type 3 injuries, tendon grafting (flexor digitorum longus tendon preferred).
- Following any surgical procedures the foot is immobilized for 3 weeks, firstly by a pressure dressing and then a posterior splint cast in plantar flexion and inversion. Passive motion is introduced to prevent adhesions forming within the surgical location.
- In severe cases, subtalar arthrodesis may be successful in restoring foot alignment and relieving symptoms.

# Flexor hallucis longus tears

## Anatomy

- Dominant flexor and inverter of the foot, with an extensive course to insert at the base of the distal phalanx of the great toe.
- Tendon runs in a fibro-osseous tunnel deep to the flexor retinaculum, along the posterior aspect of the talus which may be a site of friction leading to a tear in ballet dancers.
- Symptoms accentuated by an accessory os trigonum.

## Mechanism of injury

- Injury may occur proximally at the musculotendinous junction, usually secondary to chronic overuse at the level of the medial malleolus, as occurs in ballet dancers or distally, which is usually acute and secondary to stubbing the toe attempting to kick a football ('turf toe').
- Although peritendinous fluid is a useful marker of tendon insult and tenosynovitis, communication to the tibiotalar articulation in up to 20% of the normal population may account for the observation of fluid within the tendon sheath in the absence of symptoms.

## History and clinical findings

- Repetitive plantar- and dorsiflexion leading to tenosynovitis, e.g. foot to toe position in ballet dancers.
- Twisting ankle injury.
- Pain and swelling posterior to the medial malleolus.

## Imaging findings

### Magnetic resonance imaging

- Similar to other tendon or ligamentous injuries, intrasubstance rupture initially leads to tendon swelling prior to attenuation and rupture.
- Hyperintense fluid (STIR images) in the synovial sheath is disproportionate to the amount of fluid at the tibiotalar articulation, i.e. tenosynovitis.
- High signal in muscle if coexistent strain.
- Complete rupture is rare.



## Management

### Non-surgical

- NSAIDs, rest and immobilization.
- Modification of activity.
- Tenography with ultrasound guidance followed by tendon sheath steroid injection.

### Surgical

- Os trigonum excision if symptomatic.
- Release constricting the flexor hallucis longus tendon sheath.

# Tibialis anterior tendon tear

## Anatomy

- The tibialis anterior arises in the anterior compartment of the calf, giving rise to its tendon at the tibiotalar articulation which passes to the foot deep to the extensor retinaculum and inserts on the medial cuneiform and medial base of the first metatarsal.
- Dominant flexor and inverter of the foot.

## Mechanism of injury

- In most cases, rupture is the sequel of chronic trauma, with repeated encroachment of the tendon by the abrasive force of the extensor retinaculum over time, and in older patients especially.
- Dorsal exostoses may contribute to friction on the tendon.
- Acute rupture following forced extension and eversion (in younger patients).
- Spontaneous rupture is rare.

## History and clinical findings

- Weak dorsiflexion with or without foot drop.
- Palpable mass or gap in the tendon.

## Imaging findings

- The tendon is best visualized in the axial oblique plane with sections just distal to the medial malleolus.
- Partial or complete tears:
  - partial tear: focal high signal within enlarged tendon on STIR imaging
  - complete tear: tendon retraction with high-signal fluid-filled gap on STIR.

## Management

### Non-surgical

- Below-knee casting for older and less active patients.
- Suitable for minor tendon diastasis (<5 mm).

### Surgical

- In younger patients with higher activity levels.
- End-to-end repair.
- Tendon grafts if tendon ends are widely separated using tendons of the extensor digitorum longus or the peroneus brevis.

# Peroneal tendon injuries

## Anatomy

- The peroneal muscle bellies within the lateral compartment of the thigh give rise to the peroneus brevis and longus tendons at the ankle.
- The peroneal tendons (brevis anterior to longus) course around the lateral malleolus in a shared synovial sheath, within the slightly concave aspect of the fibular groove. Position within the fibular groove is maintained by a tight retinaculum, which prevents tendon subluxation.
- The peroneus brevis tendon passes along the lateral margin of the foot to insert at the base of the fifth metatarsal.
- The peroneus longus tendon courses beneath the cuboid to insert at the base of the first metatarsal and medial cuneiform.
- The function is to plantar flex and evert the foot and stabilize the lateral ankle joint.

## History and mechanism of injury

- The peroneus brevis tendon injury is more common than injury to the peroneus longus, suggesting that laxity of the superior peroneal retinaculum allows the brevis tendon to sublux and interpose between the peroneus longus tendon and fibrous edge of the fibula, resulting in shear-induced longitudinal tendon splits.
- Injury is usually a sequel to forced dorsiflexion or forced inversion.
- When secondary to inversion, injury is commonly accompanied by disruption of the superior peroneal retinaculum (with avulsion of a small fibular fragment at its site of attachment), fractures of the fibula, osteochondral lesions of the medial talar dome, lateral collateral ligament injury, sinus tarsi disruption and fractures of the base of the fifth metatarsal.
- Spontaneous ruptures are less common than traumatic.

## Clinical findings

- Chronic ankle pain behind and distal to the lateral malleolus and swelling of the peroneal sheath.
- ‘Popping’ and ‘clicking’ on the everting foot.
- In subluxation, snapping along the lateral ankle is present, with a sense of weakness or pain.
- Positive peroneal compression test (pain on compressing longus against brevis tendons).
- A proposed classification of tears of the peroneus brevis tendon is as follows:
  - grade 1: flattened tendon
  - grade 2: partial-thickness split less than 1 cm in length
  - grade 3: full-thickness split less than 2 cm in length
  - grade 4: full-thickness split more than 2 cm in length.

## Imaging findings

### Radiography

- The presence of an os peroneum fracture or proximal migration of the os peroneum is suggestive of peroneus longus rupture.

### Computerized tomography

- CT may also show pathology of the os peroneum.

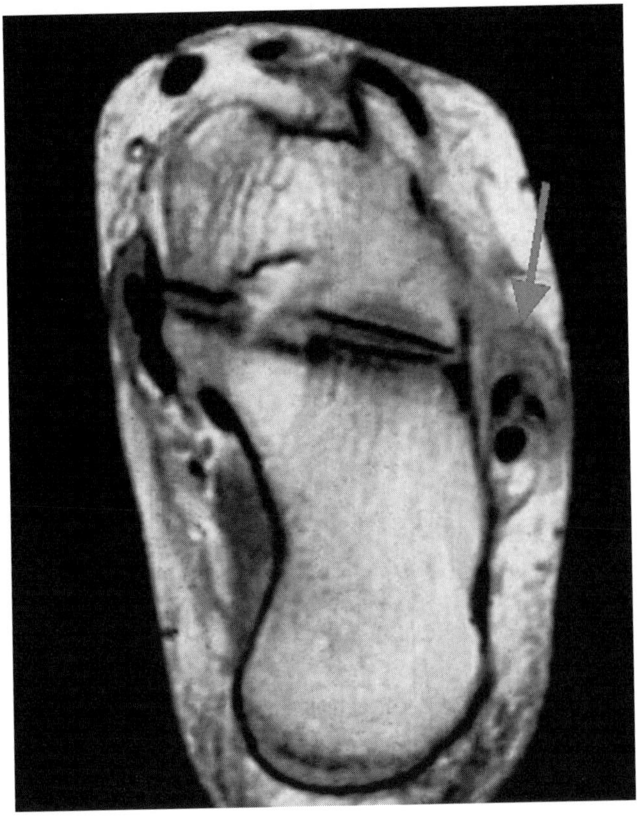

**Fig. 7.29** Following an inversion ankle sprain, an MR image shows a vertical split in the peroneus brevis tendon sheath with local inflammation.



Magnetic resonance imaging

- Tendons are best evaluated in either the axial or axial oblique planes (Fig. 7.29).
- Tendinitis manifests as peritendinous fluid and an increase in the transverse caliber.
- In most cases, reflecting mechanism, tears are longitudinal and manifest as a split or pseudo third tendon in the axial plane, although complete transverse tears are occasionally observed.
- Following retinacular disruption, tendons may sublux or completely dislocate, often only demonstrated by imaging the foot in eversion or dorsiflexion.

## Management

Non-surgical

- Antiinflammatories.
- Cast immobilization with a short leg non-weight-bearing cast for 4–6 weeks with the foot in plantar flexion and inversion for acute peroneal tendon dislocation (success rate of 50%) or tendinosis.
- Blind injection with corticosteroid is not recommended for the peroneal tendons as sural nerve damage or fat necrosis can occur. Tenography is performed with either ultrasound or fluoroscopic guidance followed by tendon sheath steroid injection.

## Surgical

- Surgery is indicated in the acute phase for peroneus brevis rupture, acute dislocation, os peroneum fracture and in peroneus longus tears associated with diminished function.
- The repair for subluxation usually involves the peroneal retinaculum, the lateral ankle ligaments and possibly the peroneal tendons. A procedure to deepen the fibular groove is also performed in many cases.
- Chronic tears of the peroneal tendons with persistent pain and instability require surgical repair. Tendinosis may cause nodules or scar tissue that may need debridement.
- Postoperatively, a short leg cast is applied for 4–6 weeks in most cases, with weight-bearing allowed after 4 weeks.
- After cast removal, return to activity with bracing is allowed once the strength and function of the ankle has been rehabilitated to 90% of that in the unaffected ankle.
- Proprioceptive rehabilitation is important.

# Anterior talofibular ligament tear

## Anatomy

- The lateral collateral ligament provides lateral stability to the tibiotalar articulation and is composed of the ATFL and PTFL, the CFL and the anterior (ATIF) and posterior tibiofibular ligaments (PTIF) ligaments, which are part of the syndesmosis.
- The ATFL runs anteromedially from the tip of the lateral malleolus (at the level of the malleolar fossa on the inner aspect of the malleolus) to the anterolateral aspect of the talus.

## Mechanism of injury

- Lateral collateral ligament injuries accompany up to 85% of ankle sprains, reflecting the commonest mechanism: inversion with plantar flexion.
- Injury tends to occur in an orderly sequence from anterior to posterior with rupture of the ATFL followed by rupture of the calcaneofibular and then, extremely rarely, the PTFL.
- ATFL taut in plantar flexion (cf. CFL taut in neutral).

## History and clinical findings

- Pain with weight-bearing and swelling around the lateral malleolus with or without hematoma.
- A sense of 'giving way'.
- Anterior drawer test (perform in 10° plantar flexion): >4 mm anterior displacement of the talus on the tibia indicates ATFL disruption. (Perform with the leg flexed and relaxed, e.g. over the side of the bed, one hand grasping the leg and the other the heel. Forward pressure is exerted to the heel with counterforce to the distal tibia and the degree of anterior translation of the talus is assessed.)
- Inversion stress test for combined ATFL and CFL instability. Place eversion stress on heel with the tibia fixed (ankle in neutral). More than 30° of tilt suggests CFL disruption. (Perform in the same position and apply varus force to the heel; this mainly tests the CFL.)
- Chapman's grading of lateral ankle sprains:
  - Grade 1: ligament stretching without a tear. There is little swelling or tenderness, minimal functional loss and no instability
  - Grade 2: partial macroscopic tear with moderate swelling and tenderness, decreased range of movement and mild or moderate instability
  - Grade 3: complete rupture with swelling, hemorrhage and tenderness, abnormal joint movement and instability.



## Imaging findings

### Radiography

- Avulsion injury or fracture.
- The role of stress radiography is controversial.

### Magnetic resonance imaging

- The ATFL is best visualized in the direct axial plane, especially $T_1$-weighted sequences (Fig. 7.30).
- In health, the ligament is a fine linear structure (5 mm wide) which is homogeneously hypointense on all sequences. Following injury, intrasubstance hemorrhage may result in ligamentous swelling and signal abnormality, often accompanied by incomplete tear of superior fibers (Fig. 7.31).

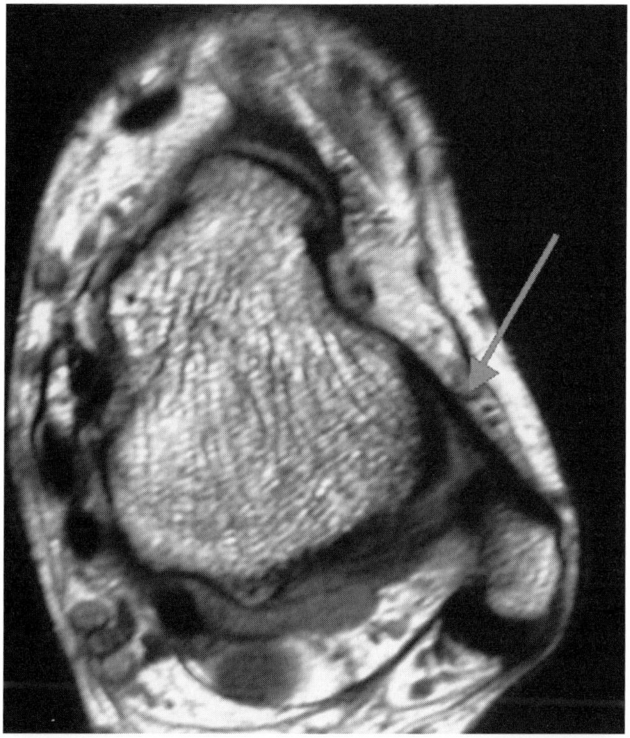

Fig. 7.30 Axial oblique MR image showing an intact talofibular ligament.

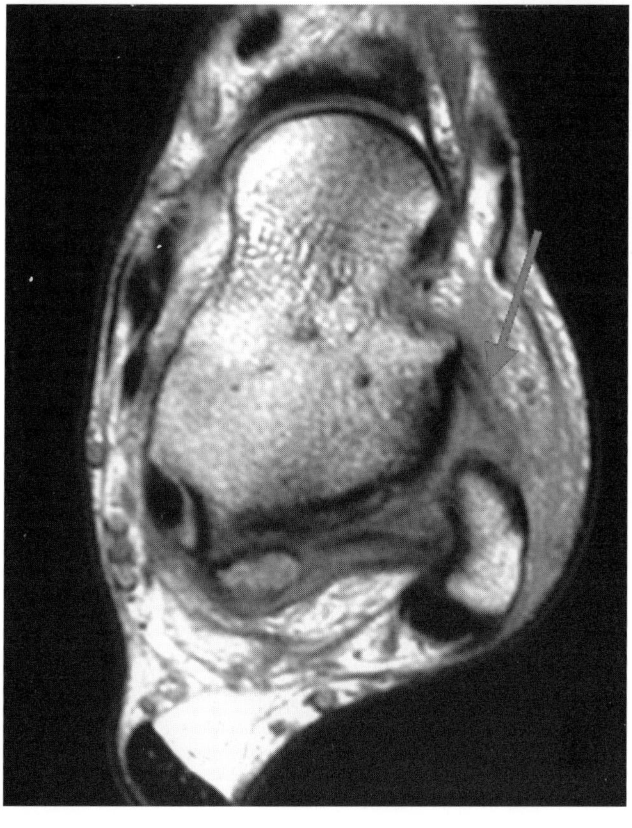

Fig. 7.31 Following inversion training ground injury in a professional soccer player, this image shows a signal abnormality and swelling of the talofibular ligament with some intact fibers secondary to sprain rather than a tear. This player returned to active training after 3 weeks.

- Complete rupture with retraction is always accompanied by joint effusion and leakage of fluid to neighboring soft tissues. The partially retracted ligament is often noted to billow freely within adjacent joint effusion.

## Management

### Non-surgical

- For grade I and grade II lateral ligament injuries: functional treatment including RICE (i.e. **r**est, **i**ce, **c**ompression, **e**levation) and short semi-rigid immobilization (for 6 weeks) followed by early motion exercises, then early weight-bearing and propioceptive ankle training.
- Of adjuvant therapies, only cryotherapy has been shown to be of benefit. Others such as ultrasound have not been shown to be beneficial.
- Treatment of grade III injuries is controversial with higher rates of chronic instability in non-surgical repair.

### Surgical

- Operative treatment produces better results than functional treatment.
- For acute grade III sprains and chronic instability.
- Surgical treatment in acute rupture employs a primary ligament repair type procedure generally.
- Currently, the Bronstrom–Gould procedure is probably the most often used.

# Calcaneofibular ligament tear

## Anatomy

- Extracapsular ligament providing lateral support to the ankle and subtalar joints.
- The CFL runs from the inferior aspect of the lateral malleolus posteriorly and distally to the lateral surface of the calcaneus (2 cm long and 5 mm wide).
- The CFL is normally taut when neutral.

## Mechanism of injury

- Twisting injury: dorsiflexion and internal rotation.
- Frequently combined with ATFL injury.

## History and clinical findings

- Pain and swelling in the lateral ankle with bruising distal to the lateral malleolus.
- Positive stress inversion (talar tilt) test: increased ankle supination; see the ATFL section above.
- Grading of injury as for the ATFL.

## Imaging findings

### Radiography

- See the ATFL section above.

### Arthrography

- Contrast leaks into peroneal tendon sheaths (for up to 1 week after a CFL tear).

### Magnetic resonance imaging

- The normal CFL is readily visualized on images acquired in an axial oblique plane prescribed perpendicular to the posterior subtalar joint or in the axial plane acquired in a plantar flexed foot.
- Fine linear structure deep to the peroneal tendons uniformly hypointense on all sequences.
- Following injury, intrasubstance hemorrhage and edema produce swelling and signal abnormality in the ligament enhancing its conspicuity (Fig. 7.32).
- Communication with peroneal tendon sheaths results in frequently identified associated peroneal tendon sheath fluid, and occasionally subluxation. Frequent peroneal retinacular thickening.
- MR arthrographic images in patients following rupture show free communication between the tibiotalar joint space and the peroneal tendon sheaths.
- Check for a coexistent ATFL tear.

## Management

### Non-surgical

- For grade I and II injuries, as for an ATFL tear.

### Surgical

- For acute grade III sprains or chronic instability.
- Primary repair is employed for acute or subacute disruption. A modified Bronstrom–Gould procedure is popular (includes a primary repair and augmentation with the extensor retinaculum).
- For chronic instability, ligament reconstruction is preferred, e.g. usually with peroneal tendons.

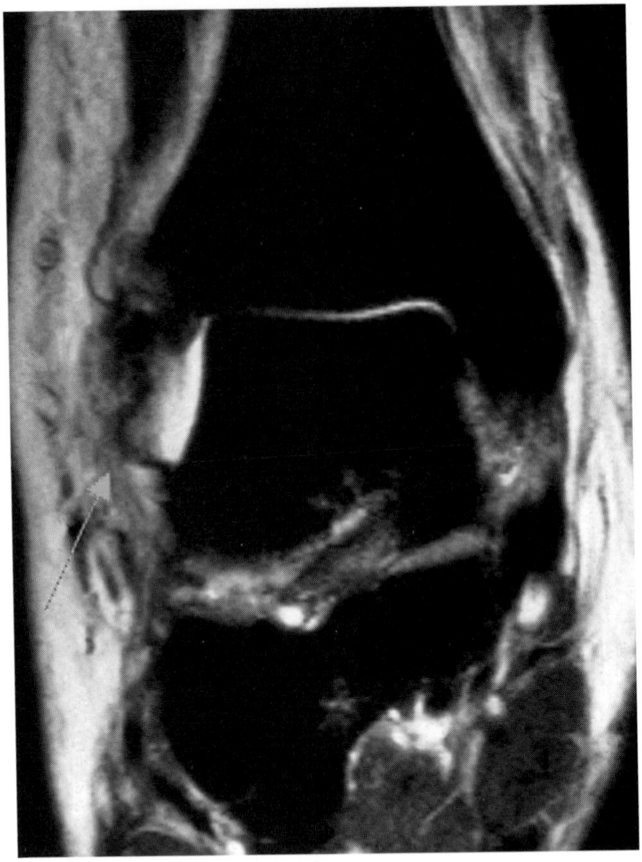

**Fig. 7.32** Coronal fat-suppressed MR image showing gross bimalleolar hemorrhage and edema accompanying a tear of the ATFL billowing in an associated joint effusion (arrow).

# Medial collateral ligament (deltoid ligament) tear

## Anatomy

- There are five components including the anterior and posterior tibiotalar, the tibiocalcaneal, the tibio spring and the tibionavicular ligaments.
- Classically, the ligament is divided into deep and superficial components, the superficial layer arising from the anterior margin of the medial malleolus and branching to the navicular, the sustentaculum, the calcaneus and to the medial tubercle of the talus; the deep layer arising from the posterior margin of the malleolus attaches to the medial aspect of the talus.

## Mechanism of injury

- Injury to the medial collateral ligament usually accompanies complex ankle trauma, invariably associated with disruption of the lateral collateral ligament or the syndesmosis; the superficial component usually fails first.
- Follows eversion or external rotation injury.
- Partial tears are more common than complete ones.

## History and clinical findings

- Swelling and tenderness at or anterior to the medial malleolus.
- Check for associated lateral ligament or syndesmosis injuries.
- Grading as before for lateral ligament injuries (1: stretching of ligament; 2: partial tear; 3: complete tear).
- The eversion test in neutral evaluates the superficial deltoid ligament complex.
- The external rotation stress test evaluates the syndesmotic ligaments and additionally the deep deltoid ligament (Fig. 7.33).

## Imaging findings

### Radiography

- Increase in the medial clear space (>4 mm) between the talus and the medial malleolus (often better seen on an anteroposterior – AP – view than a mortise view). The width of the medial clear space should equal the superomedial clear space.

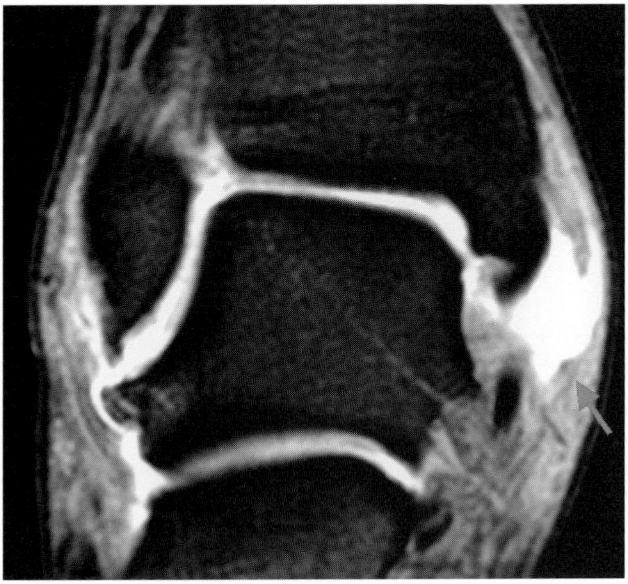

**Fig. 7.33** Coronal MR arthrogram showing complete disruption of the mid substance of the deltoid ligament with free communication to the overlying soft tissues (arrow).

- Associated bony abnormalities (malleolar or talar dome fracture, avulsion).
- Value of stress radiographs (positive if >2° of valgus tilt on valgus stress on AP view) is disputed.

Arthrography

- Rarely needed: shows the free passage of the contrast medium from the ankle joint at the medial malleolus.

Ultrasound

- Discontinuity of linear pattern of ligament fibers.
- Associated fluid around the tibiotalar articulation.

Computerized tomography

- Best for associated bony fractures.

Magnetic resonance imaging

- The fan-shaped components of the superficial medial collateral ligament are only visualized in multiple oblique planes. In contrast, the deep component is routinely identified on direct coronal images as a short striated structure.
- Interstitial hyperintensity on $T_2$-weighted images with loss of uniform hypointensity of the ligament.
- High-signal medial malleolar bone edema or associated fracture of the medial malleolus of osteochondral defect.

## Management

Non-surgical

- RICE.
- Protected weight-bearing for 3 or 4 weeks (bracing, splinting) and early functional treatment.
- Six week immobilization in a short leg cast for grade III sprains.



Surgical

- Not often used.
- Delayed primary repair.
- Want to avoid chronicity as this leads to lateral talar shift resulting from unrecognized malunited fracture of lateral malleolus or a syndesmotic injury, which widens the mortise and may produce chronic ankle instability.

# Syndesmosis sprain

## Anatomy

- The syndesmosis is the term used to describe the three stabilizing components of the inferior tibiofibular articulation: the ATIF and PTIF ligaments and the interosseous membrane.
- The ATIF ligament is a linear hypointense structure running from the anterior tibial tubercle laterally along the anterior margin of the inferior tibiofibular articulation to the fibula.
- The posterior inferior tibiofibular (PITF) ligament has a similar orientation to the ATIF and runs along the posterior margin of the tibiofibular articulation.

## Mechanism of injury

- Injury to the syndesmosis is uncommon in the absence of a fracture.
- Injury to the syndesmosis usually involves rupture to the AITF ligament and spares the PITF, which is stronger and, when stressed, results in an avulsion fracture at its insertion rather than soft-tissue rupture.
- Usually follows abduction, external rotation and dorsiflexion of the ankle.
- If untreated, chronic AITF ligament tear may produce AITF ligament thickening and fibrosis to produce a meniscoid lesion and secondary syndesmotic impingement.

## History and clinical findings

- Pain on external rotation.
- Direct palpation: palpate for tenderness over the syndesmosis.
- Squeeze test: at the mid calf, squeeze the fibula against the tibia and observe symptoms at the syndesmosis.
- External rotation test: forced external rotation may cause pain at the syndesmosis.
- Grading of syndesmotic ankle sprains:
  - 1st degree sprain: only a few ligament fibers are damaged within the interosseous membrane
  - 2nd degree sprain: more extensive damage to the interosseous membrane with some widening of the inferior tibiofibular joint
  - 3rd degree sprain: complete rupture of the interosseous ligament with gross widening of the tibiofibular joint and possible joint dislocation.

## Imaging findings

### Radiography

- Fibular fractures that begin proximal to tibial plafond are assumed to have some degree of injury of the syndesmosis.
- Dorsiflexion and external rotation will accentuate syndesmotic widening.
- Mortise view (leg internally rotated 15–20° so that the X-ray beam is nearly perpendicular to the intermalleolar line):
  1. The tibiofibular overlap should normally be >6 mm.
  2. The medial clear space should normally be <4 mm.
  3. The tibiofibular clear space (the cartilaginous space between the lateral border of the posterior tibia and the medial border of the fibula, measured 1 cm above the joint line) is normally <5?6 mm on both AP and mortise views.
  4. A tibiofibular clear space of >10 mm indicates a syndesmotic injury.
- AP view.

- Stress lateral view is more sensitive than a mortise view in determining syndesmotic injury.

**Computerized tomography**

- More sensitive than plain radiography for diastasis of less than 3 mm.

**Magnetic resonance imaging**

- The ligaments of the syndesmosis are readily visualized on direct axial images just proximal to the tibiotalar articulation (identification of the malleolar fossa on the inner aspect of the lateral malleolus is used to differentiate between the ATFL and PTFL, and the ATIF and PTIF, ligaments when any doubt exists).
- Often the AITF and PITF ligaments course slightly inferiorly and therefore can only be fully appreciated by reviewing serial images.
- ATIF ligament injury may result in intrasubstance hemorrhage and edema, or complete disruption accompanied by widening of the anterior joint space.
- Significant associations with ATFL injury, bone bruises, osteochondral lesions, tibiofibular joint congruity and height of the tibiofibular recess on MRI.

## Management

**Non-surgical**

- In the first 48–72 hours following the injury, follow the RICE protocol.
- Immobilization in a walking boot/brace for up to 1 week followed by functional exercises and strength training.
- Casting for 4 weeks is required or surgical fixation where refractory in grades 1 and 2.
- Grades 1 and 2 injuries normally take about 1 month to recover completely.
- In the early stages, ultrasound treatment is effective in encouraging the healing process and encouraging the formation of scar tissue to repair the ligament.



**Surgical**

- Open reduction, internal fixation (ORIF) in grade 3 injuries.
- Repair of the AITF ligament using the plantaris or peroneal tendons.
- Arthrodesis for severe pain and degenerative changes.

# Anterolateral impingement

**Anatomy**

- Describes soft-tissue impingement with associated pain between the anterolateral osseous structures of the ankle joint (the lateral gutter).

**Mechanism of injury**

- Follows trauma (especially plantar flexion with inversion), infection or arthritides.
- Most commonly secondary to synovitis or fibrous overgrowth following chronic tear of the ATFL or AITF ligament.
- Rarely, a tear results in a hyalinized connective tissue meniscoid lesion (a fibrocartilaginous mass extending from the AITF ligament joint capsule to the lateral gutter).

**History and clinical finding**

- Chronic pain in the anterolateral ankle following repeated ankle sprains, especially inversion injuries.
- No pain at rest with pain at push-off.
- Tender to palpation along the syndesmosis and anterior gutter with soft-tissue thickening.
- Limited and painful dorsiflexion.
- Snapping when testing for inversion stability.
- Soft-tissue thickening in the anterior aspect of the lateral gutter.

## Imaging findings

**Radiography**

- Usually not helpful but it may show anterolateral osteophytes or a loose body.

**Isotope bone scan and computerized tomography**

- May be negative.

**Magnetic resonance imaging**

- Fluid in the anterolateral gutter (bright on $T_2$-weighted images) with thickened synovium (intermediate to a low signal on $T_2$-weighted images) on axial images.
- May see an associated loose body (hypointense on $T_2$-weighted images).
- ATFL or AIFL ligament damage.
- Fibrosis (low signal on $T_1$- and $T_2$-weighted images) or an intermediate-signal meniscoid lesion.
- Talar dome chondromalacia is common (coronal $T_1$-weighted scans show thinning of the intermediate signal cartilage with subchondral bone edema).

## Management

**Non-surgical**

- NSAIDs.
- Physiotherapy, especially dorsiflexion stretching.
- Heel wedge or ankle bracing.

**Surgical**

- Arthroscopic debridement of inflammatory tissue, loose body and osteophyte removal.
- Splinting post surgery.

# Anterior impingement (footballers' ankle)

## Anatomy

- Limitation of ankle dorsiflexion secondary to osteophyte formation at the distal tibial plafond and anterosuperior talar neck.

## Mechanism of injury

- Osteophyte formation at the anterior tibial plafond where the ankle joint capsule attaches, leading to anterior inflammation and synovitis.
- Subsequent degeneration results in 'contrecoup' osteophyte formation on the anterior neck of the talus with or without localized divot formation at the talar neck.
- Follows repetitive dorsiflexion microtrauma (as in professional soccer players) or repetitive hyperflexion with traction at the joint capsule attachment.

## History and clinical findings

- Pain on foot dorsiflexion or anterior ankle pain when striking a ball.
- Anterior ankle tenderness to palpation with or without a palpable bony lump.

## Imaging findings

### Radiography

- Anterior tibial osteophyte on lateral films.
- A lateral radiograph is sometimes insufficient to detect all anteriorly located osteophytes; an oblique radiograph is a useful adjunct to detect anteromedial tibial and talar osteophytes.

### Computerized tomography

- Advocated by some parties to determine location, size, shape and number of osteophytes (Fig. 7.34).
- Inferior to MRI for soft-tissue structures.



### Magnetic resonance imaging

- Sagittal slices show low-signal osteophytes and high-signal tibiotalar joint effusion ($T_2$-weighted image) (Fig. 7.35).
- Synovial thickening of the anterior to talar neck.
- Associated subchondral edema adjacent to osteophytes.
- Cartilaginous 'divot' on the talar neck.

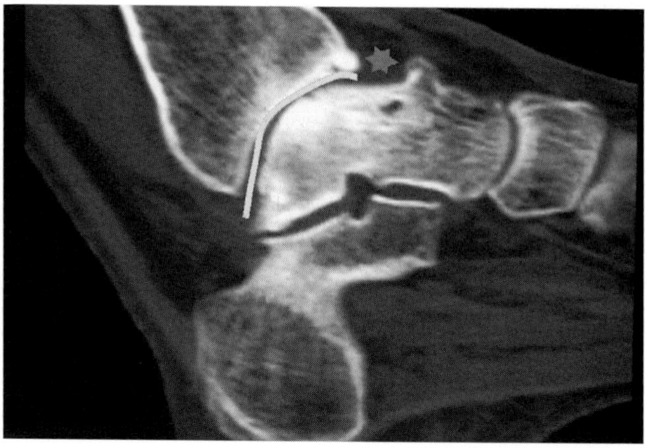

**Fig. 7.34** Sagittal reformatted CT image showing tibiotalar degenerative arthritis with contrecoup spurs from the anterior tibial plafond and the superior margin of the anterior talar process, which is typical of footballer's ankle.

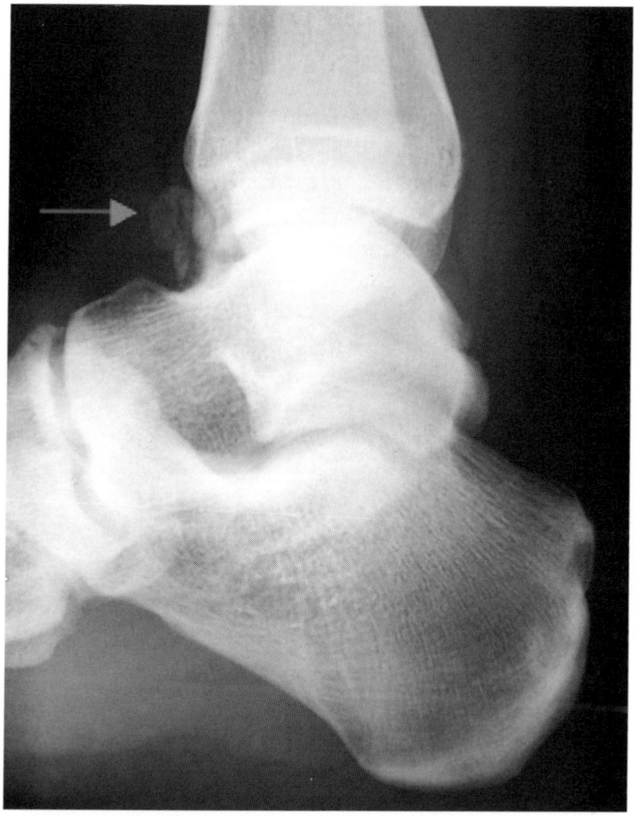

(a)

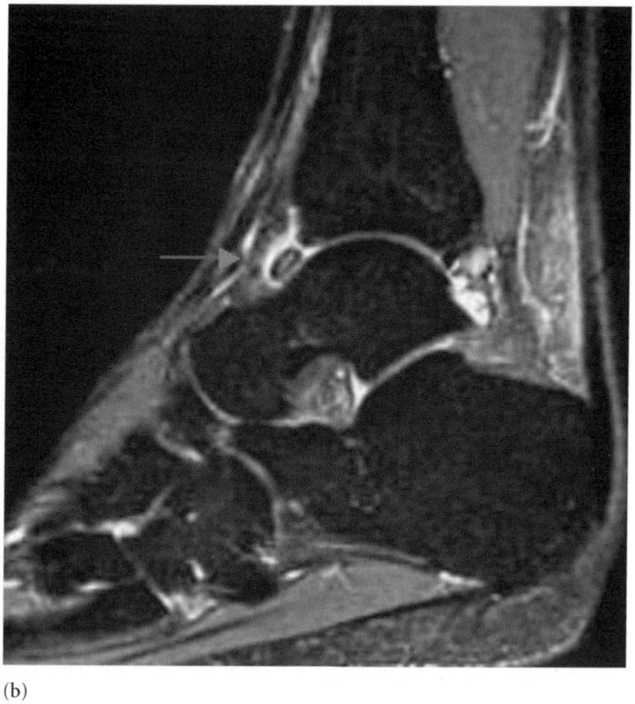

(b)

**Fig. 7.35** (**a**) Radiograph showing footballer's ankle with a secondary loose fragment in the anterior tibiotalar joint recess. This is better identified on (**b**) a sagittal fat-suppressed image of the ankle.

## Management

### Non-surgical

- Mobility, stretching and strengthening exercises.
- Wear a heat retainer or support.
- Antiinflammatories.
- Local steroid injection provides symptomatic relief.

### Surgical

- Arthroscopic osteophyte resection and removal of hypertrophic synovium.
- Open surgical resection of larger osteophytes.

## Syndesmotic impingement

**Anatomy**

- Occurs at the tibiofibular syndesmosis (composed of the ATIF and PTIF ligaments and the interosseous membrane).

**Mechanism of injury**

- Soft-tissue impingement between the osseous structures of the syndesmosis, usually manifest by thickening and synovitis at the site of a chronic tear of the AITF ligament.
- Bassett's ligament (a component of a thickened AITF ligament which encroaches on the talar dome).
- Secondary to repetitive external rotation or hyperdorsiflexion.

**History and clinical findings**

- Pain with push-off and limited dorsiflexion.
- Tenderness along the syndesmosis and the interosseous membrane.
- Sensation of 'popping' anteriorly.
- On dorsiflexion, there is anterior extrusion of the talar dome.

**Imaging findings**

- Plain radiography, isotope bone scans and CT are usually not helpful.

Magnetic resonance imaging

- Axial images show soft-tissue thickening in syndesmotic space.
- Hyperintense fluid on $T_2$-weighted images with possible low-signal intensity loose bodies.
- Associated AITF ligament tear.
- Cartilage loss and subchondral bone edema at the talar dome.

**Management**

Non-surgical

- Antiinflammatories and physiotherapy, and intra-articular steroid injection.

Surgical

- Arthroscopic resection of inflamed synovium and AITF ligament debridement.

# Posterior impingement

## Anatomy

- Impingement of posterior soft tissues between the posterolateral osseous structures of the ankle during weight-bearing with the foot in plantar flexion.

## Mechanism of injury

- In most cases, the condition reflects impingement of a hypertrophied PITF ligament on the posterior intermalleolar ligament.
- Often associated with an os trigonum (although the majority of patients with os trigonum do not have posterior impingement).
- Common in ballet dancers and gymnasts due to repeated microtrauma during plantar flexion with inversion.

## History and clinical findings

- Tenderness at the back of the ankle, which is worsened with weight-bearing in plantar flexion.
- Pain on passive ankle plantar flexion.
- Fullness in the posterior soft tissues.

## Imaging findings

### Radiography

- Os trigonum on lateral ankle X-ray may be seen (Fig. 7.36).

### Fluoroscopy

- Local steroid/anesthetic injection may relieve pain and provide diagnosis.

### Magnetic resonance imaging

- Coronal and sagittal images show a thickened synovium with fluid surrounding posterior ligaments (high signal on $T_2$-weighted images).
- May see hyperintense synovial nodules or ganglion cysts.
- Fibrotic tissue low-signal intensity on all sequences.



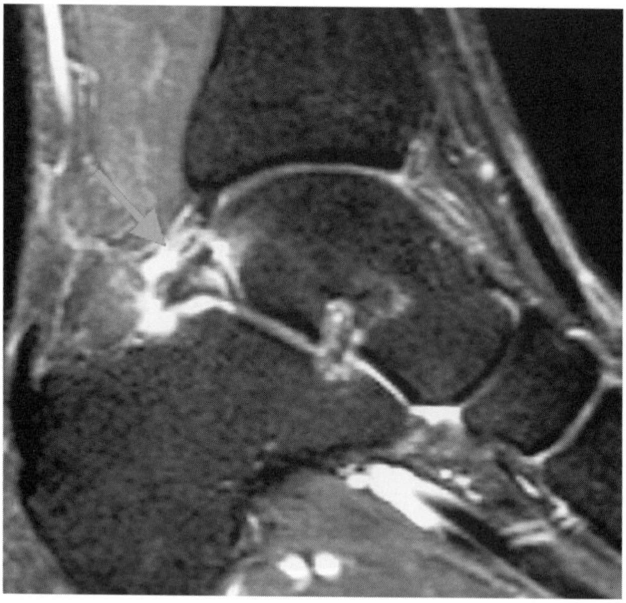

**Fig. 7.36** Sagittal fat-suppressed image showing bone edema and inflammation surrounding the os trigonum, which is typical of os trigonum syndrome. In this case, symptoms developed immediately following a forced plantar flexion injury, suggesting that the appearance actually represents an acute fracture (Shepherd's fracture). Symptoms failed to resolve and at 2 weeks a resection of the posterior fragment was performed. The player returned to professional competitive soccer 4 weeks following surgery.

## Management

### Non-surgical

- Rest and avoidance of the precipitating activity.
- Ankle muscle conditioning.
- NSAIDs.
- Steroid injection.

### Surgical

- Rarely needed: removal of the os trigonum and associated soft-tissue debridement.

# Sinus tarsi syndrome

## Anatomy

- The sinus tarsi is a cone-shaped space between the inferolateral border of the talus and superolateral surface of the calcaneus.
- Contains the interosseous talocalcaneal ligament.
- In health, the sinus tarsi is predominantly filled with fat allowing the space to narrow slightly on inversion.
- On eversion, widening of the space and hence stability between the talus and calcaneus is maintained by both the cervical and interosseous ligaments.
- It is richly vascularized, so ruptured ligaments readily heal without surgical intervention, although scarring and persistent laxity may result in long-term instability.

## Mechanism of injury

- Minor trauma (inversion or eversion) may manifest as hemorrhage, edema and secondary compression of neurovascular structures within the space, and hence acute pain.
- Acute inversion may occasionally result in disruption of ligamentous structures and gross subtalar instability.
- Never occurs as an isolated lesion but always involves rupture of the CFL or ATFL.
- Occasionally disruption of the ligaments precedes or is a part of subtalar dislocation.

## History and clinical findings

- Pain in the lateral aspect of the hindfoot at the sinus tarsi, which is worst when weight-bearing on uneven ground.
- Pain relief at rest.
- Feeling of ankle giving way.
- History of previous ankle sprain (usually significant inversion injury) in about 70% of patients.
- Possible associated subtalar and lateral ankle instability.
- Pain increases with firm palpation of the lateral opening of the sinus tarsi.



## Imaging findings

### Radiography

- Often non-contributory.
- Normal stress radiography.
- Conventional arthrography.
- Rarely performed but may show loss of sinus tarsi filling.
- May be combined with diagnostic local anesthetic injection.

### Magnetic resonance imaging

- Readily visualized on direct coronal images; fat-suppressed inversion recovery images facilitate the detection of edema and hemorrhage.
- Turbo spin echo $T_1$-weighted images allow the evaluation of interosseous and cervical ligaments; in sinus tarsi syndrome, the ligaments are poorly defined.
- Secondary subchondral edema and cystic change appear as a high signal on $T_2$-weighted sequences.
- In practice, following eversion injury, coronal imaging should be extended through the sinus tarsi to the base of the fifth metatarsal to enable evaluation of the tibiotalar articulation and to detect injury within the sinus tarsi and at the base of the fifth metatarsal.

## Management

### Non-surgical

- Physiotherapy retraining of the peroneal and calf muscles, including general strengthening and proprioception program.
- Antiinflammatories.
- Orthotics to correct foot biomechanics.
- Consecutive image-guided injection of steroid/local anesthetic into sinus: the majority respond.

### Surgical

- Sinus tarsectomy: excision of the tarsal canal contents via open or arthroscopic routes.
- More recently, subtalar arthroscopy and synovectomy have been employed successfully.
- Arthrodesis of the posterior facet of the subtalar joint if these measures fail.

# Ankle fractures

## Anatomy

- Important anatomic features include ankle mortise configuration with surrounding supporting tendons and ligaments.

## Mechanism of injury

- As below, the injury type is determined by foot position and the direction of force at impact.

## History and clinical findings

- Swelling and ecchymosis.
- Tenderness over the bone.
- Inability to bear weight.
- Fibular compression test is positive.
- Three classifications are commonly employed to describe a fracture at the ankle, based either on the mechanism of injury (Lauge–Hansen classification), radiographic anatomy (Henderson classification) or on the level of the fracture of the fibula (an attempt to triage patients into those who are and are not likely to have disruption of the syndesmosis: Danis–Weber classification).

### The Lauge–Hansen classification

- Allows a directed search for specific abnormalities when reviewing images following ankle trauma.
- Supination (inversion) injuries, which occur more frequently than eversion injuries, are associated with lateral traction and either tear of the lateral collateral ligament or transverse fracture of the distal fibula associated with oblique impaction fracture of the medial malleolus.
- When supination is accompanied by adduction (essentially simple inversion), the lateral collateral ligament usually tears while the syndesmosis remains intact.
- When supination is accompanied by external rotation (the leg internally rotates on the planted supinated foot), both the lateral collateral ligament and the anterior syndesmosis tend to rupture and torque forces tend to produce an oblique fracture extending superiorly from anteroinferior to posterosuperior. This is the most common mechanism (50–75%) of malleolar fractures.
- Pronation (eversion) injuries result in medial traction either manifest as transverse fracture through the medial malleolus or disruption of the medial collateral ligament accompanied by oblique impaction fracture through the fibula.
- When pronation is accompanied by abduction (essentially simple eversion), traction produces medial collateral disruption or medial malleolar transverse fracture accompanied by disruption of the syndesmosis. Additional lateral displacement of the talus produces an oblique fracture at or above the syndesmosis.
- When pronation is accompanied by external rotation, following medial malleolar or ligamentous injury, the anterior syndesmosis tears and the fibula fractures in a spiral or oblique manner from anteroinferior to posterosuperior. If torque forces are transmitted to the neck of the fibula, the term Maisonneuve fracture is used. Vertical forces driving the talus into the distal tibia result in an impaction fracture, the location of which is dictated by the position of the foot and the amount of loading that produces the injury.

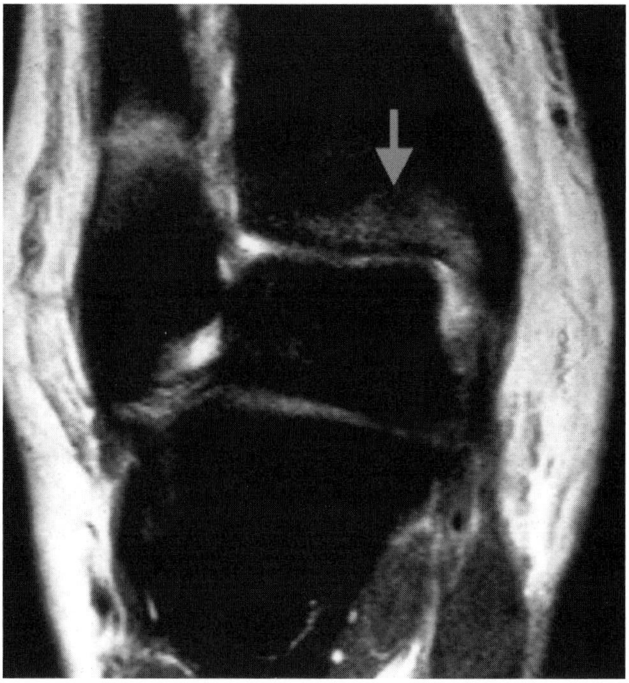

**Fig. 7.37** Coronal fat-suppressed image showing a transverse fracture of the distal fibula following an inversion injury with an associated impaction bone bruise of the tibial plafond (arrow).

### The Danis–Weber classification

- There are three types:
- Type A: the fibular fracture is below the syndesmosis secondary to supination.
- Type B: the fibular fracture begins at or near the syndesmosis secondary to supination external rotation (the syndesmosis is disrupted in 50% of cases).
- Type C: the fibular fracture begins above the syndesmosis secondary to pronation with external rotation. In type C injuries, fibular fracture may be diaphyseal or in the proximal fibula (Maisonneuve's fracture) (Fig. 7.37).

## Imaging findings

### Radiography

- AP, lateral and mortise (oblique internal rotation) views.
- Mortise view: the leg is internally rotated 10–20° so that the lateral malleolus (which is normally posterior to the medial malleolus) is at the same horizontal level as the medial malleolus and the tibia and fibula are not overlapping. This provides talar dome and joint clear space information.
- Important to image the proximal fibula.

### Isotope bone scan

- Not usually employed but can be used for occult fractures, especially of the talar dome.

### Computerized tomography

- Best for bone detail.
- With 3D reformats for possible intra-articular extension and degree of comminution.

### Magnetic resonance imaging

- Marrow edema (high signal on $T_2$-weighted images or STIR) may be diffuse or localized to the fracture site.
- Associated ligamentous and cartilage injuries are best seen with MRI.

- MR arthrography improves the evaluation of syndesmotic and collateral ligament integrity: extension of contrast 1 cm above the inferior tibiofibular articulation suggests syndesmotic injury; extravasation to the peroneal tendon sheath indicates CFL disruption.
- When clinically suspected, gradient echo sequences are used to enhance susceptibility blooming of both metal and wooden soft-tissue foreign bodies.

## Management

### Non-surgical

- Immediate treatment with RICE.
- Closed reduction followed by casting for 4–8 weeks (2–4 weeks in a long-leg cast and then 2–4 weeks in a short-leg nonwalking cast) if there is no displacement and the ankle joint is stable.
- Joint proprioceptive exercises should commence early.
- Post-reduction radiographs must show that the joint space is symmetric on a mortise view.
- Alignment important afterwards to avoid post-traumatic arthritis.

### Surgical

- If there is joint instability or displacement.
- Fractures that involve the weight-bearing surface of the plafond generally require open reduction and internal fixation in contrast to malleolar fractures.

## Specifically named ankle fractures

### Pilon fracture

- This is an impaction fracture of the distal tibia secondary to gross axial loading.
- Undisplaced fractures may be treated conservatively; displaced fractures usually require surgical reconstruction and immobilization.
- CT is routinely used in these cases to document the number and position of the fragments in severely comminuted cases.



### Triplane fracture

- Complicates external rotation of the foot at the ankle, most frequently during the 18-month period of asymmetric growth plate closure in the distal tibia (between 13–15 years of age in males and 12–14 years in females).
- Characterized by three distinct fracture planes: a vertical fracture through the epiphysis; a horizontal fracture through the physis; and an oblique fracture through the metaphysis (constituting a Salter 4 fracture).
- In most cases imaging reveals lateral displacement of the epiphyseal fragment.
- Undisplaced fractures may be treated conservatively; displaced fractures usually require screw fixation (Fig. 7.38).

### Tillaux fracture

- Described by Paul Tillaux in 1848, this fracture is a subtle avulsion from the anterolateral growth plate of the distal tibia, resulting from stress imposed by extreme external rotation.
- In adolescence, the growth plate of the distal tibia closes from medial to lateral. In such a way, traction on the ATIF ligament in external rotation (rather than rupturing the ligament) is transmitted to bone and results in an avulsion at the junction of fused and unfused growth plate (Salter 3 type fracture).

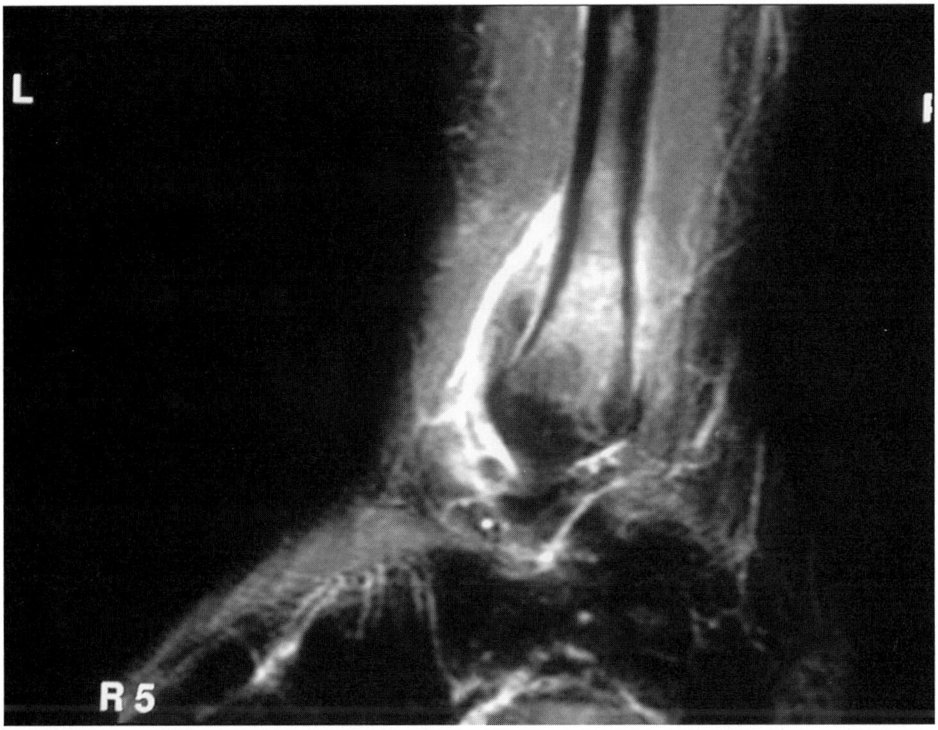


**Fig. 7.38** Fat-suppressed sagittal MR image showing extensive bone edema and inflammation at the site of an undisplaced radiographically occult fracture.



- Untreated, the fracture fails to heal as traction from the ATIF ligament draws fracture surfaces apart. Early diagnosis and either immobilization or surgical repair in displaced fractures must be undertaken.
- Diagnosis usually apparent on conventional radiographs, particularly oblique mortise views.
- Being predominantly traction rather than impaction in origin, adjacent marrow edema on MRI is usually limited.

# Calcaneal fractures

## Anatomy

- The middle third of the calcaneus supports the posterior facet.
- The tarsal canal and sinus tarsi separate the posterior from the middle and anterior facets.
- Anteriorly articulates with the cuboid.
- Böhler's angle is defined by the intersection of a line drawn from the anterior process of the calcaneus to the peak of the posterior articular surface with a line drawn from the peak of the posterior articular process to the peak of the posterior tuberosity. Normally this angle is between 25° and 40°.
- A decrease in Böhler's angle implies calcaneal fracture and subtalar joint disruption.

## Mechanism of injury

- Most commonly fractured tarsal bone (60% of tarsal bone injuries).
- The fracture, usually compression in nature, follows significant axial loading, e.g. a fall from a height. As such, fractures are sometimes bilateral (5–10%).
- May be accompanied by compression fractures at the dorsolumbar junction (10%).
- Rowe classifies calcaneal fractures 1 through 5 ranging from extra-articular (stage 1) through intra-articular comminuted (stage 5) fractures.
- Most compression fractures (75%) result in marked comminution, loss of height and extension of fracture to the articular surfaces of the posterior subtalar joint.
- In contrast, extra-articular fractures involving the margins of the calcaneus (accounting for 25% of cases) are usually a sequel to rotational injury (75% extra-articular in children).

## Clinical findings

- Ankle pain with an inability to bear weight and reduced ankle movement.
- Bruising over the heel and arch of the foot.



## Imaging findings

### Radiography

- Lateral foot and axial heel (Harris's view).
- Posterior facet visualized by dorsiflexing the foot with internal rotation.
- Böhler's angle decreased.

### Computerized tomography

- CT with reformatted images is now most frequently employed to evaluate these complex fractures. Sanders' classification is used to determine the number of fragments in the posterior facet on coronal CT.
- Specifically, tomographic imaging is undertaken to assess the amount of step-off or distraction at posterior subtalar articulations, the amount of rotation and displacement of bone fragments, and the size and position of the fixed sustentacular fragments (used for pin fixation).
- Both CT and MR imaging facilitate identification of entrapped peroneal and flexor hallucis tendons.

### Magnetic resonance imaging

- Allows the evaluation of osseous injury, except in severely comminuted cases.
- Improves the evaluation of associated soft-tissue injury (unlike many other fractures, soft-tissue injury around the calcaneus is not subtle and may be equally perceived at CT).
- Linear hyperintensity on STIR in stress fractures (Fig. 7.39).

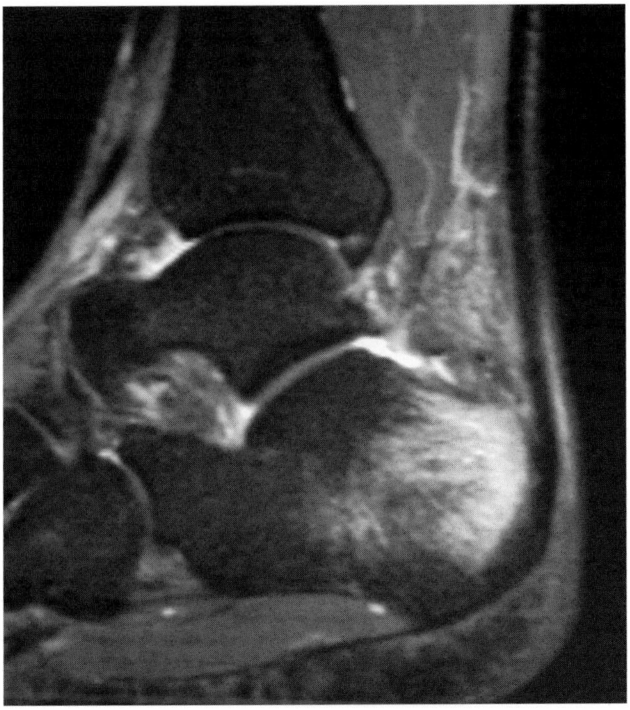

**Fig. 7.39** Sagittal image, in an elite rugby player, showing extensive calcaneal bone edema with a curvilinear orientation secondary to a stress-induced bone bruising. The player was in a competitive match 24 hours following this image despite heel pain but subsequently required 4 weeks' rest before full recovery.

## Management

### Non-surgical

- Conservative for undisplaced or minimally displaced intra-articular fractures.
- Early mobilization for non-displaced extra-articular calcaneal fractures.
- Casting is controversial. Some authorities suggest that patients wear a short-leg cast or walking boot for about 6 weeks.

### Surgical

- Most displaced fractures are managed operatively but these patients typically experience residual stiffness of their subtalar joint which may adversely affect future athletic performance.
- Arthrodesis if there is severe comminution.

# Talar fractures

## Anatomy

- The talus has the important biomechanical function of distributing weight during gait (60% of talar surfaces are covered by articular cartilage) and because of its susceptibility to ischemic necrosis following trauma.
- More than one third of fractures of the talus involve the neck. When displaced, fractures at this site disrupt supply from both the dorsalis pedis artery and the sinus tarsi (the major vascular supply to the talus), invariably resulting in osteonecrosis.
- Fractures may also involve the talar body and head, and the medial and posterior talar processes.
- Although osteonecrosis is usually self-limiting and eventually heals with non-weight-bearing, it is a significant cause of delayed union following fracture.

## Mechanism of injury

- Injury occurs secondary to axial loading on a hyperextended foot, such as occurs when drivers slam their feet onto the brakes during motor vehicle accidents. The injury was so common in World War 1 pilots that talar neck fracture was termed 'aviator's astragalus'.
- Hawkins describes three types of talar neck fracture:
  - type 1: a non-displaced fracture of the talar neck in which osteonecrosis rarely occurs
  - type 2: a displaced fracture of the talar neck with subluxation or dislocation of the subtalar joint (osteonecrosis in up to 50% cases)
  - type 3: a displaced fracture of the talar neck with complete dislocation of the body of the talus from the subtalar and tibiotalar articulations (osteonecrosis in up to 100% of cases).



## History and clinical findings

- Ankle pain and swelling with bruising.
- 15% of talar fractures are open.

## Imaging findings

### Radiography

- The most useful view is often a lateral view (for fractures of the head, neck and body and posterior process of the talus).
- Lateral process fractures are better seen on AP or mortise views.
- Supplemental views (e.g. oblique) for extent of fracture.

### Computerized tomography

- 3D reformats are useful in comminuted fractures.

### Magnetic resonance imaging

- Although identification of subchondral atrophy on a radiograph at 6 weeks (Hawkins' sign) excludes osteonecrosis, MR imaging is the only definitive diagnostic tool allowing diagnosis as early as 3 weeks.
- Imaging in three planes is used to identify marrow edema and cartilage damage in addition to this.

## Management

### Non-surgical

- Short casting.

### Surgical

- Displaced fractures require open reduction and internal fixation.

# Metatarsal stress fracture

## Anatomy

- The 2nd and 3rd metatarsal bones are the most commonly affected (the March fracture).
- The most common sites are the diaphysis or neck of the metatarsal.

## Mechanism of injury

- This fracture comprises 35% of all foot fractures.
- Stress repetitive trauma to normal bones either as a result of primary overuse or as a result of secondary overuse in an attempt to compensate for adjacent injury.
- Metatarsals are the most common sites of stress fractures (notably the 2nd metatarsal), especially in athletes triggered by impaction and are often associated with extensive marrow edema.
- Imposed stress during jogging promotes central plantar bowing of the metatarsal in the toe-off phase and initially induces acute local pain.
- Local periosteal disruption results in the development of marginal periosteal reaction with new bone formation parallel to the long axis of the bone.
- Persistent stress ultimately leads to bone fatigue and the development of a linear break traversing the shaft perpendicular to its long axis.

## History and clinical findings

- Often no recollection of injury.
- Gradual onset of pain in the forefoot, especially after activity.
- Tenderness on palpation of the affected metatarsal bone.

## Imaging findings

### Radiography

- Although changes are ultimately visualized on conventional radiographs, many patients present with symptoms in the absence of radiographic abnormality.
- May take 1–2 months to become radiographically apparent.
- Look for periosteal reaction.

### Isotope bone scan

- Positive usually within the first 2 weeks.

### Computerized tomography

- Usually not required.
- For fracture displacement, associated metatarsal dislocation.

### Magnetic resonance imaging

- Extensive marrow edema within the shafts of non-displaced fractures is readily identified on fat-suppressed MT images up to 4 weeks before the development of periosteal reaction and may be associated with an extensive mass such as circumferential soft-tissue edema (Fig. 7.40).

## Management

### Non-surgical

- Early diagnosis and enforced non-weight-bearing may promote early healing.
- Most fractures treated non-operatively with activity reduction (up to 6 weeks), icing and/or foot splinting.
- Use physical therapy in the later stages of healing.
- Occasionally a plaster cast is necessary if there is severe pain.

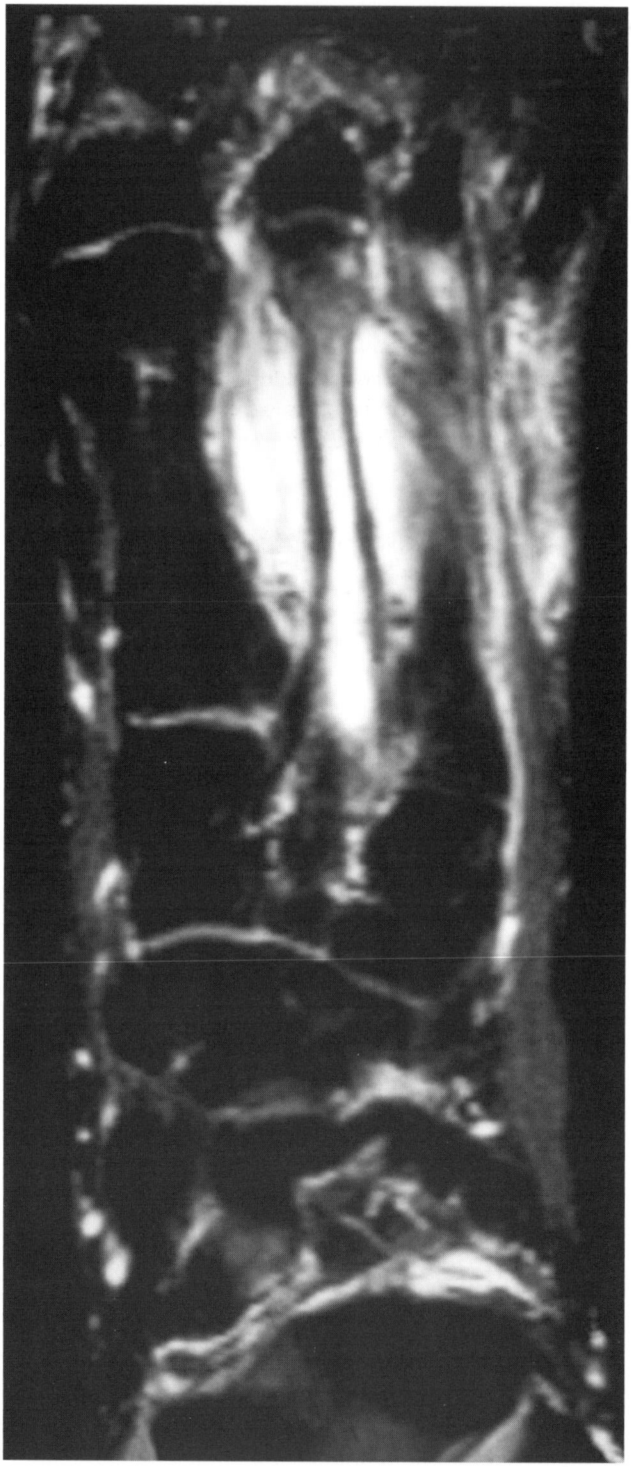

**Fig. 7.40** Coronal fat-suppressed image showing extensive bone edema within the shaft of the 2nd metatarsal secondary to a stress fracture in a long-distance runner. Radiographs showed no abnormality.



## Surgical

- Proximal 5th metatarsal stress fractures (Jones' fracture) have a propensity for non-union and malunion, and refracture.
- Fixation of these fractures with an intramedullary screw is preferred to casting to decrease healing time and facilitate an early return to activity.

## Lisfranc's (tarsometatarsal) fracture dislocation

### Anatomy

- Lisfranc's joint is the articulation between the metatarsal bases and the corresponding tarsal bones (cuboid medially and cuneiforms laterally).
- The 2nd metatarsal is important for stability. Lisfranc's ligament connects this bone to the medial cuneiform.

### Mechanism of injury

- This involves dorsal dislocation and fractures at the tarsometatarsal joints with lateral shift of the 2nd to 5th metatarsals.
- Termed homolateral if the 1st metatarsal is also laterally deviated, and divergent if it is displaced medially.
- Direct crush injury is less common, e.g. in a road traffic accident.
- Indirect mechanism involves forced plantar flexion of the forefoot on the rearfoot, e.g. a backwards fall with the toes trapped as when the foot is caught in a stirrup.

### History and clinical findings

- Midfoot pain, worse with weight-bearing.
- Foot deformity, swelling and bruising.
- Pain on palpation of the midfoot with palpable metatarsal displacement.

### Imaging findings

#### Radiography

- AP view: the medial aspect of the 2nd metatarsal should align with the medial aspect of the intermediate cuneiform (lateral metatarsal displacement in Lisfranc's fracture).
- Oblique view: the lateral aspect of the 1st metatarsal should align with the lateral aspect of the medial cuneiform (lateral metatarsal offset in Lisfranc's fracture).



#### Computerized tomography

- Superior axial visualization to check for dislocation and bone fragment number and location.

#### Magnetic resonance imaging

- Extensive soft-tissue and bone marrow edema on $T_2$-weighted axial images.
- Lisfranc's ligament irregularity, thickening and edema.
- Alignment readily demonstrated as homolateral or divergent.

### Management

#### Non-surgical

- Closed manipulation and casting may be attempted but generally management is surgical to reduce morbidity (especially subsequent post-traumatic arthritis).

#### Surgical

- ORIF to restore anatomic alignment.
- Occasionally percutaneous wire fixation is employed in undisplaced unstable fractures.
- Delayed return to sporting activity (up to 1 year).

# Osteochondral lesion of the talus

## Anatomy

- The trapezoid dome of the talus is covered by the trochlear articular surface, which supports the weight of the body.
- The anterior surface of the talar dome is wider than the posterior surface.
- The medial and lateral articular facets of the talus articulate with the medial and lateral malleoli.
- The articular surface of these facets is contiguous with the superior articular surface of the talar dome.

## Mechanism of injury

- Etiology varies with site of injury with repetitive overuse syndrome common in medial lesions, and acute traumatic events in lateral lesions.
- Lateral osteochondral lesions are invariably secondary to trauma, complicating forced inversion injuries, which result in impaction of the lateral talar dome against the fibula.
- Post-traumatic medial lesions are deeper and result from a combination of inversion, plantar flexion and external rotation forces which cause the posteromedial talar dome to impact on the tibial articular surface in a relatively more perpendicular direction.
- Berndt and Harty have staged osteochondral injuries according to relative stability of the osteochondral fragment:
  - Stage 1: subchondral bone bruise or fracture.
  - Stage 2: single rent in overlying cartilage and partial detachment of the fragment.
  - Stage 3: rents on either side of the subchondral contusion with detachment without displacement (Fig. 7.41).
  - Stage 4: presence of a displaced detached fragment.



## History and clinical findings

- Chronic ankle pain with intermittent swelling post-injury.
- Weakness, stiffness, instability and reduced range of motion may be seen.

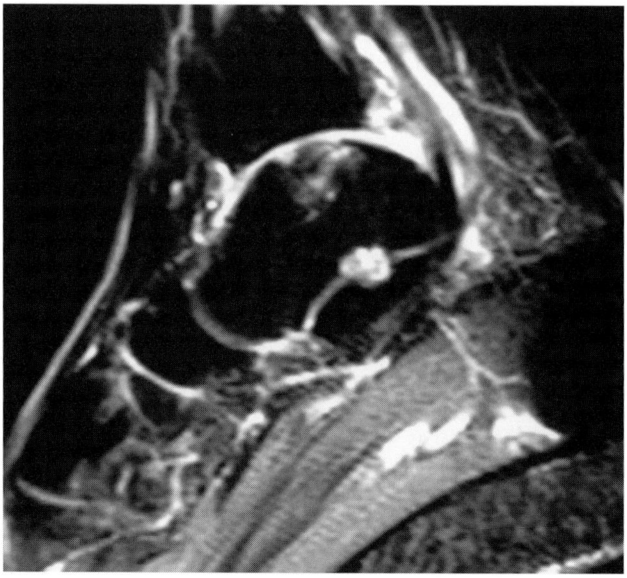

**Fig. 7.41** Sagittal image in an elite hockey player with persistent ankle pain showing a post-traumatic talar dome osteochondral lesion with a minimally displaced loose osteochondral fragment: a stage 3 lesion.

- Palpation may reveal tenderness behind the medial malleolus when the ankle is dorsiflexed (posteromedial lesion) or tenderness when the anterolateral ankle joint is palpated with the joint in maximal plantar flexion (anterolateral lesion).

## Imaging findings

### Radiography

- Weight-bearing plain radiography (AP, lateral and mortise views).
- Radiographs in varying degrees of plantar flexion and dorsiflexion may help in diagnosing posteromedial and anterolateral lesions, respectively.
- Plain radiographs of the opposite ankle should be obtained because of a 10–25% incidence of a contralateral lesion.
- Insensitive to lower grade lesions.

### Computerized tomography

- Less sensitive to chondral injury than MRI.
- Can show cystic change and displaced fragments.

### Magnetic resonance imaging

- Early identification of an osteochondral injury or subarticular bruising allows triage of patients into groups in whom additional non-weight-bearing should be undertaken to prevent progression of the injury.
- Findings include areas of focal talar dome low-signal intensity on $T_1$-weighted images and hyperintensity on $T_2$-weighted images.
- $T_2$-weighted images show marked edema surrounding an osteochondral fragment with or without low-signal loose bodies surrounded by high-signal fluid.
- A $T_1$-weighted image is the most accurate to assess sclerosis.
- Coronal and sagittal images are most useful.
- Post-treatment MRI normally reveals resolution of these findings.



## Management

### Non-surgical

- Similar to atraumatic osteochondral injury, conservative management is initially undertaken in all patients unless a free fragment is identified.
- Initial period of immobilization followed by physical therapy.
- A trial of conservative therapy does not adversely affect surgery performed after conservative therapy has failed.
- Symptoms of intra-articular derangement (catching, locking and instability) are indications for operative intervention.

### Surgical

- Technique varies according to size of defect, extent of bone and cartilage loss and patient activity levels.
- Loose-body removal with or without stimulation of fibrocartilage growth (microfracture, curettage, abrasion or transarticular drilling).
- Securing detached fragments to the talar dome through retrograde drilling, bone grafting or internal fixation.
- Stimulating the development of hyaline cartilage through osteochondral autografts (osteochondral autograft transfer system – OATS; mosaicplasty), allografts or cell culture.
- Arthroscopic intervention is associated with less surgical morbidity and joint stiffness, decreased rehabilitation time and an increased functional outcome.
- Arthrodesis if the above measures are unsuccessful.

# Plantar fasciitis

## Anatomy

- Plantar aponeurosis has its origin at the os calcis and divides distally to attach to the proximal phalanges, the base of the 5th metatarsal and the skin of the ball of the foot.
- Responsible for 50% of adult heel pain cases.

## Mechanism of injury

- Inflammation of the plantar fascia at its insertion on the medial calcaneal tuberosity, thought to be the result of repetitive microtrauma or avulsive traction forces applied at this site.
- The weakest point of the plantar fascia is its origin, not its substance, because of the high tensile strength of the fascial fibers themselves.
- Weight-bearing forces repeatedly stress the medial arch during jogging, the configuration of which is maintained by contraction of both intrinsic and extrinsic flexors and the plantar aponeurosis.

## History and clinical findings

- Pain in the medial calcaneal tuberosity, medial foot and heel, which is worse on standing for prolonged periods.
- Gradual onset of pain, generally worse in the morning and with toe dorsiflexion.
- Direct palpation of the medial calcaneal tubercle often causes severe pain, which is generally localized at the origin of the anatomic central band of the plantar fascia.

## Imaging findings

### Radiography

- Standard weight-bearing radiographs in the lateral and AP projection demonstrate the biomechanical character of the hindfoot and forefoot and associated spur formation.



### Magnetic resonance imaging

- In acute plantar fasciitis, sagittal fat suppressed turbo spin echo or turbo inversion recovery sequences show signal hyperintensity within and adjacent to the insertion of the plantar aponeurosis, often extending to adjacent subcutaneous tissues.
- In chronic plantar fasciitis, inflammatory changes extend to the mid belly of the aponeurosis, which often becomes markedly thickened, reflecting extensive fibrous replacement; signal hyperintensity is less marked (Fig. 7.42).

## Management

### Non-surgical

- This should address the inflammatory component that causes the discomfort and the biomechanical factors that produce the disorder.
- Rest, icing, NSAIDs and exercises to stretch the Achilles tendon and plantar fascia.
- Medial arch support, shoes with shock-absorbing soles or orthotic devices, e.g. a rubber heel pad.
- 90% of patients will improve significantly with only conservative management.
- Steroid injection under fluoroscopy in resistant cases.
- If symptoms persist, a walking cast for 2–3 weeks or positional splint while sleeping may be tried.

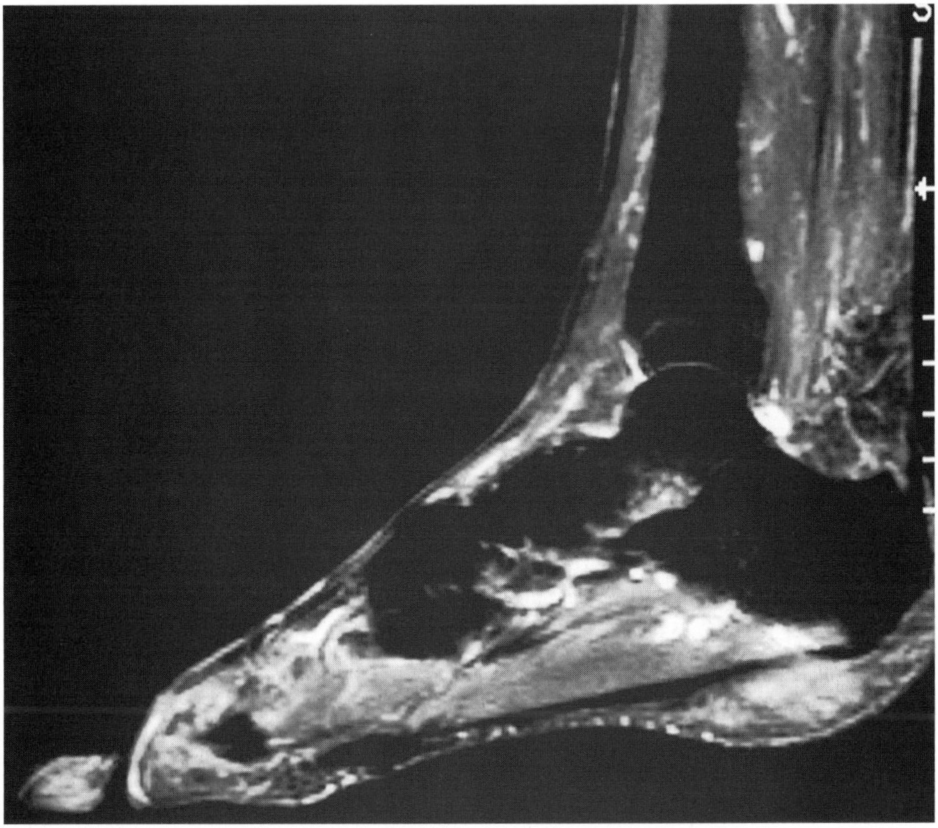

**Fig. 7.42** Sagittal fat-suppressed image showing marked inflammatory change adjacent to the plantar fascial attachment in a competitive walker with plantar fasciitis.



- Electroshock wave therapy and radiotherapy have been used for refractory cases but long-term benefit has not yet been shown.

## Surgical

- Surgical fasciotomy with or without spur removal should be reserved for use in patients in whom conservative measures have failed despite correction of biomechanical abnormalities.
- Endoscopic plantar fasciotomy is less traumatic than traditional open heel-spur surgery and is reported to allow earlier weight-bearing after surgery but may have a higher associated stress fracture incidence.

# Tarsal coalition

## Anatomy

- Rare abnormal bony, fibrous or cartilaginous union of the tarsal bones.
- Talocalcaneal and calcaneonavicular coalition more common than talonavicular.

## Mechanism of injury

- Restriction of the movement of the subtalar joint complex may cause secondary abnormal stresses on other joints and lead to pain, stiffness and ultimately degenerative arthritis.

## History and clinical findings

- Limitation of subtalar joint motion.
- Decreased inversion–eversion with pain in a younger child.
- Secondary peroneal muscle spasm and peroneal spastic flatfoot.

## Imaging findings

### Radiography

- Calcaneonavicular coalition: a 45° internal oblique view shows the protrusion of the calcaneus towards the navicular (the comma sign).
- Talocalcaneal coalition: lateral and axial views most commonly show the middle talar facet involvement with decreased joint space with beaking of the talus (Fig. 7.43).

### Computerized tomography

- 3D reformats with thin section reconstruction show coalition directly; coronal reformats useful for talocalcaneal and sagittal reformats for calcaneonavicular union (Fig. 7.44).



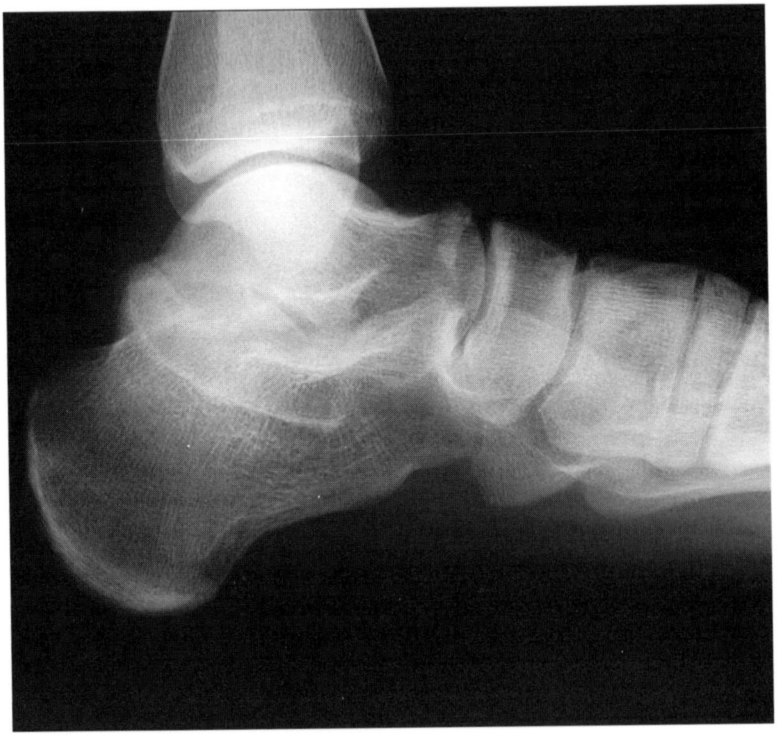

**Fig. 7.43** Lateral radiograph showing talocalcaneal fusion at a hypertrophied sustentaculum with fusion at the posterior and middle subtalar articulations.

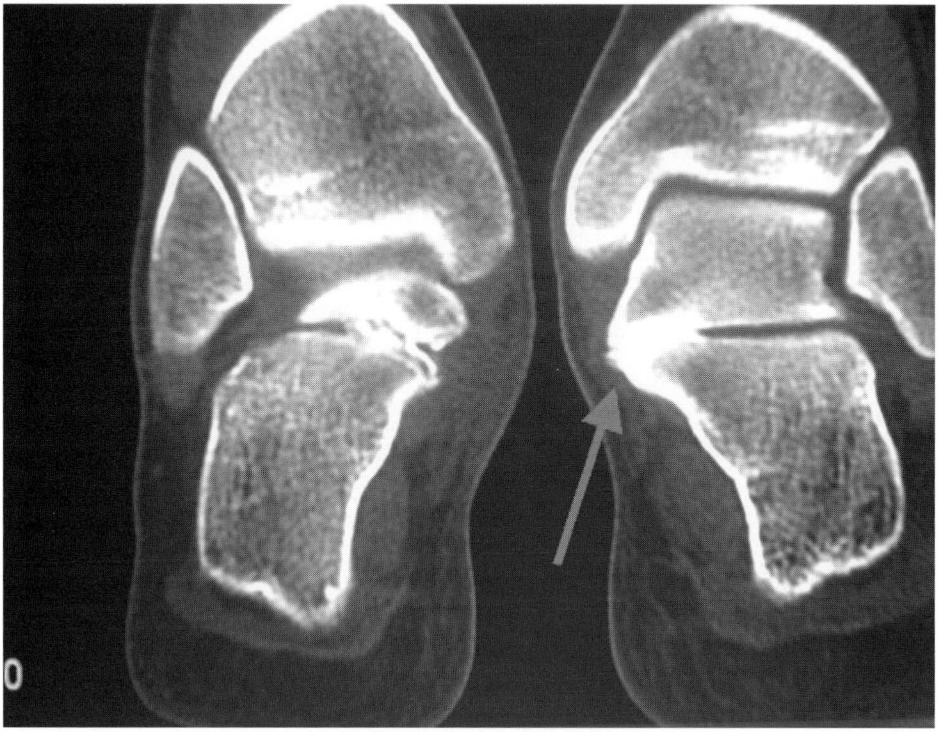


**Fig. 7.44** Coronal CT image showing fusion at the middle subtalar articulation on the left (arrow).

| | |
|---|---|
| Magnetic resonance imaging | • As with CT with additional information available regarding subchondral marrow edema and better visualization of non-osseus cartilaginous and fibrous union. |



## Management

| | |
|---|---|
| Non-surgical | • Orthotics or bracing to limit subtalar motion. |
| Surgical | • Resection of coalition.<br>• Fusion of the involved joint. |

# Os trigonum syndrome

## Anatomy

- The os trigonum represents a congenital non-union of the lateral tubercle of the posterior process of the talus, to which it remains intimately related in adulthood.
- Present in 10% of the population, bilateral in 50% and usually asymptomatic.

## Mechanism of injury

- During repetitive flexion/extension, synovial tissue may interdigitate between the os trigonum and the posterior tibia resulting in capsular entrapment, local pain and inflammation.

## History and clinical findings

- Pain in the posterior ankle, which is worse on plantar flexion.
- Tenderness and soft-tissue swelling at the posterior ankle on palpation.
- Decreased range of motion at the subtalar joint.

## Imaging findings

### Radiography

- Used to differentiate the os trigonum from a fracture of the lateral tubercle (Shepherd's fracture) by smooth edges and well-corticated bone on lateral view versus irregular edges and bony fragment separation in Shepherd's fracture.

### Magnetic resonance imaging

- Inflammatory changes are usually clearly visualized in the sagittal plane intimately related to the posterior tibiotalar joint recess, i.e. hyperintensity on $T_2$-weighted images on either side of synchondrosis.
- The relationship between the inflammatory process and the medially located flexor hallucis tendon sheath is best achieved in the axial plane.



## Management

### Non-surgical

- Rest, splinting, NSAIDs.
- Steroid injection or casting if resistant.

### Surgical

- If persistent symptoms or fracture.
- Arthroscopic resection of the os trigonum and surrounding fibrotic tissue.

# Sesamoiditis

## Anatomy

- Two sesamoid bones are located beneath the head of the first metatarsal and form an articulation with it.
- Held in position by the bands of the joint capsule and are separated by a bony bridge and by the tendon of flexor hallucis longus.
- Ossification of the sesamoids is normally complete by 11 years of age.
- In 10% of patients, one or both sesamoids (usually tibial) may exist normally as a bipartite structure, resulting from the failure of union between ossification centers, which are generally asymptomatic.

## Mechanism of injury

- Sesamoiditis generally results from repetitive microtrauma, such as in running or jumping.
- Tibial (medial) sesamoid are particularly vulnerable to impaction forces imposed by weight-bearing as forces are referred to the great toe prior to projecting the foot forwards.
- Because the sesamoids lie within the heads of the flexor hallucis brevis and tend to bowstring (with the hallucis brevis) across the first MTP joint during the toe-off phase of the gait cycle, more weight is transferred to the tibial sesamoid.
- About 1% of all running injuries involve the sesamoids (40% are stress fractures and 30% as sesamoiditis).

## History and clinical findings

- Symptoms begin as a gradual onset of vague pain in the region of the medial first MTP joint, often without history of trauma.
- Pain increases gradually if aggravating activity is continued.
- Point tenderness may be palpable beneath the affected sesamoid.
- On MTP joint dorsiflexion, the tenderness will move distally with the movement of the sesamoid.
- The passive axial compression test has been reported as a new adjunctive provocative maneuver for the clinical diagnosis of sesamoiditis.

## Imaging findings

### Radiography

- In most cases fractures are undisplaced and stellate and, in the absence of dedicated views, are radiographically occult.
- Views to visualize the sesamoids are AP, lateral, lateral oblique (fibular sesamoid) and axial (both sesamoids).

### Isotope bone scan

- Can show an increased uptake at the affected sesamoid within approximately 3 weeks and is useful in excluding fracture of the sesamoid.

### Computerized tomography

- Generally not used.

### Magnetic resonance imaging

- Inversion recovery images in the sagittal and coronal planes and turbo spin echo $T_1$-weighted images facilitate diagnosis (Fig. 7.45).
- The pattern of bone edema is used to differentiate sesamoiditis (effusion and synovitis at the 1st MTP joint) from fracture (hyperintense fracture line transversely) and bipartite sesamoid (no edema in separated fragments).

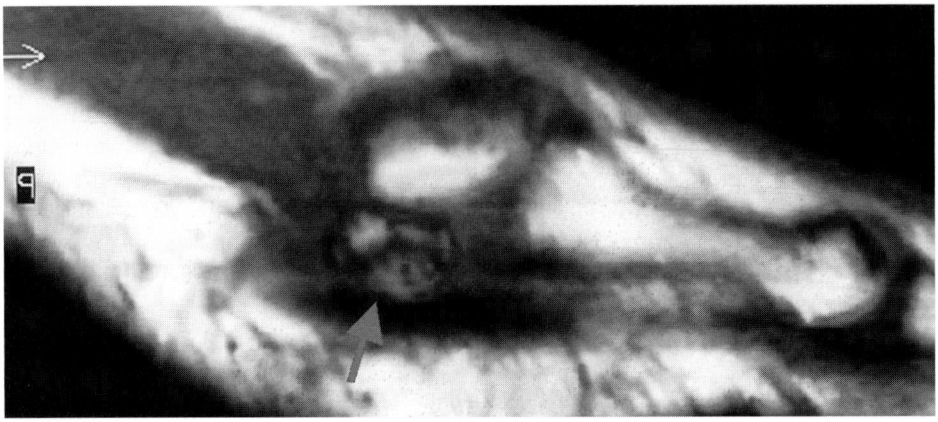

**Fig. 7.45** Sagittal $T_1$-weighted image showing an undisplaced stellate fracture of the tibial sesamoid.

## Management

### Non-surgical

- Most treatment is supportive: rest and non-weight-bearing exercise while symptoms resolve (which usually takes less than 1 month).
- U-shaped padding strapped to the region or orthotic implants to reduce sesamoid stresses.
- Antiinflammatory medication and flexibility exercises for the foot.
- Steroid injections with padding may be attempted for milder resistant cases.
- Immobilization with plaster casting below the knee for 2–4 weeks has been advocated for severe cases.
- Longstanding sesamoiditis may progress to chondromalacia of the articular surfaces, chronic synovitis and avascular necrosis; early and aggressive treatment improves outcome in problem cases.



### Surgical

- Persistent symptoms may require surgical excision.
- Untreated, stellate fractures ultimately distract at which time surgical excision is the only therapeutic option.
- Excision only of the injured sesamoid with or without silicone cushion.
- Screw fixation of sesamoid fractures is a newer technique.
- The remaining sesamoid and the tendon of the flexor hallucis longus should not be predisposed to increased stresses.

# Tarsal tunnel syndrome

## Anatomy

- Entrapment of the posterior tibial nerve or its branches as it passes deep to the flexor retinaculum at the ankle.
- The tarsal tunnel is formed by the flexor retinaculum (roof), the superior aspect of the calcaneus (floor), the medial wall of the talus and the distal medial aspect of the medial malleolus. The fibro-osseus canal contains the tendons of the flexor hallucis longus muscle, flexor digitorum longus muscle, tibialis posterior muscle, posterior tibial nerve and posterior tibial artery.
- It is analogous to carpal tunnel syndrome of the wrist.

## Mechanism of injury

- The causative factor may be extrinsic (e.g. a fractured sustentaculum tali), local causes (e.g. a soft-tissue mass) or nerve related.
- Idiopathic in 50% of cases and associated with inflammatory arthritides.
- In sports-related cases, overpronation of the foot causes inflammation of the flexor tendon sheaths at the tarsal tunnel with subsequent compression of the posterior tibial nerves.
- Hindfoot valgus deformity and external compression (e.g. lipoma) make symptoms worse.

## History and clinical findings

- Pain at the medial malleolus radiating along the medial aspect to the toes.
- Motor disturbance with resultant atrophy of intrinsic musculature, and gait abnormalities are less common.
- Focal tenderness at the flexor retinaculum.
- Eversion and dorsiflexion may cause symptoms to increase at the end-point range of motion.
- Tapping the posterior tibial nerve at the retinaculum causes burning and tingling on the plantar aspect of the foot (Tinel's sign).



## Imaging findings

### Nerve conduction studies and electromyography

- Confirms the presence of neuropathy.
- An absence of positive electrodiagnostic results does not rule out the possibility of decompression for treating symptoms of tarsal tunnel syndrome.

### Radiography

- Non-specific. May show a loss of bone density, foot structure, fractures, bony masses, osteophytes or subtalar joint coalition.

### Ultrasound

- Can aid diagnosis if a suspected soft-tissue mass is presumed to be causing symptoms.

### Magnetic resonance imaging

- Depends on the cause: soft-tissue masses at the ankle, flexor tenosynovitis, fractures, unossified subtalar joint coalitions, etc.
- May see a high signal on $T_2$-weighted scans in muscles supplied by the posterior tibial nerve.

## Management

**Non-surgical**

- Medial arch support, NSAIDs for tenosynovitis and nerve sheath inflammation.
- Steroid injections to the tarsal tunnel.
- Orthotics, physiotherapy and night splints may help.

**Surgical**

- Tarsal tunnel release of the flexor retinaculum with decompression of the posterior tibial nerve and branches.
- Removal of any coexistent soft-tissue mass.

# Epiphysiolysis: tibiotalar and calcaneal (Sever's disease)

**Mechanism of injury**

- Overuse and overtraining.

**Clinical findings**

- Ankle pain or heal pain onset during exercise with pain persisting post-exercise in severe cases. Usual onset in adolescence is during rapid growth accompanying excess pressure on the growth plate, usually due to over-participation in sport.
- The clinical history and local discomfort can be elicited on palpation.

## Imaging findings

**Radiography**

- Radiographs may show a confusing aggressive periosteal reaction in the distal tibia or calcaneum with growth-plate fragmentation and irregularity due to local trauma. Appearances may be misinterpreted as being due to tumor or infection.

**Magnetic resonance imaging**

- MRI may show aggressive-appearing bone edema, which again may lead to image misinterpretation (Figs 7.46–7.48).

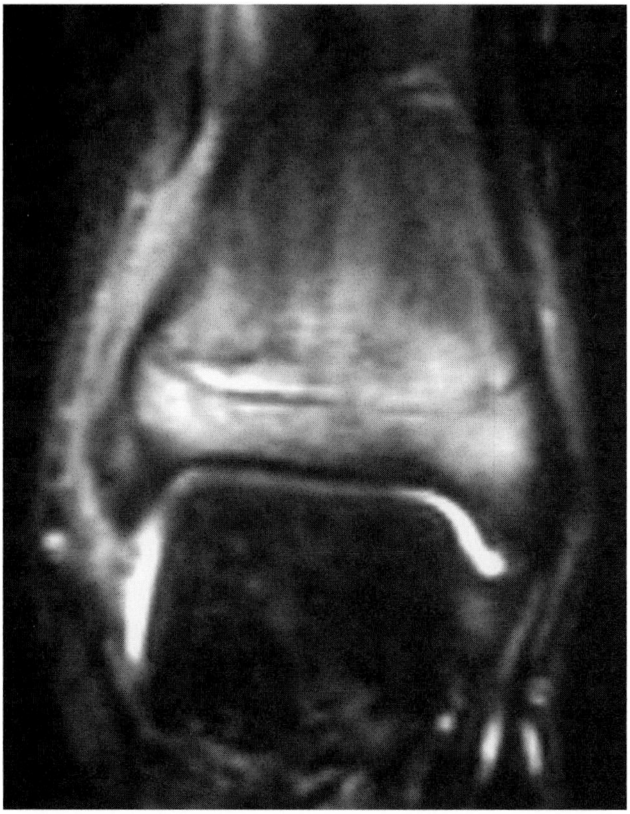

**Fig. 7.46** Coronal fat-suppressed image showing extensive bone edema on either side of the growth plate with associated periostitis and soft-tissue inflammation due to epiphysiolysis in an adolescent school girl playing sports every day.

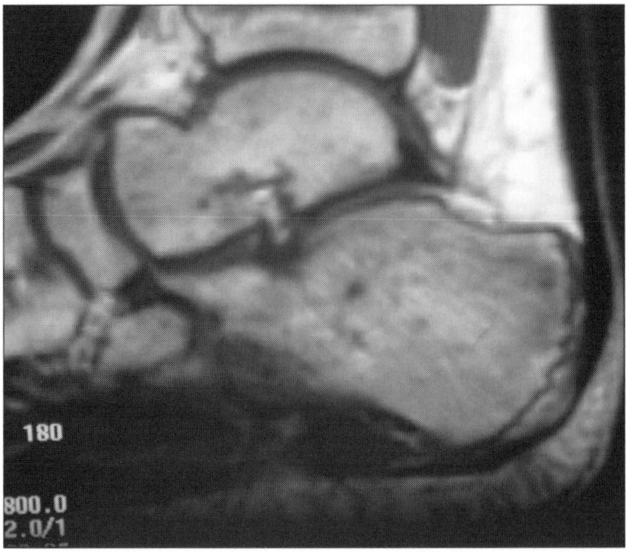


**Fig. 7.47** Sagittal $T_1$-weighted image showing focal bone edema adjacent to the calcaneal apophysis in an adolescent male with Sever's disease. He described heel pain on exertion but radiographs failed to reveal an abnormality. He returned to active participation following 4 weeks' rest.

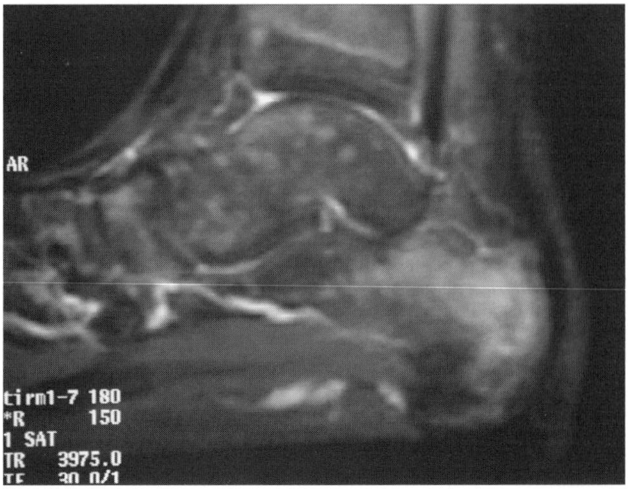


**Fig. 7.48** Fat-suppressed image showing the same condition as in Fig. 7.47 with florid edema in the region of the calcaneal apophysis.



## Management

### Non-surgical

- Conservative.
- Initial rest for 6 weeks.
- Reintroduction of modified activity, less frequent participation, in time gradual reintroduction of full activity. If symptoms recur, must consider reduced exercise for a period.

# Ankle arthritis

## Anatomy

- Ankle mortise: arthritis here is much less common than at the hip or knee.

## Mechanism of injury

- Generally only years after significant injury to the joint.
- Commonly occurs after ankle fractures, especially if alignment is suboptimal.
- Erosive arthropathies with cartilage damage.
- Advanced (stages 3 and 4) osteochondral lesions of the talus.
- Longstanding instability with cartilage damage and loss.

## History and clinical findings

- Chronic or intermittent pain.
- Grinding or popping in the ankle, which may be particularly stiff in the morning or at the beginning of activity.
- Ankle may swell up and be warm to the touch.

## Imaging findings

### Radiography

- Narrowing of the ankle joint space with osteophyte formation and subchondral sclerosis.

### Isotope bone scan

- Increased uptake may be seen with generalized sclerosis.

### Magnetic resonance imaging

- Best for cartilage visualization: thinning and focal defects on fat-suppressed proton density weighting.
- Subchondral changes vary from high signal on PD images (edema) to low signal (sclerosis).
- Loose-body visualization (especially gradient echo images).



## Management

### Non-surgical

- Weight reduction.
- Orthotics or ankle bracing may suffice in milder cases.
- NSAIDs or COX-II inhibitors.
- Steroid (antiinflammatory) or hyaluronate (increase joint space temporarily) injections may provide temporary relief.

### Surgical

- Arthroscopic debridement and loose-body removal.
- Joint distraction is a new and promising technique where the ankle load is decreased by an external frame for 3 months but long-term results are lacking.
- Total ankle replacement with a polyethylene bearing.
- Ankle arthrodesis in resistant cases; adjacent joints compensate and may allow 50% of ankle joint motion to return.

## Further reading


Aerts P, Disler DG. Abnormalities of the foot and ankle: MR imaging findings. Am J Roentgenol 1995; 165: 119–124.

Bassett FH 3rd, Gates HS 3rd, Billys JB et al. Talar impingement by the anteroinferior tibiofibular ligament. A cause of chronic pain in the ankle after inversion sprain. J Bone Joint Surg Am 1990; 72(1): 55–59.

Berkowitz JF, Kier R, Rudicel S. Plantar fasciitis: MR imaging. Radiology 1991; 179: 665–667.

Chandnani VP, Harper MT, Ficke JR et al. Chronic ankle instability: evaluation with MR arthrography, MR imaging, and stress radiography. Radiology 1994; 192: 189–194.

Daffner RH, Riemer BL, Lupetin AR, Dash N. Magnetic resonance imaging in acute tendon ruptures. Skeletal Radiol 1986; 15: 619–621.

Ferkel RD, Scranton PE Jr. Arthroscopy of the ankle and foot. J Bone Joint Surg Am 1993; 75(8): 1233–1242.

Fredericson M, Bergman AG, Hoffman KL, Dillingham MS. Tibial stress reaction in runners. Correlation of clinical symptoms and scintigraphy with a new magnetic resonance imaging grading system. Am J Sports Med 1995; 23: 472–481.

Hamilton WG. Foot and ankle injuries in dancers. New York, Raven Press, 1987; 127.

Inglis AE, Scott WN, Sculco TP, Patterson AH. Ruptures of the tendo achillis: an objective assessment of surgical and non-surgical treatment. J Bone Joint Surg Am 1976; 58: 990–993.

Liu SH, Raskin A, Osti L et al. Arthroscopic treatment of anterolateral ankle impingement. Arthroscopy 1994; 10: 215–218.

Mann RA. Biomechanics. In: Jahss MH ed. Disorders of the foot, Vol 1, 2nd ed. Philadelphia, WB Saunders, 1991.

Mann RA, Inman VT. Phasic activity of intrinsic muscles of the foot. J Bone Joint Surg 1964; 46: 469–481.

Marotta JJ, Micheli LJ. Os trigonum impingment in dancers. Am J Sports Med 1992; 20: 533–536.

Matheson GO, Clement DB, McKenzie DC et al. Stress fractures in athletes. A study of 320 cases. Am J Sports Med 1987; 15: 46–58.

Rodeo SA, O'Brien S, Warren RF et al. Turf-toe: an analysis of metatarsophalangeal joint sprains in professional football players. Am J Sports Med 1990; 18: 280–285.

Sterling JC, Edelstein DW, Calvo RD et al. Stress fractures in the athlete. Diagnosis and management. Sports Med 1992; 14: 336–346.

Thompson FM, Patterson AH. Rupture of the peroneus longus tendon. Report of three cases. J Bone Joint Surg Am 1989; 71(2): 293–295.

# 8

# The Shoulder



## CLINICAL EXAMINATION

Clinical assessment of the shoulder is a difficult and challenging exercise requiring practice and experience.

A systematic approach is required, together with a thorough knowledge of both intrinsic and extrinsic shoulder anatomy (Figs 8.2–8.4). Shoulder pain may be due to pathology in the spine, chest or visceral structures including the gallbladder. The shoulder is a complex set of articulations involving the glenohumeral joint, the subacromial articulation, the acromioclavicular (AC) joint, the sternoclavicular joint and the scapulothoracic articulation.

In an effort to arrive at the correct diagnosis, it is important not only to have knowledge of the most common conditions affecting the shoulder but also to have a more comprehensive understanding of the wide variety of differing injuries and conditions that may present with shoulder symptoms.

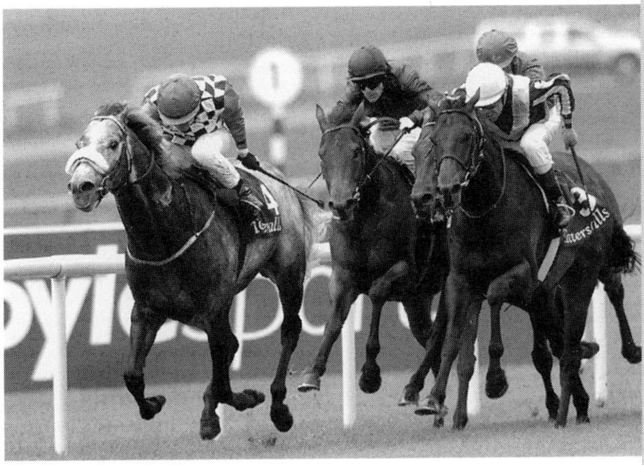

**Fig. 8.1** Sportsfile.

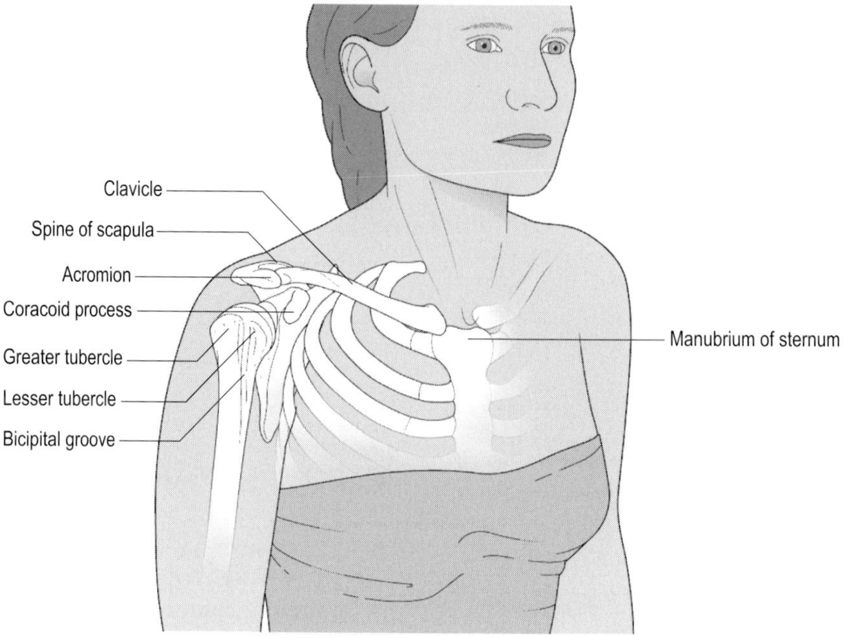


**Fig. 8.2** Anterior aspect of the shoulder's bone structure.



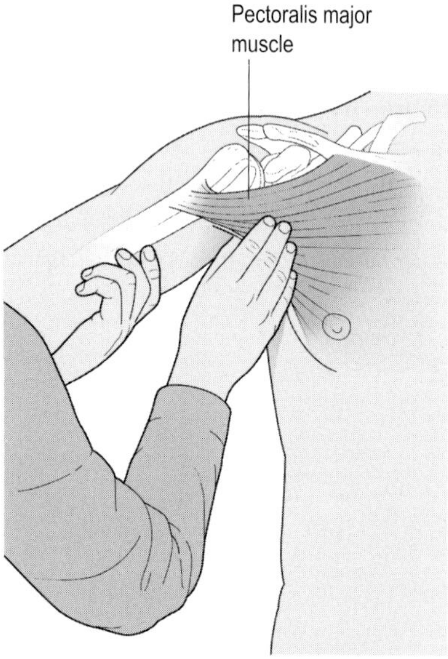


**Fig. 8.3** The anterior aspect of the axilla is formed by the pectoralis major muscle.

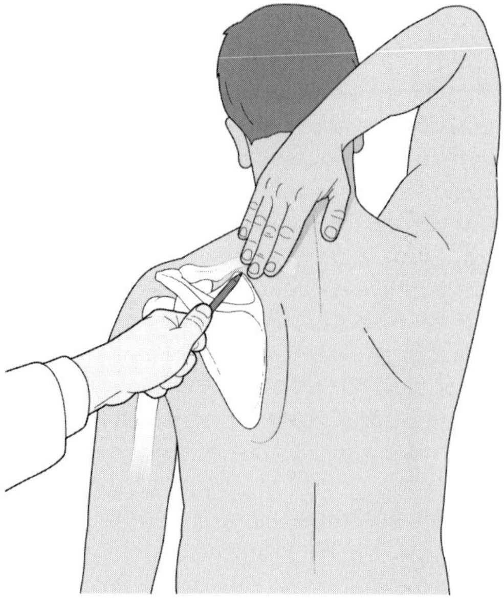

**Fig. 8.4** Evaluating range of motion at the shoulder: the Apley scratch test.

## Clinical history

First:

- Obtain a brief outline of the patient's profile including age, occupation, hand dominance and sporting pursuits.
- Establish the chief presenting complaint, which is not always pain, and define other symptoms. The most common symptoms and complaints associated with shoulder pathology include pain, instability, stiffness, deformity, locking, catching and swelling.
- It is important to understand the functional loss and to inquire about previous treatment, surgery and injury.

Pain is carefully evaluated in terms of its site, radiation, quality, onset, frequency, nocturnal occurrence, and any aggravating and relieving factors. Pain due to rotator cuff pathology and impingement is usually felt over the anterolateral part of the shoulder, often with some radiation down the upper arm, and aggravation by upper limb overhead activities, and may be symptomatic at night. Pain originating in the neck region or radiating beyond the elbow is less likely to be due to shoulder injury or pathology, particularly if associated with any sensory disturbance in the upper limb. Pain due to AC joint injury or pathology is usually well localized to the region of the joint, and there is often a clear history of recent or previous injury to this region.

Instability is very common, particularly in the younger athletic and sports populations. Glenohumeral shoulder instability may be classified according to direction (anteroposterior, inferior or multidirectional), etiology (traumatic or atraumatic), frequency (acute, recurrent or chronic) and voluntary.

Voluntary instability is precipitated by muscular contraction; involuntary instability is precipitated by arm position.

Recurrent episodes of painful dislocation, which occur during sporting activities with the arm in abduction and external rotation, strongly suggest recurrent involuntary traumatic anterior instability with a high incidence of detachment of the anterior glenoid labrum (Bankart lesion) and disruption of the anterior glenohumeral ligaments and capsule, which can usually be corrected by surgery.

Recurrent voluntary atraumatic posterior or multidirectional instability – and physiotherapy and rehabilitation exercise therapy directed at rotator cuff muscle strengthening – is the mainstay in treatment.

Glenohumeral instability may be present without any history of definite trauma or past dislocation. Throwing and 'overhead athletes' often have anterior glenohumeral instability due to chronic strain and stress on the anterior glenohumeral ligaments and capsule, and usually without a history of prior dislocation. They may present with a feeling that the shoulder partly comes out of its joint but will often complain only of pain that may be a result of secondary impingement of the rotator cuff complex. The 'dead arm syndrome', which presents with sudden onset of weakness, numbness and tingling in the upper limb, is provoked by certain activities and may be due to transient anterior subluxation of the shoulder, traction on the brachial nerve plexus or to thoracic outlet syndrome.

Stiffness or loss of motion may be the primary complaint or symptom in conditions such as adhesive capsulitis, glenohumeral osteoarthritis or missed posterior dislocation but it is more often a secondary symptom.

Deformity occurs with injuries of the AC joint and fractures of the clavicle. Sprengel's deformity and winging of the scapula may present with deformity as the primary symptom. Sprengel's deformity is the most common congenital abnormality affecting the shoulder and is characterized by the presence of a hypoplastic malrotated scapula abnormally high on the posterior chest wall. It results from failure of the normal descent of the scapula *in utero* and may be bilateral.

Winging of the scapula is due to a loss of the normal scapular stability provided mainly by the serratus anterior and trapezius muscles. Subtle forms of scapular winging occur commonly with many shoulder injuries or disorders, including glenohumeral instability, muscular imbalance or fatigue; more explicit forms occur with injury or neuropathy of the accessory or long thoracic nerves and in myopathies.

Catching, 'clunking', grinding or popping of the shoulder with various movements are usually sounds and/or sensations which may be asymptomatic and non-pathologic or may be due to some significant injury or pathology including glenoid labral disorders, rotator cuff complex tears, subacromial bursitis, acromiohumeral impingement, long head of biceps tendon disorders, glenohumeral instability, and intra-articular osseous or cartilaginous loose bodies. Sounds and/or sensations associated with shoulder pain or instability are more likely to represent a significant injury or pathologic entity.

Weakness may be the primary symptom or complaint. True mechanical weakness needs to be distinguished from weakness secondary to pain. Subacromial bursitis without a rotator cuff complex tear will often demonstrate weakness of the rotator cuff complex secondary to pain if tested with the arm positioned in the painful impingement arc but will show good strength if tested with the arm not in abduction. Significant rotator cuff complex tears usually show more profound weakness of the rotator cuff function in different arm positions. Painless weakness of shoulder function is usually due to neurologic conditions or myopathies.

It is important to understand the resultant functional loss in terms of effect of occupation work, sport, recreation, leisure and activities of daily living.

You should ascertain any previous injuries around the shoulder and what relationship, if any, they have with the present symptomatology and dysfunction. It is important to know previous treatments undertaken: physiotherapy; local anesthetic and corticosteroid injections; and surgery to outline an effective plan of management and treatment.



History is completed by an overall enquiry about general health, existing medical conditions, drug taking and allergies. This is important for the diagnosis, treatment and overall management. Adhesive capsulitis is associated with medical conditions such as diabetes mellitus and ischemic heart disease. Primary malignancy may raise the suspicion of underlying metastatic disease. Corticosteroid use causes osteoporosis and tendon degeneration atrophy, and affects wound healing.

# Physical examination

Thorough history taking and symptom profile analysis will probably suggest the diagnosis. The experienced clinician will focus accordingly on the physical examination.

Examination of the shoulder joint and region should be systematic and organized in every patient with:

- inspection
- palpation
- ranges of motion
- strength tests
- neurologic tests
- special shoulder tests.

Physical examination should include a thorough assessment of the cervical spine and the remainder of the upper extremity.

Cervical injury and pathology is common, with pain often referred to the shoulder and upper arm region. Cervical radiculopathy, particularly affecting the fifth cervical nerve root, will often be associated with shoulder pain but it can be differentiated from true shoulder injury or pathology by the physical findings on cervical spine examination, with the lack of physical findings on examination of the shoulder joint and region.

## Inspection

Inspection begins by careful observation. The examination begins with a more formal inspection but it cannot be adequately performed unless the shoulder region is adequately (but appropriately) undressed. Males should be undressed to the waist and for females a garment wrap around the upper chest should be placed so as to ensure adequate visualization. The shoulder is systematically inspected from the anterior, lateral and posterior positions. The presence of scars, color changes, swelling, muscle atrophy, asymmetry and deformity are observed.

### Anterior inspection

Deformity, swelling and asymmetry anteriorly may represent sternoclavicular, clavicular, or AC injury or pathology. Anterior dislocation of the shoulder leads to squaring of the shoulder region as the deltoid is no longer rounded out over the head of the humerus. Rupture of the long head of biceps can be noticed by the change in contour of the anterior arm with bunching of the muscle (the 'Popeye' appearance).

### Posterior inspection

Posteriorly, the position and attitude of the scapula is observed. A high and often small scapula is seen in

Sprengel's deformity and is often bilateral. Winging of the scapula usually suggests underlying scapulothoracic dysfunction and may be associated with shoulder instability, muscle imbalance or fatigue, and not necessarily secondary to long thoracic nerve injury. Wasting of the supraspinatus and infraspinatus is commonly seen with massive rotator cuff tears but may also be observed in suprascapular nerve entrapment or other neuropathies or myopathies.

## Palpation

Palpation must also be systematic and focus on specific anatomic structures. The sternoclavicular joint is palpated and compared with the contralateral side. Sternoclavicular dislocation is rare but frequently a delayed diagnosis. Trauma to the shoulder girdle may cause a sternoclavicular dislocation, which is more common and visible when it occurs in the anterior direction. Posterior dislocation is rarer but is potentially a very serious injury due to the proximity of the trachea and blood vessels. Palpate along the clavicle noting any deformity, swelling or areas of tenderness. Isolate and palpate the AC joint. Injuries and arthritis of the AC joint are common, and focal tenderness is an important sign. Proceed with palpation of the subacromial bursa and the various tendons of the rotator cuff tendon complex. The subscapularis tendon can be palpated at its insertion to the lesser tuberosity of the humerus by positioning the arm in external rotation and palpating just lateral to the coracoid process of the scapula. The supraspinatous tendon can be brought out from beneath the acromion by extension and external rotation of the arm and palpation just distal to the anterolateral corner of the acromion. The infraspinatus portion of the rotator cuff complex is best palpated just distal to the posterolateral aspect of the acromion with the arm in slight flexion and internal rotation. The tendon of the long head of the biceps brachii tendon is palpated anteriorly in the bicipital groove with the arm held in neutral rotation.

## Range of motion tests

Assess the total active and passive range of elevation in the plane of the scapula which lies approximately 20°–30° forward of the coronal plane. The normal range is 150°–170°. External rotation is assessed with the arms to the side and elbows flexed to 90°. Loss of motion relative to the opposite side is the most significant finding as there is quite a large variation in range of motion among normal subjects. (Most people will achieve between 50° and 70°.) It is important to assess active and passive ranges of motion as loss of active ranges of motion with normal ranges of passive motion may indicate muscular weakness. Active external rotation should also be tested with the arm in 90° of abduction with most subjects having approximately 80°–100° in this position but it may be abnormally increased at the expense of internal rotation, particularly in throwing or overhead athletes. Internal rotation is assessed by the position reached by the extended thumb up the thoracic spine with normal subjects reaching the T5 to T10 level. Loss of internal rotation in young patients may be an important finding suggestive of posterior capsular contracture that is often associated with subtle glenohumeral instability. It is also important to note if pain occurs and during what arc of the range when testing the range of motion.

Impingement classically causes a painful arc during elevation between 60° and 120° as the rotator cuff tendons are compressed against the anterior acromion and coracoacromial ligament of the coracoacromial arch. Compressive forces across the AC joint occur mainly in the terminal 60° of abduction; this often causes pain during this range if pathology exists at the AC joint. It is also important to assess the rhythm of shoulder glenohumeral and scapulothoracic motion. Normal elevation of the arm involves 120° of glenohumeral motion and 60° of scapulothoracic motion, with most of the glenohumeral motion in the early stage of elevation and scapulothoracic motion in the latter stage of elevation. Acromiohumeral impingement, rotator cuff tendon complex injury and pathology, glenoid labral tears and glenohumeral instability can all cause interference with normal shoulder motion rhythm.



## Strength tests

Muscle testing should be performed with the aim of specifically isolating certain muscles or muscle groups. Subscapularis function is best assessed using the lift-off test described by Gerber and Krushell. This test is performed with the arm in internal rotation so that the dorsal surface of the hand rests on the lower back. Active lifting of the hand away from the back and against resisting force suggests integrity of the subscapularis muscle. A modified test can be performed by positioning the palm of the hand against the anterior abdominal wall and then resisting further internal rotation if there is loss of internal rotation. External rotators – teres minor and infraspinatus muscles – can be tested by active and resisted external rotation with the arm by the side and elbow flexed to 90°. Large and massive tears of the rotator cuff tendon complex will demonstrate significant weakness with the arm in this position. The biceps brachii and brachialis muscle function can be tested by resisted flexion in external rotation, and a long head of biceps rupture will become more obvious. Deltoid muscle function is best tested with the arm in 90° of abduction and neutral rotation.

Supraspinatus muscle function is best tested with the arm in 90° of abduction brought forward 30° into the scapular plane and into maximal internal rotation. Dropping of the arm is a sign of a significant tear or weakness of supraspinatus muscle function as the other rotator cuff muscles are relatively inactive in this position. Pain alone without weakness may be suggestive of supraspinatus tendinitis.



## Impingement tests

'Impingement' refers to the encroachment on the rotator cuff tendons by a rigid and tight coraco-acromial arch.

### Neer's test

Impingement can occur during the functional arc of elevation (in the plane of the scapula) against the anterior acromion and coracoacromial ligament. Neer's test is a passive test performed by placing one hand on the top of the shoulder girdle while elevating the arm in the scapular plane with the other hand that involves forced elevation of the humerus against the coracoacromial arch, which causes pain that may be abolished by the instillation of local anesthetic into the subacromial space.

### Hawkins–Kennedy test

Hawkins and Kennedy described a further test for impingement performed by forward flexing the shoulder to 90° and then forcibly internally rotating the shoulder. Pain is a positive test and is due to impingement of the supraspinatus tendon and greater tuberosity under the coracoacromial ligament and anteroinferior acromion.

## Instability tests

Shoulder instability may be anterior, posterior, inferior or multidirectional. It may be very obvious and easy to demonstrate or it may be very subtle and difficult to diagnose. In the shoulder, it is difficult to know if translation felt is subluxation to an abnormal position or relocation to a normal position. The normal shoulder has a degree of physiologic laxity and can translate significantly. Comparison to the contralateral shoulder is vital. Actual subluxation, apprehension and the reproduction of pain are all positive physical examination findings. Some of the tests are best performed in the standing, sitting and supine lying positions.

### Load and shift test

With the patient comfortably seated with hands in the lap, one can perform the anteroposterior (AP) translation or load and shift test. To perform this, the right humeral head is grasped with the right hand while the left hand is positioned over the top of the shoulder girdle so that the scapula can be stabilized. Simultaneously, the posterior joint line is palpated with the thumb while the anterior shoulder is palpated with the index and middle fingers. The right hand then loads the joint to ensure concentric reduction and then applies anterior and posterior shearing forces. The direction and translation can then be determined and graded using a scale of 0 to 3 (0 for no instability; 1 for mild translation of less than 1 cm; 2 for moderate translation of 1–2 cm or to the glenoid rim; and 3 for severe translation of greater than 2 cm or over the glenoid rim). The fingers of the left hand should be positioned with the middle finger on the coracoid and index finger on the humeral head. In this way, abnormal anterior translation can be appreciated as the index finger moves forward of the middle finger. To perform the apprehension test, move the right hand to the patient's right wrist and keep the left hand on the shoulder. With the arm in adduction and internal rotation, the shoulder will not be anteriorly subluxated. From this position, bring the arm into abduction and external rotation while using the left hand to palpate any anterior subluxation. Using the left thumb to push the humeral head forward can augment the test.

### Apprehension (crank) test and relocation test

The tests are best performed with the patient supine with the shoulder brought just beyond the edge of the examination table.

The apprehension or crank test is performed by external rotation and abduction at 90°, the angle of which can be varied to stress different portions of the glenohumeral ligament complex. One hand rotates and abducts the arm while the other is used to palpate the anterior and posterior shoulder region to reference the direction of any translation, and augmented by pushing the humeral head anteriorly from behind with the thumb.

The relocation test can be performed in the supine lying position. The test is positive if the symptoms of apprehension or pain produced by the apprehension test are relieved, thereby allowing further external rotation before re-emergence of the symptoms. Patients with impingement will often experience pain on the apprehension test but it is not relieved by performing the relocation test.

Sulcus sign inferior instability is assessed by applying inferior traction to the arm. Gross instability is demonstrated by visible widening of the subacromial space with a sulcus appearing in the adjacent area just distal to the lateral acromion (the sulcus sign). It is important to remember that normal shoulders can translate significantly. The significance of generalized ligamentous laxity must be appreciated, particularly in those patients with multidirectional instability, and the examiner should test for this by looking for elbow, finger and thumb hyperextension, with knee recurvatum and increased ankle dorsiflexion and inversion.

### Posterior apprehension test

Posterior apprehension is elicited by maximally internally rotating the humerus with the shoulder in 90° of abduction and then applying a posteriorly directed force on the humeral head. In a positive test, the patient feels as if the shoulder is about to dislocate. O'Driscoll has found this test to be highly sensitive and specific for posterior shoulder instability. It can be differentiated from impingement by the absence of relief after an injection of local anesthetic into the glenohumeral space. Often, however, posterior instability is not associated with pain or apprehension so most clinical tests rely upon the detection of the subluxation that occurs in certain arm positions.

### Posterior subluxation test

Posterior subluxation usually occurs with the arm in adduction and internal rotation combined with some degree of flexion. Abduction and external rotation will relocate the subluxated shoulder. To assess the right shoulder, the examiner stands to the side of the patient, who is supine with the right shoulder off the edge of the bed. The examiner's right hand takes the elbow and positions the arm in a position of adduction, internal rotation and 70°–90° of flexion. From this position, a posteriorly directed force is applied to accentuate any posterior instability. The examiner's left hand is positioned over the top of the shoulder with the thumb on the anterior shoulder and fingers on the posterior joint line. With the shoulder subluxated, the humeral head fills the normal hollow that is present below the acromion. From this position, the arm is brought out slowly into abduction and external rotation and will at some point relocate with a 'clunk', which is palpable with the left hand.



### Flexion rotation pivot test

Another test the authors have found particularly useful in assessing for the presence of posterior instability is the flexion rotation pivot test. In this test, the patient's arm is positioned in 90° of abduction and neutral rotation with the elbow flexed at 90°. The examiner holds the patient's elbow with one hand and places the opposite hand on the patient's elbow on the ipsilateral anterior axillary fold while stabilizing the acromion and clavicle. The examiner then forward flexes and adducts the patient's arm while exerting a posteriorly applied force on the humeral head. In a positive test, the glenohumeral joint subluxates posteriorly, reproducing the patient's symptoms and occasionally producing a palpable 'clunk'. A similar test can be performed by moving the shoulder in a similar way with the other hand positioned posterior to the shoulder joint. In this way, subtle posterior subluxation and relocation can be palpated.

## The tendon of the long head of biceps brachii and the superior glenoid labrum

The long head of biceps tendon runs up the bicipital groove under the transverse humeral ligament and then runs through the shoulder joint to attach to the superior glenoid tubercle via the superior glenoid labrum. The biceps tendon and superior labrum can be involved in various pathologic processes including bicipital tendinitis, biceps rupture, biceps tendon subluxation or dislocation, and tears of the superior labrum. Since the advent of arthroscopy, lesions of the superior labrum and biceps anchor have been more clearly defined and classified. Although this is a difficult area to assess clinically, various tests may help to make these diagnoses.

### Yergason's test

Yergason's test is performed with the elbow in flexion to 90° and the forearm in pronation with active and resisted supination by the patient. Pain in the tendon of the long head of the biceps brachii and bicipital groove is a positive test and indicates possible wear or tendinitis of the tendon of the long head of biceps brachii (Fig. 8.5).



### Speed's test

Speed's test is performed with forward flexion against resistance with the elbow in extension and the forearm in supination. Pain or tenderness in the tendon of the long head of biceps brachii in the bicipital groove may indicate bicipital tendinitis but can cause nonspecific shoulder pain with superior glenoid labral lesions suggesting that tests for the competence of the biceps anchor.

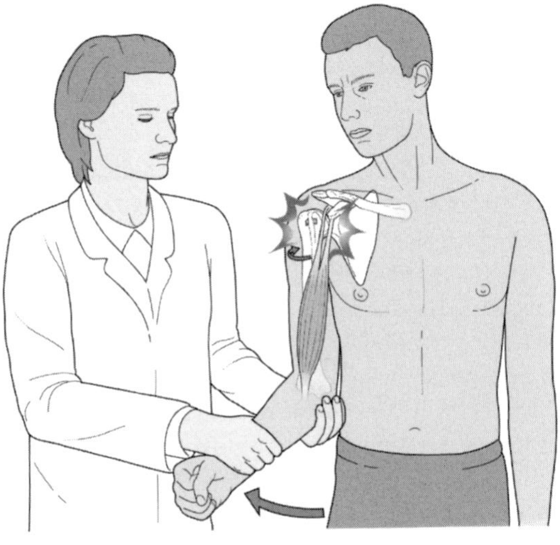

**Fig. 8.5** Assessing the stability of the long head of the biceps tendon in the bicipital groove: the Yergason test.

### Clunk test

During this test the arm is rotated and loaded from a position of extension to one of forward flexion. A clunk-like sensation may be felt if a free labral fragment is caught in the joint. This test is similar to McMurray's test of the knee. Clinical studies have found that a click on manipulation of the glenohumeral joint was a common finding in patients with labral tears even in the absence of joint instability.

### Anterior slide test

This test is another clinical test designed to stress the superior labrum. The patient stands with hands on the hips such that the thumbs are positioned posteriorly. One of the examiner's hands is placed over the shoulder and the other hand behind the elbow. A force is then applied anteriorly and superiorly, and the patient is asked to push back against the force. The test is considered positive if pain is localized to the anterosuperior aspect of the shoulder, or if there is a pop or a click in the anterosuperior region.

## Helpful clinical tests

### Painful arc

- Painful arc is found on active glenohumeral abduction between 60° and 120°.
- Performed in the standing position.
- Injury or condition in the subacromial/subdeltoid bursa or the tendons or teno-osseous attachments of the rotator cuff muscles with impingement on passing under the coracoacromial arch. Not found in isolation, and specific positive findings on other tests may reveal underlying structural injury or condition more clearly.

### Scapular winging

- Scapular winging is usually associated with dysfunction of the serratus anterior and/or trapezius muscles.
- Performed in the standing position.

- Serratus anterior dysfunction is characterized by prominence of the inferior angle of the scapula and loss of scapular protraction during shoulder elevation; flexion is limited (80°–120°).
- Trapezius dysfunction is characterized by a marked drooping of the affected shoulder and lateral displacement of the scapula, and a weak and asymmetric shoulder shrug.
- If normal passive glenohumeral movements are absent, the scapular winging is probably secondary to glenohumeral joint stiffness: adhesive capsulitis or osteoarthrosis.
- Scapular winging can also be associated with instability of the shoulder joint; the apprehension test is performed to confirm this.

## Empty can test

- Tests the supraspinatus muscle.
- Performed in the standing or sitting position.
- Abduct the upper limb to 90° then forward 30° into the scapular plane and maximally internally rotate with the thumb pointing downwards towards the floor; then resisted adduction of the arm in the scapular plane.
- This test is positive if there is pain or weakness.

## Resisted external rotation

- This tests the infraspinatus and teres minor muscles.
- Performed in the standing position.
- Upper arm by the side with the elbow in flexion to 90° and resisted internal rotation of the upper limb.
- Positive if there is pain or weakness.

## Yergason's sign

- Tests the long head of biceps brachii muscle.
- Performed in the standing or sitting position.
- Upper arm by the side with elbow in flexion to 90°and full pronation of the forearm; resisted active supination.
- Positive when pain is localized to the tendon of the long head of biceps brachii and/or the bicipital groove.

## Speed's test

- Tests the long head of biceps brachii muscle.
- Performed in the standing position.
- Shoulder flexion (elevation anteriorly) with the elbow in full extension and the forearm in full supination against resistance.
- Positive when pain is localized to the tendon of the long head of biceps brachii and/or the bicipital groove.

## O'Brien's test

- Tests the superior labral anteroposterior (SLAP) lesion or biceps anchor tear.
- Performed in the standing position.
- Resisted shoulder flexion to 90°, elbow in full extension, upper limb adducted to 10°–15° in internal rotation with the thumb pointing downwards; repeated in external rotation with the thumb pointing downwards.
- Positive when pain and/or weakness occurs with the thumb pointing downwards, which is reduced or eliminated with the thumb pointing upwards.
- Pain localized to the AC joint or the top of the shoulder region suggests an AC injury or pathology.

## Gerber's lift-off test

- Tests the subscapularis muscle.
- Performed in the standing or sitting position.
- Internal rotation of the shoulder and upper limb: the dorsal surface of the hand rests on the lumbar spine with active and resisted lifting of the dorsum of the hand off the lumbar spine.
- Positive if there is pain or weakness.

## Sulcus sign

- Tests for inferior glenohumeral instability.
- Performed in the standing position.
- Downward traction of the humerus and upper arm.
- Positive when a depression or sulcus is observed between the lateral edge of acromion and the greater tuberosity of the humerus.

## Hawkin's test

- Tests for acromiohumeral impingement.
- Performed in the standing position.
- Elevation of the upper arm to 90° and forward 30° in the scapular plane with the scapula

stabilized, and internal rotation of the upper arm.
- Positive if pain during internal rotation due to the greater tuberosity of the humerus impinging under or against the coracoacromial arch.
- Anterior pain is due to acromiohumeral impingement; posterior pain may be due to a tight posterior glenohumeral joint capsule.

## Neer's test
- Tests for acromiohumeral impingement.
- Performed in the standing position.
- Flexion of the upper arm into an overhead elevated position with the elbow in extension, and the scapula stabilized by other hand.
- Positive if there is pain, which is due to impingement of the greater tuberosity of the humerus against the coracoacromial arch.

## Scarf test
- Tests the AC joint injury or pathology.
- Performed in the standing position.
- Upper arm placed into forced horizontal adduction applying overpressure to the AC joint.
- Positive if there is pain in the AC joint.



## Apprehension test
- Tests for anterior glenohumeral instability.
- Performed with patient sitting, standing or lying in supine positions.
- Passively move the shoulder into maximum external rotation in varying degrees of abduction and apply forward pressure to the posterior aspect of the humeral head.
- Positive if the patient becomes apprehensive and/or complains of pain in the shoulder (Fig. 8.6).

## Relocation test
- Tests for anterior glenohumeral instability.
- Performed in the lying supine position.
- Upper arm in abduction and external rotation. This may produce apprehension sometimes coupled with pain in recurrent dislocations, and

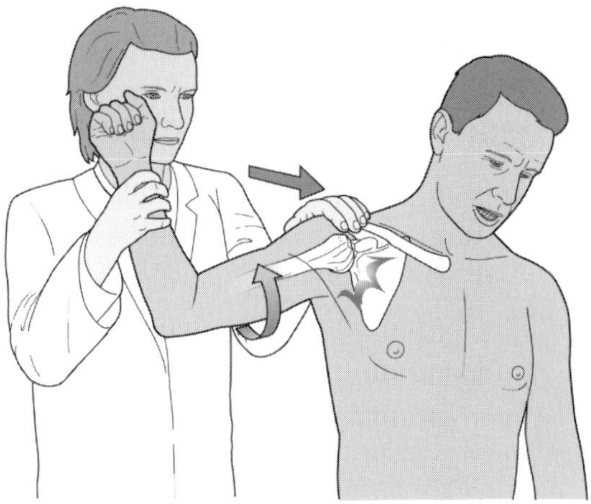

**Fig. 8.6** Testing for chronic shoulder dislocation: the apprehension test.

pain but not apprehension in anterior subluxation.
- This test is then performed by applying a posteriorly directed force on the humeral head or proximal humeral shaft.
- Positive if this maneuver relieves the pain or apprehension.
- Note that patients with primary impingement will have pain unchanged by the relocation maneuver.

## Posterior subluxation test
- Tests for posterior glenohumeral joint instability.
- Performed in the lying supine position.
- Shoulder placed over the edge of the examination couch, flexion of the elbow, upper arm into adduction, internal rotation, and 70°–90° of flexion; the other hand over the shoulder with the thumb on the anterior shoulder and fingers on the posterior joint line, while a posterior force is applied to accentuate any posterior instability. The test is then performed by bringing the arm slowly into abduction and external rotation.
- Positive if the head is felt to relocate with a 'clunk'.

# PATHOLOGIES

## Subacromial impingement

- 'Primary impingement' is used to describe extrinsic compression of the rotator cuff by structures of the coracoacromial arch as a result of either congential or acquired coracoacromial outlet narrowing, leading to cuff tendinopathy, attenuation and tear.
- 'Secondary impingement' is used to describe dynamic narrowing of the coracoacromial outlet as a result of shoulder instability, as a sequel to labral, capsule or, most frequently, rotator cuff tear.
- According to Neer, three distinct stages are observed following cuff injury each of which is accounted for by primary impingement.
  - stage 1, which occurs between 20 and 30 years of age, follows acute injury and is characterized by the development of reversible cuff edema (Fig. 8.7).
  - stage 2, which occurs between 30 and 45 years of age, is the sequel to repetitive trauma and is characterized by the development of irreversible tendon scar and fibrosis (Fig. 8.8).
  - stage 3, which occurs from 45 years onwards, follows further shoulder trauma and results in the development of degenerative tear (Fig. 8.9).

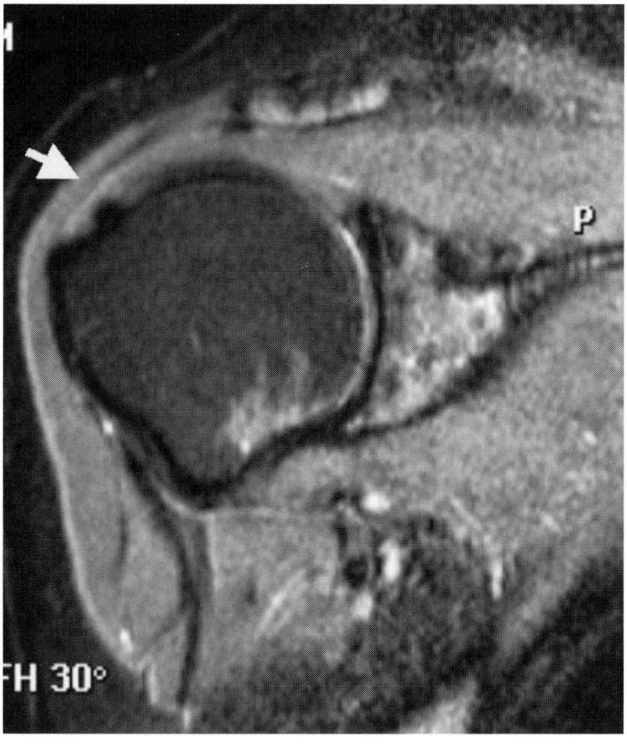


**Fig. 8.7** In a 23-year-old transatlantic swimmer with shoulder pain, this MR image shows subtle subacromial inflammation secondary to impingement. Immediate symptom relief was provided by image-guided bursography with an associated injection of 40 mg of steroid and 1 mL of 0.25% bupivocaine.

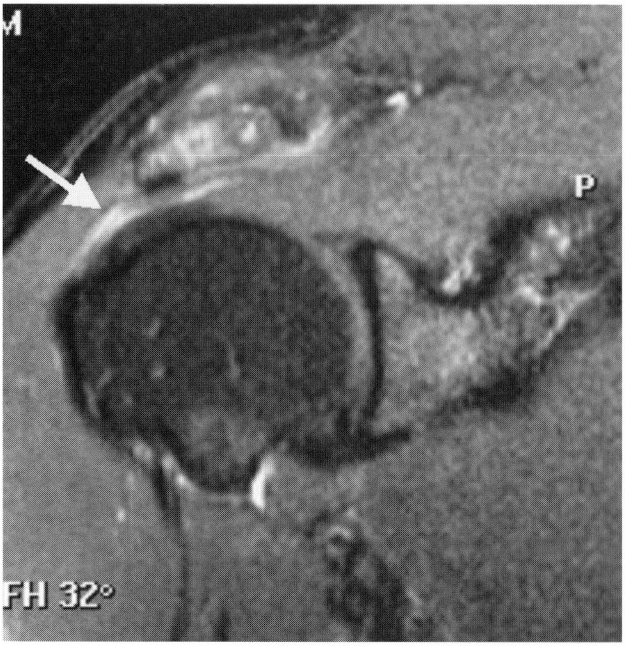


**Fig. 8.8** In a 39-year-old recreational golfer with intractable shoulder pain, this coronal oblique fat-suppressed image shows inflammation in the acromioclavicular articulation with associated subacromial bursal inflammation secondary to impingement. There is a normal rotator cuff. Symptom relief was provided by image-guided injection into the AC joint and subacromial bursa.



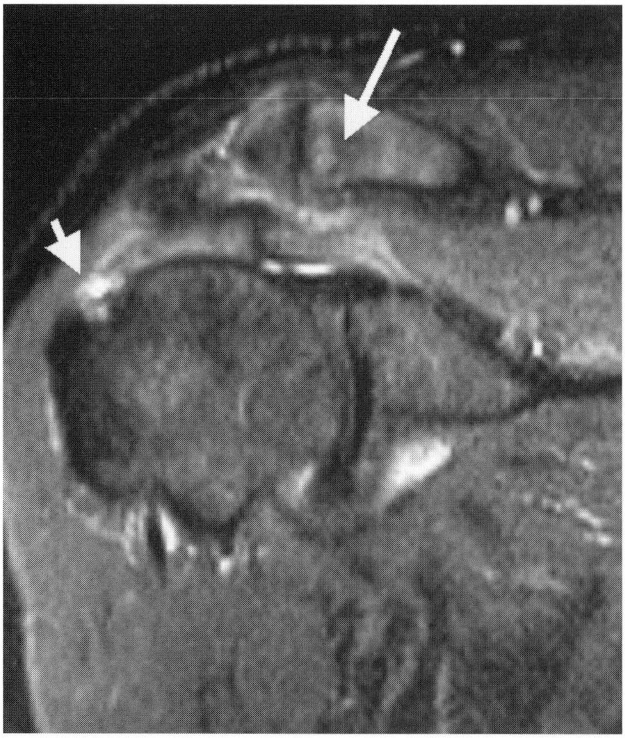

**Fig. 8.9** In a 55-year-old recreational golfer with intractable shoulder pain (which was worse at night lying on the affected shoulder), this coronal oblique fat-suppressed image shows hypertrophic degenerative change in the acromioclavicular joint with secondary impingement producing subacromial bursitis and incomplete tear of the supraspinatus tendon at its attachment to the superior facet of the humeral head. Bursography and steroid injection failed to resolve the symptoms and the golfer subsequently underwent acromioplasty and cuff repair.

- Neer previously proposed that primary impingement accounted for almost 95% of recognized cuff tears.
- It is now clear that cuff tears may occur without impingement, and that narrowing of the coracoacromial space producing an appearance of impingement may be a secondary phenomenon, so-called secondary impingement.
- The coracoacromial arch is formed by the coracoid, the coracoacromial ligament and the acromion process. Several studies have reviewed anatomic variations in the arch contributing to or promoting impingement.
- Morrison and Bigliani described three variations in the shape of the acromion:
  - type 1: flat
  - type 2: curved
  - type 3: hooked.
- Several authors have demonstrated an association between the type 3 shape and rotator cuff impingement and tear.
- The acromion arises from the fusion of three ossification centers, which occurs by 25 years of age. Unfused segments – termed os acromiale – occur in up to 3% of the population, and being unstable and pulled inferiorly by the coracoacromial ligament are associated with cuff impingement and tear.
- Pathologic thickening of the coracoacromial ligament as a degenerative process or the development of traction osteophytes at its insertion (enthesopathy of the coracoacromial ligament).
- Similarly, osteoarthritis of the AC joint, with formation of inferior osteophytes from the distal clavicle may result in cuff impingement.
- Identification of each pathology is crucial as surgical intervention is tailored to mechanism.
- Anterior acromioplasty is undertaken in patients with the type 3 hooked acromion.
- Resection of the distal clavicle is undertaken in patients with inferior osteophytes at the AC articulation.
- Resection of the coracoacromial ligament is undertaken in patients with thickening or enthesopathy involving the ligament.
- Fusion or resection is undertaken in patients with os acromiale.

## Subcoracoid impingement

- Subcoracoid impingement may be secondary to altered anatomic configuration following coracoid or lesser tuberosity fracture, or reflect dynamic narrowing secondary to anterior instability.
- In chronicity, impingement leads to attenuation and tear of the subscapularis, often accompanied by biceps tendon subluxation (Fig. 8.10).

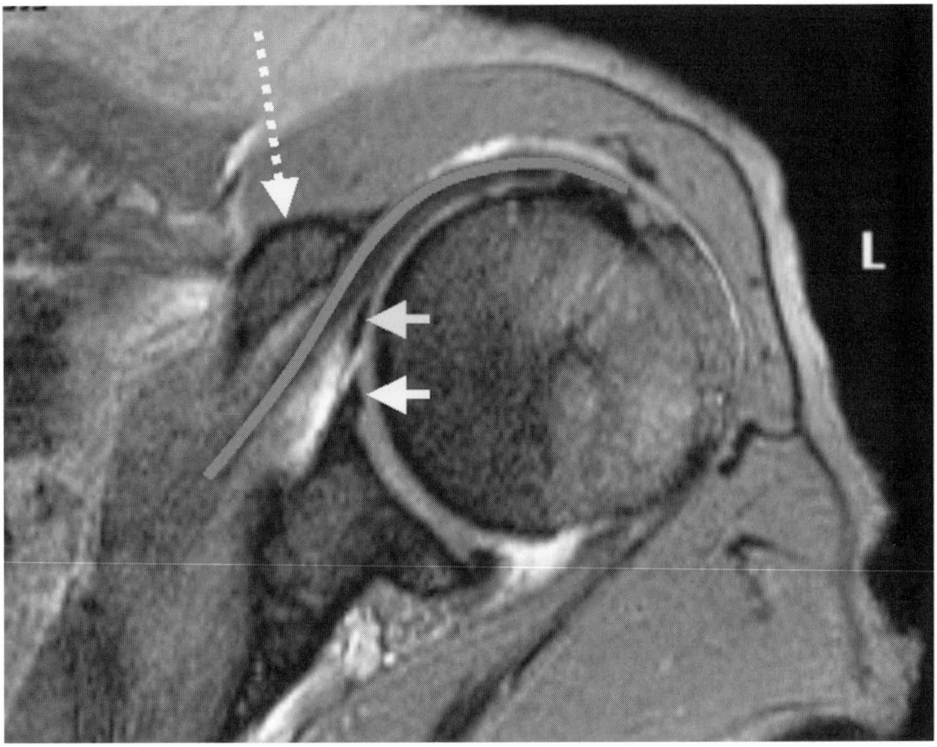


**Fig. 8.10** Axial MR image showing the structures of the subcoracoid space, the coracoid process (dotted arrow), the subscapularis (solid line), the middle glenohumeral ligament (small arrow) and the anterior glenoid labrum (arrow).

# Posterosuperior glenoid impingement

- Posterosuperior impingement is uncommon and is only generally seen in professional athletes such as pitchers, in whom coracoacromial impingement with tear of the posterior fibers of the supraspinatous and superior fibers of the infraspinatus occurs in the late cocking phase or internal rotation accompanying tear of the posterosuperior glenoid labrum (Boxes 8.1 and 8.2).

**Box 8.1 Contributors to primary cuff impingement**

- Acromial downslope
- Acromial shape: hooked type 3 acromion
- Unfused acromion: os acromiale
- Thickened coracoacromial ligament
- Coracoacromial enthesopathy
- Abnormal scapula motion

**Box 8.2 Contributors to secondary impingement (coracoacromial outlet narrowing)**

- Rotator cuff tear
- Bicipitolabral tear

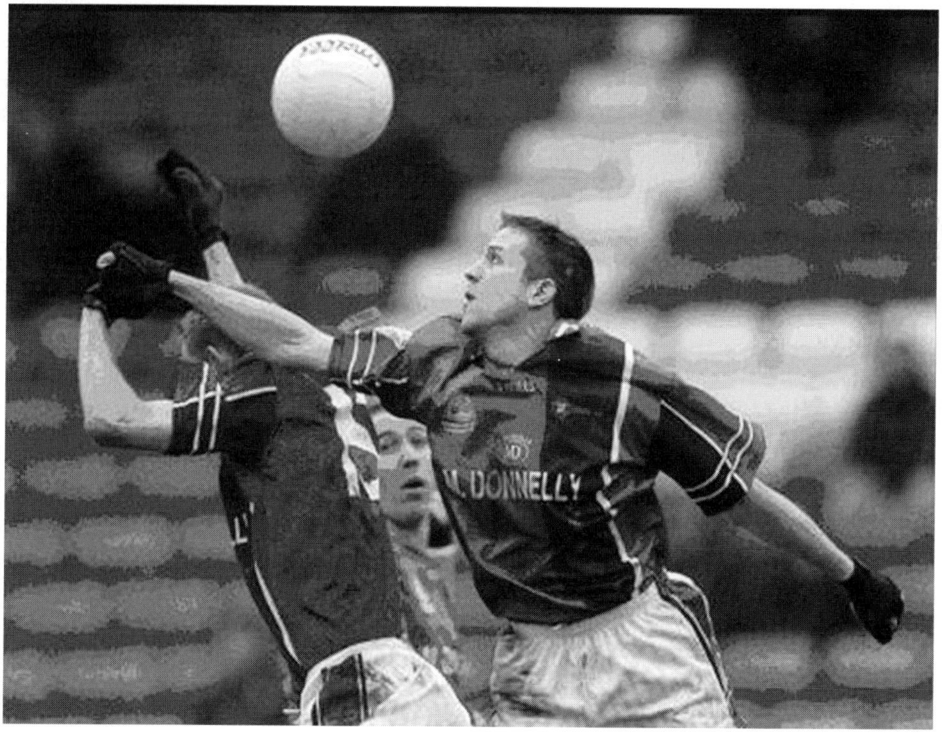

**Fig. 8.11** Sportsfile.

## Subacromial bursitis

### Anatomy and pathogenesis

- The subacromial bursa interposed between the acromion and the muscles of the rotator cuff functions to allow unopposed gliding of the contracting muscles of the rotator cuff between the humeral head and acromion during abduction.
- The subacromial space remains preserved during abduction by scapular tilt but narrows in maximal abduction resulting in physiologic impingement of the muscles of the rotator cuff, particularly the supraspinatus and infraspinatus muscles and of the bursa itself.
- Either due to overuse, repeated abduction with repeated physiologic impingement or secondary to pathologic impingement of the bursa and cuff by either acromial osteophytes, hypertrophic AC changes, downsloping acromion, os acromiale or impaired scapula tilt, the bursa becomes inflamed (Fig. 8.12).
- Bursitis with associated synovial inflammation results in overproduction of bursal fluid and secondary distension of the bursa. In this setting, abduction further irritates the bursa resulting in pain and restricted shoulder movement, particularly abduction.

### History and clinical findings

- Affected individuals typically complain of shoulder pain aggravated by abduction. Pain is often worse at night time aggravated by laying on the shoulder at night.
- On examination, affected individuals have restricted active and passive shoulder motion, particularly full abduction.

### Imaging findings

- Ultrasound employing high-frequency probes allows identification of subacromial fluid and an assessment of the integrity of the rotator cuff.
- MRI coronal oblique images show hyperintense fluid within the subacromial bursa and may show either hypertrophic AC joint change, a downsloping acromion, an acromial osteophyte or an os acromiale, each of which might cause or promote impingement. The degree of scapula tilt during abduction is not assessed (Fig. 8.13).

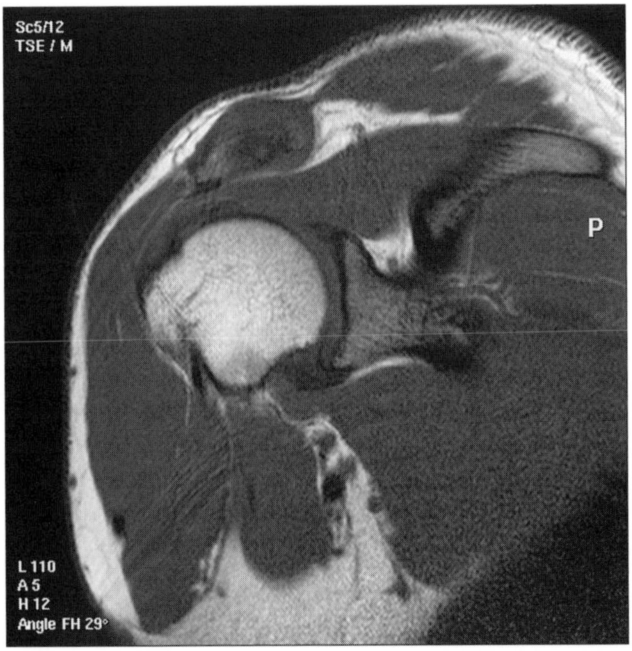


(a)

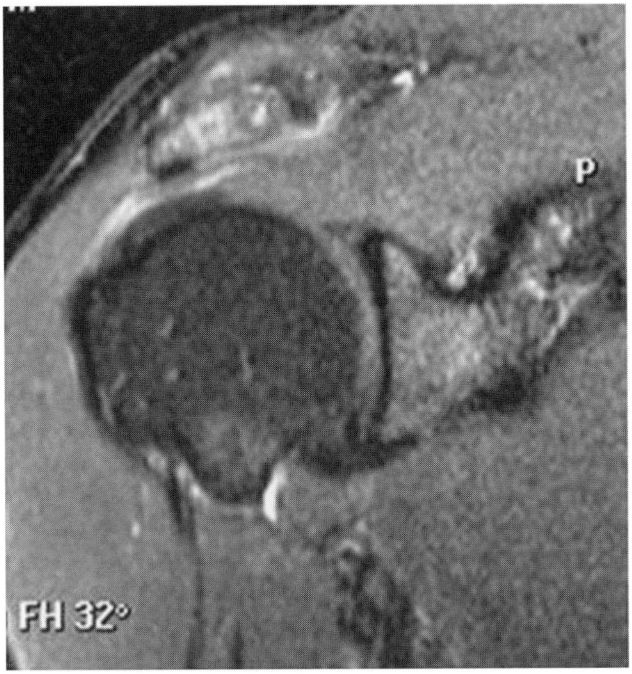


(b)

**Fig. 8.12** (**a**) Coronal oblique $T_1$-weighted and (**b**) fat-suppressed images showing hypertrophic inflammatory change in the acromioclavicular joint with secondary subacromial inflammatory change, and bursitis. The rotator cuff is intact.

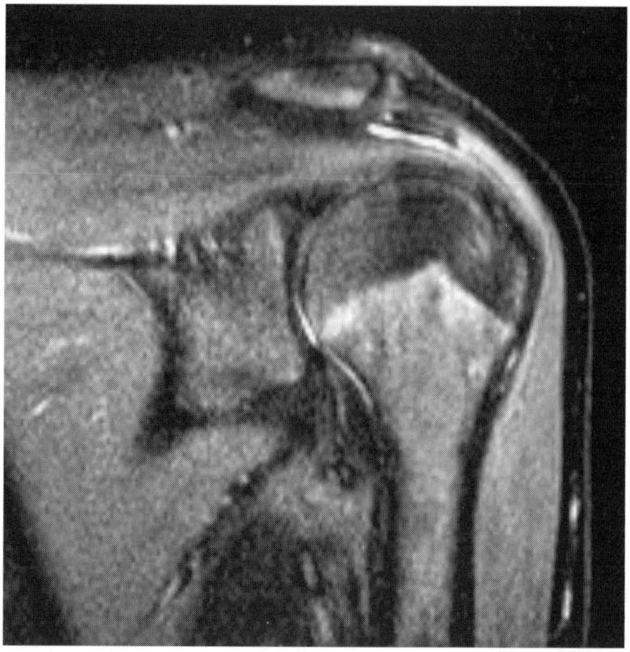

(a)

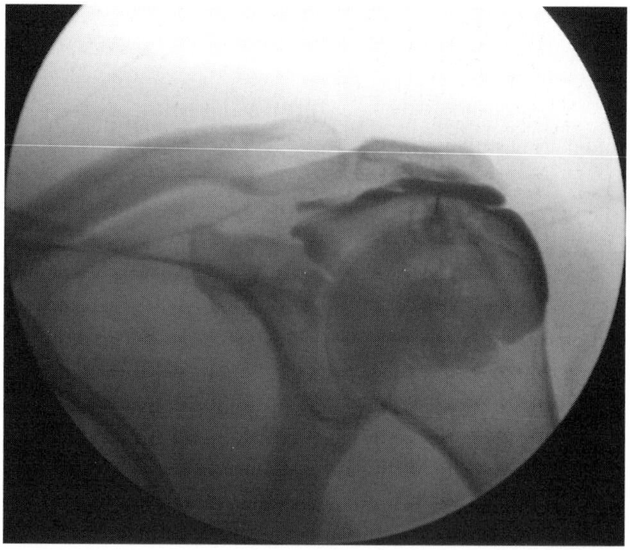

(b)

**Fig. 8.13** (**a**) Coronal oblique fat-suppressed image shows subacromial bursitis. Symptoms of impingement were immediately resolved by an injection of bupivacaine hydrochloride to the bursa as part of image guided bursography. (**b**) Contrast injected into the subacromial bursa.

## Management

### Non-surgical

- Oral antiinflammatories may reduce subacromial inflammation.
- Image-guide bursography: the injection of contrast to the subacromial bursa and of therapeutic steroid (± bupivacaine hydrochloride) injection frequently leads to the rapid resolution of the subacromial inflammation. Many patients complain of accelerated pain in the 24 hours following bursography after which symptoms usually resolve (Fig. 8.14).
- Physiotherapy: ultrasound and heat may reduce inflammation and associated pain. Rehabilitation and re-education exercises are employed during recovery including exercises to improve scapular tilt.

### Surgical

- Resistant bursitis provoked by impingement may require subacromial decompression. This may take the form of acromioplasty (curetting the inferior surface of the acromion and associated osteophytes), acromioclavicular joint debridement or incision of a thickened AC ligament.

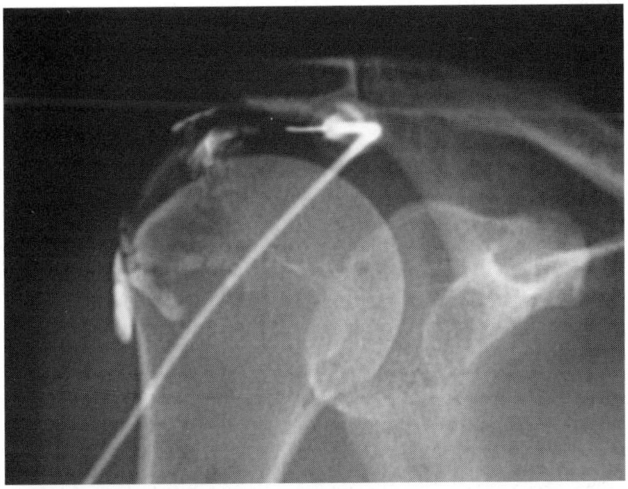

(a)

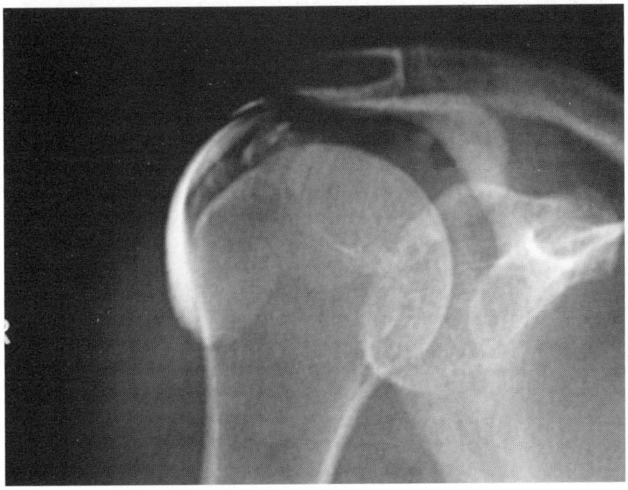

(b)

**Fig. 8.14**
**(a, b)** Radiographs showing needle placement in the subacromial bursae with contrast filling of the space prior to placement of steroid and bupivacaine hydrochloride.

# Rotator cuff (supraspinatus) tendinitis

## Anatomy

- The supraspinatus, infraspinatus and teres minor tendons insert on the greater tuberosity; the subscapularis tendon inserts on the lesser tuberosity. Together they comprise the rotator cuff.

## Mechanism of injury

- Injury to the supraspinatus may be secondary to direct trauma exacerbated by intrinsic factors such as diminished vascularity (the 'critical zone,' 5 mm proximal to the tendon insertion, is thought to be a zone of relative ischemia), overuse or failure of the tendon's normal healing mechanism or may occur secondary to chronic impingement.
- Irrespective of the cause, tendon injury may manifest as tendinosis, partial (incomplete thickness) or full (complete) thickness tears.

## Definition of terms

- The term tendinopathy (rather than tendinitis) is used to describe minor tendon injury, as biopsy in these cases often fails to reveal inflammatory cells.
- Rotator cuff tear can be defined as partial when disruption of the tendon fibers involves only a part of the tendon, the superior surface, the inferior surface or the mid substance of the tendon.
- Full-thickness tendon tears are characterized by complete superoinferior disruption of the tendon fibers.
- A full-thickness tear is incomplete if it fails to extend from anterior to posterior. A complete full-thickness tear extends from the anterior tendon margin to the posterior tendon margin allowing complete tendon retraction.

## History and clinical findings



- Patients frequently complain of chronic shoulder pain often radiating to the neck, lateral arm and elbow. Affected individuals often give a history of chronic shoulder pain which is worse at night when laying on the affected shoulder.
- On inspection, patients with chronic tendinopathy may have evidence of muscle wasting. Both passive and active abduction are limited, particularly above 90°, up to which point abduction reflects deltoid contraction.

## Imaging findings

### Ultrasound

- Ultrasound allows clear visualization of the supraspinatus tendon. The normal tendon shows uniform echogenicity. In tendinitis, the tendon becomes swollen and shows a reduction in echotexture at the affected site due to a relative increase in water content.

### Magnetic resonance imaging

- At MRI, tendinitis manifests as an increase in signal within the otherwise hypointense healthy tendon. (The magic angle phenomenon describes an artefactual change in tendon signal at 55° to the main magnetic field simulating tendinitis) (Fig. 8.15).
- Tendinopathy is traditionally graded 1, 2A or 2B:
  - grade 1 tendinopathy, reflecting mild tendon disruption, is manifest as subtle signal abnormality on short TE $T_1$- and proton density-weighted images
  - grade 2A tendinopathy, reflecting more marked tendinosis, is manifest by both signal change and smooth tendon swelling
  - grade 2B tendinopathy, the more severe form, is manifest as signal change and tendon swelling with slightly irregular surfaces (Fig. 8.16).

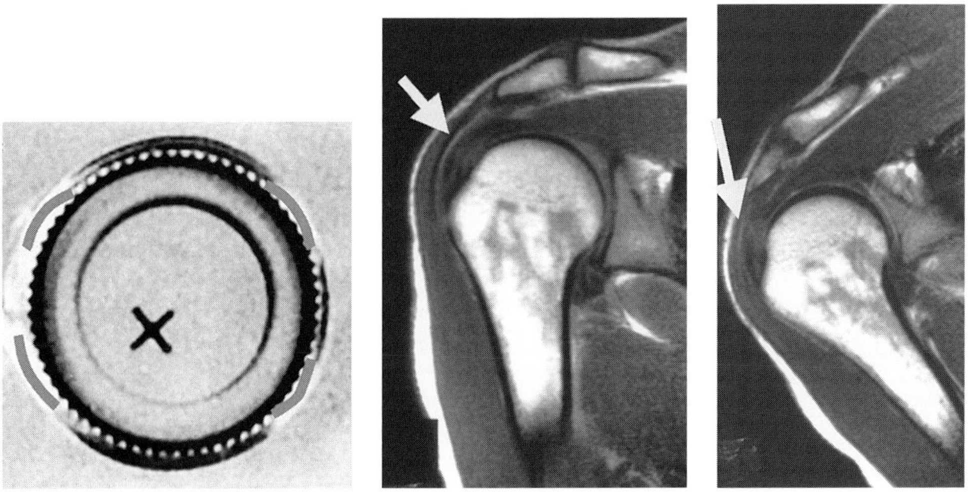

(a) (b) (c)

**Fig. 8.15** (**a**) This image shows signal hyperintensity at four points in a cadaveric tendon wrapped around a Petri dish, each point at 55° to the main magnetic field. This is the so-called magic angle phenomenon. (**b**) This image shows signal abnormality in the supraspinatus tendon either due to tendinopathy or the magic angle phenomenon. (**c**) This image shows persistent signal abnormality despite a change in patient position, indicating supraspinatus tendinopathy.

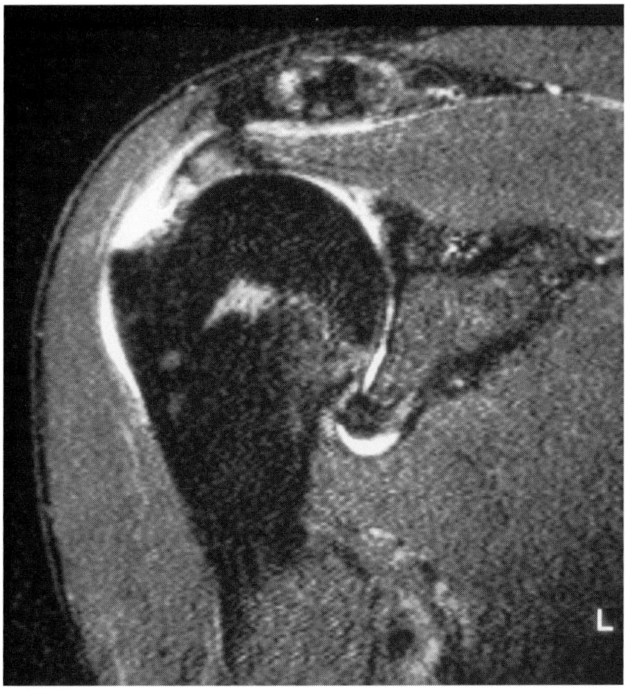


**Fig. 8.16** A full-thickness supraspinatus tendon with 2 cm retraction and gap at the site of a tear.

## Management

### Non-surgical

- Rest.
- Physiotherapy.
- Antiinflammatories.
- Intra-articular steroids and subacromial bursal steroids.

### Surgical

- Surgery addresses the cause of tendinopathy, in particular the causes of impingement: acromioplasty, AC joint debridement and coracoclavicular ligament incision may all be undertaken to reduce impingement.

# Rotator cuff (supraspinatus) partial tears

## Mechanism of injury

- Partial tears of the rotator cuff most frequently arise from the articular surface, particularly along the anterior margin of the tendon. Alternatively, partial tears may involve the bursal surface, involve the central substance of the tendon (so-called intrasubstance tears) or occur at the attachment of the tendon to the superior facet of the greater tuberosity.
- Bursal surface partial tears are less common and identification in the absence of bursal contrast (bursography) is difficult. Conspicuity of these lesions is enhanced by the presence of effusion in the subacromial subdeltoid bursa.
- At arthrography, partial tears are considered to be:
  - grade 1: extending through less than a quarter of the tendon
  - grade 2: extending through less than half of the tendon
  - grade 3: extending through more than half of the tendon (Fig. 8.17).
- Partial supraspinatus tendon tears (Box 8.3).

(a)
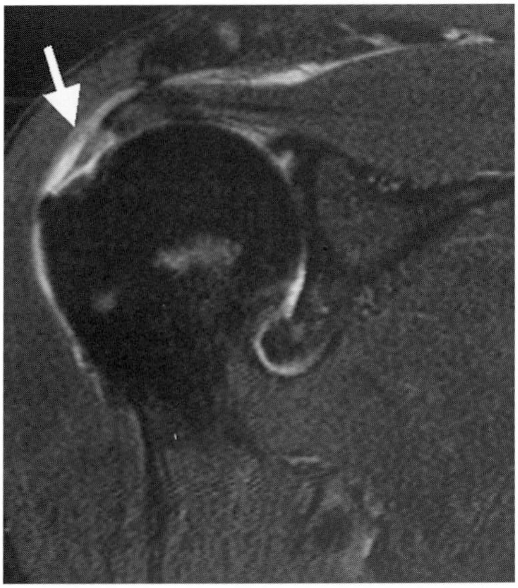
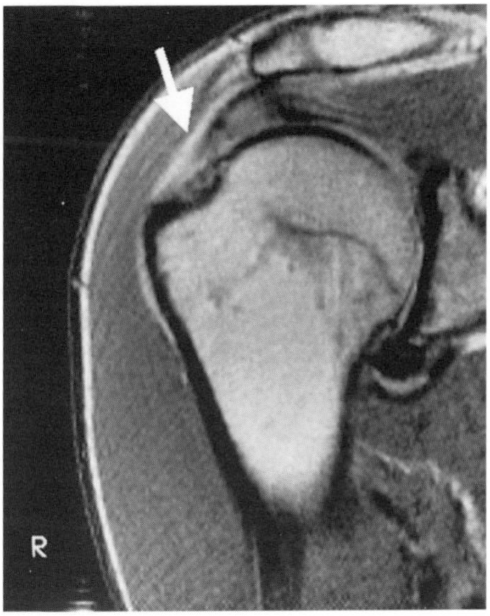

(b)

**Fig. 8.17** MR images. (**a**) Fat-suppressed and (**b**) $T_1$-weighted images showing a partial supraspinatus tendon tear with some intact fibers preventing retraction.

**Box 8.3 Partial supraspinatus tendon tears**

- Articular surface
- Bursal surface
- Intrasubstance
- Superior facet avulsion

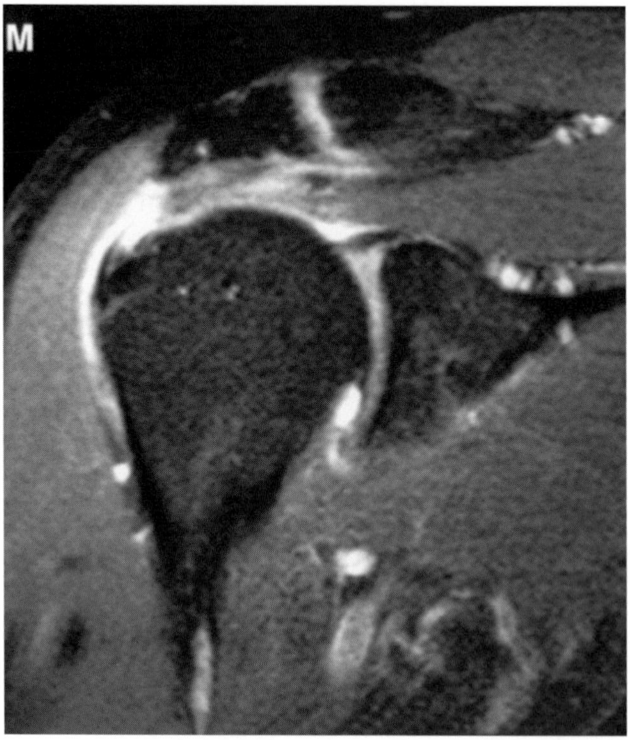


**Fig. 8.18** Coronal oblique fat-suppressed image showing signal hyperintensity within the supraspinatus tendon secondary to an intrasubstance tear.



- Occasionally articular surface partial tears occur at the posterior rotator interval at the junction of the supraspinatus and infraspinatus secondary to impaction against the posterosuperior glenoid in internal rotation, in throwing athletes such as baseball pitchers.
- In this setting, cuff tears are often associated with the development of cysts in the humeral head, posterosuperior labral tears and posterior capsular ossification (Bennet's lesion) (Fig. 8.18).

## History and clinical findings

- Pain exacerbated by cuff stress induced by tendon contraction in abduction.
- Affected individuals often complain of pain at night radiating to the neck and down the outer arm to the elbow.
- Examination: similar to tendonitis.

## Imaging findings

- These may be identified at both ultrasound and MRI. At MRI, tears are manifest by the presence of local hemorrhage and fluid at the site of the tear.

## Management

### Non-surgical

- Similar to tendonitis.

### Surgical

- Treatment of impingement (see 'Supraspinatus tendonitis' above).
- Primary debridement and tendon repair.

# Full-thickness rotator cuff (supraspinatus) tears

## Definition of terms

- Similarly to partial tears, complete tears tend to extend posteriorly from the anterior margin of the tendon.
- Detachment of the distal anterior aspect of the supraspinatus tendon from the greater tuberosity is often the earliest sign of a full-thickness tear.
- Uninterrupted tendon fibers are retracted in time leaving an obvious gap in the tendon.
- Tears are considered to be small when the retraction is less than 1 cm, medium when the retraction is 1–3 cm and massive when the retraction is greater than 5 cm. See Box 8.4.

## History and clinical findings

- Similar findings to other forms of impingement with bursitis, tendinopathy and partial tears. On inspection there may be obvious muscle atrophy and limitation of passive movement on examination.

## Imaging findings

### Ultrasound

- High-frequency probes may reveal full-thickness tendon tears with the hand and arm held in external rotation.

### Magnetic resonance imaging

- Full-thickness cuff tears (see Fig. 8.19) allow free communication between the shoulder joint space and the subacromial subdeltoid bursa and are therefore manifest by signal abnormality on $T_1$-, proton-density and $T_2$-weighted scans.

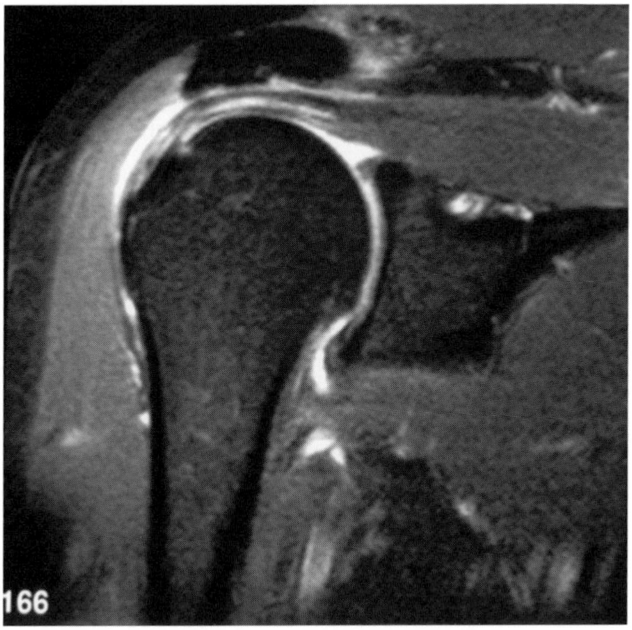


**Fig. 8.19** Coronal oblique fat-suppressed MR image showing a full-thickness tear of the supraspinatus tendon.

**Box 8.4 Grades of tendon tear**

**Partial tear**

- Grade 1: less than $^{1}/_{4}$ tendon thickness
- Grade 2: less than $^{1}/_{2}$ tendon thickness
- Grade 3: more than $^{1}/_{2}$ tendon thickness

**Full thickness**

- Small: 1 cm
- Medium: 1–3 cm
- Massive: 5 cm

**Box 8.5 Tendinosis (no inflammatory infiltrate)**

- Grade 1: signal abnormality at MRI
- Grade 2A: signal abnormality at MRI with associated swelling
- Grade 2B: signal MRI with swelling and surface irregularity
- Grade 3A: signal abnormality with definite partial defect.
- Grade 3B: signal abnormality with full-thickness defect.

Uninterrupted signal abnormality traversing the tendon on $T_2$-weighted scans allows the differentiation of partial and complete injuries.

- Both the AP extent of the tear and the amount of retraction are usually recorded, being useful predictors of outcome following surgical intervention.
- In chronicity, atrophy of the muscle belly commonly accompanies tendon injury. Secondary elevation of the humeral head with coracohumeral arch impingement results in biceps tendon impaction, shear and secondary tendinosis (Boxes 8.4 and 8.5).

## Management



### Non-surgical

- In early cases, causes of impingement should be addressed. In chronic cases attempts should be made to provide symptom relief by combining physiotherapy, oral antiinflammatories and intra-articular steroid injections.

### Surgical

- In chronic rotator cuff tears, associated muscular atrophy precludes primary tendon repair as suture material tears through devitalized muscle fibers resulting in re-tear at sites of attempted treatment.

## Subscapularis injury

- Subscapularis tendon injury is uncommon but when it occurs is usually as a sequel to anterior dislocation, injury to the shoulder in abduction with external rotation or chronic subcoracoid impingement. Being inserted in the biceps tendon sheath groove, rupture is often accompanied by biceps tendon subluxation, tear or dislocation.

## Infraspinatus

- Isolated infraspinatus tendon injury is extremely uncommon, rarely complicating posterior shoulder dislocation.

# Biceps brachii: tendinitis and tear

## Anatomy

- The biceps brachii muscle is composed of a long head and short head.
- The two muscle bellies share a single tendon insertion on the bicipital tuberosity of the radius.
- The short head arises from the apex of the coracoid.
- The long head arises from the supraglenoid tubercle of the scapula.
- Stabilization of the long head of biceps tendon within the joint space is by the coracohumeral ligament (the coracohumeral ligament fuses with the supraspinatous tendon).
- Extra-articular stabilization outside the joint within the biceps tendon sheath groove is by the transverse humeral ligament and subscapularis proximally, and by the pectoralis major distally.

## Mechanisms of injury

- Injury involving the biceps muscle more often involves the tendons than the muscle bellies, and of the tendons injury most frequently affects the tendon of the long head in the shoulder.
- Injury occurs at either the shoulder or elbow. Shoulder injury is divided into long or short head. Long-head injury is divided into intra-articular and extra-articular forms.
- Long-head tears are common as part of age-related attrition. Tear of a healthy long-head tendon in sportsmen is uncommon. Dislocation is considerably more common in this setting and accompanies traumatic subscapularis tears during shoulder dislocation.
- Shoulder: intra-articular long-head tendon injury occurs secondary to impingement accompanying chronic supraspinatous tendon tears.
- Shoulder: extra-articular long-head tendon injury, either tear or dislocation, occurs secondary to chronic subcoracoid impingement with subscapularis tear.
- Elbow: at the elbow biceps tendon tear typically occurs at the attachment to the radial tuberosity or at the musculotendinous junction. Partial tears are common and should be differentiated from inflammation in the adjacent bicipitoradial bursa.
- Biceps injury at the elbow is often encountered in weightlifters. Musculotendinous junction tears are often encountered following the use of anabolic steroids where muscle belly bulk and contraction cannot be supported by the adjacent tendon and musculoskeletal junction.

## History and clinical findings

- Affected individuals often describe an acute 'giving way' either at the shoulder or elbow. Intra-articular tendon rupture often occurs innocuously and is followed by discomfort rather than pain. Similarly extra-articular rupture or subluxation occurs innocuously with discomfort rather than acute pain. Individuals describe a subjective loss of power over the following weeks.
- Tendon rupture at the elbow frequently occurs as an acute event in response to a forced extension during attempted flexion or muscle belly contraction as in weightlifting or tackling in rugby. The injury is typically acutely painful.

### Examination

#### Biceps shoulder injury

- Passive examination reveals an apparent defect in the upper arm, becoming more marked during contraction. Similarly, retraction during muscle belly contraction results in the development of a gross lump in the mid arm.

- Active examination reveals significant weakness when compared to the unaffected side.

Biceps elbow injury

- Passive examination is often unremarkable. Active examination reveals weakness and pain during elbow flexion.

## Imaging findings

### Ultrasound and magnetic resonance imaging

- These readily allow identification of the normal long-head tendon in the bicipital groove and hence allow detection of tear and subluxation.
- Short-head biceps tendon injury is less readily identified. At MRI injury is best identified on sagittal images.
- Tendon injury in the elbow can be readily detected at both ultrasound and MRI. Both modalities allow the differentiation of tendon tear (partial or complete) from pain induced by inflammation in the associated bicipitoradial bursa.

## Management

### Non-surgical

- Collar and cuff immobilization.
- Shoulder injuries are frequently managed conservatively with the use of antiinflammatories and intra-articular steroids.
- Because the biceps sheath communicates with the shoulder joint space, intra-articular steroids are often employed to treat long-head tendinosis.
- In the elderly, physiotherapy is employed to help improve strength and mobility of the residual biceps unit.
- Ultrasound-guided steroid injection to the bicipitoradial bursa is often an effective treatment of bicipitoradial bursitis.



### Surgical

- Primary tendon repair is employed in young patients following acute sports-related biceps tendon tears of the short head and of the musculotendinous junction at the elbow.
- Acute tear of the long head during sport is uncommon; dislocation is considerably more common and is treated by relocation within the bicipital groove and repair of the stabilizing intertubercular ligament and of the associated tear of the subscapularis.

# Parsonage–Turner syndrome (brachialis neuritis)

## Definition

- A brachial plexus neuronitis thought to be related to a viral infection.
- May affect any branch of the brachial plexus (most commonly the suprascapular nerve) manifest as a neuropathy with denervation of the affected muscles of the rotator cuff, typically the supraspinatous and the infraspinatous muscles.
- Muscle weakness may be incorrectly attributed to muscle tear.

## Clinical findings

- Clinical features of rotator cuff tear.

## Imaging findings

- MRI allows the identification of muscle edema in affected muscle groups particularly on fat-suppressed images. Abnormalities are not detected on any other imaging modality. This most frequently involves the suprascapular nerve and associated musculature but may affect any branch of the brachial plexus including the interosseous nerve in the forearm (Fig. 8.20).

## Management

- Physiotherapy.
- Antiinflammatories.
- Antiviral therapy.
- Resolution is between 6 months and 2 years, frequently with complete recovery and occasionally with residual deficit producing winging of the scapula.

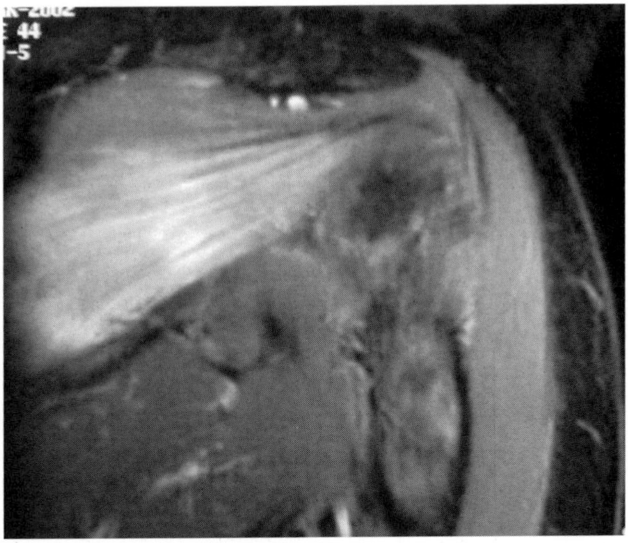

**Fig. 8.20** Coronal oblique fat-suppressed image of the left shoulder showing signal hyperintensity diffusely through the infraspinatus muscle belly, secondary to muscle edema, typical of Parsonage–Turner syndrome.

# Suprascapular notch ganglion cyst

## Anatomy

- Thought to be secondary to an occult superior labral tear, impaired healing is complicated by the formation of a ganglion cyst which tracks along the path of least resistance to the suprascapular notch. Within the notch the enlarging cyst compresses the suprascapular nerve. Secondary nerve palsy produces marked rotator cuff weakness often incorrectly thought to be secondary to a muscular tear.

## Clinical findings

- Patients present with features of a rotator cuff tear.

## Imaging findings

- MRI allows the identification of a ganglion cyst within the notch (Fig. 8.21).

## Management

- CT or ultrasound-guided aspiration with steroid injection.
- Surgical decompression.



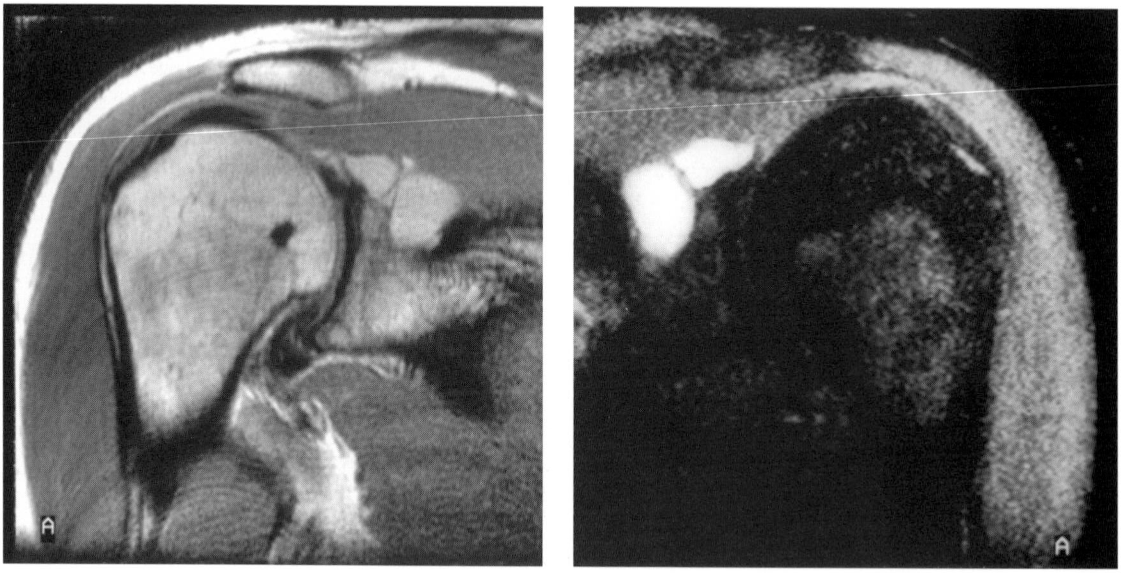


(a) (b)

**Fig. 8.21** (**a**) Coronal oblique $T_1$-weighted and (**b**) fat-suppressed image showing a suprascapular notch ganglion cyst compressing the suprascapular nerve.

# Glenohumeral instability: the labral–ligamentous complex

## Anatomy

- The labral–ligamentous complex, which includes the glenoid labrum, and the superior, middle and inferior glenohumeral ligaments, functions to anchor the humeral head to the osseous glenoid.
- The superior and middle glenohumeral ligaments originate together from the superior labrum immediately anterior to the labral–bicipital anchor. The superior ligament courses anteriorly to merge with the coracohumeral ligament; the middle ligament courses inferiorly to merge with the subscapularis.
- The inferior glenohumeral ligament has three components including anterior and posterior bands and intervening axillary pouch. The anterior band is thicker than the other glenohumeral ligaments and has a broader glenolabral origin, therefore being the dominant contributor to shoulder stability (between 3 and 9 o'clock).
- Although the middle glenohumeral ligament is usually broad, merging with the subscapularis laterally, it is associated with considerable variation in form, ranging from absence, to a cord-like configuration.
- A cord-like middle glenohumeral ligament is often associated with absence of the anterosuperior glenoid labrum, the Buford complex.
- Variations in the structure of the middle glenohumeral ligament are thought to account for six reported variations in the pattern of synovial recesses within the joint space. According to De Palma, a type 1 joint is characterized by one recess above the middle glenohumeral ligament, a type 2 joint is characterized by one recess arising below the middle glenohumeral ligament, a type 3 joint is characterized by two recesses above and below the middle glenohumeral ligament, a type 4 joint is characterized by one large recess and an absent glenohumeral ligament, a type 5 joint is characterized by division of the middle glenohumeral ligament into two synovial folds and a type 6 joint has no synovial recesses.



### Box 8.6 Variations in labral anatomy

**Bicipito–labral complex (BLC)**

- Type 1: BLC adherent to the superior pole of the glenoid
- Type 2: BLC attaches to the superior labrum
- Type 3: meniscoid labrum with large sulcus

**Absent middle glenohumeral ligament**

**Cord-like middle glenohumeral ligament with an absent anterosuperior labrum (Buford complex)**

**Anterior capsule insertion**

- Type 1: capsule arises from the labrum
- Type 2: capsule arises from the scapular neck
- Type 3: from the neck 1 cm medial to the labrum

- There are three variations in the pattern of insertion of the tendon of the long head of the biceps to the labrum, the bicipitolabral complex. Most commonly, the biceps inserts at the junction of the superior margin of the labrum and glenoid itself. Less frequently, the biceps inserts to the superior labrum. Also less frequently, the biceps inserts to the body of the superior labrum in a meniscoid form.
- Articular cartilage normally undercuts the labral fibrocartilage; particularly marked undercutting commonly forms sulci at the labral bicipital junction (the sublabral sulcus and foramen) and between the origins of the middle and inferior glenohumeral ligaments. In old age, sulci become more prominent and frequently mimic labral tears.

## Variations in labral anatomy

- See Box 8.6.

## Definition of terms

- Traumatic unidirectional anterior, inferior or posterior instability with a Bankart lesion usually considered to be correctable by surgical reconstruction. (TUBS: traumatic, unidirectional, Bankart, surgical.) **OR**
- Multidirectional atraumatic instability, which is rarely correctable by surgical intervention. (AMBRI: atraumatic, multidirectional, bilateral instability). Multidirectional instability is most frequently characterized by osteoarthritis, osteophytes and both tear and attenuation of the labrum.

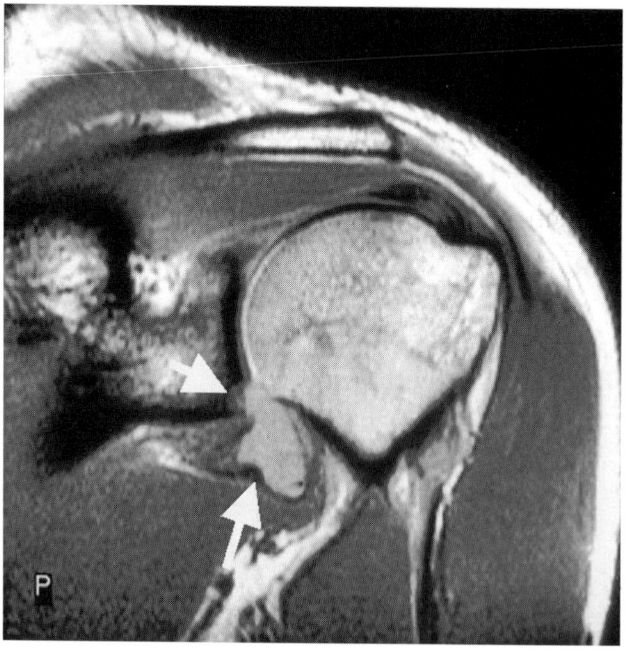


**Fig. 8.22** Coronal oblique image showing an impaction fracture of the anteroinferior glenoid with a displaced labral fragment attached to the inferior glenohumeral ligament (arrow) in a Gaelic footballer following multiple dislocations.

## Isolated labral tears: superior labral anteroposterior tear

### Anatomy

- Isolated tears of the anterosuperior, superior and posterior labrum (SLAP lesions) following shoulder trauma may occasionally present with shoulder pain or impaired shoulder movement.
- Snyder described four types of superior labral tear following trauma:
  - type 1: simple fraying of the articulating surface of the labrum
  - type 2: fraying and stripping of the labrum and biceps anchor
  - type 3: bucket handle tear with displacement of the central portion
  - type 4: bucket handle tear with longitudinal extension to the biceps tendon.
- Neviaser described the glenolabral articular disruption (GLAD) lesion, which refers to a partial labral tear associated with articular cartilage divot that follows acute forced adduction, as seen when one athlete or professional footballer falls on another. The lesion typically involves the anterosuperior labrum and does not result in instability.

### Mechanism of injury

- Injury to the superior labrum is usually secondary to traction effect imposed on the labrum at the long head of biceps attachment. Such traction occurs when the arm is in the overhead position as in javelin throwing, baseball pitching, tennis serving or diving.

### History and clinical findings

- Affected individuals complain of shoulder pain on abduction with onset following a traction episode. Mechanical locking occurs following a Snyder grade 4 bucket handle tear.
- Multidirectional pain without a discernable loss of either active or passive motion and power.

### Imaging findings

#### Magnetic resonance imaging

- Coronal oblique MRI scans show a focal linear signal abnormality in the superior labrum.

#### Computerized tomography

- CT or MRI arthrography improve assessment of intra-articular soft tissues. Axial CT arthrography scans allow the detection of GLAD lesions, and in the reformatted coronal oblique plane allow the detection of SLAP lesions. MRI arthrograms allow the direct visualization of the superior labrum in the coronal oblique planes (Fig. 8.24).

### Management

- Collar and cuff immobilization.
- Arthroscopic repair or debridement of the superior labrum.

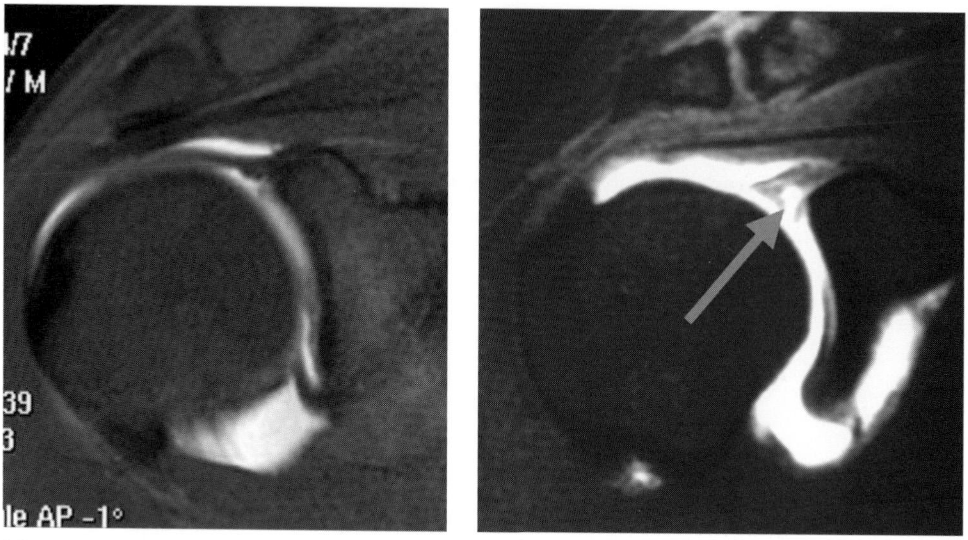

(a) (b)

**Fig. 8.23** (**a**) Coronal oblique fat-suppressed image shows the normal attachment of the long head of biceps to the superior labrum. (**b**) This image shows a tear in the superior labrum (arrow) – a SLAP injury.

# Anterior dislocation: isolated or recurrent

## Mechanism of injury

- Reflecting the anterior obliquity of the glenoid, injury to shoulder in abduction external rotation or by direct impaction yields either anterior subluxation or frank anterior dislocation.
- Tendancy to sublux is prevented predominantly by the anterior labrum and inferior glenohumeral ligament.
- Anterior capsular structures tear as a result of extreme forces imposed by a dislocating humeral head; most frequently at the glenoid (Bankart lesion and variants), less frequently at the attachment of the capsule to the lesser tuberosity (HAGL: humeral avulsion of the glenohumeral ligament).
- Impaction of the posterolateral surface of the greater tuberosity of humeral head on the inferior margin of the glenoid results in an impaction fracture termed a Hill–Sachs lesion (see Fig. 8.24).

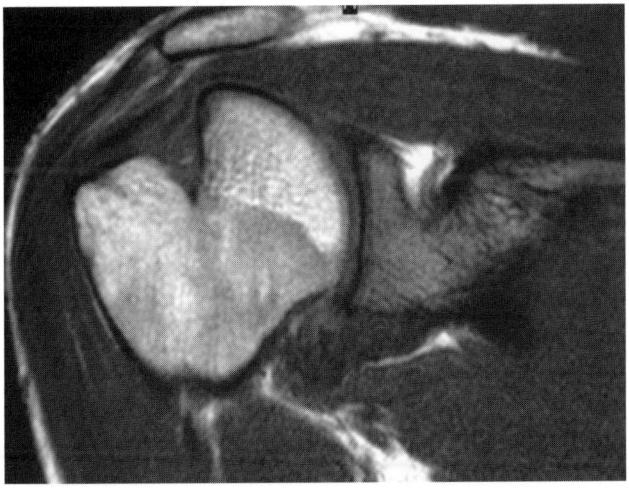

(a)

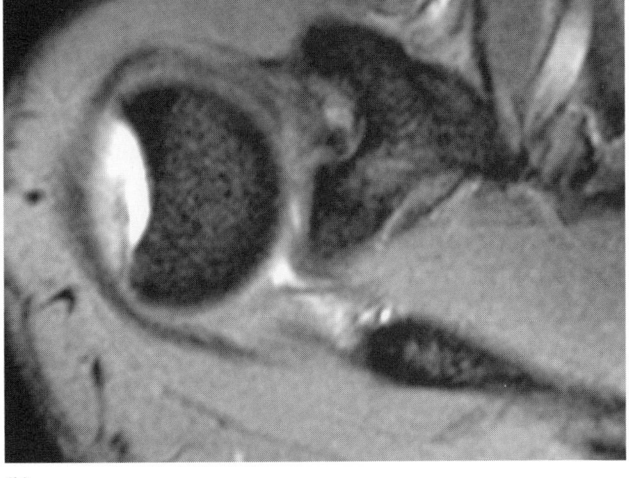

(b)

**Fig. 8.24** (**a**) Coronal oblique and (**b**) axial images showing a hatchet defect in the humeral head, the so-called Hill–Sachs lesion occurring in a patient with recurrent shoulder dislocations.

## History and clinical findings

- Dislocation usually complicates a fall directly on the shoulder.
- At the time of injury, examination reveals a fixed contour deformity with limited passive and active motion. The shoulder may be relocated by internal rotation and posterior pressure.

## Imaging findings

### Radiography

- Radiographs confirm acute anterior dislocation manifest as anteroinferior displacement of the humeral head to overlap the glenoid. Radiographs often fail to assess the anteroinferior labrum. Labral injury is best detected by either CT or MRI.

### Computerized tomography and magnetic resonance imaging

- At both CT and MRI, acute injuries are usually evaluated without exogenous contrast because of the intrinsic contrast afforded by intra-articular joint effusion.
- Subacute injuries following recurrent dislocation are best evaluated with intra-articular contrast, either CT arthrography or MRI arthrography (MRI is favored).
- At imaging, both CT arthrography and at MRI arthrography the following terms are used to describe labral injuries:
  - Perthes' lesion: injury to the anteroinferior labral fibrocartilage without osseous injury. These lesions may reapproximate and synovialize and may only become identified by imaging with the inferior glenohumeral ligament stretched in the ABER position (abducted externally rotated), in such a position the torn labrum becomes redetached and is readily identified
  - Bankart lesion: injury to fibrocartilage and underlying bone. Rowe and Zarins have classified Bankart lesions into type 1 (characterized by a small detachment of the capsulolabral complex without glenoid stripping), type 2 (characterized by moderate detachment with glenoid stripping), type 3 (characterized by severe detachment) and type 4 (in which both labrum and bone are detached)
  - occasionally the underlying scapular periosteum remains intact and the torn labral–ligamentous complex rolls up and displaces medially. This is termed an ALPSA lesion (anterior labral periosteal sleeve avulsion). As this lesion heals, fibrous tissue heaps up over the displaced labrum and may make detection difficult despite clinical instability
  - HAGL (humeral avulsion of the glenohumeral ligament) is employed to describe avulsion of the inferior glenohumeral ligament from the lesser tuberosity of the humerus.

## Management

### Non-surgical

- Antiinflammatories.
- Collar and cuff.
- Physiotherapy.

Surgery

- Surgery ranges from repair of the anterior capsule to reinforcement of the anterior glenoid by bone graft. In high-performance sportsmen, a return to high-level activity occurs as early as 6 months following surgery (mean 9 months).

### Outcome

- Sequelae following anterior dislocation in patients over the age of 35 differ from those in younger patients. In patients over 35, approximately one third of patients develop tears of the rotator cuff, one third sustain a fracture of the greater tuberosity (usually treated conservatively) and one third tear the anterior capsule and subscapularis (usually requiring surgical repair).

## Posterior dislocation

### Mechanism of injury

- Reflecting anteromedial obliquity on the glenoid, posterior dislocation can occur when injury is to the internally rotated adducted shoulder, such as occurs following a fall on an outstretched hand. Altered glenoid angulation or scapula inclination may predispose to such an injury.
- In addition to disruption of the posterior labrum (a reverse Bankart injury) and occasionally the posterior capsule, anterior stress on the subscapularis and impaction may lead to avulsion of the lesser tuberosity (Fig. 8.25).

### Management

Non-surgical

- Reduction and immobilization with collar and cuff, antiinflammatories and physiotherapy.

Surgery

- Posterior capsular repair with or without repair of the posterior glenoid with K wire and bone graft.



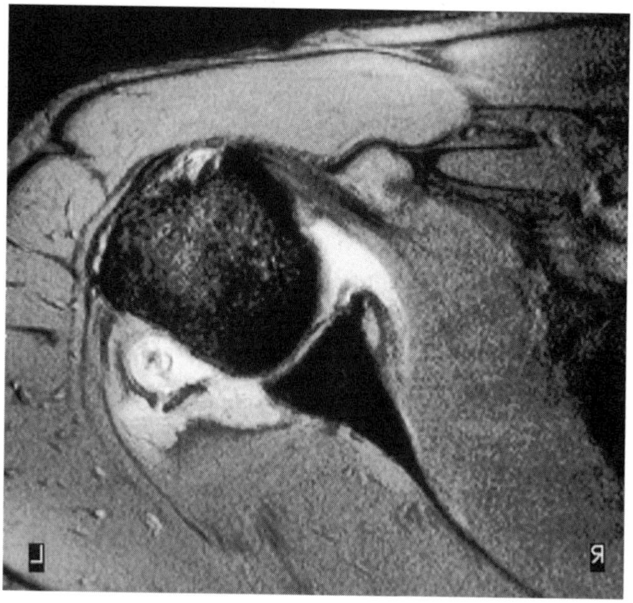

**Fig. 8.25** Axial MR image showing an avulsion fracture of the posterior glenoid following a posterior shoulder dislocation (arrow).

# Fractures of the proximal humerus and head

## Definition of terms

- Neer's modified classification of fractures of the head and neck of humerus (dividing the proximal shaft into four segments, greater tuberosity, lesser tuberosity, anatomic and surgical necks) is widely used for the extent of injury and to plan operative intervention (Box 8.7).
- According to Neer's classification, a fracture dislocation describes a fracture in which the head is displaced outside the joint space (not merely rotated). A head splitting fracture is an intra-articular fracture involving more than 15% of the articular surface.
- The Academy of Orthopaedics' classification of fractures of the proximal humerus specifically addresses the likelihood of a fracture developing avascular necrosis (AVN):
  - type A fracture is extracapsular and involves two of the primary four segments; AVN is unlikely
  - type B fracture is a partially intracapsular fracture involving three of the four primary segments; AVN is uncommon
  - type C fracture is intra-articular and involving all four segments; AVN is likely.
- In one study, AVN occurred in 14% of patients with three-part fractures and in 34% of patients with four-part injuries.

## Imaging findings

- Radiography.
- Computerized tomography.
- Dynamic contrast-enhanced MRI: early identification of ischemia results in humeral head replacement at the time of injury rather than as a delayed event when severe AVN is manifest or non-union is evident (Fig. 8.26).



### Box 8.7 Neer's classification

- One-part fractures have minimal (<1 cm) or no displacement, and have minimal (<45°) or no angulation (they are common, occurring in approximately 85% of cases)
- Two-part fractures have one fracture segment displaced or angulated
- Three-part fractures have two fracture segments displaced or angulated
- Four-part fractures have three segments displaced including the greater and lesser tuberosities and the surgical neck, with displacement or angulation of all four major fragments

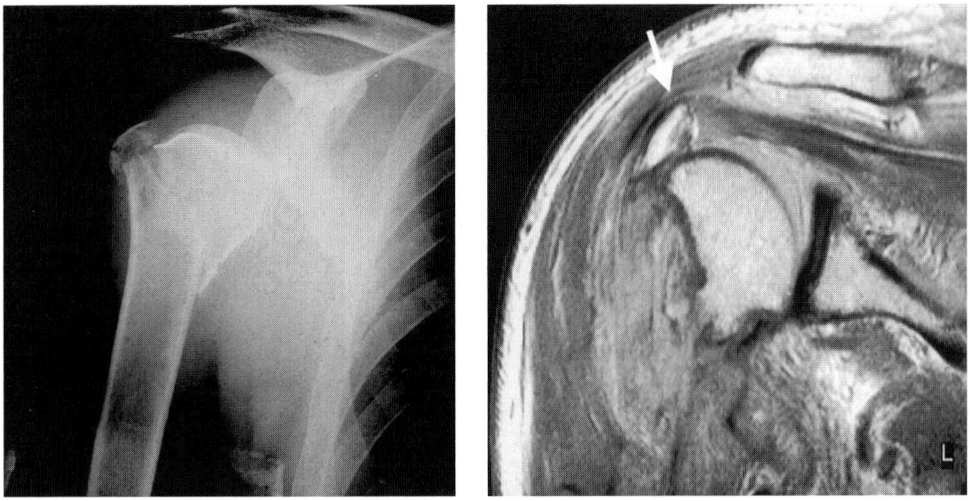

(a) (b)

**Fig. 8.26** (**a**) Radiograph showing a comminuted fracture of the humeral head. (**b**) In the same patient as in (a), an MR image showing an intact supraspinatous tendon attached to the avulsed superior facet fragment.

## Management

### Non-surgical

- When the fracture fragments are not displaced or there is minimal angulation, fractures are treated conservatively with collar and cuff immobilization.

### Surgery

- Surgery is undertaken when the fracture fragments are displaced or there is marked angulation at the fracture margin. Surgery is undertaken to restore anatomic alignment with either internal or external fixation; humeral head replacement is undertaken in patients with complex comminuted fractures or in patients with definite avascular fragments.

# Fracture of the humeral diaphysis

## Anatomy

- At the level of the mid humeral diaphysis, the radial nerve crosses the bone posteriorly from medial to lateral within the spiral groove, its proximity accounting for frequently encountered radial nerve palsy in fractures at this site.
- Up to 18% of humeral shaft fractures have an associated radial nerve injury, most commonly neuropraxia or axonotmesis; 90% resolve in 3–4 months.
- Although commonly associated with oblique fractures of the distal third of the humerus (Holstein–Lewis fracture), the injury also accompanies fractures of the mid diaphysis.

## Management

- While angulation and displacement of fragment may be corrected by manipulation and cast fixation or delayed internal fixation, operative intervention is undertaken acutely in patients with associated nerve palsy in whom MR images show impaction of the nerve within the fracture margins.
- In contrast, delayed operative fixation or conservative management is undertaken if the radial nerve is demonstrated remote from fracture margins, displaced by either hematoma or soft-tissue edema, in whom palsy is presumed to be secondary to reversible contusion.

# Acromioclavicular subluxation

## Mechanism of injury

- A fall on an outstretched hand or directly onto the shoulder.

## Clinical findings

- Affected patients complain of pain, impaired range of shoulder motion and of a palpable lump over the joint.

## Imaging findings

- Acromioclavicular subluxation or dislocation is usually readily identified on conventional radiographs with or without the stresses of weight bearing. Occasionally, patients are referred with suspected injury to the rotator cuff in whom pain relates to unrecognized AC joint disease. MRI, although generally unnecessary, may be used to determine the integrity of the coracoclavicular ligament in patients in whom surgical intervention is being considered (Fig. 8.27).

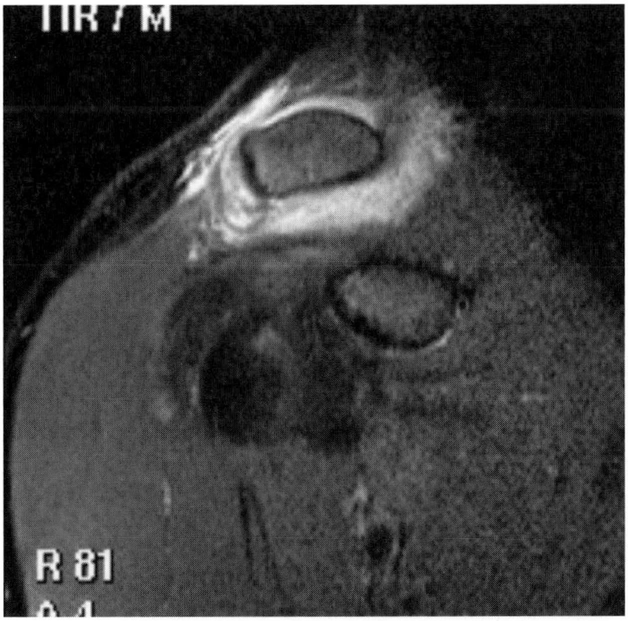


**Fig. 8.27** Coronal oblique fat-suppressed image showing hemorrhage and edema at the AC joint following a recent subluxation during a rugby training ground accident during a tackle.

# Recurrent acromioclavicular joint subluxation: post-traumatic osteolysis/stress osteolysis of the clavicle

## Mechanism of injury

- Osteolysis after trauma most commonly occurs at the lateral aspect of the clavicle, distal ulna and pubis. Osteolysis of the outer clavicle may follow a single episode of blunt trauma (post-traumatic osteolysis) or recurrent minor trauma (stress osteolysis) such as occurs following bench pressing.
- Although poorly understood, similar to algodystrophy, autonomic dysfunction is thought to induce vascular changes in the outer clavicle resulting in bony resorption. Soft-tissue or synovial overgrowth is accompanied by swelling, hyperemia, demineralization and finally resorption.

## Clinical findings

- Pain, crepitus and impaired motion. Pain, which is often worse at night, prevents the affected patient lying on the affected shoulder.

## Imaging findings

### Magnetic resonance imaging

- In affected patients, repeated subluxation results in the development of para-articular marrow edema readily identified at MRI usually many weeks prior to radiographic changes.
- At MRI, osteolysis is noted to be hypointense on $T_1$-weighted and heterogeneous on $T_2$-weighted images. Fat suppression often reveals marrow edema long before osseous change is apparent (Fig. 8.28).

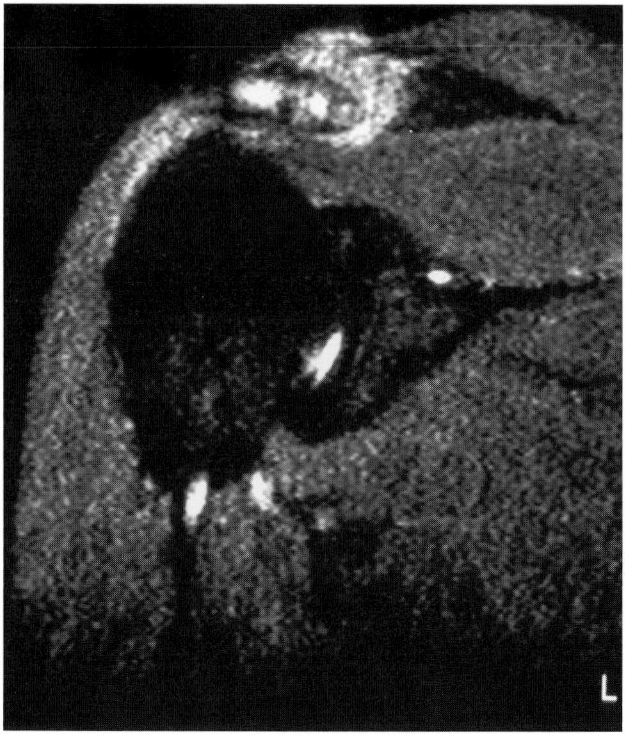


**Fig. 8.28** Coronal oblique fat-suppressed image showing extensive edema in the outer clavicle with evolving osteolysis secondary to recurrent AC joint subluxations in a bench presser.

**Management**

- The process is self-limiting over 18 months and followed by bony reconstitution. However, surgery and early immobilization may decrease symptoms and the amount of bone loss.

## Fractures of the clavicle

**Mechanism of injury**

- Direct impaction trauma following blunt trauma to the shoulder during a fall directly on the shoulder.
- Classification:
  - fractures of the clavicle are readily identified on conventional radiographs. Fractures are classified as fractures of the middle third (in 80% of cases), fractures of the distal third (15%) and fractures of the inner third (5%).
  - commonly accompanying severe trauma to the upper thorax, fractures of the clavicle are often associated with rib fractures, parenchymal lung contusion and occasionally brachial plexopathy.

**Clinical findings**

- On examination, affected patients describe severe local discomfort on palpation and often reveal associated deformity.

**Imaging findings**

- Radiography.

Magnetic resonance imaging

- Employed in patients with associated brachial plexopathy.
- Used to differentiate compression of the brachial plexus by post-traumatic hematoma requiring evacuation and displaced fracture fragment requiring decompression from simple neuropraxia, which may be treated conservatively. When it occurs, direct injury to the plexus usually involves the lateral cord. Late-compression neuropathies usually involve the middle cord and produce ulnar neuropathy, which is particularly common in fractures of the mid clavicle with complicating hypertrophic non-union.
- Vascular injury to the subclavian artery and vein is uncommon, primarily because the inner fracture segment is elevated by the action of the sternocleidomastoid away from the vessels. Occasionally downward traction on the inner segment by the pectoralis muscles impacts on vessels resulting in either spasm or less frequently laceration.

# Sternoclavicular dislocation

- Sternoclavicular dislocation is uncommon.

## Mechanism of injury

- In most cases dislocation is anterior and follows a fall on the shoulder; the medial clavicle subluxes anteriorly and is readily apparent clinically.
- Occasionally – either secondary to direct impaction trauma in motor vehicle accidents or secondary to a sharp blow to the back of the shoulder, in which torque is transmitted to the medial clavicle – the subluxation or dislocation is posterior.

## Imaging findings

### Computerized tomography

- CT with multislice 3D reconstractions is of considerable value in diagnosis and operative management.

# Scapula fractures

- Fractures may be confined to the coracoid, the neck of the acromion or extend through the scapular body to the glenoid articular surfaces (Fig. 8.29 and Box 8.8).

## Imaging findings

### Computerized tomography

- Multislice CT scanning allows reformatting of images in all planes.

## Management

- Type 3 fractures are considerably more difficult to treat and are often associated with other injuries, including pneumothorax in up to 30% of patients, pulmonary contusion, rib fractures and injuries to the brachial plexus and vascular structures.

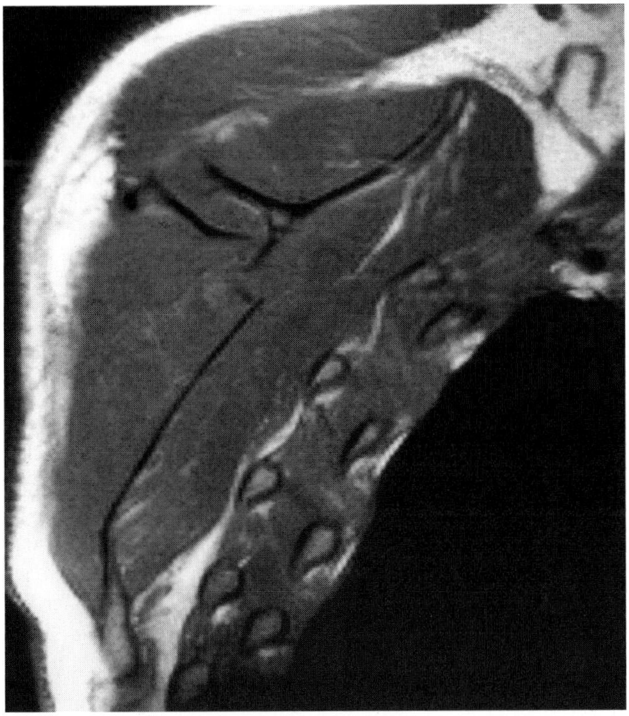

**Fig. 8.29** Sagittal oblique MR image showing a complex fracture of the scapula.

**Box 8.8 Zdravkovic and Damholt classification of fractures**

- Type 1: fractures of the body
- Type 2: fractures of the apophysis including the coracoid and acromion
- Type 3: fractures of the superior lateral angle including the neck and glenoid

## Complications

- Fractures of the acromion are frequently associated with rotator cuff tears.
- Intra-articular glenoid frcatures are frequently associated with labral tears.
- Coracoid fractures frequently accompany AC separations.
- Body fractures altering scapula inclination are often associated with the development of primary rotator cuff impingement.
- Coracoid fractures predispose patients to subcoracoid impingement and subscapularis tear.

# Further reading

Eustace S. MRI of orthopaedic trauma. Philadelphia, Lippincott Williams & Wilkins, 1999.

Fritz RC, Stoller DW. MR imaging of the rotator cuff. MRI Clinics of North America, 1997; 5: 735–754.

Fu FH, Harner CD, Klein AH. Shoulder impingement syndrome. A critical review. Clin Orthop Relat Res 1991; 269: 162–173.

Iannotti JP, Zlatkin MB, Esterhai JL et al. Magnetic resonance imaging of the shoulder. Sensitivity, specificity, and predictive value. J Bone Joint Surg Am 1991; 73: 17–29.

Post M, Silver R, Singh M. Rotator cuff tears. Diagnosis and treatment. Clin Orthop 1083; 173: 78–91.

Rafii M, Firooznia H, Sherman O et al. Rotator cuff lesions: signal patterns at MR imaging. Radiology 1990; 177: 817–823.

Stoller DW. MR imaging in orthopedics and sports medicine, 2nd edn. Philadelphia, Lippincott Raven, 1997; 674.

Walch G, Boileau P, Noel E et al. Impingement of the deep surface of the supraspinatous tendon on the posterosuperior glenoid rim. An arthroscopic study. J Shoulder Elbow Surg 1992: 1: 238–245.

Zlatkin MB, Iannotti JP, Roberts MC et al. Rotator cuff disease. Diagnostic performance of MR imaging: comparison with arthrography and correlation with surgery. Radiology 1989; 172: 223–229.

# 9 The elbow



## CLINICAL EXAMINATION

The elbow joint consists of the humeroulnar, humeroradial and proximal radioulnar joints. The capitellum of the humerus articulates with the head of the radius and the lochlea articulates with the ulna.

Flexion and extension occur at the humeral articulations while the normal function of the radioulnar joint is important for forearm supination and pronation.

The medial collateral ligament contributes to valgus stability, particularly the anterior band. Varus stability is provided by the lateral collateral ligament (LCL), anconeus and the extensor origin.

The normal carrying angle is 5° in men and 15° in females. The normal flexion/extension is 0°–150°, 70° pronation and 90° supination.

Examination should begin with inspection of the carrying angles, for muscle wasting and olecranon bursitis.

Palpation should include the medial epicondyle and lateral condyle, and the humeroradial articulation and the radial head while pronating and supinating. Soft tissues palpated should include the common extensor origin over the lateral aspect of the elbow joint, the ulnar nerve as it passes below the medial epicondyle, the flexor origin on the medial epicondyle. The olecranon bursa and triceps should be palpated posteriorly.

Range of motion – passive and active – should be assessed.

Assess elbow stability by applying a varus and valgus stress with the elbow flexed at approximately 30°.

Applying resistance to the dorsum of a dorsally extended clenched fist will usually cause pain if the patient has tennis elbow. Neurologic examination of the upper limb and examination of the cervical spine should complete the elbow examination (Figs 9.1–9.6).

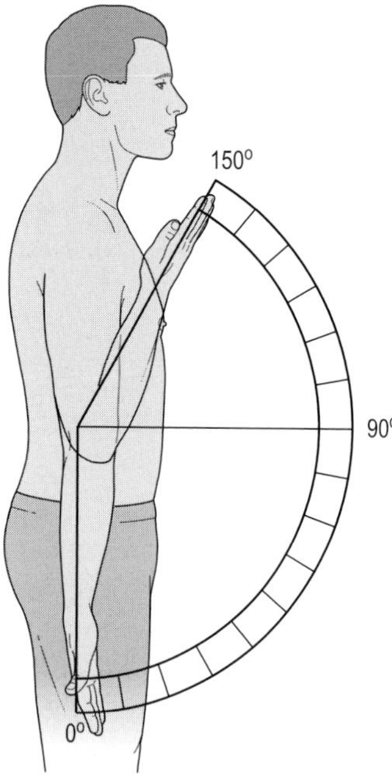


**Fig. 9.1** The normal range of motion at the elbow from extension to flexion.

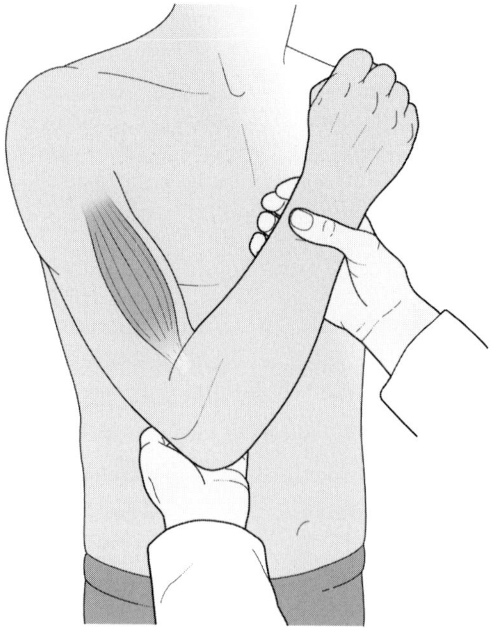

**Fig. 9.3** Assessing flexion strength at the elbow.



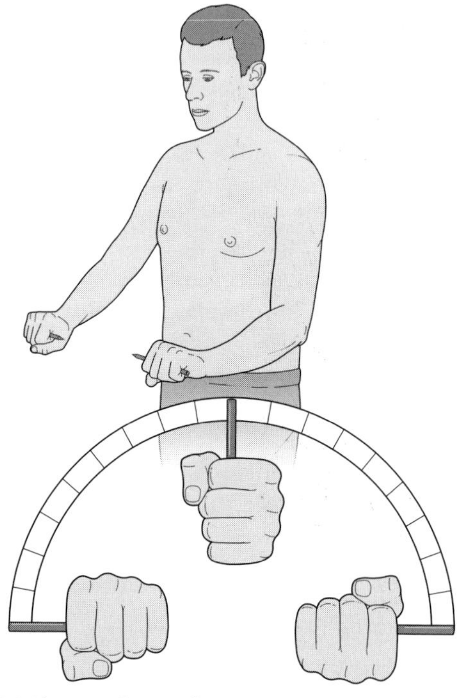

**Fig. 9.2** The normal range of supination and pronation at the elbow.

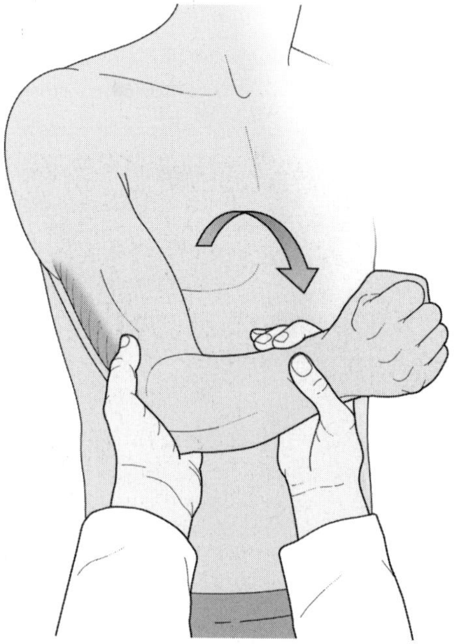

**Fig. 9.4** Determining the strength of extension.

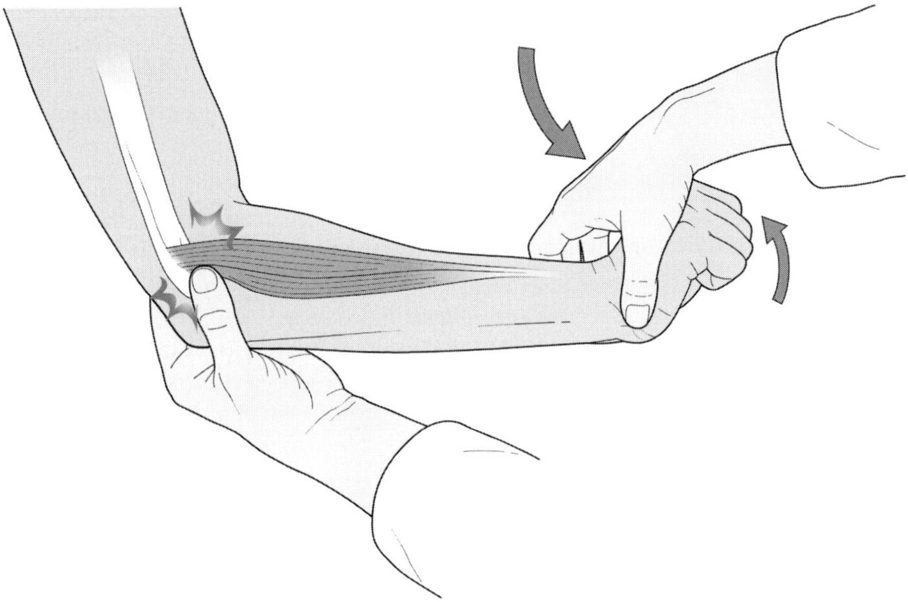

Fig. 9.5 Examination for tennis elbow.

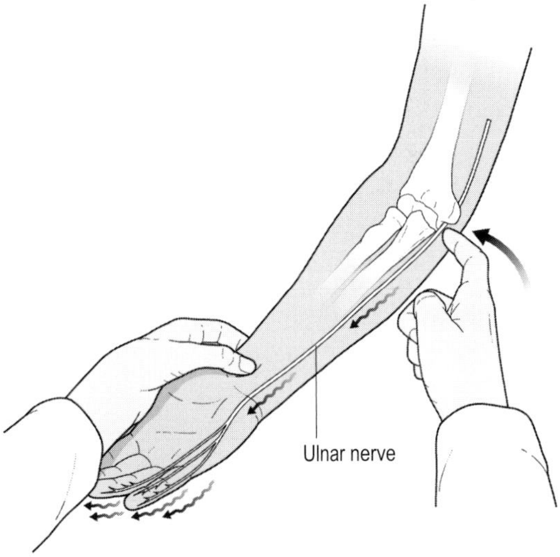


Fig. 9.6 Eliciting Tinel's sign at the elbow.

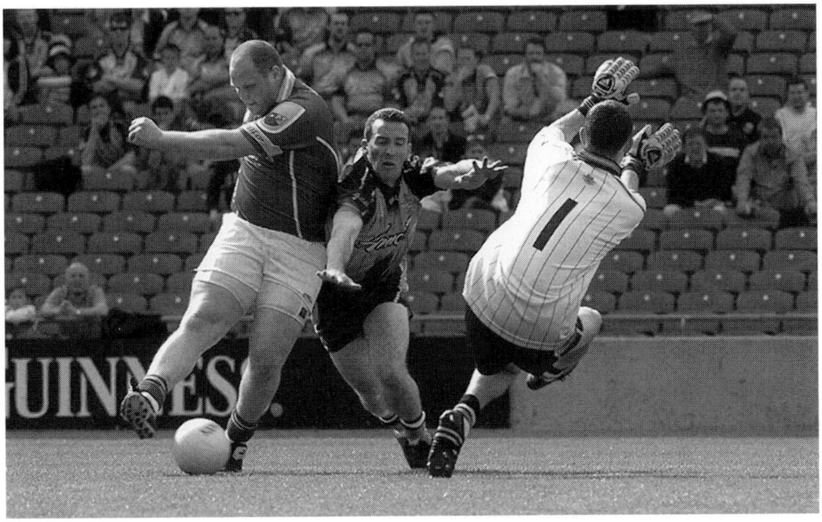


Fig. 9.7 Sportsfile.

## INJURIES AND PATHOLOGIES

# Acute soft-tissue injuries. Ulnar collateral ligament: collateral ligament injury

- Similar to the knee, injury to the medial or ulnar collateral ligament (UCL) occurs considerably more frequently than injury to the LCL or radial collateral ligament.

### Anatomy

- The UCL is responsible for medial elbow joint stability and resistance to valgus strain. It is composed of three discrete tendon bundles, the anterior bundle, the posterior bundle and the transverse bundle. Despite anatomic complexity, the anterior bundle is the most important contributor to stability and is therefore most frequently injured.
- The anterior bundle (i.e. the A-UCL) is taut in the extended elbow position running from the undersurface of the medial epicondyle just deep to the common flexor tendon origin, distally to its attachment to the medial aspect of the ulnar coronoid process. The anterior bundle blends with the fibers of the overlying flexor digitorum superficialis muscle.
- The posterior and transverse bundles form the floor of the cubital tunnel.

### Mechanism of injury

- Applied valgus strain in contact sports such as rugby may overload and tear the ligament. Ligament sprain may occur following overuse as in pitching in baseball.
- Elbow dislocation.



### Clinical findings

- Affected patients complain of medial joint line pain and swelling.
- On examination, applied valgus stress demonstrates joint line laxity.

### Imaging findings

#### Radiography

- Radiographs are usually normal.

#### Ultrasound

- Ultrasound allows the dynamic assessment of the medial joint line during applied valgus stress.

#### Magnetic resonance imaging

- At MR imaging, similar to other tendons with organized structure, the UCL is hypointense on all sequences. Following injury, intrasubstance hemorrhage and edema result in localized signal changes or loss of hypointensity. Tendon strain following valgus injury results in associated edema both within and without the collateral ligament, often extending to the overlying flexor digitorum superficialis muscle belly. In severe injury, complete rupture occurs, which is most frequently mid substance (87%). Avulsion is extremely uncommon (Fig. 9.8).
- The sensitivity of MR imaging to complete collateral ligament injury is reported to be as high as 100%. The sensitivity to partial tears, particularly undersurface tears, is considerably less; surgically proven undersurface partial tears are

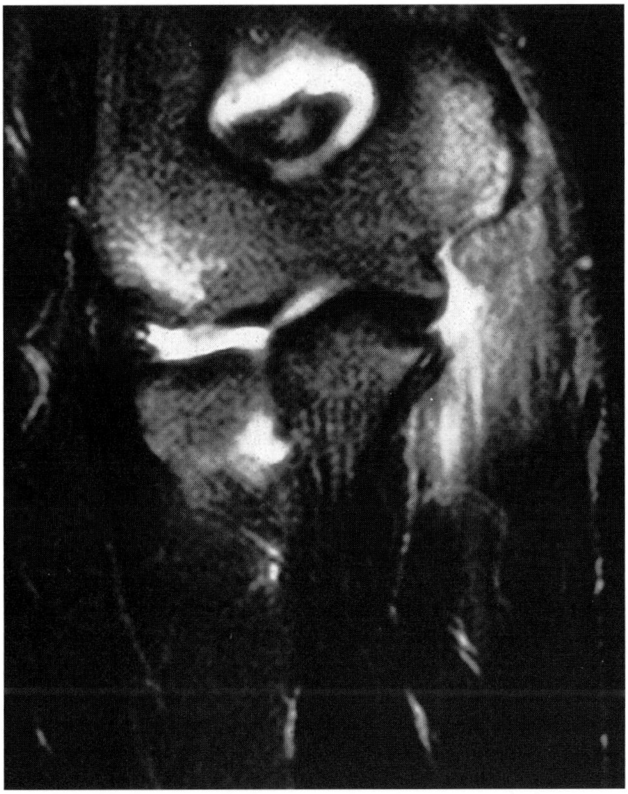

**Fig. 9.8** Following a valgus sprain injury in a rugby professional, there is disruption of the medial collateral ligament, hemorrhage and edema in the common flexor tendon attachment with an impaction bone bruise of the capitellum.



identified in as few as 14% of cases. When partial tears are suspected, MR arthrography dramatically improves the sensitivity to almost 86%; partial tears manifest by the extension of fluid along the medial margin of the coronoid process.

## Management

### Non-surgical

- Antiinflammatories.
- Rest.
- Physiotherapy.
- Support bandage.

### Surgical

- When repair is undertaken in proven cases, a graft is usually harvested from either the palmaris longus or Achilles tendons.

# Acute soft-tissue injuries. The lateral or radial collateral ligament

## Anatomy

- The LCL has four components: the radial collateral ligament, which is primarily responsible for lateral joint line stability; the lateral UCL, primarily responsible for posterolateral stability; and the annular and accessory annular ligaments, which are responsible for stability of the proximal radioulnar joint.
- The radial collateral ligament remains taut throughout elbow flexion. The lateral UCL is obliquely oriented, running from the lateral epicondyle to the posterolateral aspect of the ulnar. It is taut when varus strain is applied.
- Injury to the annular ligaments should be suspected in patients with either acute or repeated radial head subluxation or dislocation.

## Mechanism of injury

- Applied varus strain.

## Clinical findings

- Lateral joint line inflammation and palpable discomfort.
- Laxity on applied varus strain.

## Imaging findings

### Radiography

- Radiographs are usually normal.

### Ultrasound

- Ultrasound diagnosis is technically difficult as the anatomy is complex.

### Magnetic resonance imaging

- At MRI similar to the UCL as injury ranges from subtle signal abnormality through peritendinous edema to complete tendon disruption. Radial collateral ligament injury because it often reflects long-term overuse, is commonly accompanied by extensor tendon injury, epicondylitis or tennis elbow (most frequently accompanied by partial tear of the extensor carpi radialis brevis) (Fig. 9.9).
- The sensitivity of MR imaging in the detection of LCL complex injury is currently unclear as injury is less common than injury to the UCL and therefore surgery, allowing correlation, is infrequently undertaken.

## Management

### Non-surgical

- Antiinflammatories.
- Rest.
- Physiotherapy.
- Support bracing.

### Surgical

- Rarely undertaken.

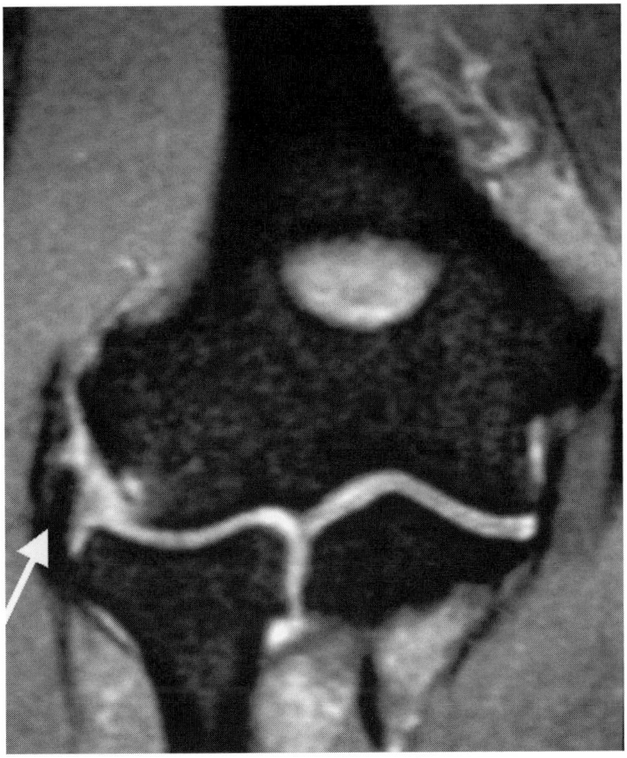

**Fig. 9.9** Following varus injury, MR shows disruption of the lateral collateral ligament and of the common extensor tendon attachment.

# Soft-tissue injury accompanying chronic repetitive trauma: lateral epicondylitis

## Definition

- Lateral epicondylitis ('tennis elbow') is the commonest cause of elbow pain in the adult population. However, the term 'epicondylitis' is misleading as the disorder is often characterized by soft-tissue changes in the absence of epicondylar bony edema or inflammation.

## Mechanism of injury

- It is thought to reflect degeneration and tearing of the common extensor tendon as a result of chronic microtrauma secondary to traction forces, as it is most frequently identified in tennis players.
- Resected specimens show fibrillary, hyaline and myxoid degeneration with angiofibroblastic proliferation within the tendon origin with minimal associated inflammatory change.

## Clinical findings

- Pain referred from the outer elbow to the hand or from the hand to the lateral epicondyle during resisted hand extension.
- Pain is induced over the lateral epicondyle during resisted extension of the middle finger. In moderate and severe cases, patients describe local pain at the lateral epicondyle on palpation.

## Imaging findings

### Radiography

- Radiographs may show subtle mineralization within the common extensor tendon at its attachment to the lateral epicondyle in chronic cases.

### Ultrasound



- Ultrasound may show common extensor tendon thickening and peritendinous fluid. Doppler may reveal hyperemia secondary to local inflammation.

### Magnetic resonance imaging

- Reflecting tendon degeneration, MR images show local tendon thickening with low to intermediate signal change.
- Acute injuries are less common, but manifest as local edema and hemorrhage, both visible as poorly defined increased signals on $T_2$-weighted images.
- More often, acute partial tears are superimposed on chronic tendon thickening, particularly of the extensor carpi radialis brevis muscle tendon unit.
- Occasionally, edema is identified in the adjacent anconeus (posterolateral) muscle belly unit.

## Management

### Non-surgical

- Rest.
- Antiinflammatories.
- Physiotherapy.
- Peritendinous steroid injection.
- Lithotripsy: a number of studies have advocated its use with or without a period of subsequent elbow immobilization although recent data do not support the use of lithotripsy for this ailment.

### Surgical

- Tenotomy, usually of tendon fibers of a single extensor muscle group, most frequently the extensor carpi radialis.

## Soft-tissue injury accompanying chronic repetitive trauma: medial epicondylitis

**Definition**

- Medial epicondylitis or golfers' elbow is considerably less common than lateral epicondylitis. Similarly to lateral epicondylitis, the descriptive term is misleading as the injury is primarily to the common flexor tendon rather than to the underlying bone.

**Mechanism of injury**

- Repetitive valgus stress at the elbow, in overhead racquet games, in golfers and in adolescent baseball pitchers, results in chronic microtrauma to the common flexor tendon with secondary degenerative rather than inflammatory changes. Swelling of the flexor carpi ulnaris within the cubital tunnel may lead to secondary ulnar nerve compression.

**Imaging findings**

Radiography

- Radiographs may show subtle mineralization within the common flexor tendon at its attachment to the medial epicondyle.

Ultrasound

- Ultrasound may reveal common flexor tendon thickening and peritendinous fluid adjacent to the medial epicondyle. Doppler may reveal local hyperemia due to inflammation.

Magnetic resonance imaging

- At MRI, medial epicondylitis is manifest as tendon swelling with associated intermediate signal abnormality within the common extensor tendon, superficial to the UCL, on all sequences. Superimposed partial tears, which frequently accompany medial epicondylitis, generate foci of signal hyperintensity on $T_2$-weighted sequences.



**Management**

Non-surgical

- Rest.
- Antiinflammatories.
- Physiotherapy.
- Peritendinous steroid injection.
- Lithotripsy: there are no significant data to support its use here.

Surgical

- Tenotomy: the incision of a single component of the common flexor tendon, usually the flexor carpi radialis brevis.

## Biceps tendon injury

**Mechanism of injury**

- Tendon injuries at the elbow most frequently follow forced eccentric contraction. They are more common in patients with connective tissue diseases on long-term steroids, in patients debilitated by chronic renal impairment or hyperparathyroidism, or in individuals on anabolic steroids. In the latter group, with excessive muscle strength, additional stress is transmitted to the tendon unit.

# Biceps muscle injury

## Anatomy

- The biceps brachii muscle is composed of a long head and a short head. The two muscle bellies share a single tendon insertion on the bicipital tuberosity of the radius. The short head arises from the apex of the coracoid, the long head from the supraglenoid tubercle of the scapula.

## Mechanism of injury

- Injury involving the biceps muscle most frequently involves the tendons more than the muscle bellies, and of the tendons, most frequently affects the tendon of the long head.
- Injury to the distal biceps tendon is less common but and when it does occur it is usually secondary to acute macrotrauma or eccentric overload, as occurs when attempting to catch or carry a heavy object.
- In such a way, attempted elbow flexion through the biceps tendon is counterposed by forced extension induced by the object. The resulting tear occurs most frequently at or just proximal to the tendon insertion on the radial tuberosity. Following rupture, the main muscle belly retracts proximally to the mid arm with extensive residual hemorrhage and edema at the site of the tear.

## Clinical findings

- Although such an injury is usually clinically apparent (manifesting as an obvious mass), compensatory flexion incurred by the brachialis may obscure the diagnosis.

## Imaging findings

### Ultrasound

- Ultrasound allows the clear visualization of the superficial biceps tendons and therefore readily allows diagnosis of biceps tendon rupture.



### Magnetic resonance imaging

- When apparent, MRI is favored prior to surgical repair to determine the extent and site of the retracted tendon.
- The distal biceps tendon is best visualized in the axial and sagittal planes, the axial images clearly depicting the normal insertion site on the radial tuberosity, the sagittal images allowing an appreciation of the extent of retraction (Fig. 9.10).
- Partial tears of the distal biceps or tendinosis are less common and are usually a sequel to overuse, often induced by weight lifting. MRI is helpful as it allows the differentiation of primary tendon abnormality, manifest as tendon thickening or partial tear from either brachialis tendon injury or bicipitoradial bursitis, which may accompany or occur in isolation in overuse syndromes (Fig. 9.11).

## Management

### Non-surgical

- Ultrasound-guided steroid injection to the bicipitoradial bursa.
- Physiotherapy in partial tears or tendinosis.
- Antiinflammatories.

### Surgical

- Primary tendon suture repair allows early recovery and resolution of contact sport within 4 weeks of injury.

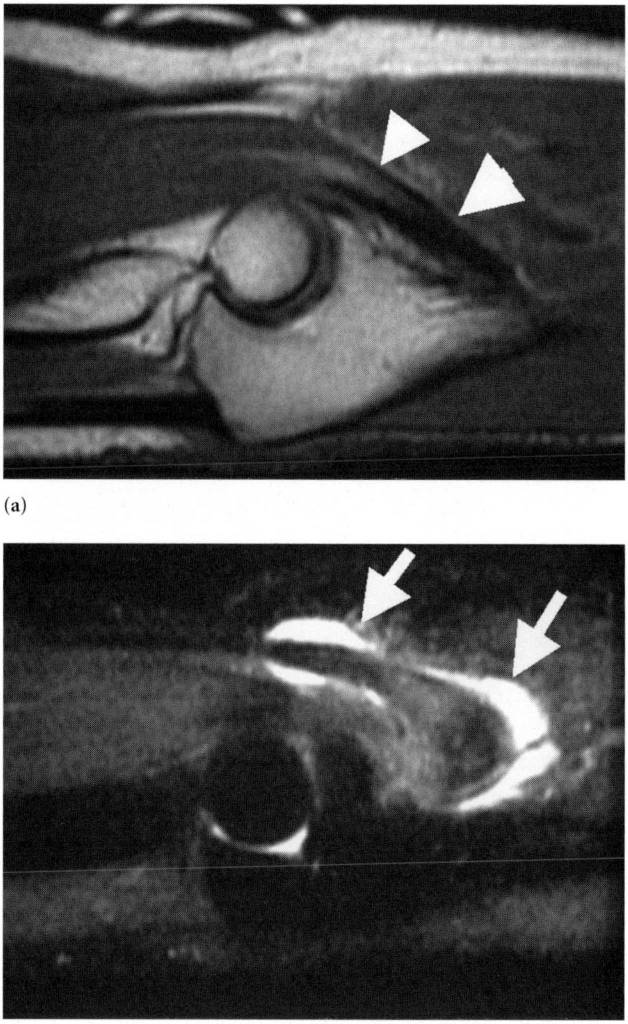

(a)

(b)

**Fig. 9.10** (**a**) Sagittal $T_1$-weighted and (**b**) fat-suppressed images showing inflammation around the distal biceps tendon within the bicipitoradial bursa, producing pain on resisted elbow flexion secondary to bicipitoradial bursitis.

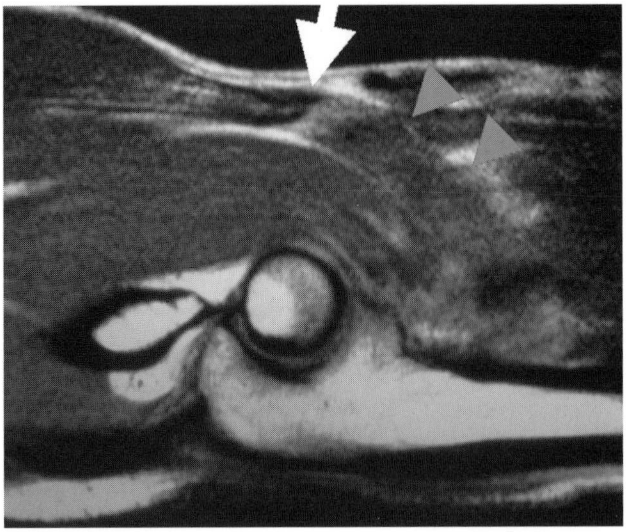

(a)

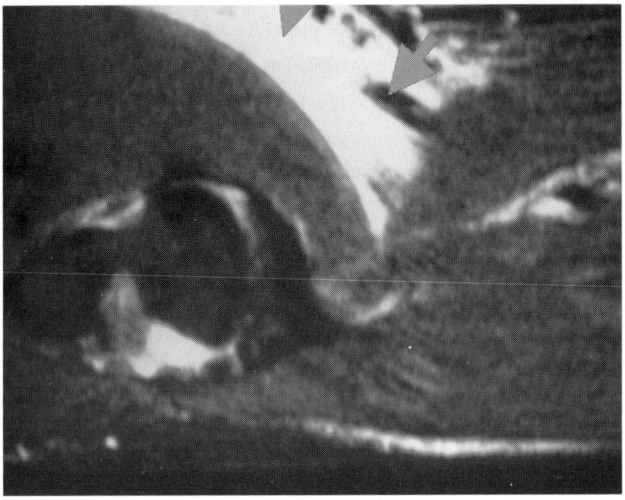

(b)

**Fig. 9.11** (**a**) Sagittal $T_1$-weighted and (**b**) fat-suppressed MR images showing a complete rupture of the distal biceps tendon with retraction and hemorrhage (arrows).

# Triceps tendon injury

## Anatomy

- The triceps muscle lies in the posterior compartment of the arm and is composed of three heads, the long head arising from the infraglenoid tubercle, the lateral head from the lateral and posterior aspect of the humerus, and the medial head distally from the medial and posterior aspect of the humerus. The three heads unite to form the triceps tendon in the mid arm, the tendon being composed of a dominant deep component, which merges with a superficial component before inserting on the posterosuperior surface of the olecranon.

## Mechanism of injury

- Triceps tendon injury is extremely uncommon, and most frequently occurs secondary to forced flexion against a contracting muscle (attempting to extend the elbow) as occurs following a fall on an outstretched hand (forced eccentric contraction).
- Rarely, injury may follow a direct blow or complicate olecranon bursitis where steroid injections, synovitis and superimposed infection conspire to weaken the tendon.

## Clinical findings

- Impaired passive extension of the forearm.

## Imaging findings

### Radiography

- In most cases, the tear is complete and associated with the avulsion of a small fragment of bone from the posterior aspect of the olecranon, which is readily visualized on conventional radiographs. Rupture of the muscle belly or at the myotendinous junction, in the absence of an avulsion, is extremely uncommon (Fig. 9.12).

### Ultrasound

- Ultrasound allows the clear identification of the superficial triceps tendon at the olecranon.

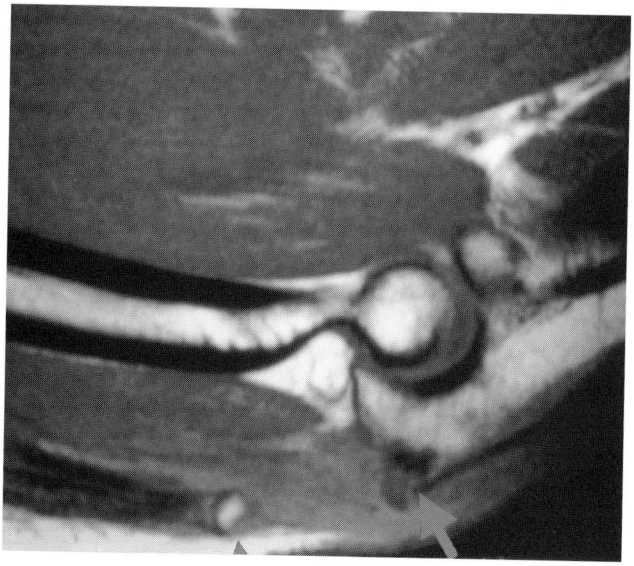

**Fig. 9.12** Sagittal $T_1$-weighted image showing a triceps avulsion from the olecranon (arrows).

Magnetic resonance imaging

- Acute rupture of the triceps tendon is readily visualized in both the sagittal and axial planes at MRI, manifest by both morphologic and signal changes of hemorrhage and edema.
- Tendinosis secondary to overuse is manifest by tendon thickening with loss of normal signal hypointensity.
- Partial tear, which is extremely uncommon, is manifest by the disruption of fibers usually within the middle third of the tendon.

### Management

Non-surgical

- Antiinflammatories.
- Physiotherapy in partial tears.
- Immobilization in extension in partial tears.

Surgical

- Primary suture repair or reattachment of bone fragment to the olecranon with K wire.

## Osseous injury

- The ages at which ossification centers appear are shown in Box 9.1.

**Box 9.1 Appearances of ossification centers**

| | |
|---|---|
| Capitellum | 1–2 years |
| Radial head | 3–6 years |
| Inner (medial) epicondyle | 4 years |
| Trochlea | 8 years |
| Olecranon | 9 years |

# Pediatric elbow fractures

## Classification

- Salter and Harris originally classified growth-plate injuries in 1963. Although the understanding of growth-plate injury has improved since that time, these injuries have continued to present special problems in both diagnosis and management.

## Mechanism of injury

- The growth plate is considerably weaker than both adjacent ligaments and bone, making it susceptible to injury, particularly during growth spurts at puberty. In most cases, callus formation and subsequent healing of fractures is uneventful.

## Complications

- Rarely, persistent motion at the fracture margins or the development of bone bridges impairs healing and leads to long-term complications such as growth arrest or deformity. It is only by complete and accurate imaging, allowing appropriate orthopedic intervention, that these complications may be avoided.

## Imaging findings

### Radiography

- Radiographs fail to identify unossified cartilage within the growth plate.

### Ultrasound

- Ultrasound allows the identification of unossified cartilage but is an operator-dependent modality and the images are in a form often not readily interpreted by referring clinicians.

### Scintigraphy

- Scintigraphy, although widely used in adults with suspected fractures, is not widely favored for this purpose in children, as an intense physiologic osteoblastic response concentrating radiopharmaceutical at the margin of the growth plate can mask an underlying fracture.

### Computerized tomography

- Although many radiologists employ spiral CT to evaluate growth-plate injuries, on the premise that the displacement of fracture fragments is the principal issue in treatment planning, this modality affords limited evaluation of unossified cartilage.

### Magnetic resonance imaging

- When employed, this allows the evaluation of injury to bone and unossified cartilage. The visualization of unossified cartilage is important as the identification of fracture extension through unossified cartilage changes the fracture description from Salter 2 to Salter 4 (Fig. 9.13). Type 2 supracondylar fractures are treated conservatively whereas type 4 fractures generally require open reduction and internal fixation.

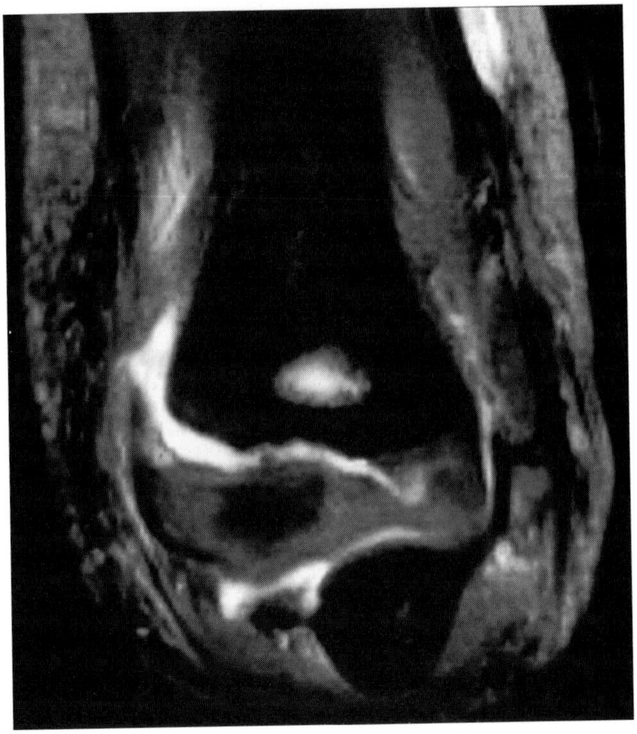

**Fig. 9.13** Coronal $T_2$-weighted MR image shows a type 4 Salter–Harris fracture extending through unossified cartilage.

## Supracondylar fractures



- Supracondylar fractures account for up to 60% of pediatric fractures of the distal humerus, most frequently complicating a fall on the outstretched hand with the elbow in extension (although a significant number of fractures complicate a fall in flexion).
- They occur most frequently between 3 and 10 years of age.

### Imaging findings

Radiography

- Supracondylar fractures are easily diagnosed on conventional radiographs as they extend through the ossified metaphysis and are usually associated with dorsal angulation of the distal fragment.

### Management

Non-surgical

- Reduction – Realignment – Immobilization.
- Inadequate reduction and malunion predispose to subsequent deformity, posterior elbow dislocation and occasionally nerve injury.

# Epiphyseal fractures: lateral condylar fractures

- Lateral condylar fractures are the commonest of the epiphyseal fractures of the elbow, occuring between 5 and 10 years of age.

## Mechanism of injury

- Similar to supracondylar fractures, they most frequently complicate a fall on the outstretched hand in both extension and varus.

## Imaging findings

- Fractures extending through unossified cartilage are inadequately evaluated by conventional radiographs and, in this setting, ultrasound, arthrography or direct visualization of cartilage with MRI are of particular value.

### Magnetic resonance imaging

- The Rutherford system classifies fractures using MRI into:
  - type 1, in which the distal articular cartilage is intact and the fragment is hinged
  - type 2, where the fracture extends to involve the distal articular surface, although the fragment remains undisplaced
  - type 3, in which the fragment is both displaced and rotated.
  - type 4, in which there is more than 2{ts}mm displacement, which requires surgical fixation (Fig. 9.13).

## Management

### Non-surgical

- Collar and cuff immobilization for 6 weeks

### Surgical

- Surgical realignment with K wire fixation.



# Epiphyseal fractures: medial epicondyle fractures

- Medial epicondylar avulsions represent 10% of pediatric elbow fractures, which are third in frequency after supracondylar and lateral condylar fractures.

## Mechanism of injury

- This injury is a complication of acute valgus stress either in isolation or accompanying elbow dislocation.
- The avulsion usually involves the growth plate of the medial epicondyle and may extend through the physis of the distal humerus, the latter defining whether it is a Salter 3 or 4 injury.

## Management

### Non-surgical

- Most cases are minimally displaced and can be treated conservatively.

### Surgical

- Displaced fractures require surgical fixation.

# Medial condylar fracture: trochlear fractures

- Medial condylar fractures are uncommon, and often unrecognized, as the fracture extends through the unmineralized trochlear cartilage and is not perceived on conventional radiographs.
- Management of these fractures is usually surgical.

# Capitellar fractures

- Capitellar fractures are uncommon and classified types 1–3.
- Types 1 and 2 described by Kocher and Lorenz are readily visualized as they involve the mineralized capitellar ossification center, displacement of which is readily identified on radiographs.
- Type 3 fractures described by Wilson are chondral and are characterized by subtle fractures of the cartilage of the articular surface only identified at MRI or arthography. These fractures generally complicate impaction and shear transmitted through the radial head.

## Management

Non-surgical

- For undisplaced fractures.
- Collar and cuff immobilization for 6 weeks.

Surgical

- Displaced fractures.
- Realignment and K wire fixation.

# Distal humeral epiphyseal separation: transcondylar fractures

## Mechanism of injury

- The physis between the distal humerus and the unossified epiphysis represents a plane of potential weakness. Until 2 years of age, the fracture may extend through this plane alone (Salter type 1); after 2 years the fracture may also involve the metaphysis (Salter type 2).

## Imaging findings

### Radiography

- Although the diagnosis is readily made on conventional radiographs by analyzing the anterior humeral line and by comparison with the asymptomatic elbow, difficulty obtaining a true lateral film may create diagnostic difficulty.

### Ultrasound

- Ultrasound allows the visualization of the osseous and cartilaginous components.

### Magnetic resonance imaging

- MRI provides a 'map', which can be readily employed by referring surgeons (Fig. 9.14).

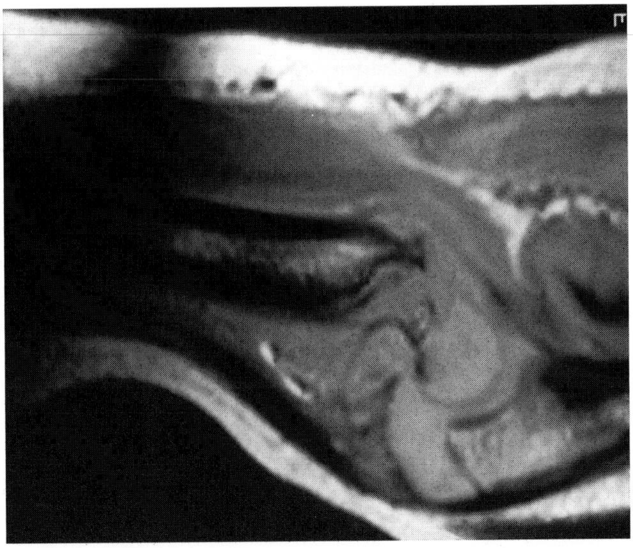

**Fig. 9.14** Sagittal image showing a transphyseal fracture of the distal humerus in a 2-year-old.

# Radial head fractures

- Radial head fractures are uncommon in childhood but when they do occur they most commonly complicate posterior dislocation when they are often associated with fracture of the coronoid. Displaced fractures may be complicated by avascular necrosis (Fig. 9.15).

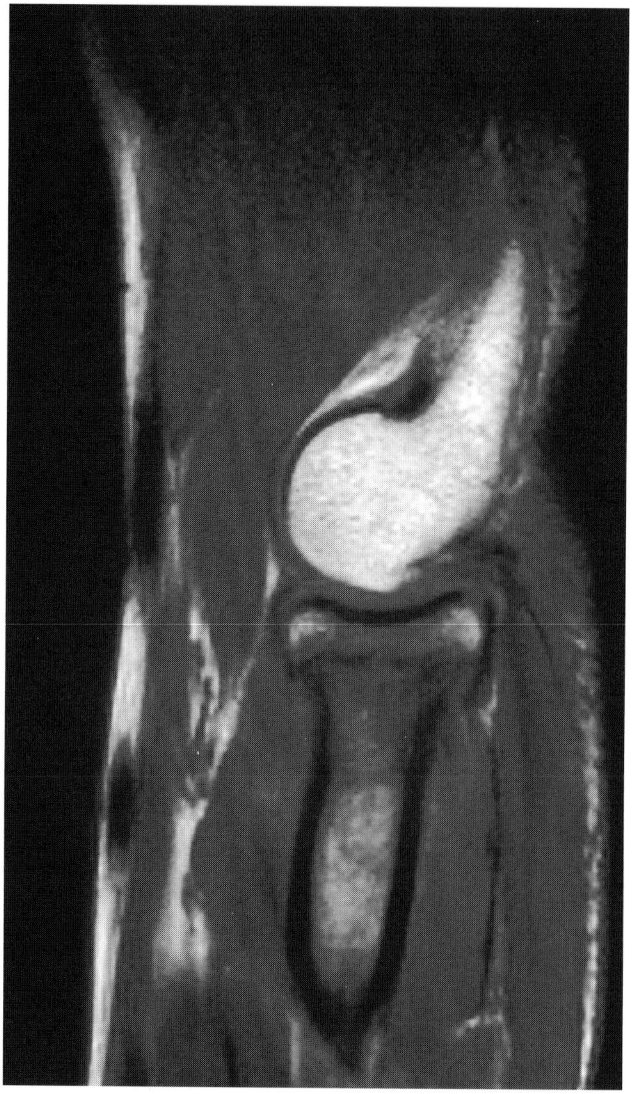

**Fig. 9.15** Sagittal image showing an impaction fracture of the radial head following a fall on an outstretched hand.

## Elbow fractures in adulthood: fractures of the coronoid

**Mechanism of injury**

- The coronoid process is responsible for anterior joint stability. Fracture, although uncommon, usually complicates elbow dislocation or subluxation.

**Classification**

- Type 1 fractures are small shear fractures and do not lead to joint instability.
- Type 2 fractures involve less than 50% of the coronoid but generally require fixation.
- Type 3 fractures involve greater than 50% of the coronoid and despite fixation are often associated with long-term instability.

## Elbow fractures in adulthood: condylar fractures

**Mechanism of injury**

- Fractures of the condyles in adulthood usually complicate trauma in hyperextension with superimposed abduction or adduction forces.

**Classification: medial condylar**

- Milch classifies medial condylar fractures according to whether or not the fracture involves the lateral trochlea ridge:
  - type 1 fractures spare the ridge therefore maintaining ulnohumeral stability
  - type 2 fractures involve the ridge resulting in ulnohumeral instability and subluxation, which is often associated with disruption of the LCL and capsular disruption.

**Classification: lateral condylar**

- Fractures of the lateral condyle are divided into types 1 and 2 on the basis of preservation or disruption of the lateral trochlea ridge:
  - type 2 fractures – extending from the lateral condyle through the trochlea ridge – are usually associated with medial collateral ligament tears.



## Elbow fractures in adulthood: olecranon fractures

**Mechanism of injury**

- Fractures of the olecranon complicate either direct trauma and impaction.

**Classification**

- Fractures are divided into two types according to Colton:
  - type 1 fractures are non-displaced: non-displaced fractures show no change in position on gentle flexion–extension and less than 2 mm articular step-off.
  - type 2 fractures are displaced.

# Elbow fractures in adulthood: posterior elbow dislocation

- Elbow dislocation is the second most common major joint dislocation in adults and the most common dislocation in children under 10 years old, most frequently accompanying a fall on an outstretched hand in hyperextension.

## Mechanism of injury

**Posterior dislocation**

- Posterior forces imposed by a fall are opposed by ossified coronoid in adulthood, which is invariably fractured in such an injury. In childhood, constraining forces of the mineralized coronoid are absent up to the age of 10 years, allowing dislocation and often accompanying spontaneous reduction in childhood.

**Anterior dislocation**

- This rarely occurs, complicating a blow to the dorsal aspect of the olecranon or forearm in the flexed position.

**Medial and lateral dislocations**

- These complicate condylar fractures, secondary to applied abduction or adduction forces in extension.

# Radioulnar dislocation

## Mechanism of injury

- Isolated dislocation of either the ulna or radius may occur in patients with combined injury to collateral ligaments, specifically the annular ligaments of the radioulnar articulation.
- If the radial head is dislocated anteriorly, a Monteggia fracture should be suspected (associated fracture of the proximal ulna).
- If the radial head is dislocated posteriorly, disruption of the lateral UCL should be suspected.

# Panner's disease and Little Leaguers' elbow

## Mechanism of injury

- Osteochondral injury to the radial head and capitellum commonly accompanies repetitive valgus strain with impaction in adolescent baseball pitchers in the USA or direct impaction in young female gymnasts.
- Trauma-induced osteochondral injury may be isolated and self-limiting but when recurrent is often accompanied by disruption of a tenuous blood supply to the capitellum resulting in osteochondritis.
- Persistent ischemia results in infarction and fragmentation of the capitellum with the development of articular cysts and loose bodies. Up to 50% of affected individuals ultimately develop osteoarthritis.

## Imaging findings

### Radiography

- Radiographs may show osseous irregularity of the capitellum.

### Magnetic resonance imaging

- MRI in the coronal plane reveals local edema, manifest as a loss of $T_1$ signal and as signal hyperintensity on inversion recovery sequences, adjacent to the articular surface of the capitellum often prior to any radiographic abnormality.

## Management

- Rest and splinting may result in resolution of the changes over 6 weeks.
- Abrasion chondroplasty is occasionally undertaken to promote vascular reperfusion and a healing response at the site of injury.
- When fluid is identified encircling fragments on $T_2$-weighted MR scans, surgery is undertaken either to fix or remove fragments and occasionally to reconstruct with bone grafts.
- Panner's disease is an osteochondrosis that occurs before ossification of the capitellum between 5 and 11 years of age. Unlike post-traumatic osteochondritis ('Little Leaguers' elbow') cartilagenous fragmentation occurring in Panner's disease resolves during mineralization of the capitellum without sequelae.

# Further reading


Bourne MH, Morrey BF. Partial rupture of the distal biceps tendon. Clin Orthop 1991; 271: 143–148.

Brogden BG, Crow NE. Little leaguer's elbow. Am J Roengenol 1960; 83: 671–675.

Childress HM. Recurrent ulnar nerve dislocation at the elbow. J Bone Joint Surg Am 1956; 38: 978–984.

Colton CL. Fractures of the olecranon in adults: classification and management. Injury 1973; 5: 121–129.

Foster DE, Sullivan JA, Gross RH. Lateral humeral condyle fractures in children. J Pediatr Orthop 1985; 62: 1159–1163.

Ho CP. Sports and occupational injuries of the elbow. MR imaging findings. Am J Roengenol 1995; 164: 1465–1471.

Knight RA. Fractures of the humeral condyles in adults. South Med J 1955; 70: 1165–1173.

Kuroda S, Sakamaki K. Ulnar collateral ligament tears of the elbow joint. Clin Orthop 1986; 208: 266–271.

Morrey BF, An KN. Articular and ligamentous contributions to the stability of the elbow joint. Am J Sports Med 1983; 11: 315–319.

Morrey BF, An KN. Functional anatomy of the ligaments of the elbow. Clin Orthop 1985; 201: 84–90.

Ogden JA. The evaluation and treatment of partial physeal arrest. J Bone J Surg Am 1987; 69A: 1297–1302.

Potter HG, Hannafin JA, Morwessel RM et al. Lateral epicondylitis: correlation of MR imaging surgical and histopathologic findings. Radiology 1995; 196: 43–46.

Regan W, Morrey BF. Fractures of the coronoid process of the ulna. J Bone Joint Surg Am 1989; 71A: 1348–1354.

Rogers LF, Poznanski AK. Imaging of epiphyseal injuries. Radiology 1994; 191: 297–308.

Salter RB, Harris WR. Injuries involving the epiphyseal plate. J Bone Joint Surgery Am 1963; 45A: 587–622.

Schwartz ML, Al-Zahrani S, Morwessel RM et al. Ulnar collateral ligament injury in the throwing athlete. Evaluation with saline enhanced MR arthrography. Radiology 1995; 197: 297–299.

Tarsney FF. Rupture and avulsion of the triceps. Clin Orthop 1972; 83: 177–183.

Timmerman LA, Andrews JR. Undersurface tears of the collateral ligament in baseball players. A newly recognized lesion. Am J Sports Med 1994; 22: 33–36.

Wilson PD. Fractures and dislocations in the region of the elbow. Gynecol. Obstet 1933; 56: 335–359.

# 10

# The Wrist and Hand



## CLINICAL EXAMINATION

### Clinical history

As with other anatomic sites it is critical to record a detailed history. Mechanism of injury, pattern of debility, pain or loss of function, aggravating and relieving factors and so on should all be noted as for other sites.

### Physical examination

The wrist consists of the distal radioulnar joint, the radiocarpal joint, and eight carpal bones in proximal

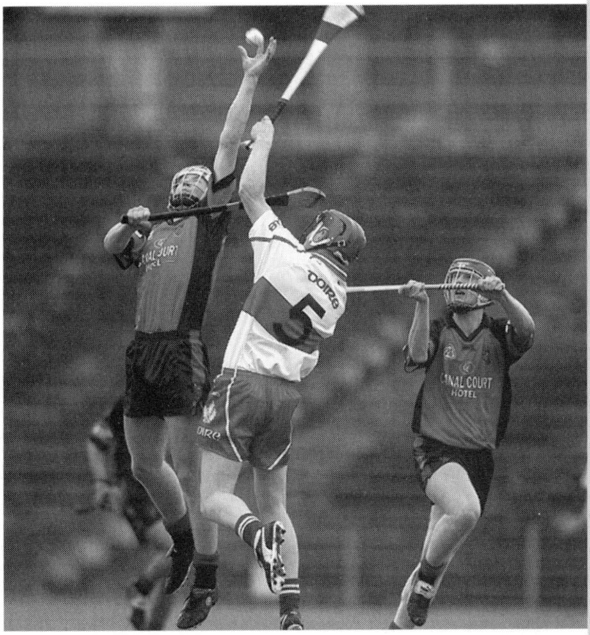

**Fig. 10.1** Sportsfile.

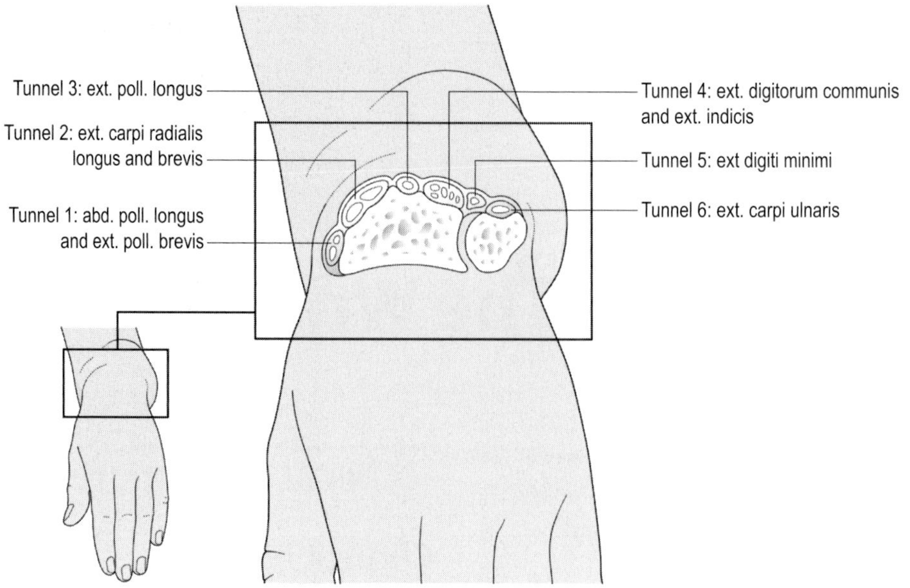


**Fig. 10.2** There are six extensor compartments. The short tendons to the thumb are separated from the long extensors to the thumb by Lister's tubercle, which can be readily palpated over the dorsum of the radius.



and distal rows. The palpable bony areas are the radial styloid, more distally the scaphoid in the anatomical snuffbox, trapezium, then the base of the first metacarpal. Posteriorly, the tubercle of the radius is the nodule just dorsal to the radial styloid. The lunate and capitate are palpable distal to this. The ulnar styloid process is the prominent bone palpable on the dorsal aspect on the ulnar side. On the volar aspect, the pisiform is palpable on the ulnar side, and the lunate radially. The anatomical snuffbox is bound by the extensor pollicis longus tendon dorsally and the abductor pollicis longus (APL) and extensor pollicis brevis (EPB) volarly (Figs 10.2–10.5).

The soft tissues on the volar aspect include the radial artery, flexor carpi radialis and ulnarly flexor carpi ulnaris.

**Tinel's test**: tapping over the carpal tunnel to elicit median nerve symptoms if the nerve is compressed in a tight canal (Fig. 10.6).

Phalen's test: hyperflexion of the wrist for 30 seconds leads to medial nerve symptoms (Fig. 10.7).

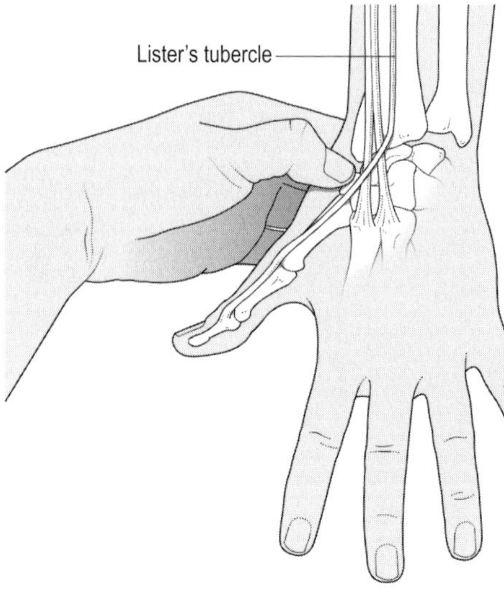


**Fig. 10.3** The extensor radialis tendons are palpated on the radial side of Lister's tubercle.

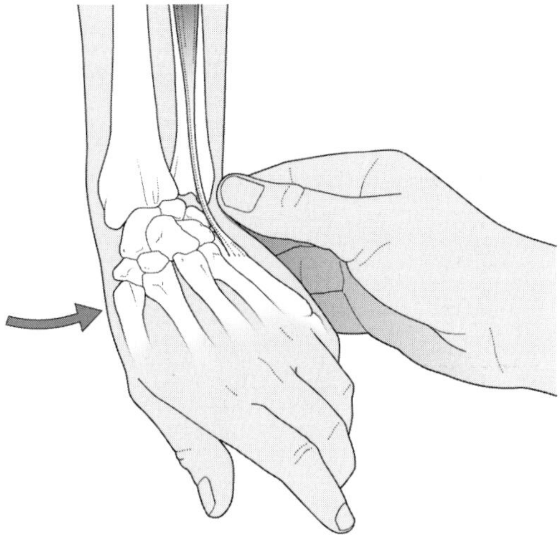

Fig. 10.4 The extensor carpi ulnaris tendon is readily palpated in ulnar deviation.

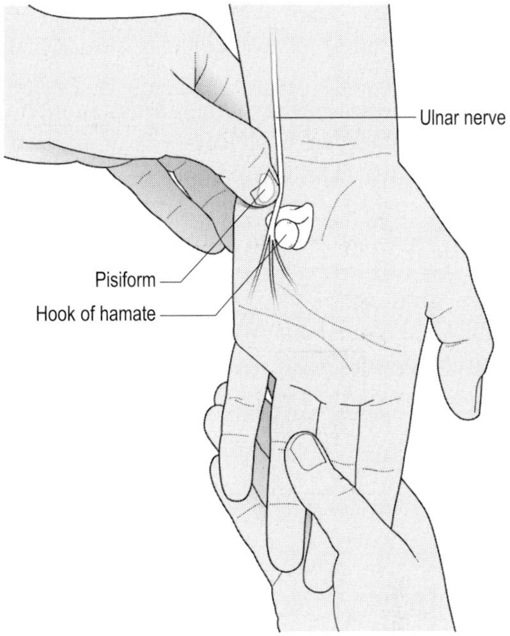


Fig. 10.5 The palmaris longus tendon is visualized and palpated with the thumb and little finger in opposition.



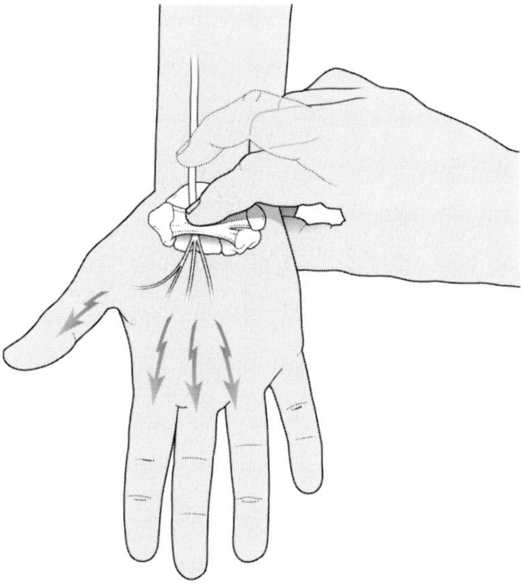

Fig. 10.6 Tinel's sign ('pins and needles' in the palm of the hand) is induced by tapping over the flexor retinaculum.

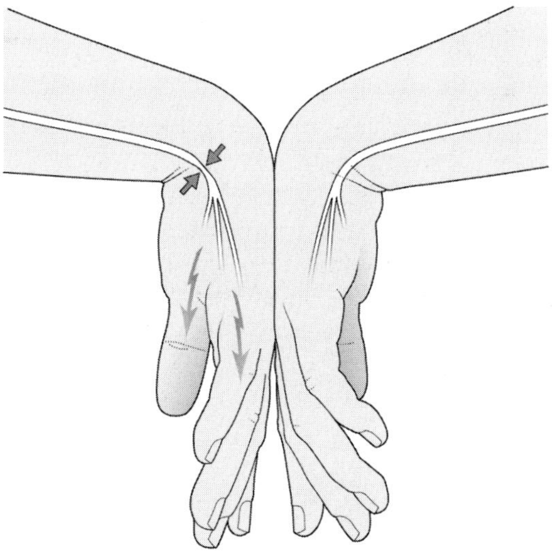

Fig. 10.7 Forced palmar flexion may also be used to produce symptoms of carpal tunnel syndrome: Phalen's test.

Pain aggravated by ulnar deviation occurs in patients with injury to the triangular fibrocartilage complex (TFCC).

Pain aggravated by passive and active pronation and supination occurs in patients with injury to the distal radioulnar joint, where injury is often accompanied by a palpable 'clunk' on rotation as the distal ulnar subluxes into and out of the distal radioulnar joint.

Loss of sensation over the ulnar side of the 4th digit and throughout the 5th digit suggests ulnar nerve compression, which may occur in Guyon's canal adjacent to the hook of the hamate in the wrist (Fig. 10.8).

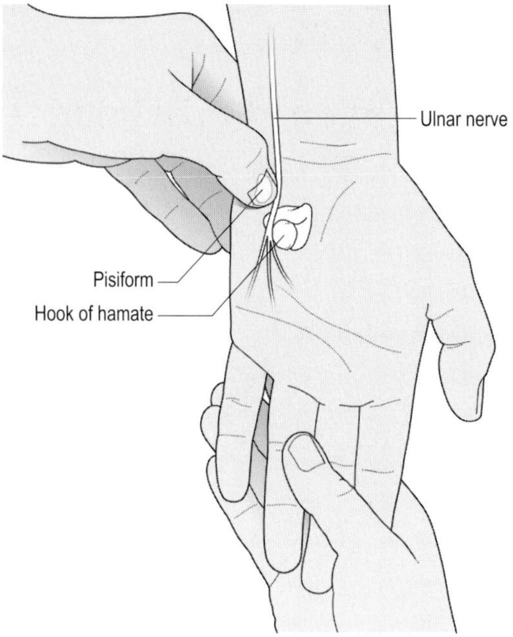


**Fig. 10.8** Guyon's canal is palpated over the pisiform and contains the ulnar nerve, artery and vein.

## PATHOLOGIES

# Classification of wrist injuries

- Injury to intrinsic ligaments (scapholunate and lunatotriquetral ligaments) disrupts coordinated movement of carpal bones within intercalated segments and is considered to be dissociative: carpal instability dissociative (CID).
- Injury leading to disruption of extrinsic ligaments or bones also results in instability although movement of intercalated segments remains coordinated: carpal instability non-dissociative (CIND).
- Wrist injuries can be classified as:
  - perilunar (perilunate and lunate dislocations)
  - midcarpal
  - proximal carpal instabilities.
- Further, perilunate injuries can be subdivided into greater and lesser arc injuries:
  - greater arc injuries are divided into scaphoid fractures, scaphoid fracture with perilunate dislocation and transcaphoid transtriquetral perilunate dislocation
  - lesser arc injuries involve disruption of the scapholunate and lunatotriquetral ligaments and complete perilunate instabilities.
- Midcarpal instability is classified as intrinsic or extrinsic in origin. Intrinsic instabilities include:
  - palmar midcarpal instability secondary to laxity of the volar arcuate ligament, which leads to an audible 'clunk' in the clenched fist position as the capitate subluxes over the volarly angulated lunate to the space of Poirier
  - dorsal midcarpal instability secondary to malunion of a distal radial fracture with persistent dorsal angulation.
- Proximal carpal instabilities include:
  - ulnar translocation of the carpus in which more than 50% of the lunate is medial to the radius
  - dorsal instability (secondary to a dorsal rim fracture of the radius – CIND – or secondary to scapholunate ligament disruption – CID
  - volar instability secondary to a volar rim fracture (volar Barton) (non-dissociative) or lunatotriquetral ligament disruption (dissociative).

# Wrist biomechanics

- The biomechanics of the wrist are complex and involve the integrated motion of two intercalated segments (carpal bones linked by intercarpal ligaments), the proximal and distal row of carpal bones, which articulate with the bases of the metacarpals and the distal radius at the radiocarpal articulation, facilitating wrist flexion and extension, ulnar and radial deviation, and minimal pronation and supination (although this is most marked at the distal radiocarpal articulation) (Fig. 10.9).
- Within the proximal carpal row there is a delicate balance between the opposing forces of the volarly angulated scaphoid and the mildly dorsally angulated lunate, transmitted through the scapholunate ligament (Fig. 10.10).
- In the sagittal plane the scapholunate angle (i.e. the angle between the volarly angulated scaphoid and mildly dorsally angulated lunate) is from 30° to 60°, while the angle between the lunate and capitate is from 0° to −30° (Fig. 10.11).

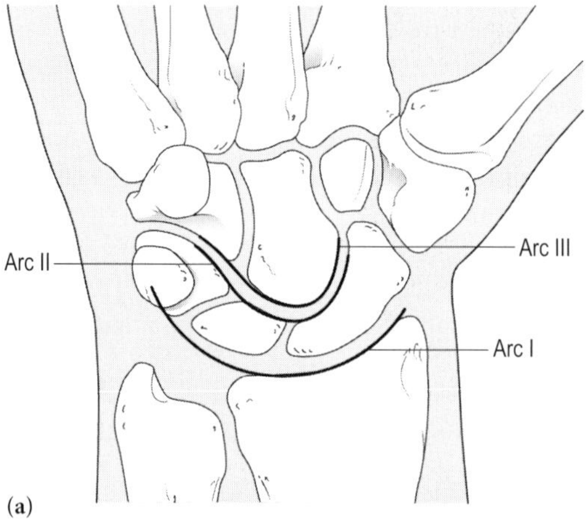


(a)

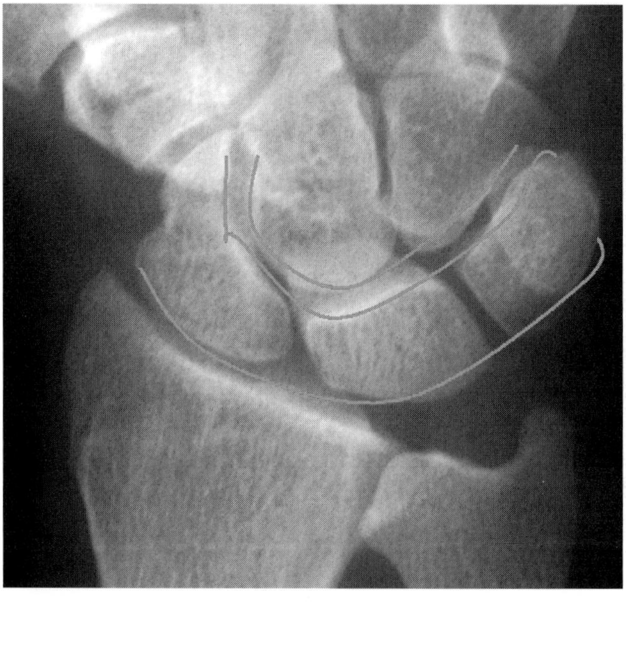

(b)

**Fig. 10.9** (**a**) Diagram and (**b**) radiograph showing normal anatomy and three recognizable lines created by congruity of the small bones of the wrist: the Gilula's arcs.

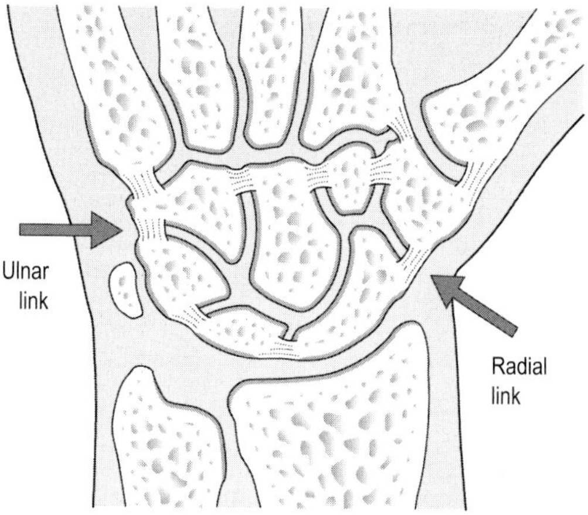


**Fig. 10.10** Carpal bones are linked by ligaments resulting in two biomechanical intercalated segments.

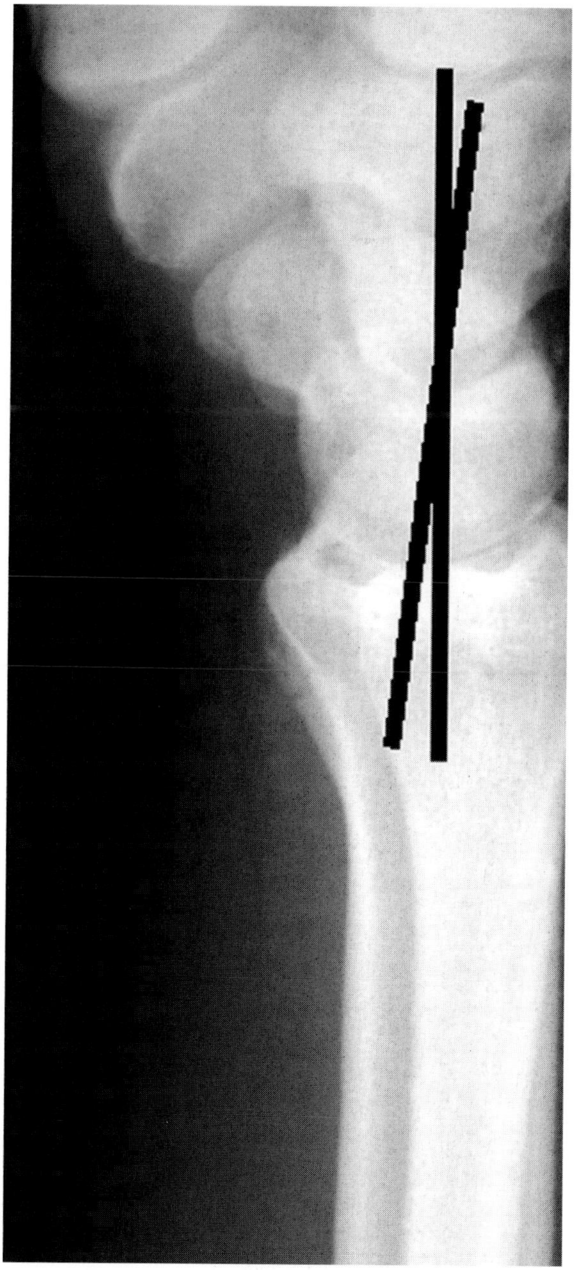

(a)

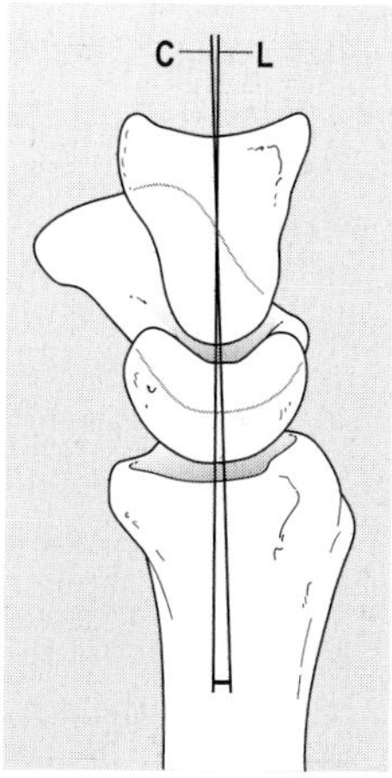


(b)

**Fig. 10.11** (**a, b**) Lateral radiographs showing the normal alignment of the lunate relative to the capitate: the lunatocapitate angle of 0° to −10°.

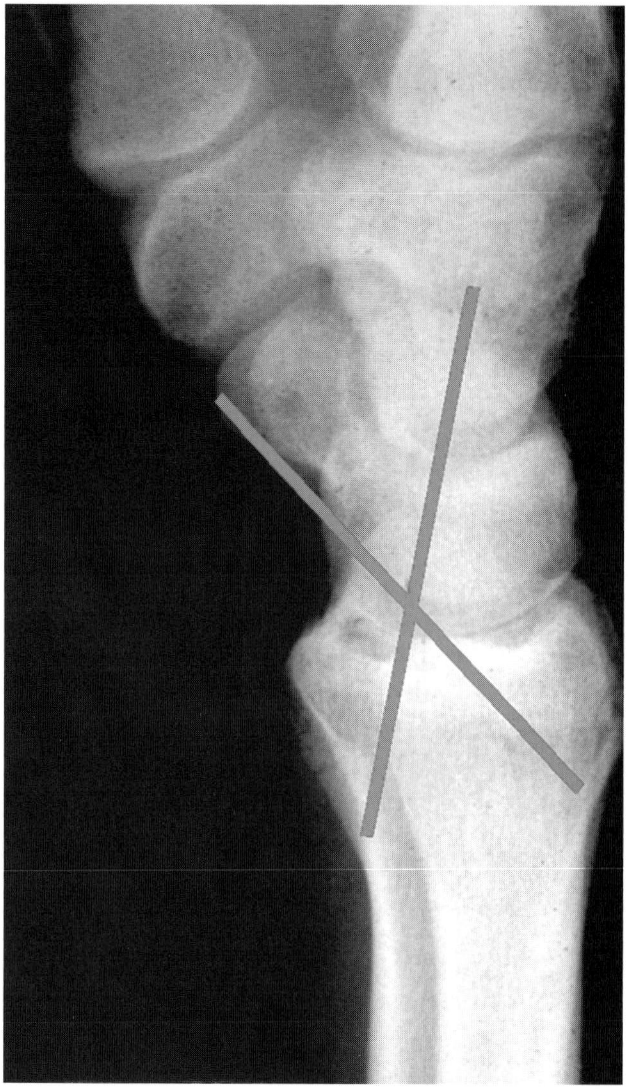
(a)

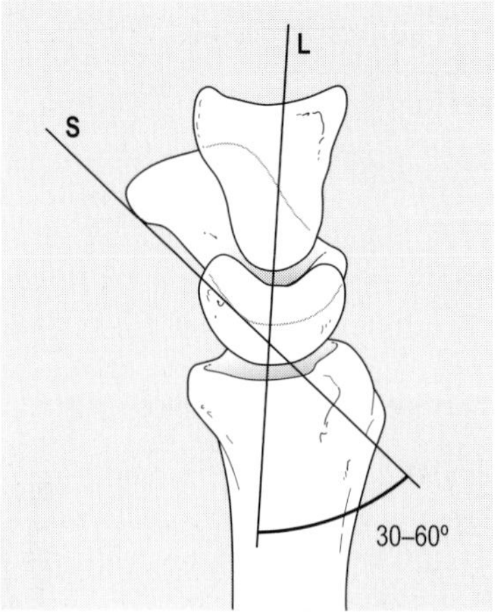

(b)

**Fig. 10.12** (**a, b**) Lateral radiographs showing the normal alignment of the scaphoid relative to the lunate: the scapholunate angle.



- The angle of the distal radial articular surface is 10° volar angulation. Although slightly decreasing the range of dorsiflexion at the radiocarpal articulation, it is an evolutionary attempt to stabilize the radiocarpal articulation and limit the tendency to dislocate dorsally at the radiocarpal articulation following a fall and dorsally oriented impaction forces (Fig. 10.12).
- When forces are applied to the wrist, induced deformity may be constrained by osseous and soft-tissue ligamentous plasticity, so that following the removal of forces the original alignment is restored; this is called stable equilibrium.
- If either osseous or soft-tissue structures fracture or rupture, the original alignment is not restored following the removal of applied forces, but forces induced by the deformity displace osseous structures even further from equilibrium: unstable equilibrium.

# Scapholunate ligament disruption

## Anatomy

- In health, the scapholunate ligament balances opposing forces of the volarly angulated scaphoid and the dorsally angulated lunate. The ligament is delta shaped in 75% of cases and linear in 25%.
- The ligament is usually less than 3 mm in maximal transverse diameter in the coronal plane, and is interposed between the scaphoid and lunate in the axial plane as thick dorsal (responsible for stability) and volar fibers, and an interposed membranous portion.

## Mechanism of injury

- Following a fall on an outstretched hand, impaction forces through the long axis of the capitate are transmitted to the scapholunate interspace and the scapholunate ligament. Under the action of such forces, the scapholunate ligament may acutely rupture, most commonly from the proximal pole of the scaphoid, or may stretch before rupture, in both cases resulting in widening of the scapholunate interspace.

## History and clinical findings

- Affected patients complain of pain on wrist motion, which is often worse on ulnar and radial deviation. On examination, affected patients may reveal local tenderness on palpation over the proximal pole of the scaphoid.

## Imaging findings

### Radiography

- In the absence of restraint, the scaphoid tilts volarly, the lunate tilts dorsally. Induced changes in biomechanics following ligament rupture result in previously described radiographic signs:
  - widening of the scapholunate interspace greater than 4 mm: the 'Terry-Thomas sign'
  - volar angulation and flattening of the scaphoid producing the ring sign (the distal pole of the scaphoid projected over the waist and proximal pole)
  - dorsal tilt of the lunate relative to both the capitate (a lunatocapitate angle greater than −30°) and scaphoid (scapholunate angle greater than 60°) producing a dorsal intercalated segmental instability pattern (DISI) (Fig. 10.13).

### Magnetic resonance imaging

- Following injury, the delta configuration of an intact ligament is lost as the ligament elongates prior to rupture; frequently intra-substance edema results in apparent swelling or thickening of the ligament. The lunate attachment has more Sharpey's fibers and hence, when it occurs, a tear is usually from the base of the scaphoid. Following rupture, hyperintense fluid is noted to pass freely between the radiocarpal and mid carpal joint spaces. Induced instability promotes further deformity before establishing the DISI pattern, considered to be unstable equilibrium.

## Management

### Non-surgical

- Most patients are treated conservatively combining the use of antiinflammatories with wrist support bracing.

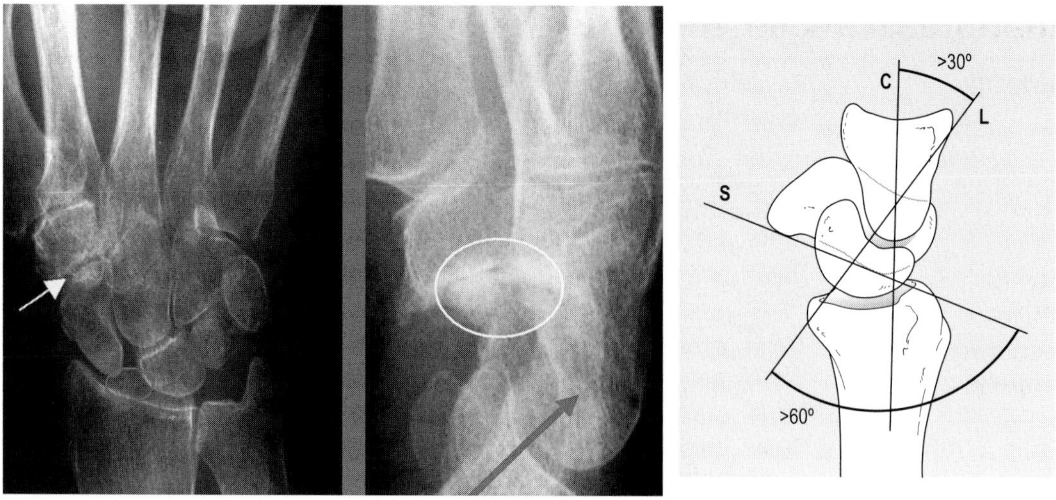


(a) (b) (c)

**Fig. 10.13** **(a, b, c)** Scapholunate ligament disruption is manifest by widening of the scapholunate interspace, arthritis at the scapho-trapezio-trapezoid articulation, and by dorsal tilt of the lunate relative to the scaphoid, widening the scapholunate angle; this is called DISI (i.e. dorsal intercalated segmental instability).

## Surgical

- Acute scapholunate ligament disruption when identified within 4 weeks of initial injury is treated operatively with primary repair.
- In addition to primary repair, dorsal capsulodesis (Blatt's procedure) is often employed to re-establish stability.
- In chronicity, when surgery is undertaken, some resolution of symptoms may be achieved by scapho-trapezio-trapezoid fusion or implant arthroplasty. However, the results are inconsistent and although pain is often reduced, it is at the expense of wrist mobility.

# Lunatotriquetral ligament disruption

## Anatomy

- The lunatotriquetral ligament, similar to the scapholunate, is comprised of both volar and dorsal components that attach directly to bone rather than to hyaline cartilage overlying carpal bones. The ligament establishes continuity between radial and ulnar structures of the proximal carpal row of bones or intercalated segment.

## Mechanism of injury

- Following a fall in ulnar deviation, impaction forces are transmitted through the ulnar side of the wrist with acute shear manifest as rupture of the lunatotriquetral ligament, disruption of components of the TFCC, as subluxation of the distal radioulnar joint or as fracture.

## Imaging findings

### Radiography

- In an attempt to establish unstable equilibrium, the lunate tilts volarly under the influence of unapposed volar tendency of the scaphoid, establishing a volar intercalated segmental instability pattern. The scapholunate angle decreases to an angle often less than 30° while the lunatocapitate angle increases to as much as 30° (Fig. 10.14).

### Magnetic resonance imaging

- Shearing forces lead to acute tear of the lunatotriquetral ligament, which, in contrast to the scapholunate ligament, does not stretch and widen the interspace before actual rupture. The sensitivity of MRI in this setting is as low as 50%.

## Management

### Non-surgical

- In most patients lunatotriquetral ligament injury is managed conservatively, combining antiinflammatories and bracing if symptomatic.

### Surgical

- Although the results of surgical repair are inconsistent, when undertaken, direct suture repair of the ligament and lunatotriquetral fusion are undertaken.

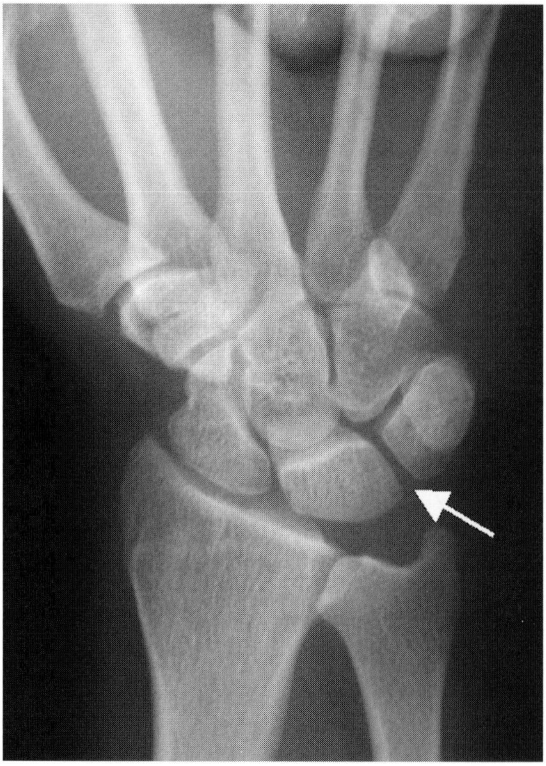

(a)

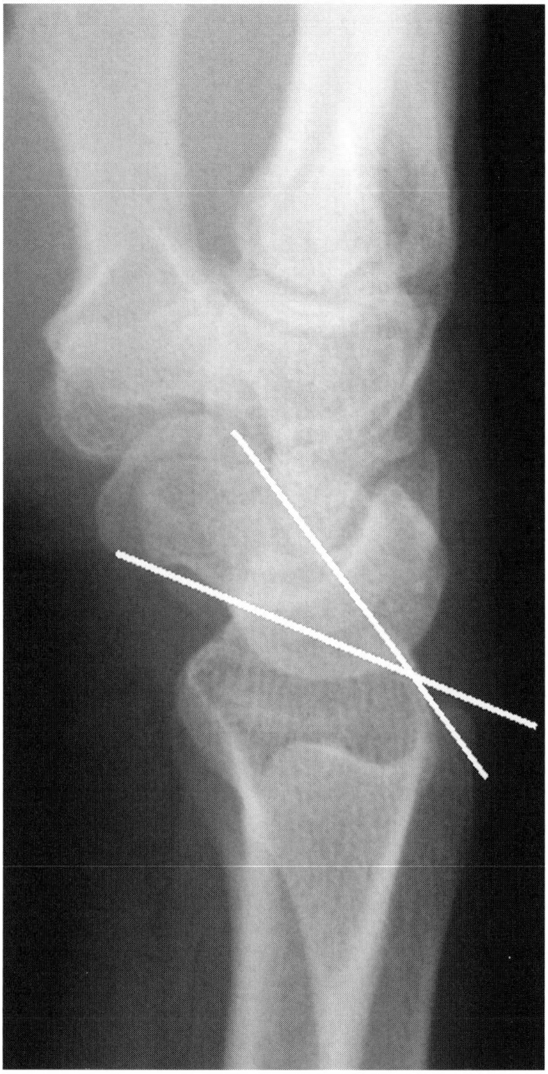

(b)



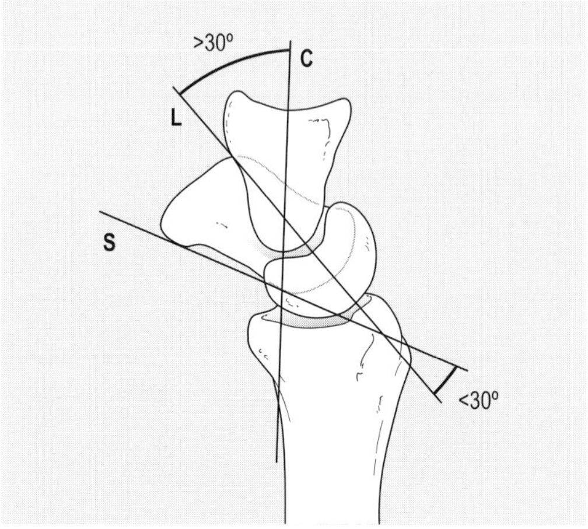


(c)

**Fig. 10.14** (**a, b, c**) Disruption of the lunatotriquetral ligament is manifest by volar tilt of the lunate relative to the scaphoid; this is called VISI (volar intercalated segmental instability).

## Triangular fibrocartilage complex

### Anatomy

- The TFCC is a complex anatomic structure composed predominantly of a triangular wedge-shaped fibrocartilaginous disk bridging the distal radioulnar joint supported thus:
  - anteriorly and posteriorly by radioulnar ligaments
  - distally by attachments to the lunate through the volar ulnocarpal ligaments (the ulnolunate and ulnotriquetral ligaments)
  - laterally by the ulnar collateral ligament and the extensor carpi ulnaris.
- The TFCC is completed by an additional fold in the lateral capsule interposed between the ulnar styloid and the triquetrum: the meniscal homolog.

### Mechanism of injury

- En bloc, the TFCC functions to buttress forces transmitted to the distal ulnar and distal radioulnar articulations secondary to impaction during ulnar deviation. Following a fall on the outstretched hand, impaction forces lead to shear through the triangular fibrocartilage attachments, most frequently at the attachment to the radius.
- Degenerative tears of the triangular fibrocartilage occur most commonly at the ulnar attachment and most likely reflect a combination of both chronic impaction and age-related ischemia. In such a way, degenerative tears are most frequently identified in patients with positive ulnar variance or positive ulnar impaction syndrome and are often accompanied by disruption of the lunatotriquetral ligament.

### Classification

- TFCC tears may be either traumatic (Palmer class I), subdivided according to site of tear, or degenerative (Palmer class II), subdivided according to extent of degeneration.
- Traumatic tears most commonly occur within 1–2 mm of the radial origin of the fibrocartilage where vascular supply is poor. In contrast, reflecting microvascular supply, tears at the ulnar attachment, where vascular supply is rich, have a greater propensity to heal.
- Fortuitously, MRI is accurate in the detection of radial tears which heal poorly but is relatively inaccurate in the detection of ulnar-sided tears which frequently heal without intervention.



### History and clinical findings

- Injury is usually manifest as atypical pain and tenderness localized to the region of the ulnar styloid, which is often worse in ulnar deviation. Such discomfort often limits pronation and supination at the distal radioulnar articulations.
- In old age, as a result of cartilage degeneration, asymptomatic tears of the triangular fibrocartilage are common (Fig. 10.16).

### Imaging findings

#### Radiography

- No radiographic abnormality.

#### Magnetic resonance imaging

- MRI has a reported sensitivity of 72–100% in the detection of tears of the triangular fibrocartilage, with associated specificity of 89–100%.

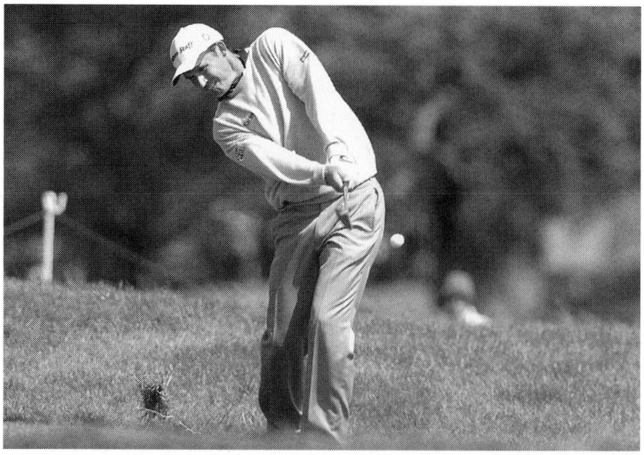

**Fig. 10.15** Sports file.

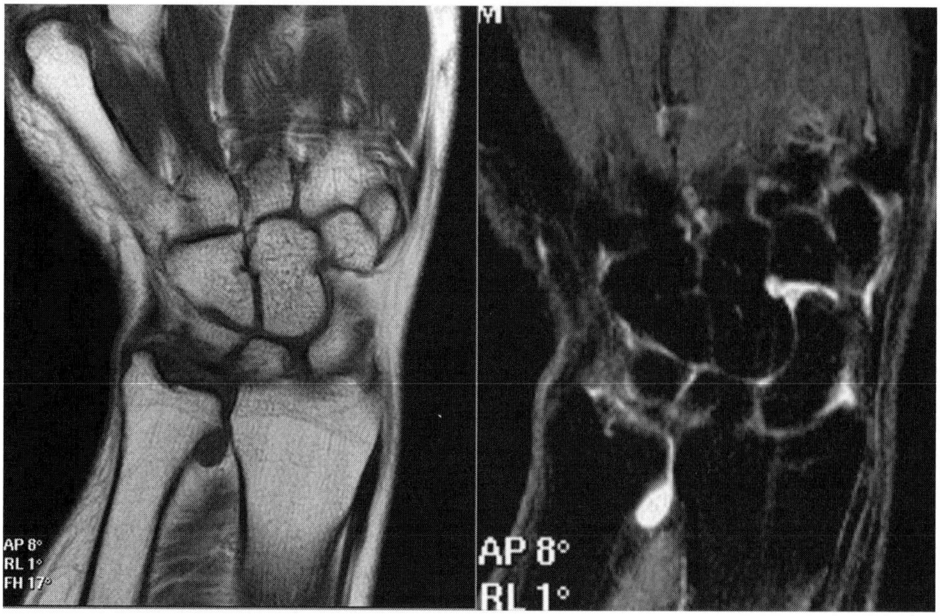


(a) (b)

**Fig. 10.16** (**a**) Coronal $T_1$-weighted and (**b**) fat-suppressed images show a chronic tear of the triangular fibrocartilage at its ulnar attachment allowing communication between the radiocarpal and distal radioulnar joints.

## Management

### Non-surgical

- Antiinflammatories.
- Wrist support bracing.
- Intra-articular steroid injection.

### Surgical

- In acute symptomatic tears in young patients, surgical repair is often undertaken with success. In this setting, surfaces are either debrided or reconstructed.
- In patients with positive ulnar variance, ulnar shortening or osteotomy is often undertaken.

## Extensor carpi ulnaris syndrome

**Mechanism of injury**

- Extensor carpi ulnaris tenosynovitis usually complicates chronic occupational overuse.

**History and clinical findings**

- Typically presenting as ulnar-sided wrist pain mimicking a TFCC tear, in chronicity commonly accompanying a TFCC tear.

**Imaging findings**

Ultrasound

- Ultrasound allows the identification of tendon thickening with peritendinous fluid.

Magnetic resonance imaging

- At MRI, the tendon sheath is noted to be thickened, associated with peritendinous hyperintense fluid on $T_2$-weighted sequences.
- In chronicity, foci of mineralization within the tendon are often noted to be hyperintense. Extension of chronic synovitis at the level of the radiocarpal articulation often leads to TFCC degeneration in chronicity.

**Management**

- Immobilization.
- Antiinflammatories.
- Ultrasound-guided tendon sheath steroid injections.
- Surgery unnecessary; rarely tendon sheath debridement.

## First extensor compartment syndrome: de Quervain's tenosynovitis



**Mechanism of injury**

- Repetitive wrist flexion and extension, particularly repetitive extension of the thumb may promote chronic tenosynovitis within the first dorsal compartment or fibro-osseous tunnel at the level of the radial styloid surrounding the EPB and APL tendons.

**History and clinical findings**

- Local tenderness on palpation.
- Pain exacerbated by flexion and extension of the thumb.

**Imaging findings**

Magnetic resonance imaging

- At MRI, there is focal peritendinous fluid and apparent soft-tissue thickening.

**Management**

- Immobilization.
- Antiinflammatories.
- Rarely ultrasound-guided tendon sheath steroid injections.

# Intersection syndrome: peritendinous crepitans; abductor pollicis longus bursitis; oarsman's wrist

- Intersection syndrome involves the abductor longus bursa 4–5 cm proximal to Lister's tubercle. When rarely encountered it occurs in golfers and oarsmen.

## Mechanism of injury

- Friction during flexion extension produces a bursitis of the bursa at the intersection of the APL, the EPB and the radial wrist extensors. In effect, friction produces a stenosing tenosynovitis of the second extensor compartment.

## Clinical findings

- Localized pain, swelling, crepitus and distal forearm swelling.

## Management

- Thumb spica splinting.
- NSAIDs.
- Corticosteroid injection.
- 4–6 weeks' restricted activities and rest.
- Excision of the bursa undertaken in refractory cases, followed by delayed reintroduction of offending activity and preconditioning including reverse wrist curls with progressively greater weights.

# Fractures of the distal radius

## Classification

- Traditional classifications of fractures of the distal radius are based on early clinical descriptions by Abraham Colles (1814), John Barton (1838) and Robert Smith (1854).

### Colles

- Colles described the most common fractures of the distal radius, characterized by fracture through the distal radial metaphysis within 2 cm of the distal articular surface. They are associated with dorsal angulation and displacement and radial angulation and shortening, and often with fracture of the ulnar styloid, thought to be secondary to TFCC avulsion or traction effect (Fig. 10.17).

### Smith

- Smith described a fracture of the distal radius with volar angulation with or without intra-articular extension (Fig. 10.18).

### Barton

- Barton described a fracture of the dorsal rim of the distal radius with radiocarpal subluxation, and fracture of the volar rim of the distal radius (reverse Barton) with radiocarpal subluxation.

Two further types of fracture are commonly specifically described:

### Chauffeur's fracture (Hutchinson's fracture)

- This describes an intra-articular fracture through the base of the radial styloid, often associated with disruption of the scapholunate ligament or scaphoid fractures.

### Die punch fracture

- This describes an isolated intra-articular fracture through the lunate facet with variable degrees of displacement, depression and comminution.



## Universal classification

- This was proposed by Rockwood and Green, a modification of the Frykman and of the Mayo and Melone classifications:
  - type 1: fractures are non-displaced and stable
  - type 2: fractures are displaced and unstable
  - type 3: undisplaced intra-articular
  - type 4: displaced intra-articular type 4a reducible stable; type 4b reducible unstable; type 4c complex irreducible (Fig. 10.19)
  - instability is defined as more than 20° of dorsal angulation, marked dorsal comminution and radial shortening of 10 mm or more
  - primary external fixation is recommended for all universal type 3 and 4 fractures (except 4c)
  - percutaneous pinning is recommended to restore articular integrity in type 2, 3, and 4a fractures
  - open reduction is recommended in intra-articular fractures with more than 2 mm distraction
  - bone graft reconstruction is recommended when there is more than 5 mm residual impaction following attempted restoration of alignment.

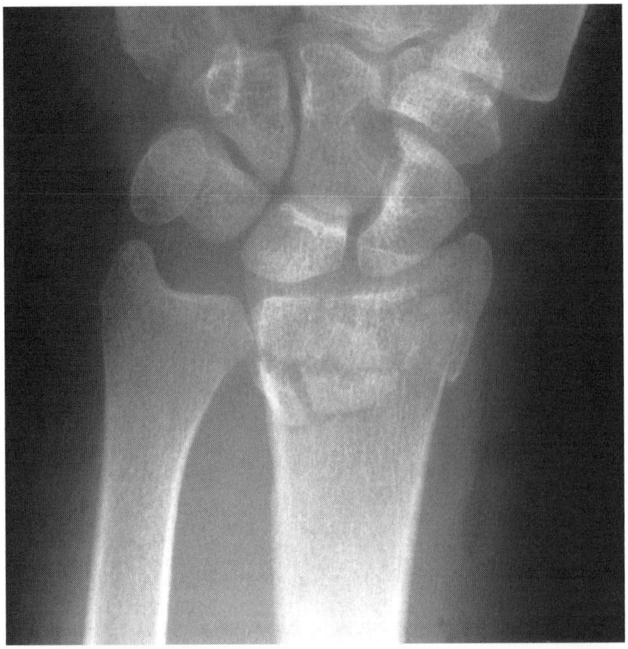

(a)

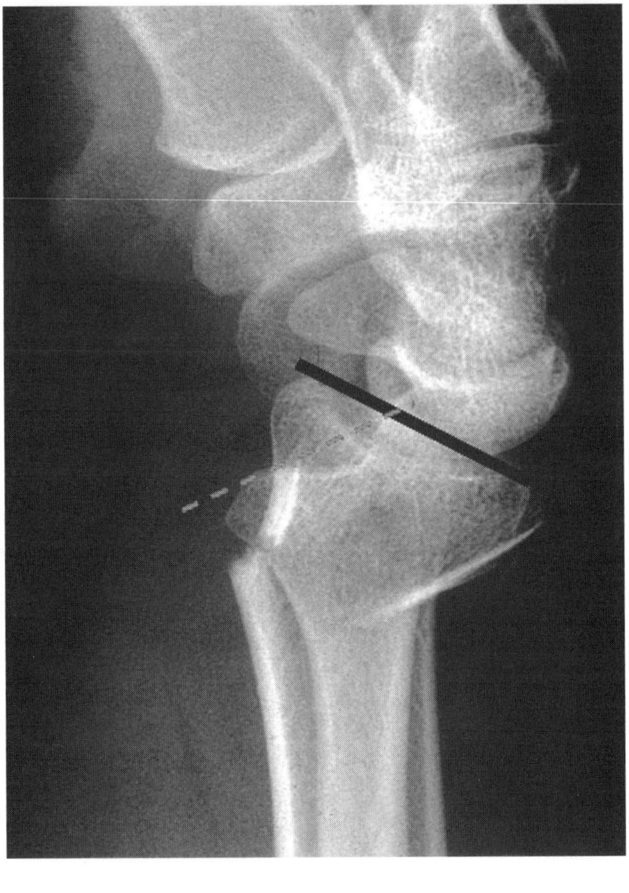

(b)

**Fig. 10.17** (**a, b**) Colles' fracture: AP radiographs showing a comminuted impaction fracture of the distal radius with dorsal tilt and angulation of the distal radius.

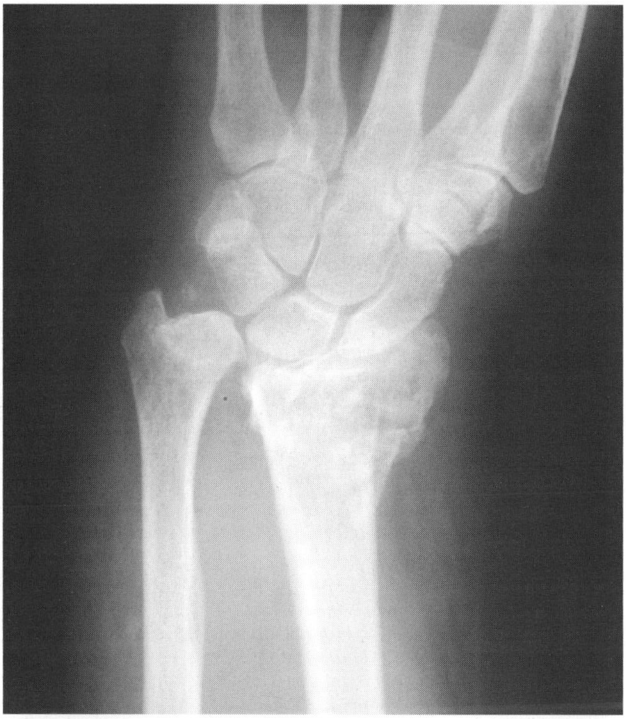

(a)

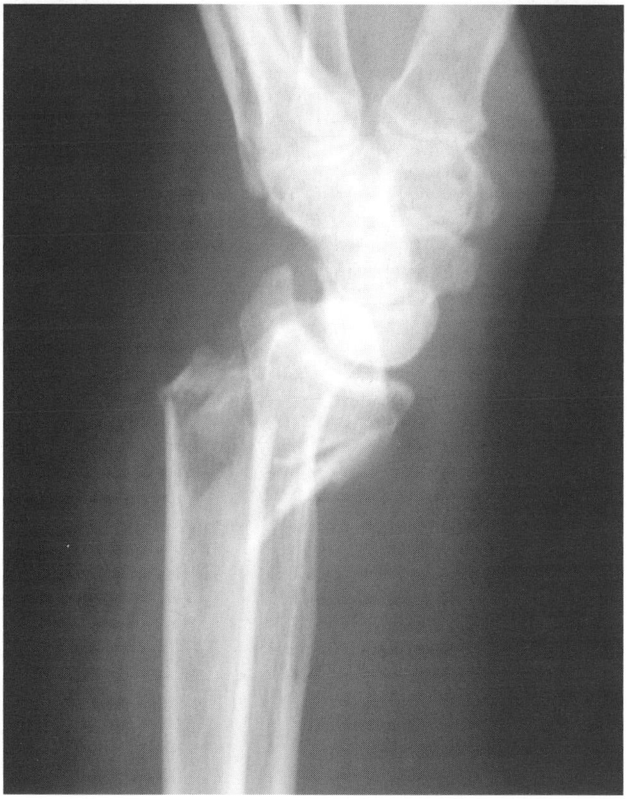

(b)

**Fig. 10.18**
**(a, b)** Radiographs showing a comminuted fracture of the distal radius with volar tilt and angulation of the distal radial fragment.

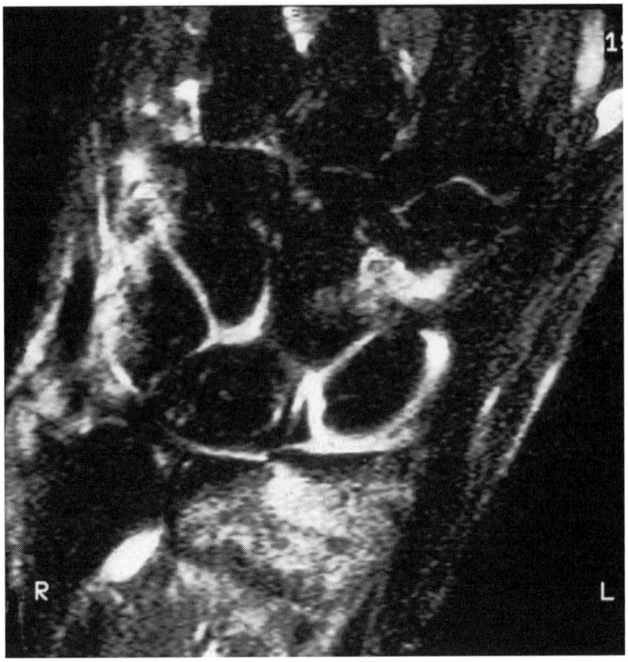


**Fig. 10.19** Coronal radiograph showing an intra-articular impaction fracture of the distal radius extending to the junction of the scaphoid and lunate articular facets of the distal radius with disruption of the scapholunate ligament.

## Median nerve injury

- Median nerve injury commonly accompanies distal radial fractures either secondary to the tension of forceful hyperextension or secondary to direct impaction by fracture fragment in forced flexion injury. This is Smith's fracture.
- Chronic median neuropathy was identified in 23% of 536 patients with fractures of the distal radius in one study.
- Median neuropathy is also identified in patients with acute and chronic DISI with compression of carpal tunnel structures by the body of the lunate, which displaces volarly as it angulates dorsally. (Such an injury is often occupationally acquired or the sequel to recreational overuse as occurs in oarsmen.)

## Post-traumatic epiphysiolysis

### Mechanism of injury

- Injury to the developing growth plate may follow repetitive minor trauma such as occurs to the radial and ulnar epiphyses in adolescent gymnasts. Repeated minor trauma may lead to physeal widening, metaphyseal irregularity and sclerosis without epiphyseal displacement.

### Imaging findings

#### Radiography

- Radiographs show sclerotic change and osseous irregularity along the margins of the growth plate

#### Magnetic resonance imaging

- MRI allows an earlier and more detailed evaluation of the growth plate. MR images show irregularity of the growth plate with periarticular marrow edema reflecting chronic stress and microtrabecular trauma.

### Management

- Usually reversible by removing the stressor.

# Distal radioulnar joint injury

## Mechanism of injury

- Distal radioulnar joint (DRUJ) injury may follow either pronation or supination injury, either accompanying fracture of the distal radius or the radial shaft (Galeazzi's fracture). Pronation results in disruption of the dorsal radioulnar ligament while supination results in disruption of the volar radioulnar ligament.

## Imaging findings

### Radiography

- Radiographs acquired in pronation and supination may show widening and displacement at the DRUJ.

### Computerized tomography

- CT allows the detailed evaluation of DRUJ congruity in pronation, neutral and supinated positions.

### Magnetic resonance imaging

- MRI also allows assessment of DRUJ congruity by axial images acquired in pronation, neutral and supinated positions (Fig. 10.20).

## Management

### Non-surgical

- This is undertaken in the majority of patients.
- Support bracing.
- Antiinflammatories/targeted steroid injection.

### Surgical

- Surgery is undertaken in resistant cases with persistent discomfort despite conservative approaches.
- Fusion via K wire results in a loss of pronation and supination at the wrist.
- Osteotomy.



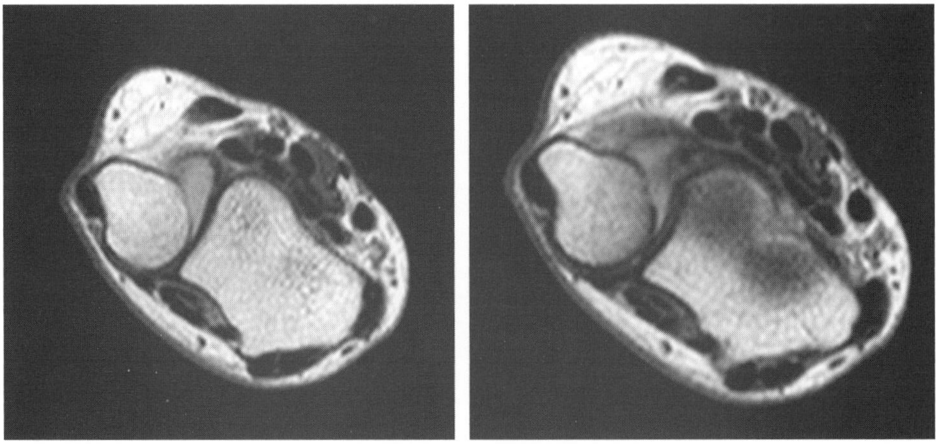

(a) (b)

**Fig. 10.20 (a, b)** Axial $T_2$-weighted MR images showing disruption of the distal radioulnar joint with tear of the volar radioulnar ligament and associated subluxation of the ulnar.

# Scaphoid fractures

**Mechanism of injury**

- The scaphoid bone is the second most commonly fractured bone of the wrist, typically complicating a fall on a dorsiflexed hand.

**Classification**

- Fractures are classified by site and orientation into those affecting the proximal pole, the waist and the distal pole. Fractures of the distal pole rarely develop either non-union or avascular necrosis (AVN). In contrast, fractures of the proximal pole develop non-union in almost all cases. Healing of fractures through the mid zone or waist is variable. Complications are more common in fractures with displacement or humpback angulation at the fracture margin.
- Undisplaced fractures heal without complication in up to 95% of cases. Displaced fractures occur in up to 30% of cases and when displacement is greater than 1 mm, approximately 50% of cases develop either non-union, AVN or both.

## Imaging findings

Radiography

- Radiographs with specific scaphoid views often allow the identification of subtle fractures (Fig. 10.21).

Scintigraphy

- A scintigraphy (Tc 99m methylene diphosphonate) scan may show osteoblastic activity manifest as a hot spot at the fracture margins (Fig. 10.22).

Magnetic resonance imaging

- MRI has two specific roles in the evaluation of scaphoid fractures: in the detection of radiographically occult fractures and in the evaluation of vascular integrity (Fig. 10.23).

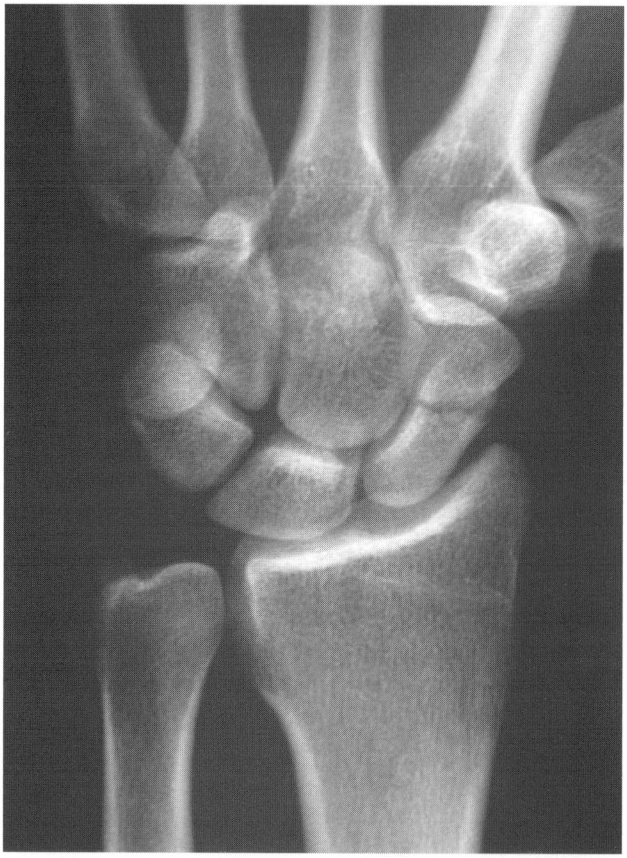

(a)



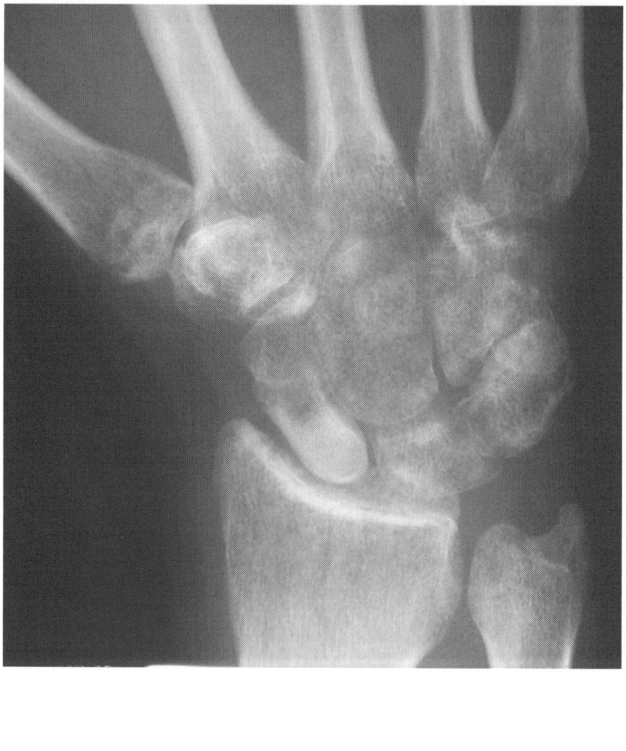

(b)

**Fig. 10.21**
(**a**) Radiograph showing an undisplaced fracture of the waist of the scaphoid with normal density in the proximal fragment.
(**b**) Radiograph of the wrist showing sclerotic change in the proximal pole of the scaphoid secondary to AVN complicating wrist fracture.

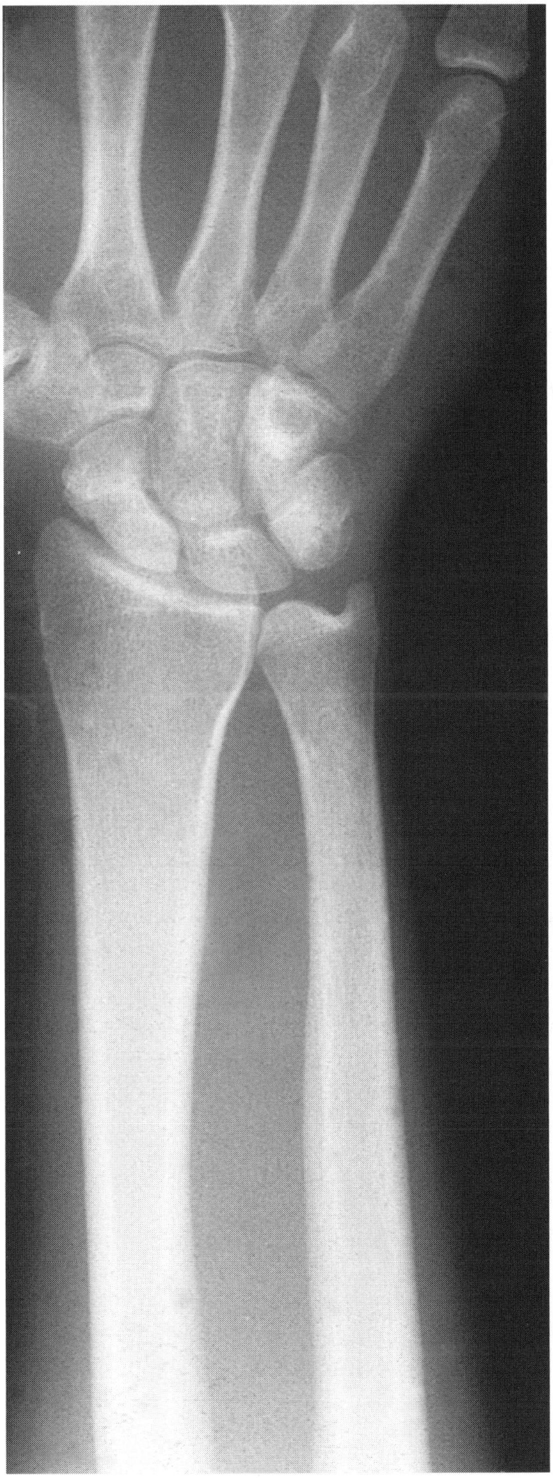

(a)

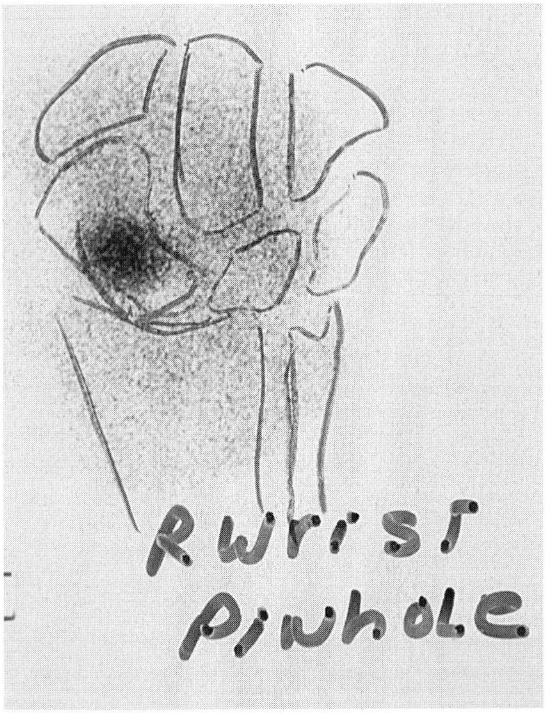


(b)

**Fig. 10.22** (**a**) Radiograph showing a linear sclerotic band through the scaphoid waist, which is worrisome for an impaction fracture. (**b**) Isotope bone scan showing the concentration of radiotracer over the scaphoid waist indicating fracture.

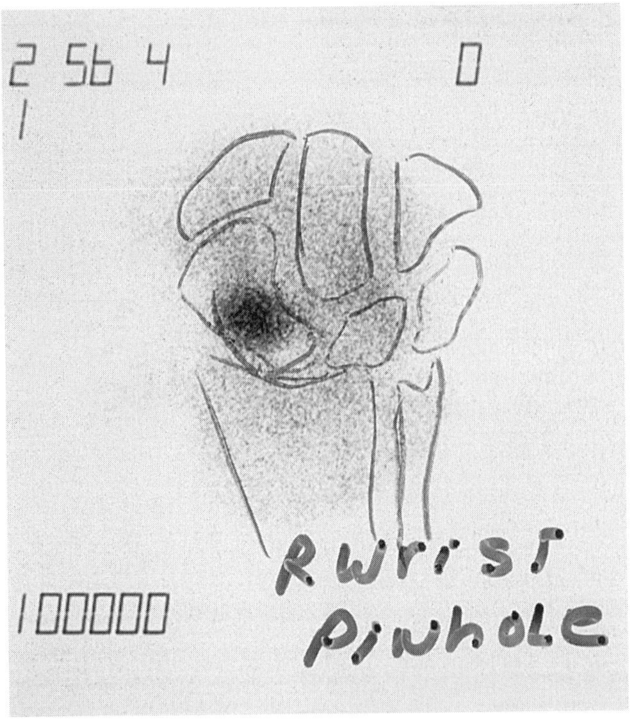


(a)

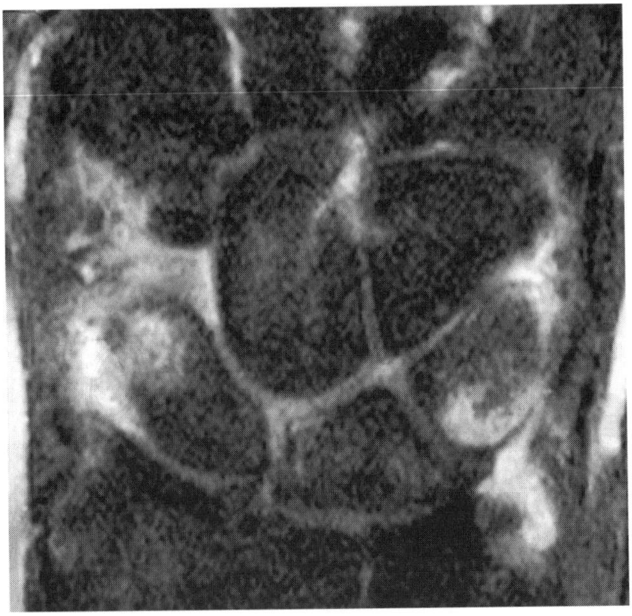

(b)

**Fig. 10.23** (**a**) Isotope bone scan showing the concentration of radiotracer in the scaphoid waist. (**b**) Fat-suppressed MR image in the same patient as in (a) showing focal bone edema in the distal pole of the scaphoid indicating undisplaced fracture.

## Occult fracture detection

- Using scintigraphy, fractures are only detected if there is an attempt at bone healing, or reactive marginal osteoblastic activity with secretion of hydroxyapatite. In health, the healing response is often delayed to 48 hours, while in the elderly the response may be delayed as long as a week. In effect, using scintigraphy, a result may not be yielded at the time of injury. Similarly, using scintigraphy, uptake by overlying inflamed soft tissues may be misleading and generate inaccuracy.
- Induced bone edema may be detected within hours of injury using MRI and confirm the presence of a fracture.

## Vascular integrity of fracture fragments

- The proximal 70–80% of the scaphoid is supplied by the dorsal branch of the radial artery. Disruption of this vessel invariably occurs in fracture through the proximal pole and occasionally in fracture through the wrist resulting in ischemic necrosis. (Atraumatic interruption of vascular supply to the proximal pole is called Preiser's disease.) The tuberosity and distal pole are supplied by the volar branches, rarely interrupted by fracture.
- Following fracture, a relative increase in density is identified in the ischemic portion between 4 and 8 weeks. Such a change is readily manifest at MRI with loss of normal marrow signal, and replacement by signal hypointensity on both $T_1$- and $T_2$-weighted sequences.

### Management

- Untreated, non-union results in altered carpal equilibrium and the development of a DISI configuration. As a result, radiocarpal arthitis is commonly identified within 5 years in affected patients, midcarpal arthritis is commonly identified at 5–10 years and generalized arthritis is identified at 20 years.

#### Non-surgical

- Management: employed in undisplaced fractures.
- Cast fixation for 6 weeks.
- Antiinflammatories.

#### Surgical

- Surgery is employed in minimally displaced fractures.
- Herbert screw fixation with cast immobilization.
- Herbert screw fixation with a bone graft harvested from the dorsal surface of the distal radius. This is employed in patients with delayed non-union in the absence of AVN.

# Lunate fractures and Kienböck's disease

## Mechanism of injury

- Acute trauma to the lunate may manifest as dislocation or rarely fracture. When they occur, fractures may involve the palmar or dorsal surfaces or extend through the body.

## Imaging findings

### Radiography

- Radiographs with AP, lateral, oblique and carpal tunnel projections.

### Computerized tomography

- CT may allow the identification of subtle fractures of the dorsal or volar surfaces of the lunate.

### Magnetic resonance imaging

- MRI allows similar tomographic imaging and the ability to detect bone edema, which allows the identification of subtle bone injuries.

## Outcome

- Being poorly vascularized, ischemic necrosis may complicate fracture, particularly fractures extending through the body and proximal pole. Ischemia may also follow repetitive minor trauma, enhanced by increased lunate axial loading induced by a short ulnar (negative ulnar variance). This is Kienböck's disease. This most frequently occurs in young male manual laborers, affects the dominant hand and is most frequently unilateral.
- At MRI, Kienböck's disease is staged according to pattern and extent of signal changes. In stage 1 disease, focal signal changes are observed, hypointense on $T_1$-weighted images and hyperintense on $T_2$-weighted images. In stage 2 disease, signal changes progress to involve the entire lunate. In stage 3 disease there is collapse of fragments, while in stage 4 disease there is complicating osteoarthritis.



## Management

- Stage 1 disease is treated by cast immobilization for 6 weeks.
- Stages 2 and 3 may be treated by ulna lengthening.
- Stage 4 disease is treated by either excision or carpal fusion (Figs 10.24 and 10.25).

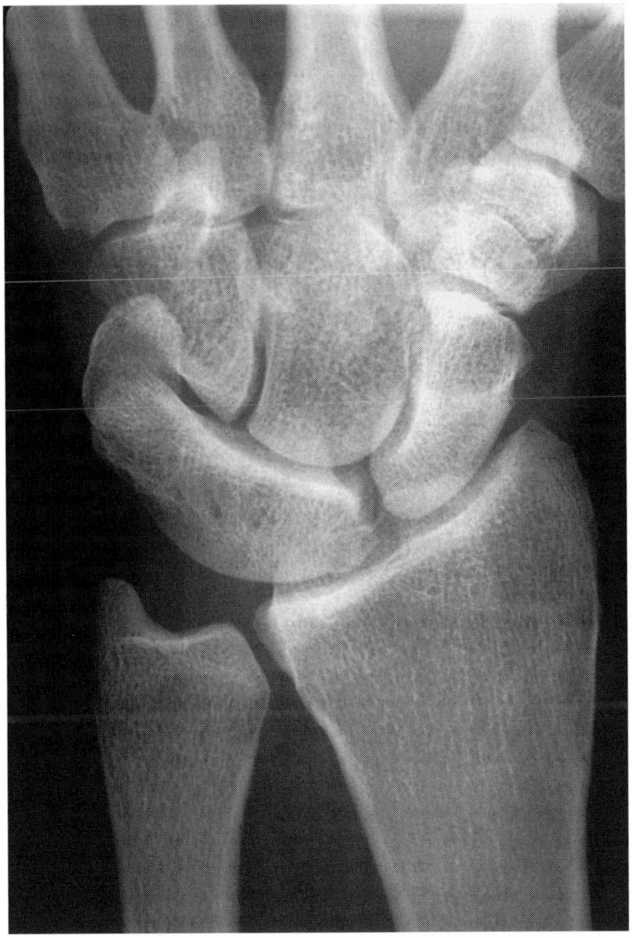

**Fig. 10.24**
AP radiograph showing lunatotriquetropisiform coalition; the remainder of the bone outlines are normal. Coalition in either the proximal or distal row of carpal bones is usually sporadic, while coalition between the proximal and distal row of carpal bones is usually secondary to a syndrome.

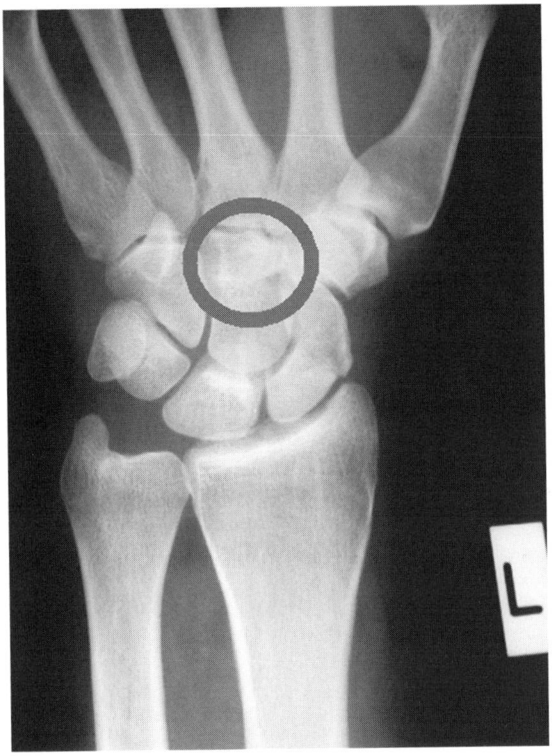


(a)

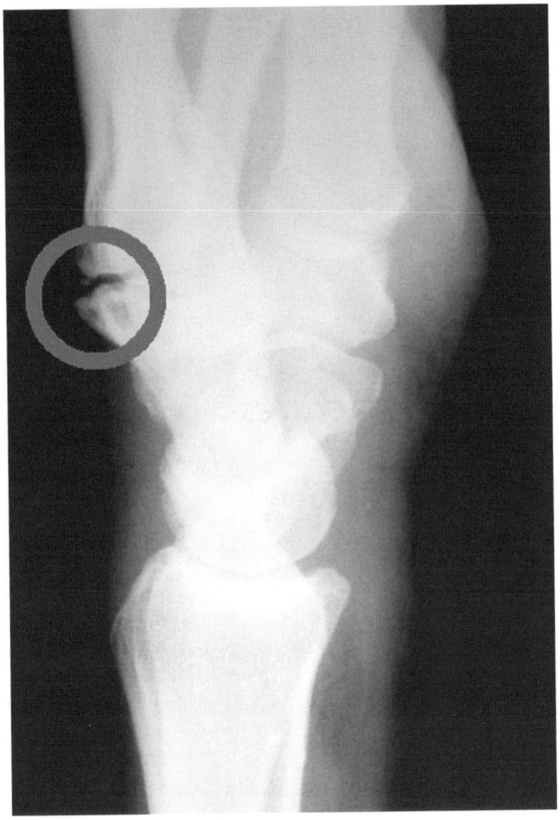

(b)



**Fig. 10.25** (**a**) AP radiograph showing accessory bone over the distal capitate, which is shown (**b**) as dorsal bossing on the lateral radiograph.

## Triquetral fractures

- Dorsal avulsions of the triquetrum are the second most common fracture of the carpal bones. They arise from an avulsion of the dorsal radiotriquetral ligament in hyperflexion or rarely from an avulsion of the ulnotriquetral ligament with hyperextension.

## Pisiform fractures

- Fractures of the pisiform are rare and most commonly follow a direct blow to the volar ulnar aspect of the wrist.

## Capitate fractures

- Capitate fractures are usually transverse in orientation and extend through the carpal wrist and are therefore readily identified on conventional radiographs. Complex intra-articular fractures occasionally accompany fractures through the bases of the 3rd and 4th metacarpals. Occasionally, radiographically occult capitate fractures are identified accompanying impaction fractures of the distal radius at MRI, particularly using fat-suppressed inversion recovery sequences.

## Hamate fractures

### Mechanism of injury

- Hamate fractures are uncommon. They are now occasionally identified following motorcycle accidents and in professional cyclists.

### Classification

- Three types of hamate fracture are recognized: sagittal split; fracture of the dorsal articular surface accompanying carpometacarpal fracture dislocation; and fracture of the hook.

### Imaging findings

- Conventional radiographs allow the visualization of fractures using oblique and carpal tunnel projections.
- Improved detection is yielded by tomographic imaging using either CT or MRI.

## Guyon's canal and ulnar neuropathy

- Guyon's canal is a fibro-osseous canal superficial to the flexor retinaculum, and intimately related to both the pisiform and the hook of hamate. The canal contains the ulnar nerve, artery and vein.
- At the level of the hook of hamate the nerve divides into a superficial palmar branch and a deep motor unit such that fracture may disrupt either or both branches by direct contusion or persistent compression.

# Gamekeeper's thumb

- This condition acquired its name from an injury to the metacarpophalangeal articulation acquired by Scottish gamekeepers attempting to kill rabbits by strangulation. A contemporary term – skier's thumb – is now more frequently employed as it is in this group that the injury is now more frequently recognized.

## Anatomy

- The injury is characterized by disruption of the ulnar collateral ligament at the base of the thumb, integrity of which dictates the ability to successfully appose the thumb and digits.

## Classification

- Two forms of injury are recognized, one in which a small ossific fragment is avulsed at the insertion of the ligament (type 1), which is readily identified on radiographs, and type 2, which is radiographically occult and characterized by intrasubstance rupture without avulsion of bone.

## Imaging findings

- Both forms of the injury result in instability and complete rupture indicated by more than 35° of abduction on stress.

### Radiography

- Radiographs may reveal a small ossific fragment along the ulnar border of the base of the thumb at the site of avulsion.

### Magnetic resonance imaging

- At MRI, the normal ulnar collateral ligament is band-like and is uniformly hypointense, lying deep to the adductor aponeurosis. Following injury, fluid is noted to bridge the site of tear. In patients with a Stener lesion, the proximal ligament is noted to be retracted with interposition of lax adductor aponeurosis at the site of tear.



## Management

### Non-surgical

- In practice, most injuries are now treated conservatively by immobilization within a splint.

### Surgical

- Surgery is undertaken in a minority of patients.
- In type 1 injuries, surgery is undertaken when the avulsed fragment is displaced. Here, healing can only be achieved by surgically restoring apposition at the site of the avulsion with fragment fixation using hooked K wire.
- In type 2 injuries, surgery is undertaken when the margins of the torn ulnar collateral ligament are retracted (Stener lesion). Classically, the term 'Stener lesion' is only used when the proximal portion of the torn ligament is retracted sufficiently to allow the adductor aponeurosis to lie between the torn edges of the collateral ligament. Surgical repair must be undertaken within 3 weeks of injury if successful reconstruction is to be achieved (Fig. 10.26).

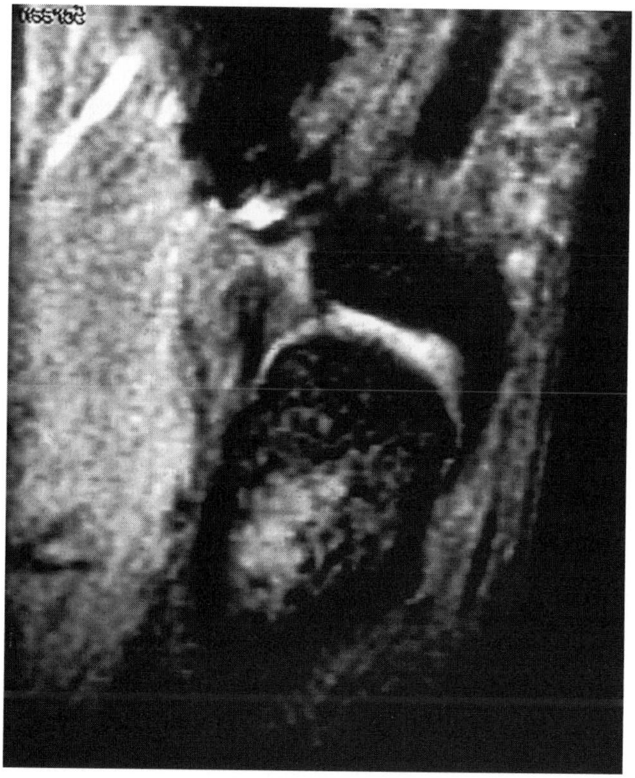


**Fig. 10.26** Coronal image of the thumb showing disruption of the ulnar collateral ligament secondary to a soft-tissue gamekeeper's thumb-type injury in a downhill skier.

## Radial collateral ligament injury

- This injury is considerably less common than injury to the ulnar collateral and diagnosis is usually late. Affected patients often complain of local tenderness immediately following attempted opening of a large jar lid or car door.
- In suspected cases, radiographs, arthrography, ultrasound or MRI may be used to confirm diagnosis.
- Similar collateral ligaments are responsible for radial and volar stability in all the interphalangeal joints and using MRI may be imaged following suspected trauma.

## Thumb dislocation and proximal interphalangeal joint dislocation

- Dorsal dislocation at the proximal interphalangeal joint (PIP) is the most common articular injury in the hand.
- Dislocation at the base of the thumb is less common, occurring either in isolation or accompanying intra-articular fractures (Bennet's fracture: simple intra-articular; Rolando's fracture: comminuted intra-articular).
- The thumb and phalanges dislocate dorsally more often than volarly.
- Diagnosis is by clinical examination.

### Management

- Following dislocation, reduction is often difficult, and when this occurs interposition of the volar plate or flexor pollicis longus or digitorum tendons should be suspected. Volar dislocation is invariably associated with collateral ligament disruption and interposition of the dorsal capsule to the joint space impairing reduction.
- Following reduction splinting, immobilization is achieved by strapping the injured phalanx to the adjacent uninjured digit.



## Volar plate injuries

### Anatomy

- The volar plate represents the ligamentous thickening of the volar capsule bridging and stabilizing the volar aspect of the interphalangeal and metacarpophalangeal joints. The volar plate is primarily responsible for passive resistance to hyperextension at these articulations, active resistance being provided by the contraction of flexor muscle groups.

### Diagnosis

- Volar pain on induced hyperextension with local tenderness suggests the injury, which can be clearly visualized in both passive and stressed sagittal views of the digits using MRI.

### Management

- Most patients are treated conservatively with immobilization via splinting to an adjacent uninjured digit.
- In symptomatic cases, volar capsulodesis, ligamentous reconstruction and arthrodesis are occasionally undertaken.

## Sesamoid and volar plate injuries of the thumb

### Anatomy and mechanism of injury

- Two sesamoids are identified adjacent to the volar aspect of the metacarpophalangeal joint of the thumb in almost all patients where they reside within the volar plate. The tendon of the adductor pollicis inserts into the ulnar sesamoid, and the tendon of the flexor pollicis brevis into the radial seamoid, accounting for loss of tendon function and distraction of fragments following sesamoid injury.

### Management

- In the majority of patients with injury without displacement, simple support strapping is employed.
- In patients with volar plate injury and evidence of distraction, primary surgical repair is undertaken.

## Extensor tendon injury: mallet finger

- 'Mallet finger' is used to describe the flexion deformity of the distal interphalangeal (DIP) joint resulting from loss of extensor tendon continuity to the distal phalanx. 'Mallet finger of bony origin' is used to describe the same deformity occurring secondary to an intra-articular fracture of the dorsal lip of the distal phalanx.

### Classification

- Three patterns of tendon-related mallet finger are recognized:
  - type 1 injury resulting from stretching of the ligament
  - type 2 injury characterized by rupture of the tendon at its insertion
  - type 3 injury characterized by a subtle avulsion at the site of tendon insertion.



### Management

Non-surgical

- When uncertainty exists and surgical repair is contemplated, MRI is occasionally used to differentiate between tendon stretching and complete tear.
- In practice, conservative management is undertaken if lacerations involve less than 60% of tendon cross-sectional area.

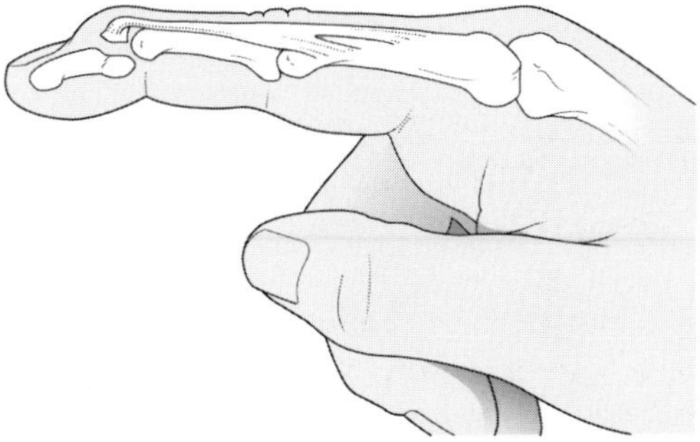

**Fig. 10.27** Flexion deformity at the distal interphalangeal articulation due to extensor tendon rupture produces a mallet finger.

# Extensor tendon injury: boutonnière deformity

## Anatomy

- Boutonnière deformity (or buttonhole deformity) is caused by disruption of the central slip of the extensor tendon combined with tearing of the triangular ligament on the dorsum of the middle phalanx, allowing the lateral bands of the extensor tendon to slip below the axis of the PIP articulation.

## Diagnosis

- Clinical examination.
- Although clinically apparent, MRI allows detailed evaluation of tendon position and integrity, triaging patients into surgical and non-surgical groups.

## Management

### Non-surgical

- Non-surgical splinting for 6 weeks allows scar formation and stabilization.

### Surgical

- In failed conservative management, primary surgical repair of the extensor tendon may be undertaken.

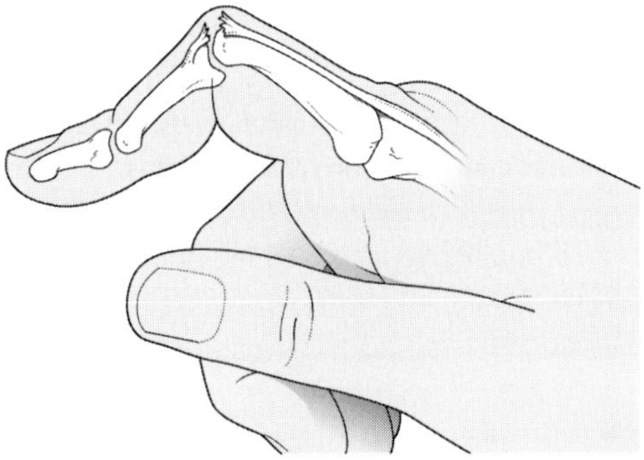

**Fig. 10.28** Flexion deformity at the proximal interphalangeal joint due to extensor tendon rupture produces a boutonnière deformity.

# Flexor digitorum profundus tendon injury: jersey finger

## Definition and mechanism of injury

- Avulsion of the flexor digitorum profundus tendon from its insertion into the base of the distal phalanx is a relatively uncommon injury, usually occurring during active sports, typically when a football or rugby player attempts to tackle the opposition but ends up grabbing at a handful of jersey, hence the term 'jersey finger'.

## History and clinical findings

- Affected patients complain of an inability to flex at the DIP articulation. However, the injury is often overlooked unless specifically sought.

## Classification and management

- Leddy and Packer have identified three patterns of injury:
  - type 1 injury is characterized by retraction of the tendon to the palm, severing all blood supply and necessitating repair within 7 days
  - in type 2 injury the tendon retracts to the PIP articulation where it becomes entangled with the flexor digitorum superficialis
  - in type 3 injury a large bony fragment is avulsed and becomes trapped at the site of the distal pulley.

## Imaging findings

### Magnetic resonance imaging

- Recognizing the importance of localizing the position of the avulsed tendon stump prior to surgical exploration, MRI in the sagittal plane is frequently employed in preoperative evaluation of these patients.

# Further reading

Andrews JG, Youm Y. A biomechanical investigation of wrist kinematics. J Biomech 1979; 12: 83–93.

Berger RA, Blair WF, Crowninshield RD, Flatt AE. The scapholunate ligament. J Hand Surg (Am) 1982; 7: 87–91.

Gilula LA. Carpal injuries: analytic approach and case exercises. Am J Roentgenol 1979; 133: 503–517.

Lavernia CJ, Cohen MS, Taleisnik J. Treatment of scapholunate dissociation by ligamentous repair and capsulodesis. J Hand Surg (Am) 1992; 17: 354–359.

Linscheid RL. Kinematic considerations of the wrist. Clin Orthop Relat Res 1986; 202: 27–39.

Linscheid RL, Dobyns JH, Beckenbaugh RD et al. Instability patterns of the wrist. J Hand Surg (Am) 1983; 8(5 Pt 2): 682–686.

Linscheid RL, Dobyns JH, Beabout JW, Bryan RS. Traumatic instability of the wrist: diagnosis, classification, and pathomechanics. J Bone Joint Surg Am 1972; 54: 1612–1632.

Mayfield JK. Patterns of injury to carpal ligaments. A spectrum. Clin Orthop Relat Res 1984; 187: 36–42.

Palmer AK, Werner FW. The triangular fibrocartilage complex of the wrist: anatomy and function. J Hand Surg (Am) 1981; 6: 153–162.

Smith DK. Scapholunate interosseous ligament of the wrist: MR appearances in asymptomatic volunteers and arthrographically normal wrists. Radiology 1994; 192: 217–221.

Taleisnik J. The ligaments of the wrist. J Hand Surg (Am) 1976; 1: 110–118.

Thorson E, Szabo RM. Common tendinitis problems in the hand and forearm. Orthop Clin North Am 1992; 23: 65–74.

Viegas SF, Patterson RM, Hokanson JA, Davis J. Wrist anatomy. Incidence, distribution, and correlation of anatomic variations, tears, and arthrosis. J Hand Surg (Am) 1993; 18: 463–475.

# 11

# The Spine



## CLINICAL EXAMINATION

### Cervical spine examination

Neck injuries encountered during sports range from mild neck spasms to catastrophic injuries with cervical spine fractures and dislocations with paralysis. Chronic neck pain can be associated with degenerative spondylosis.

*Inspection* Note the position of the head as the patient moves, and during history taking and undressing.

*Palpation* The bony landmarks anteriorly are the hyoid bone at the angle of the chin and neck. This corresponds to the 3rd cervical vertebra. The 'Adam's apple' is the thyroid cartilage and corresponds to the 4th cervical vertebra. The first cricoid ring is just below the thyroid cartilage. Emergency tracheotomies are performed just below this ring. Posterior palpation reveals the inion, which is the bump in the occipital region on the midline. The spinous process beginning at C2 should be palpated. The C7 and T1 processes are more prominent than C2–C6. Palpate gently for loss of alignment or a palpable interspinous defect. Palpate the trapezius muscle for muscle spasm or tenderness. Anterior neck examination should include palpation of the sternomastoid muscle and adjacent lymph node chain. The thyroid gland and carotid pulse should also be examined.

The range of motion of the neck is then examined. Almost half of the flexion/extension occurs between the skull and the atlas and half the rotation occurs between the atlas (C1) and the axis

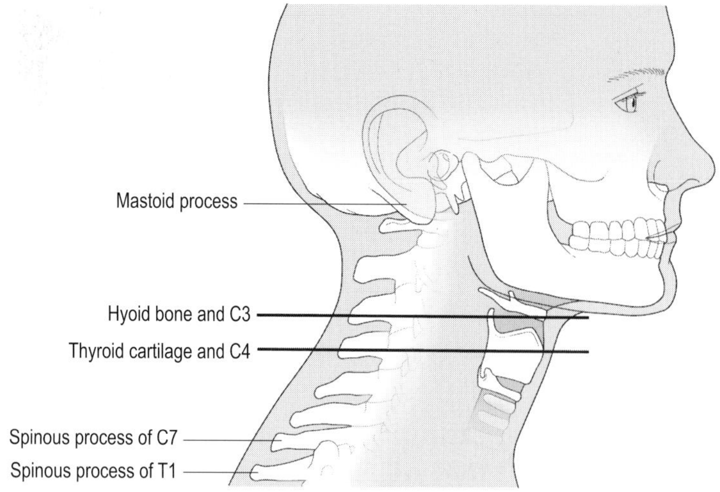


**Fig. 11.1** Examination of the cervical spine.

**Table 11.1** The cervical spine

| Root | Muscle(s) | Sensation | Reflexes |
|---|---|---|---|
| C5 | Deltoid; biceps | Lateral arm | Biceps |
| C6 | Wrist extension | Lateral forearm | Brachioradialis |
| C7 | Wrist flexors; triceps | Middle finger | Triceps |
| C8 | Finger flexion | Medial forearm | – |
| T1 | Intrinsics | Medial arm | – |



(C2). The remainder of the range of motion, including lateral flexion, occurs evenly along the rest of the cervical spine.

The neck examination then involves a full neurologic examination of the upper limbs with motor, sensory and reflex examination.

Distraction and compression tests can identify pathology of the facet joints (Fig. 11.1 and Table 11.1).

# Lumbar spine examination

## Back pain

The patient's history of back pain is crucial and includes mechanisms of injury, onset, distribution, radiation, patterns, relieving and aggravating factors, and any associated neurologic symptoms.

The examination should occur during the history taking by noting the patient's gait, deportment and posture.

Inspection of the painful lumbar spine most frequently reveals a loss of lumbar lordosis with associated muscle spasm. Listing to one side may be a compensatory scoliosis in an attempt to relieve nerve root compression in a patient with sciatica. Hyperlordosis and 'heart-shaped' buttocks can indicate an underlying spondylolisthesis.

Gait should be addressed for antalgic or ataxic features.

## Bony palpation

Palpate the interspinous spaces. The top of the posterior iliac crests usually approximates to the L4–5 level. A 'step-off' may be felt in spondylolisthesis.

The paraspinal muscles may exhibit tenderness, spasm or wasting. Anterior abdominal muscles may be weak and trunk posture may contribute to back pain.

## Movement

More movement occurs at L5–S1 than in the upper lumbar spine. Therefore it is not surprising that there is more pathology at these levels. Flexion and extension can be easily assessed as can lateral bending and rotation. The lower limb neurologic examination should follow your looking at each nerve root level, including the sacral roots The superficial and deep reflexes should be tested. Babinski's test should also be performed.

## Straight leg raise test

The patient lies supine with the hips and knee extended. Place one hand under the calcaneus and the other hand on the front calcaneus. If the patient says they cannot lift the leg and there is no downward pressure under the opposite calcaneus, this may indicate a lack of effort. This is Hoover's test.

Occasionally, a patient may exhibit reduced forward flexion of the lumbar spine on standing and may describe agonizing pain at 20° on the straight leg raise test. However, the same patient may clearly be able to sit up on the couch with hips flexed and knees extended and reach forward without difficulty. These physical findings are inconsistent.

Milgram's test involves asking the supine patient to elevate both heels 6 cm from the couch. Intrathecal pathology is unlikely if this can be maintained.

## Sacroiliac joint examination

The pelvic rock test involves forced compression of the pelvis on a supine patient.

### Gaensten's test

With the patient supine, allow one buttock and lower limb to hang over the side of the couch while the other lower limb is flexed at the hip and knee.

### Fabere's test

This test externally rotates, flexes and abducts the hip of the side being examined. With the lower limb in the 'figure four' position compression is applied to the flexed knee and the opposite hemipelvis.

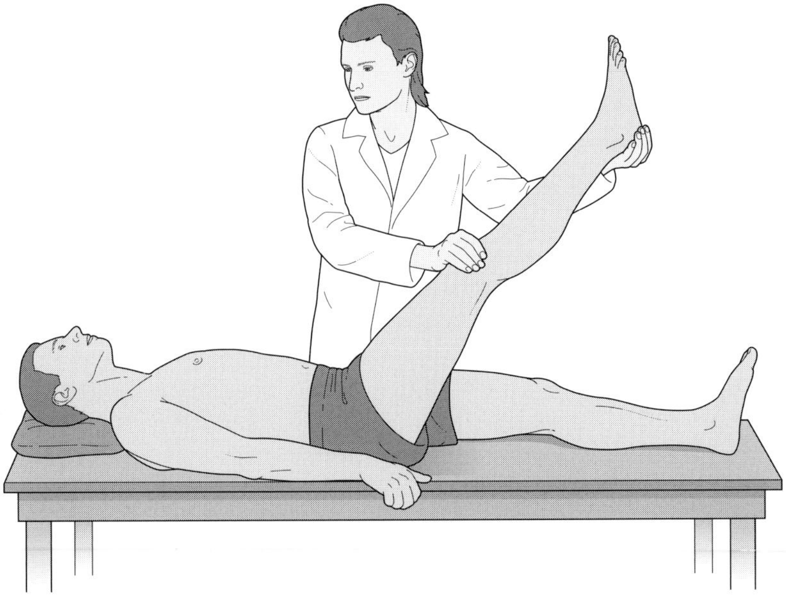

**Fig. 11.2** The straight leg raise test.

Pathology of the hip, pelvis and intrapelvic structures may present as low back pain and these areas should also be assessed (Figs 11.2 and 11.3, and Table 11.2).

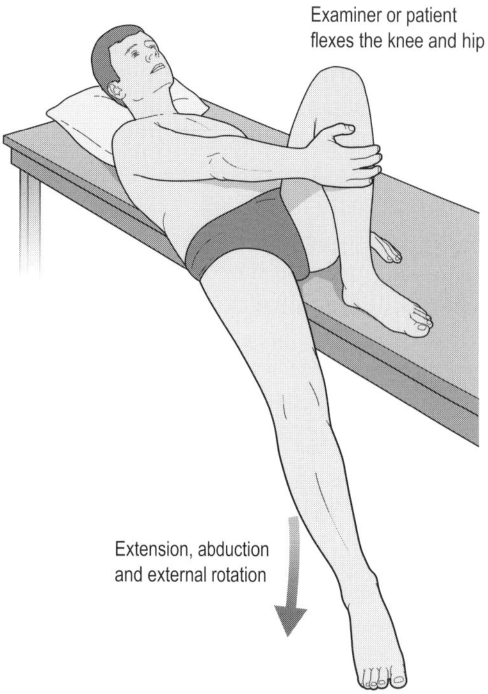


Fig. 11.3 Examination of the sacroiliac joint.

**Table 11.2** Examination of the spine

| Root | Muscle(s) | Sensation | Reflex |
|---|---|---|---|
| L4 | Tibialis anterior | Medial leg and foot | Patellar tendon |
| L5 | Extensor hallucis longus | Lateral leg and dorsum of foot | – |
| S1 | Peroneus longus and brevis | Lateral foot | Ankle |

# PATHOLOGIES

## Cervical spine trauma

### Anatomy

- Components of the three columns of the cervical spine are shown in Table 11.3.

### Mechanism of injury

- Most cervical spine injuries result from motor vehicle accidents, recreational sports, rugby and diving-related accidents. The mechanism of injury has an important role in the type of injury sustained (Table 11.4).

**Table 11.3** Components of the three columns of the cervical spine

| Column | Components |
|---|---|
| Anterior | Anterior longitudinal ligament<br>Anterior annulus fibrosis<br>Anterior vertebral body |
| Middle | Posterior vertebral body<br>Posterior annulus fibrosis<br>Posterior longitudinal ligament |
| Posterior | Posterior elements<br>Facet capsules<br>Interlaminar ligaments (flava)<br>Supra-/Interspinous ligaments |

NB Instability requires disruption of at least two columns.

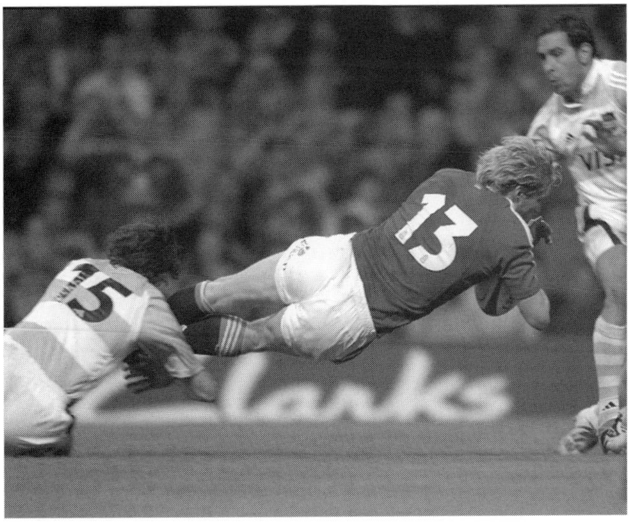

**Fig. 11.4** Sportsfile.

**Table 11.4** The relationships between the mechanism of injury and the type of injury sustained

| Mechanism of injury | Type |
| --- | --- |
| Hyperflexion | Anterior subluxation (sprain)<br>Bilateral interfacetal dislocation<br>Simple wedge fracture<br>Clay shoveler's fracture<br>Tear-drop fracture |
| Hyperextension | Dislocation (sprain or strain)<br>Avulsion fracture of the anterior arch of C1<br>Fracture of the posterior arch of C1<br>Tear-drop fracture of C2<br>Laminar fracture<br>Hangman's fracture<br>Fracture/dislocation |
| Vertical compression | Jefferson fracture<br>Burst fracture |
| Hyperflexion and rotation | Unilateral interfacetal dislocation |
| Hyperextension and rotation | Pillar fracture |
| Lateral flexion | Uncinate process fracture |
| Indeterminate | Atlanto-occipital disassociation<br>Odontoid fractures |



## History and clinical findings

- Cervical spine and spinal cord injuries have been classified based on neurologic deficits, type of injury (blunt versus penetrating trauma), mechanisms of injury and anatomic location (craniocervical junction versus lower cervical spine).
- Using these various classification schemes as guidelines, there are two fundamental issues unique to the spine that need to be addressed prior to planning appropriate therapy and judging prognosis: characterization of direct injury to the spinal cord; and identification of spinal instability and associated spinal cord damage.

## Imaging findings

### Radiography

- Under ideal circumstances, conventional radiographs detect up to 93% of cervical spine fractures, including flexion wedge and tear-drop fractures, extension tear-drop fractures, unilateral and bilateral facet dislocations, and most injuries around the craniocervical junction.
- Of the 7% of fractures missed on plain radiographs, odontoid peg, hangman's and facet fractures are the most frequent although these are often better evaluated with axial CT. MRI may be employed, especially for improved soft-tissue visualization.

### Computerized tomography

- When MRI is used as a standard of reference, CT has approximately a 33% and 44% sensitivity for the detection of post-traumatic spinal cord compression and disk herniation, respectively.

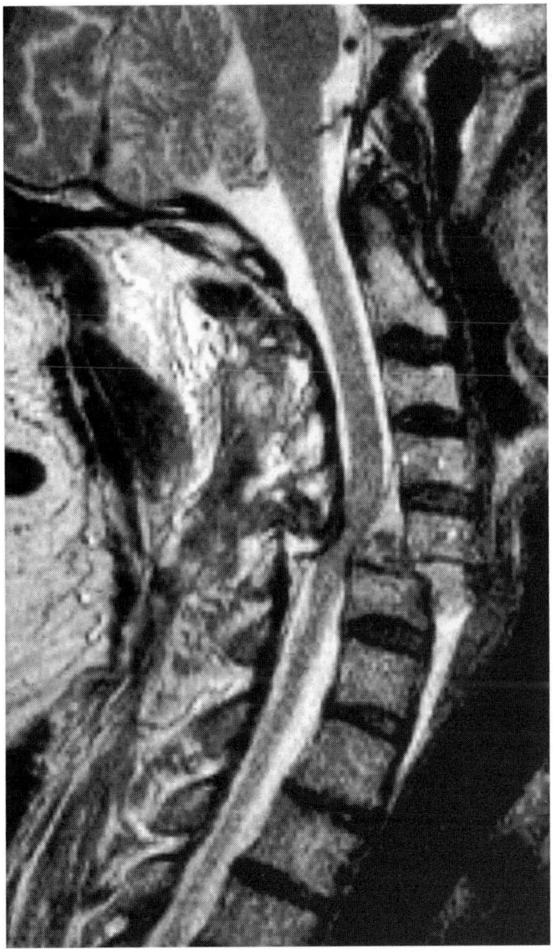

(a)

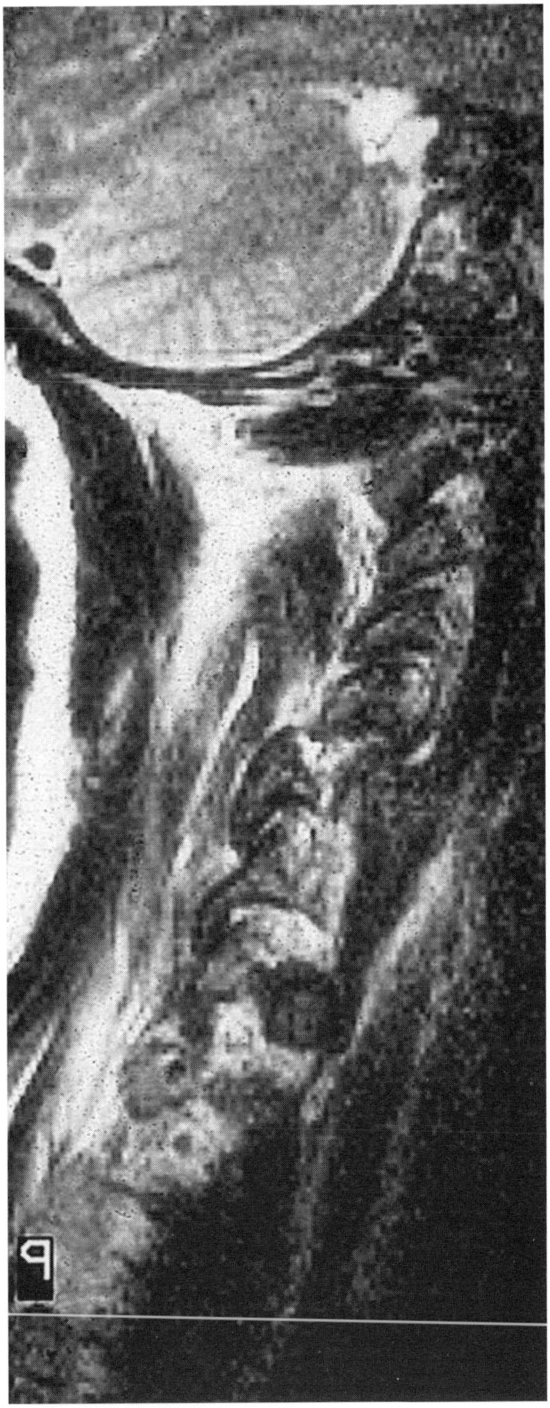

(b)

**Fig. 11.5** (**a**) Sagittal midline image showing acquired spinal stenosis at the C5–6 level secondary to (**b**) hyperflexion injury with bilateral jumped facets.



## Magnetic resonance imaging

- Fractures within the vertebral body are readily detected as a result of intense edema induced within cancellous bone.
- Posterior elements lack cancellous bone and therefore generate less edema following injury; these fractures are often localized by the presence of edema in the adjacent soft tissues.

- The analysis of MR images and correlation with other available imaging modalities (plain radiographs and CT) as well as the patient's neurologic examination should be performed (Fig. 11.5).
- MRI is superior in the depiction of spinal cord abnormalities.
- Cord injury relates to site, intensity and distribution of impact, and can be categorized as concussion, contusion and compression.

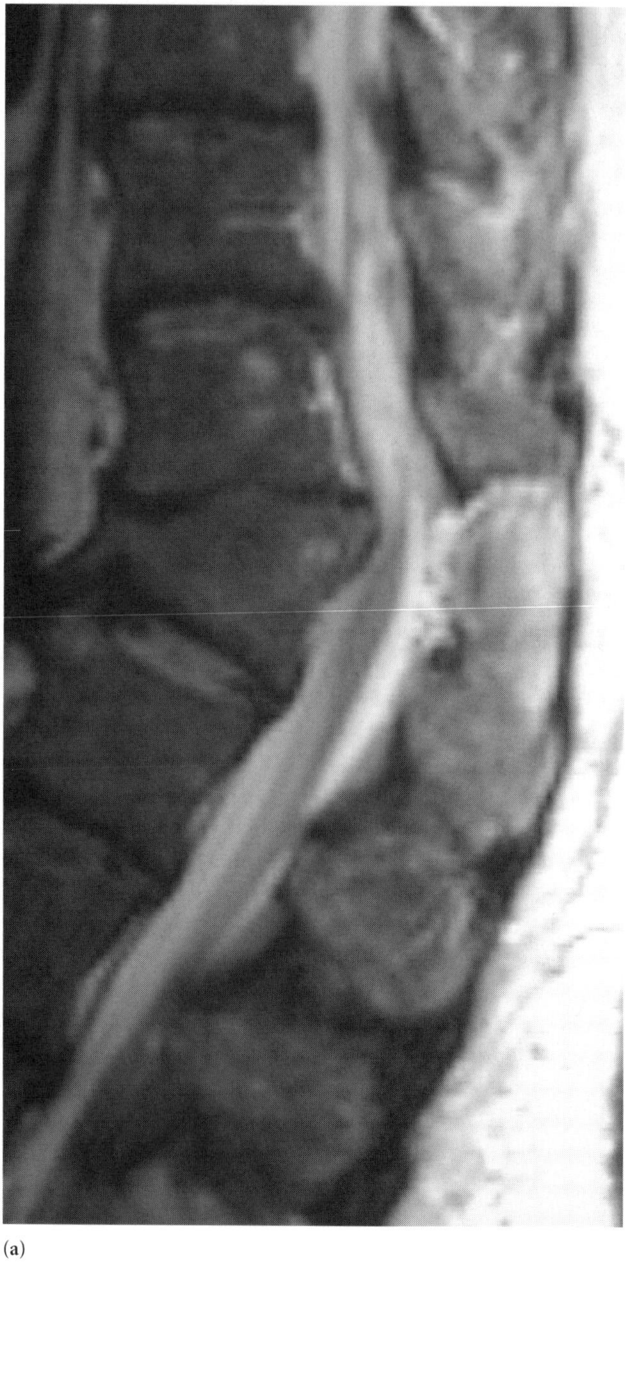

(a)

**Fig. 11.6** (**a**) Sagittal image showing an image of a 10-year-old wedge compression fracture at the L1 level, which occurred following a climbing accident.

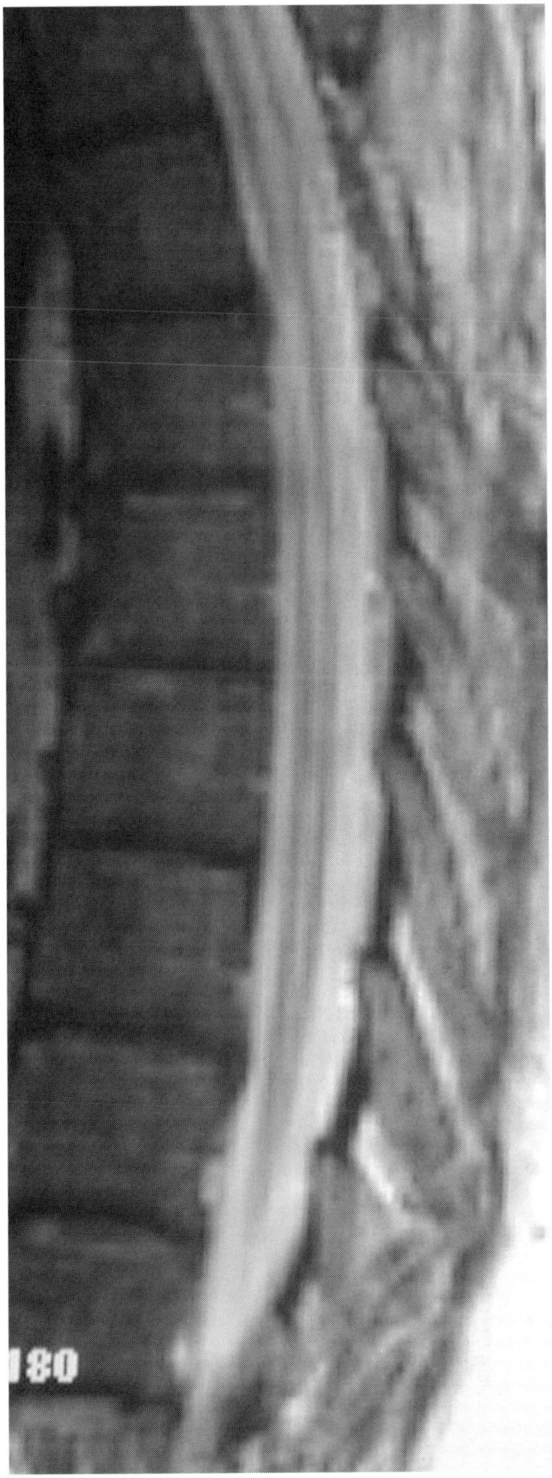


(b)

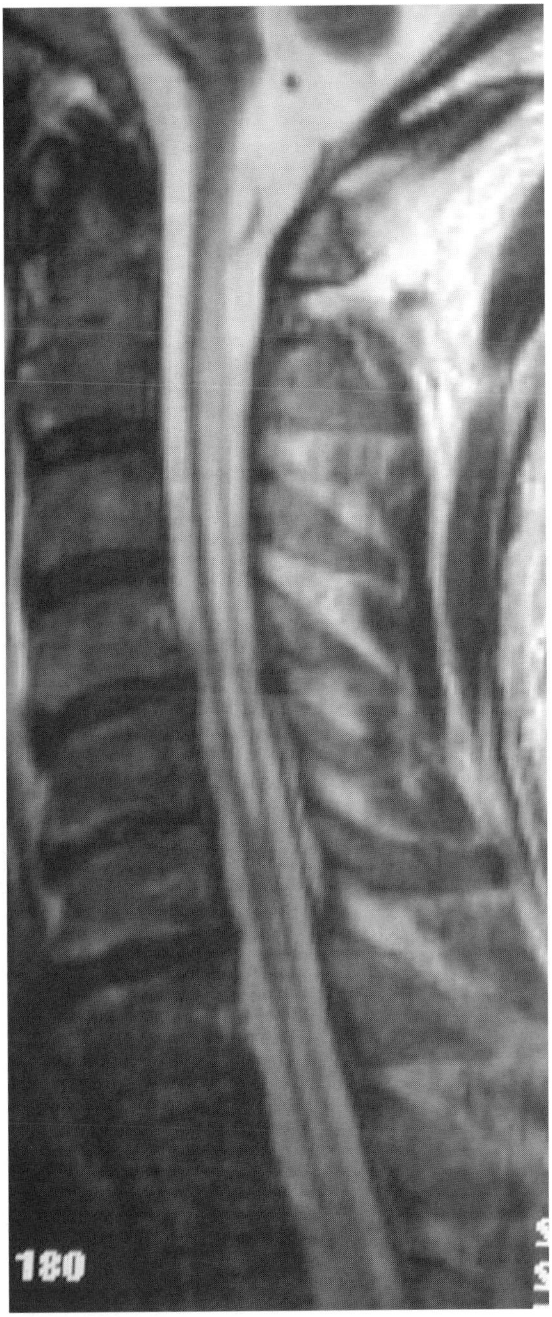


(c)

**Fig. 11.6** (**b, c**) The patient represented with dysarthria, and sensory loss in both hands secondary to acquired syringobulbia. Images show an extensive syrinx extending through dorsal spine (**b**) to the brainstem (**c**).

- Concussion of the cord is a purely functional and fully reversible derangement which has been attributed to transient deficiencies in the cord's microcirculation.
- The demonstration of cord edema on $T_2$-weighted images is uncommon and transient.
- Cord contusion has a spectrum extending from simple edema to petechial hemorrhage to severe hemorrhagic necrosis and even complete transection. See Figure 11.12.
- Subsequent demyelination, micro- and macrocystic myelomalacia, and arachnoiditis are common. Contusion can result from transient compression or stretching of the cord.
- Cord compression results from the same spectrum of injury to the cord as contusion with the additional demonstration of the compressive lesion (bone fragment, subluxation/dislocation, disk herniation, epidural hematoma and spondylotic spicule).
- A 50% or greater reduction in AP dimension of the spinal canal has been suggested as a necessary condition for cord compression.
- The identification of an acute compressive lesion is of utmost clinical importance because its identification mandates immediate surgical intervention (Fig. 11.6).
- MR signal patterns correlate well with neurologic functionality of injured patients. Pattern I is associated with the highest degree of acute neurologic deficit and the least degree of improvement; the second and third patterns are associated with less acute neurologic deficit and most improvement (Table 11.6).



**Table 11.5** Functional classification of spinal cord injury

| Grade | Neurologic deficit |
|---|---|
| A | Complete motor and sensory loss |
| B | Preserved sensory function |
| C | Preserved motor activity (non-functional) |
| D | Preserved motor activity (functional) |
| E | Complete neurologic recovery |

After Frankel.

**Table 11.6** Magnetic resonance signal pattern in acute spinal cord injury

| | MR pattern | $T_1$-weighted images *Central* | $T_2$-weighted images *Peripheral* |
|---|---|---|---|
| I | Heterogeneous signal with focal cord swelling | Large area of hypointensity at gray/white matter junction | Thin rim of hyperintensity at gray/white matter junction |
| II | Normal | Hyperintensity spindle shaped | Hyperintensity spindle shaped |
| III | Normal | Small area of hypointensity | Thick rim of hyperintensity |

After Kulkarni.

- The importance of distinguishing cord contusion from direct cord compression is based on evidence showing improvement of neurologic deficits following surgical decompression.
- Although the benefit of emergency spine decompression is somewhat controversial, most authorities agree to the need for immediate intervention in patients with acute cord compression regardless of the severity of neurologic deficit.
- MRI optimally demonstrates non-osseous causes of cord compression, e.g. disk herniation or epidural hematoma.

# The role of MRI in the identification of spinal instability

- Instability of the cervical spine is defined as the inability to maintain normal association between vertebral segments while under a physiologic load.
- Instability in the setting of trauma results from the loss of structural integrity of the bony spine and ligaments, which may lead to damage to the spinal cord and nerve roots or to pain and incapacitating deformity of the spinal column.
- Several clinical criteria have been established to suggest spinal instability. By dividing the spine into three columns, Denis defines instability as disruption of at least two of these columns.
- Other more objective criteria, which are completely reliant on imaging, include the displacement of two adjacent vertebrae by more than 3.5 mm and at an angulation greater than 11°.
- The role of MRI in the evaluation of spinal instability is less well defined.
- Patients with clear evidence of instability on plain radiographs, without signs of spinal cord injury, or patients in whom reduction of misalignment is not contemplated, do not require MRI.
- On the other hand, if the clinical evaluation and plain radiographic/CT findings are inconclusive but suggest instability, then MRI may become necessary for confirmation.
- The superiority of MRI in the detection of ligamentous injuries or tears and the questionable reliability of cervical spine flexion/extension radiography in the acute setting have rendered MRI the imaging method of choice for the confirmation of instability.
- The reported sensitivity of MRI, using high-resolution CT as standard, in the demonstration of cervical spine fractures, is variable and ranges from 25% to 100%. This wide range reflects significant differences in the ability of MRI to demonstrate vertebral body versus posterior element fractures and variability in the MRI techniques implemented.
- Subtle bony fractures of the posterior elements, which may be the only evidence of a second column disruption, can be missed with current MRI.
- At present, this limitation secures the role of high-resolution CT in the evaluation of cervical spine trauma (Fig. 11.7).



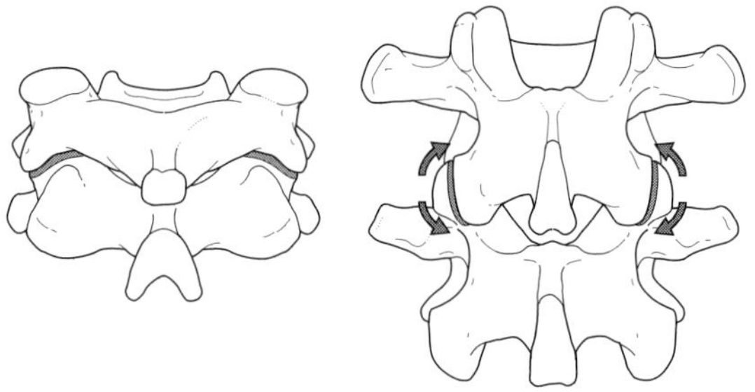

**Fig. 11.7** (**a**) Obliquely oriented facets in the cervical spine, which allow anterior vertebral body subluxation following hyperflexion injury. (**b**) Vertically oriented facets in the lumbar spine, which prevent subluxation following hyperflexion but lead to vertebral body wedging and wedge compression fractures at this site.

# Classifications of cervical spine injuries

**Penetrating trauma**

- Penetrating trauma to the cervical spine can be further divided into missile injuries and puncture wounds.
- In peace time, the most common missile injuries are the result of bullet fragments. Spinal cord damage from missile injuries can be due to direct passage of the missile through the cord or more commonly due to displaced bone fragments and blast effects.
- On the other hand, puncture wounds are the result of stabbing with a sharp instrument. Because of the protective nature of the bony posterior elements, especially the laminae and spinous processes, most entry sites are off-midline through the interlaminar ligaments and most injuries involve the dorsolateral aspect of the cord.
- MRI plays an important role in the evaluation of penetrating trauma. Victims of puncture wounds, in whom the injury is frequently limited to the soft tissues and spinal cord, may have a completely negative plain radiographic and CT examination. MRI can provide critical information regarding location, extent and type of cord injury as well as precise correlation with the level of neurologic deficit. In contrast, MRI for the evaluation of direct missile injuries may be limited by ferromagnetic susceptibility artifacts.

**Blunt trauma**

- Blunt trauma to the cervical spine is classified according to anatomic location of injury (cervicocranial junction versus lower cervical spine).
- Injuries at the cervicocranial junction are further divided into those involving the atlanto-occipital articulation and the atlantoaxial articulation.
- Lower cervical spine injuries are more common because of increased mobility and are commonly classified according to underlying mechanism.



**Atlanto-occipital disassociation**

- This injury is commonly fatal and describes any separation of the atlanto-occipital articulation. The separation may be complete (dislocation) or partial (subluxation) with posterior, anterior or superior (distraction) displacement of the skull.
- The primary injury is ligamentous with disruption of the ligaments that provide structural support to the cervicocranial junction, namely the atlanto-occipital capsular ligaments, anterior and posterior atlanto-occipital membrane ligaments, paired lateral atlanto-occipital ligaments, the longitudinal component of the cruciate ligament, apical ligament, paired alar ligaments and tectorial membrane.
- Multiplanar capability and sensitivity to ligamentous injury render MRI the best imaging modality for the demonstration of the relationship between the basion/opisthion and the tip of the dens, between the occipital condyle and the superior facets of the atlas, and the disruption of the supporting ligaments. Also, commonly existing cord injuries are well demonstrated on MRI.

**Atlantoaxial disassociation**

- This disassociation can be either secondary to distraction with superior displacement of the atlas and skull or secondary to odontoid fractures with resultant anterior or posterior displacement of the atlas.
- The former is commonly associated with atlanto-occipital disassociation and is primarily the result of ligamentous disruption.

**Table 11.7** Classification of odontoid fractures

| Type | Description |
|---|---|
| I | Avulsion fracture of the tip of the dens |
| II | Transverse fracture of the dens above the body of C2 |
| III | Fracture of the superior body and the superior articulating facets of C2 |

After Anderson and D'Alonzo.

- Conversely, in odontoid fractures, the bony injury predominates. Generally, the mechanism of injury in odontoid fractures is not well understood although hyperflexion is suspected to represent a dominant component. These fractures are typed by Anderson and D'Alonzo based on the location of the fracture in the axis.
- Again, the disruption of the supporting ligaments, and the relationship of the atlas to the axis is well demonstrated on MRI.
- In addition, spinal cord injury and compression are best shown on MRI.
- With respect to odontoid fractures, MRI may often demonstrate the fracture lines and associated bone-marrow edema (especially when implementing fat-saturation techniques).
- However, high-resolution CT, plain film tomography, or Tc 99m methylene diphosphonate bone scan may be better than MRI for the detection of subtle cortically based fractures, e.g. type I.



## Hyperflexion injuries

- Flexion injury of the cervical spine results in the forward rotation or translation of the vertebra in the sagittal plane.
- This injury is caused by direct trauma to the head and neck in the flexed position or by forces that cause hyperflexion of the neutral cervical spine.
- There are several subtypes of flexion injuries with associated different degrees of cord injury and instability depending on the severity of the traumatic force and the position of the neck at the time of impact. The injury tends to be more severe if the cervical spine is flexed at the time of impact (Fig. 11.8).
- Anterior subluxation of the vertebral body, reversal of cervical lordosis, anterior narrowing and posterior widening of the intervening disk space, anterior displacement of the superior facets, and fanning of the spinous processes are common features of flexion injury. These are the result of disruption of the posterior ligament complex (inter- and supraspinous ligaments), the interlaminar ligaments, the facet capsules, the posterior longitudinal ligament, and the posterior portion of the annulus fibrosis.
- The degree of anterior displacement may be minimal (hyperflexion sprain) or obvious (bilateral interfacetal dislocation and tear-drop fracture).
- The clay shoveler's fracture and the simple wedge fracture tend to be stable.
- In contrast, the bilateral interfacetal dislocation and the tear-drop fracture are unstable fractures. The hyperflexion sprain result in delayed instability. Also, the bilateral interfacetal dislocation and the tear-drop fracture frequently result in cord injury and compression.

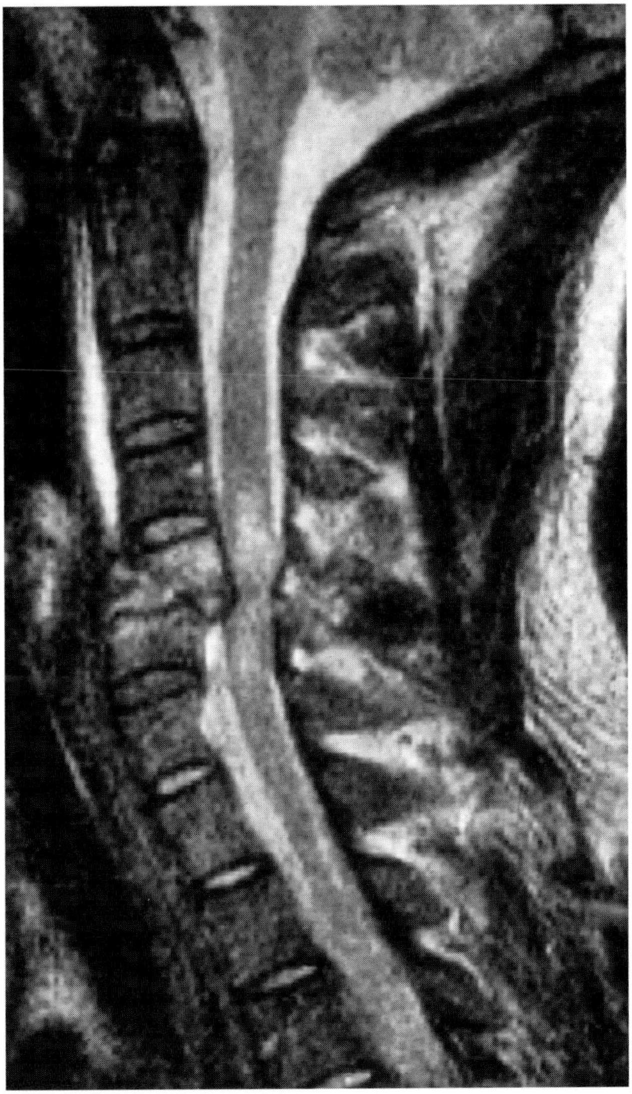

**Fig. 11.8** Sagittal $T_2$-weighted image following a diving hyperflexion injury shows a fracture of the anteroinferior corner of the C5 vertebral body (hyperflexion tear drop) with retropulsion of the remaining body of C5 to the spinal canal and cord. The image shows secondary cord hemorrhage.



- Most flexion injuries are well demonstrated on MRI. In addition to the demonstration of alignment abnormalities and fractures, MRI provides unique information regarding ligamentous injury, cord abnormalities and acute disk herniations commonly associated with hyperflexion injury.
- The importance of MRI is highlighted by its ability to differentiate between anterior subluxation due to chronic spondylotic changes and that due to hyperflexion sprain.
- In the acute setting, because of the questionable reliability of flexion/extension radiography, MRI becomes a valuable alternative capable of demonstrating posterior ligamentous injury and hence confirming the presence of hyperflexion sprain.

## Hyperextension injuries

- Extension injury of the cervical spine results in the backward rotation or translation of the vertebra in the sagittal plane. It is often the result of an anterior force impacting on the mandible, face or forehead, or it is due to a sudden decelaration.
- There are several subtypes of extension injuries with associated different degrees of cord injury and instability depending on the direction and magnitude of the hyperextensive force.
- The different subtypes can be further categorized into stable and unstable fractures.
- An avulsion fracture of the anterior arch of the atlas and extension tear-drop fracture are limited to the anterior column of the cervical spine.
- Conversely, an isolated fracture of the posterior arch of the atlas and laminar fractures are limited to the posterior column.
- This limited involvement renders these fractures relatively stable.
- On the other hand, in more severe types of hyperextension injuries – such as hangman's fracture, hyperextension/dislocation and hyperextension fracture/dislocation – at least two columns are disrupted with resultant instability.
- Hangman's fracture or C2 traumatic spondylolisthesis is a fracture involving the pars interarticularis or adjacent structures.
- This fracture is categorized into three types:
  - type 1 is defined as an isolated hairline fracture of the pars without displacement of the body or facets of C2
  - type 2 is defined as a fracture of the pars with anterior displacement of the body of C2
  - type 3 is defined as a fracture of the pars with anterior displacement of the body of C2 in a position of flexion and associated bilateral facet dislocation.
- It is felt by some investigators that type 3 hangman's fracture is not a pure hyperextension injury but rather results from a combination of hyperflexion followed by rebound hyperextension.
- A hyperextension/dislocation injury is a predominantly ligamentous injury resulting in distraction of the anterior column, buckling of the middle column (posterior longitudinal ligament) and transient posterior intervertebral dislocation, which is usually reduced immediately after impact.
- Plain radiographic findings can be subtle despite commonly associated serious neurologic deficits, and include prevertebral soft-tissue swelling, avulsion fracture arising from the inferior end-plate of the distracted vertebra, widening of the disk space and a vacuum disk.
- MRI plays a critical role in defining the type of spinal cord injury responsible for the neurologic deficit and extent of ligamentous injury, and identifying an associated acute compressive herniated disk.

## Vertical compression injuries

- Axial loading injury of the cervical spine result from forces transmitted through the skull and occipital condyles to a voluntarily straightened spine. This type of injury gives rise to the well-described Jefferson's fracture of the atlas and the bursting fracture in the lower cervical spine.
- Jefferson's fracture consists of simultaneous disruption of the anterior and posterior arches of C1 with or without disruption of the transverse atlantal ligament. Identification of transverse ligament disruption, with resultant atlantoaxial instability, is crucial in the evaluation of this injury.
- MRI, with its superior multiplanar capability and sensitivity to ligamentous injury, nicely demonstrates the lateral displacement of the lateral masses of C1 on the coronal images, the increase in the atlantodental interval on the sagittal images, and disruption of the transverse ligament on the axial images.
- As the vertical force is transmitted to the lower cervical spine, it is dissipated by compression of the intervertebral disk. The build up of pressure within the disk results in either an acute herniated disk or a comminuted fracture in the adjacent vertebral body with associated retropulsion of the posterior body fragments (bursting fracture). In either case, MRI plays an important role in defining the relationship of the herniated disk or retropulsed fragment to the spinal cord and in demonstrating cord injury (Table 11.7).

## Management

### Non-surgical

- Immobilization, hard collar, soft collar, etc.
- Intravenous steroids are employed in patients with cord edema in whom an antiinflammatory effect may improve neurologic function. The impact of steroids on cord hemorrhage is thought to be negligible.

### Surgical

- Surgical spinal canal decompression is undertaken in patients with neurologic symptoms in whom decompression may conceivably lead to improvement in function within 24 hours of injury.

# Intervertebral disk degeneration and herniation

## Anatomy

- The intervertebral disk functions as a shock absorber to cushion the impaction forces imposed by weight bearing. Composed predominantly of water and polysaccharide, the intervertebral disk is composed of a central nucleus pulposus surrounded by the outer annulus fibrosus.
- Water within the intervertebral disk accounts for $T_1$ signal hypointensity and $T_2$ signal hyperintensity at MRI in healthy subjects.
- In adulthood, as disk degeneration develops (which is thought to be related to biomechanical trauma and changes in vascular supply through lumbar arteries), the disk loses water resulting in loss of $T_2$ signal hyperintensity.
- Loss of water and mucopolysaccharide content in maturity results in morphologic changes, loss of height and annular bulging of the disk.

## Disk degeneration

- The precursor to disk degeneration is thought to be tearing of the outer annular fibers either anteriorly, laterally or posteriorly.
- Annular tears are conspicuous on heavily $T_2$-weighted scans as foci of hyperintensity (high-intensity zones or HIZs) secondary to the presence of edema and granulation tissue (Fig. 11.9).



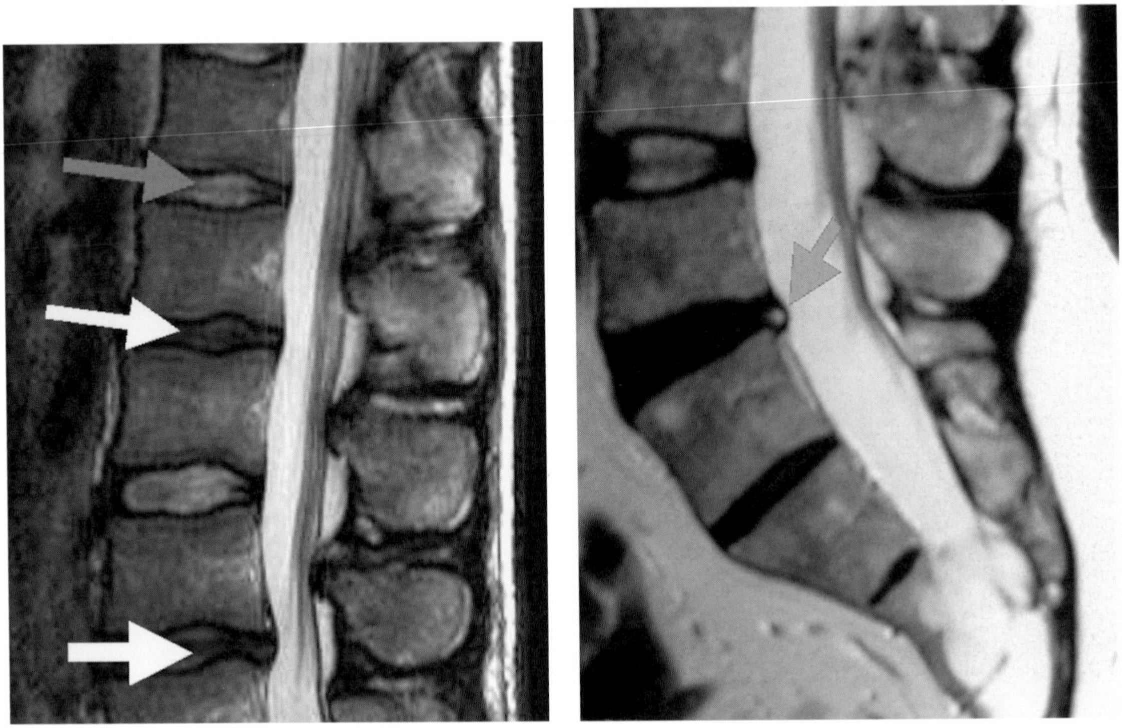

(a) (b)

**Fig. 11.9** **(a)** Sagittal $T_2$-weighted image showing signal hyperintensity within a healthy hydrated disk (red arrow) with loss of signal due to loss of water in early disk degeneration, progressing to mild disk bulging (lowest disk). **(b)** This image shows a focal high-intensity zone at the site of an annular tear.

- Nerve endings are known to exit in the periphery of the annulus and may be irritated by a tear accounting for a documented correlation between HIZs and low back pain.
- Somatic fibers of the recurrent meningeal nerve of Luschka supply fibers of the posterior longitudinal ligament, the meninges, blood vessels, posterior outer fibers of the annulus and the vertebral body periosteum.
- As tears extend, morphology of the disk in the sagittal and axial planes is lost, with loss of height and bulging (Figs 11.10 and 11.11).

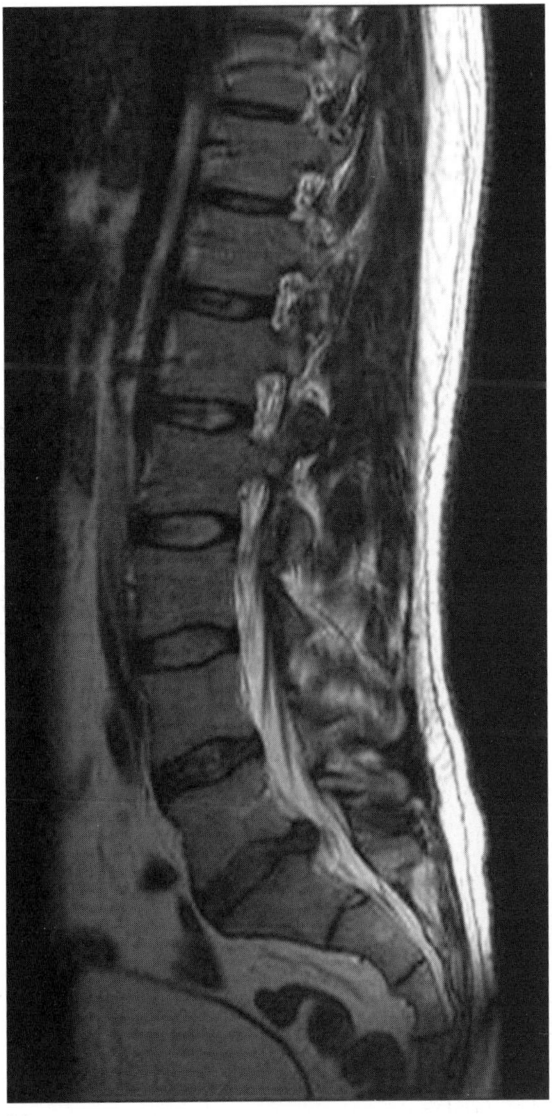

(a)

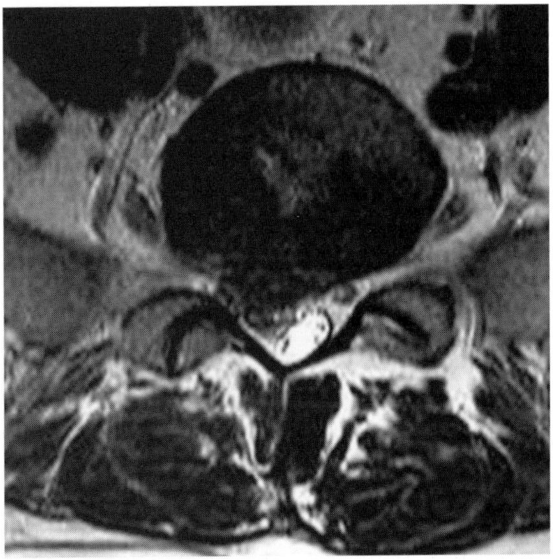

(b)

**Fig. 11.10** (**a**) Sagittal MR image showing a disk protrusion at L5–S1. (**b**) Axial image at this level showing disk protrusion to the right lateral recess where there is compression of the exiting right S1 nerve root.

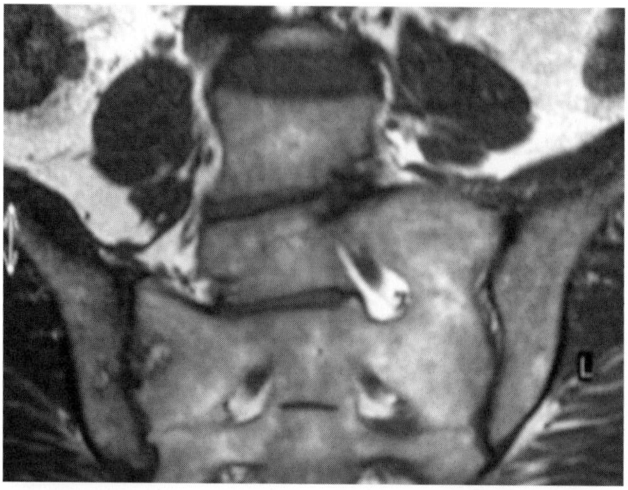

(a)

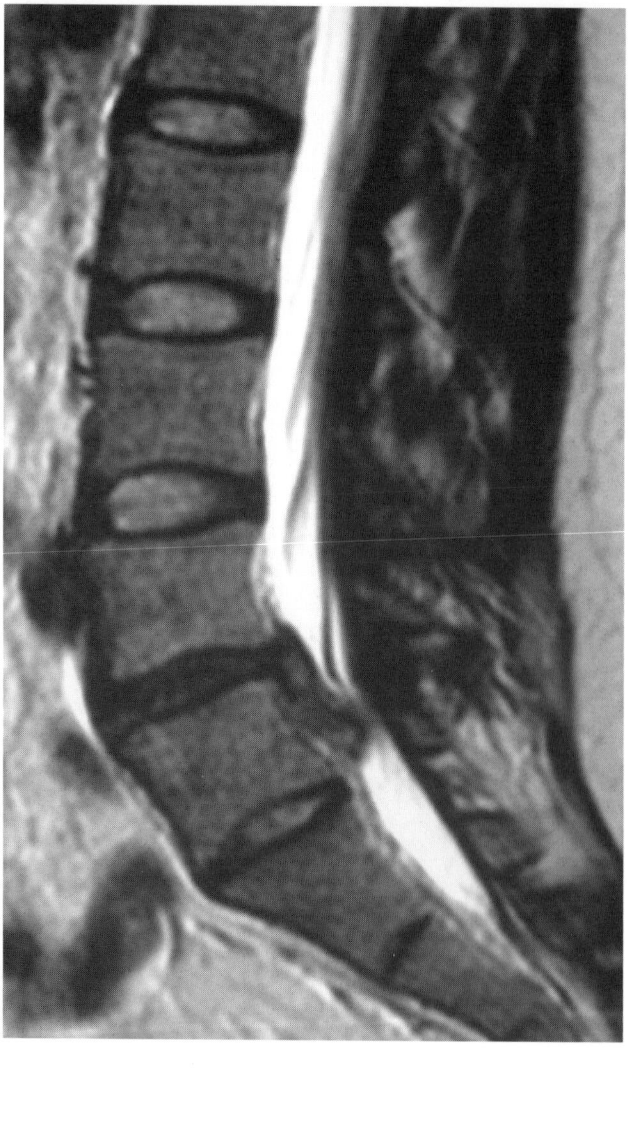

(b)

**Fig. 11.11** Coronal $T_1$-weighted image shows fusion between the transverse process of L5 and the sacral ala with acquired premature disk disease and protrusion at the L4–5 disk space. Segmental fusion leads to increased motion at L4–5 with secondary early acquired disk degeneration at this level.

- As annular fibers are stretched, traction effects promote the development of osteophytes at the insertion of the outer annular Sharpey's fibers.
- Using MRI, signal abnormalities are noted in the marrow immediately adjacent to the vertebral body end-plate adjacent to the degenerating disk, preceding radiographic evidence of end-plate sclerosis.
- Early in discogenic degeneration (type 1 change) marrow is characterized by end-plate $T_1$ signal hypointensity and with $T_2$ signal hyperintensity.
- In chronicity (type 2 change), marrow adjacent to the end-plate appears to become fatty with $T_1$ signal hyperintensity and persistent although slightly less marked $T_2$ signal hyperintensity.
- In end-stage disease, marrow becomes replaced by dense bone, obvious on radiographs, and hypointense on both $T_1$- and $T_2$-weighted scans at MRI.
- Modic marrow changes:
  - type 1: blood like; $T_1$ dark; $T_2$ bright; enhance with gadolinium (Gd)
  - type 2: fat like; $T_1$ bright; $T_2$ bright; enhance with Gd
  - type 3: fibrous; $T_1$ and $T_2$ dark; no enhancement.

## Disk bulging

- As the disk degenerates, annular tears, either posterolateral or in the midline allow herniation of central content (the nucleus pulposus).
- Loss of water content accounts for the development of signal hypointensity at MRI within the disk on $T_2$-weighted scans.
- Loss of both water and mucopolysaccharide from the disk promotes diffuse disk bulging.
- Superimposed discrete annular tears result in focal extension of the central nucleus pulposus through the defect; this is disk protrusion.
- Disruption of the outer fibers of the annulus (Sharpey's fibers) allows disk extrusion.
- When extrusion is followed by fragment migration at, above or below the disk level, the term disk sequestration is applied (Table 11.8).
- Virtually all lumbar and thoracic disk herniations are associated with loss of $T_2$ signal (disk degeneration). Nevertheless, only a minority of degenerating disks progress to protrusion or extrusion.
- The hallmark feature of a herniated disk is a focal contour abnormality (contiguous with the intervertebral portion of the disk by a narrow waist) along the posterior disk margin with a soft-tissue mass displacing epidural fat, nerve root, epidural veins or thecal sac.
- Loss in vertebral disk height secondary to degeneration may lead to abnormal facet joint motion with both secondary osteoarthritis and compensatory hypertrophy of the ligamentum flavum (an attempt to resist abnormal motion).

**Table 11.8** The reasons for the four types of disk problem

| Disk problem | Reason |
|---|---|
| Bulging | Loss of water and polysaccharide |
| Protrusion | Herniation of nucleus through an annular tear |
| Extrusion | Herniation beyond disrupted Sharpey's fibers |
| Sequestration | Migration of disk fragment at, above or below level |

- The combination of hypertrophic change at the facet joint, ligamentous hypertrophy and disk prolapse may lead to marked central canal stenosis (AP diameter of less than 11.5 mm and area less than 1.5 cm).
- In patients with congenital 'short pedicles', the effect of these changes is magnified.
- Asymmetric facet overgrowth (particularly of the superior facet) leads to osseous encroachment of the lateral recesses, and foramina with compression of lateral nerve roots (foraminal stenosis, which is defined as a distance of less than 4 mm between the superior facet and the vertebral body) (Fig. 11.12).

## History and clinical findings

- Back pain and early morning stiffness. Back pain exaggerated by coughing suggests an annular tear with disk prolapse. Also radicular pain.
- Local discomfort exacerbated by palpation. Straight leg raise test is positive (Fig. 11.2).

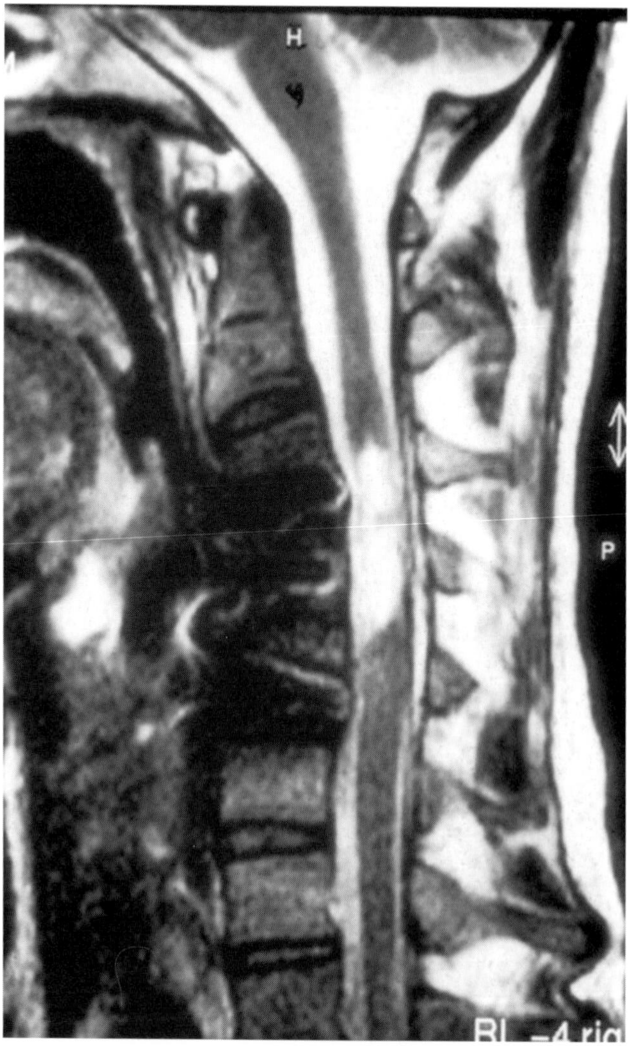


**Fig. 11.12** Sagittal $T_2$-weighted image showing persistent cord hemorrhage in a patient following plate and screw stabilization of the C3–5 segment.

## Imaging findings

Radiography

- AP, lateral, oblique radiographs.

Diskography

- Contrast injection to the interverterbal disk to provoke discogenic back pain. Undertaken to absolutely confirm that symptoms relate to a particular disk prior to surgery. Rarely undertaken as MRI allows non-invasive assessment.

Lumbar myelography

- Contrast injection to the thecal sac to identify contrast filling of the exiting nerve root sheaths. Extrinsic compression of the nerve root sheath by a disk bulge impairs nerve sheath filling. Infrequently undertaken with the advent of MRI.

Facet arthrography

- Contrast injection to facet joints usually undertaken for anatomic localization prior to steroid bupivacaine hydrochloride injection (Fig. 11.13).

Epidural nerve root block

- The injection of steroid bupivacaine hydrochloride to the fat space surrounding the exiting nerve roots. This is undertaken both as a diagnostic maneuver and to a greater extent as part of therapy (Fig. 11.14).

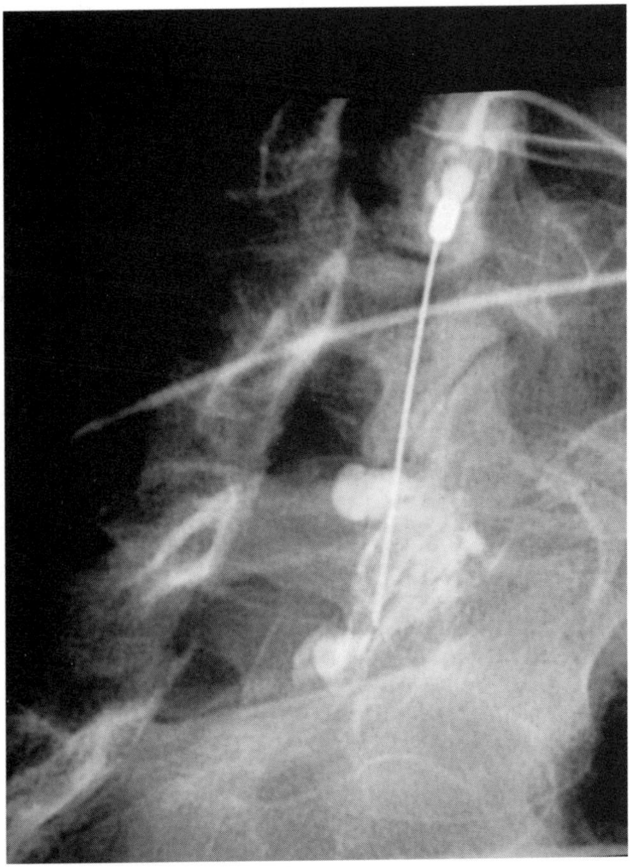

**Fig. 11.13** Facet arthrogram showing contrast injection to the facet joint revealing the characteristic S-shaped configuration prior to steroid bupivacaine hydrochloride injection.

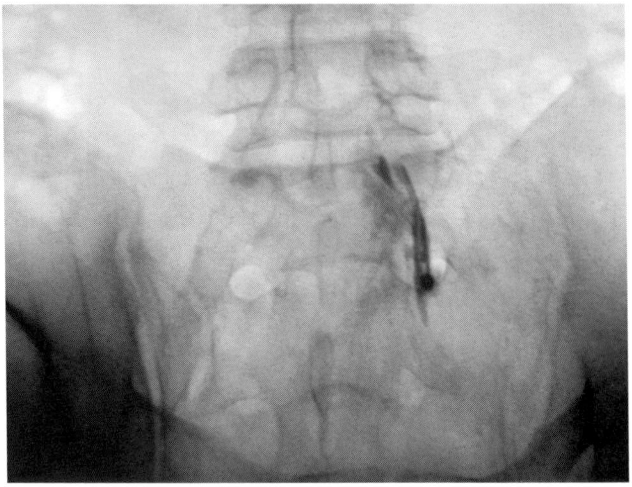

**Fig. 11.14** Contrast outlines the exiting S1 nerve root (linear filling defect) following contrast injection to the epidural space prior to steroid bupivacaine hydrochloride injection in a selective S1 epidural nerve root block.

## Caudal epidural

- Injection of steroid in a non-selective manner to the epidural space employed as a therapeutic maneuver.

## Magnetic resonance imaging

- Discussed above (Fig. 11.15).



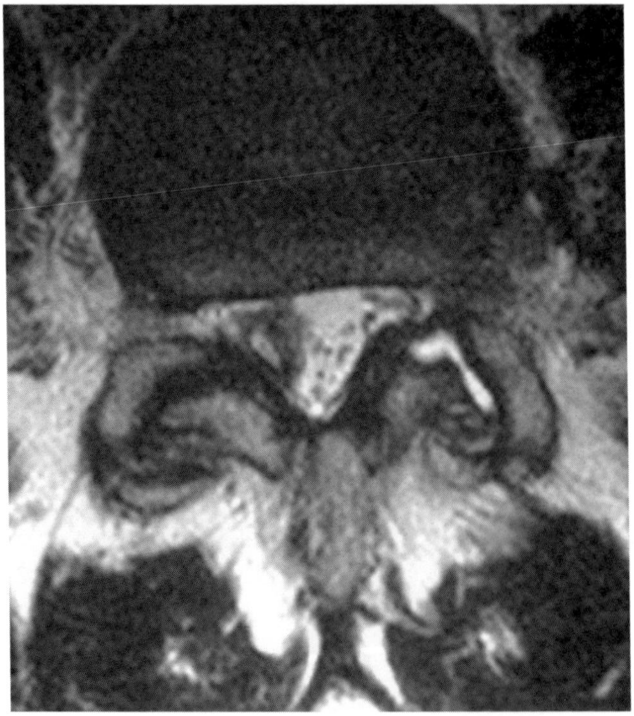

**Fig. 11.15** Axial $T_2$-weighted MR image showing hypertrophic degenerative change within the facet joints bilaterally, narrowed on the left, widened on the right.

**Box 11.1 Back pain differential**

- Discogenic back pain: back pain due to tear of outer annular fibers
- Radicular back pain: back pain due to nerve root compression by disk bulge
- Facet disease back pain: back pain due to facet joint degenerative arthritis
- Modic marrow back pain: back pain secondary to end-plate bony impaction

### Electromyography

- See Chapter 2

## Management

### Non-surgical

- Weight reduction.
- Lifestyle changes, e.g. avoid lifting heavy objects.
- Physiotherapy.
- Analgesia/antiinflammatories (see Chapter 3).
- Oral steroids.
- Epidural steroid.
- Selective nerve root block.
- Facet joint steroid bupivacaine hydrochloride injection.

### Surgical

- Microdiskectomy: shaving the disk bulge via a hemilaminotomy (Figs 11.16 and 11.17).
- Diskectomy: undertaken in conjunction with verterbral body fusion now with disk replacement via an intervertebral body prosthesis.
- Spinal fusion: undertaken in patients with pseudoarthrosis secondary to chronic end-stage disk disease.
- Posterior decompression: laminectomy undertaken in patients with spinal stenosis.



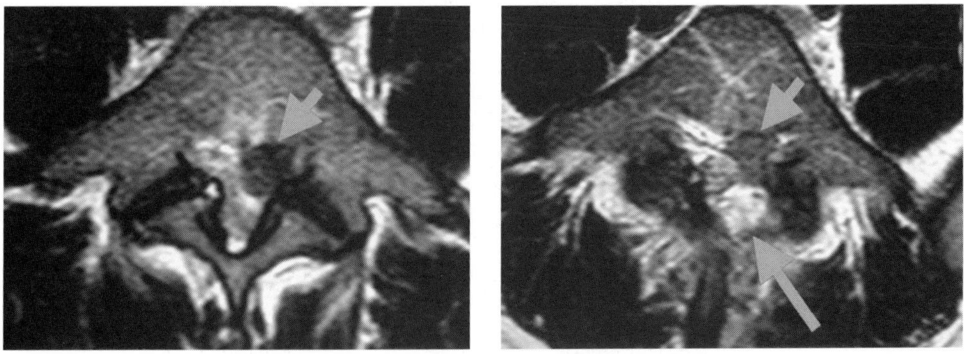

(a) (b)

**Fig. 11.16** **(a)** A disk protrusion to the left lateral recess compressing the left L4 nerve root in a patient with left radiculopathy. **(b)** Post surgery with left laminectomy, showing compression of the thecal sac as the laminectomy defect is packed by fat, in the same patient with post operative right radiculopathy.

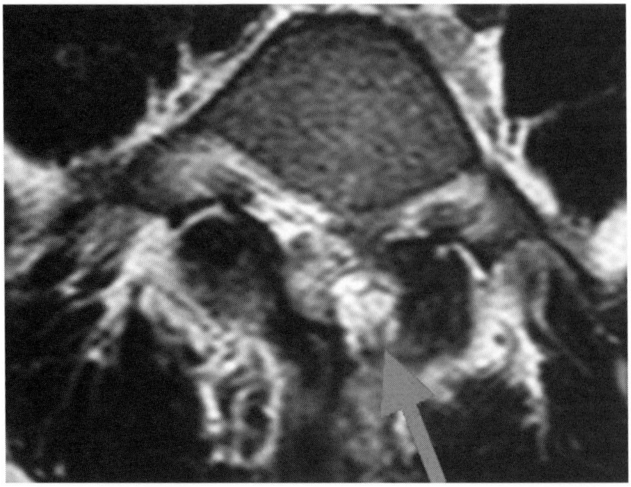

(a)

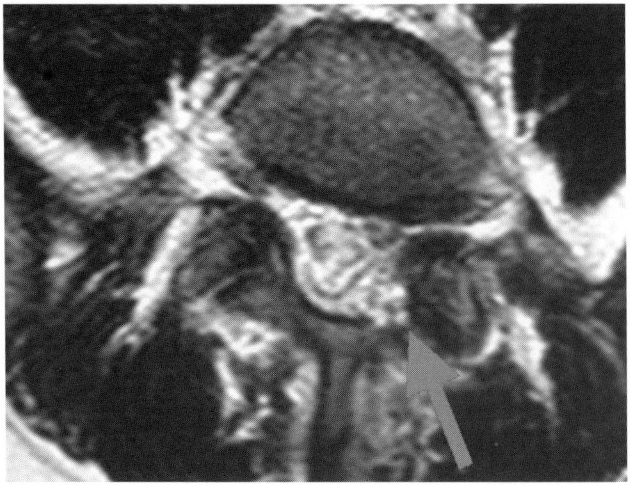

(b)

**Fig. 11.17** (**a**) Image showing fat in the laminectomy defect in a patient with postoperative right radiculopathy. (**b**) Image showing restoration of thecal sac dimension following removal of the excess fat, with ultimate resolution of symptoms.

# Spondylolisthesis and spondylolysis

- Spondylolysis is the term used to describe an abnormality of the spine in which a defect or cleft is found in the pars interarticularis (Figs 11.18 and 11.19).

## Mechanism of injury

- Although the etiology of spondylolysis is unclear, most believe it results from repeated trauma during adolescence and that it represents a form of stress fracture.
- Rapid growth during adolescence in conjunction with weight gain places significant stress on the lower lumbar spine, maximally at L5. Repeated flexion/extension leads to the development of microtrauma with disruption of internal trabeculae, which progresses to disruption of the cortex and the development of a true fracture or lysis.
- Spondylolysis is not identified in children with neuromuscular diseases who never walk.
- Although spondylolysis is occasionally identified following local isolated macrotrauma, this is extremely uncommon.
- Reflecting onset in childhood, the recorded prevalence of between 3% and 10% is noted to be the same in both children and adults.
- Although any vertebra can be involved, the L5 posterior element is involved in up to 95% of cases; bilateral involvement occurs in 90%.

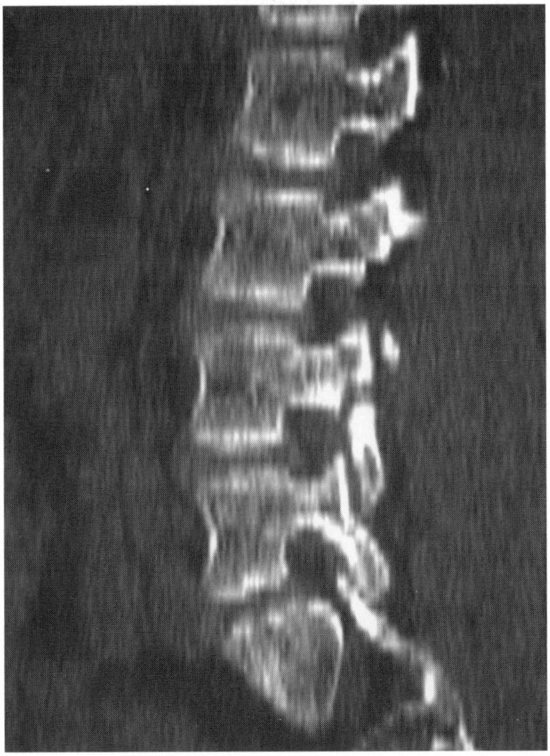

(a)

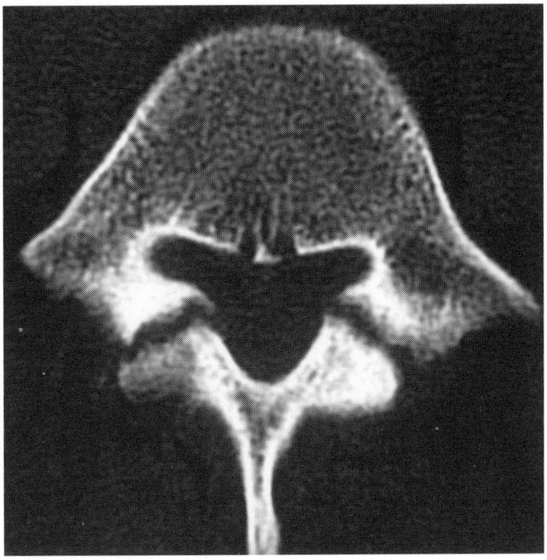

(b)

**Fig. 11.18** Sagittal reformatted CT image showing a spondylolysis of the L4 pars, identified on both sides in the axial image.

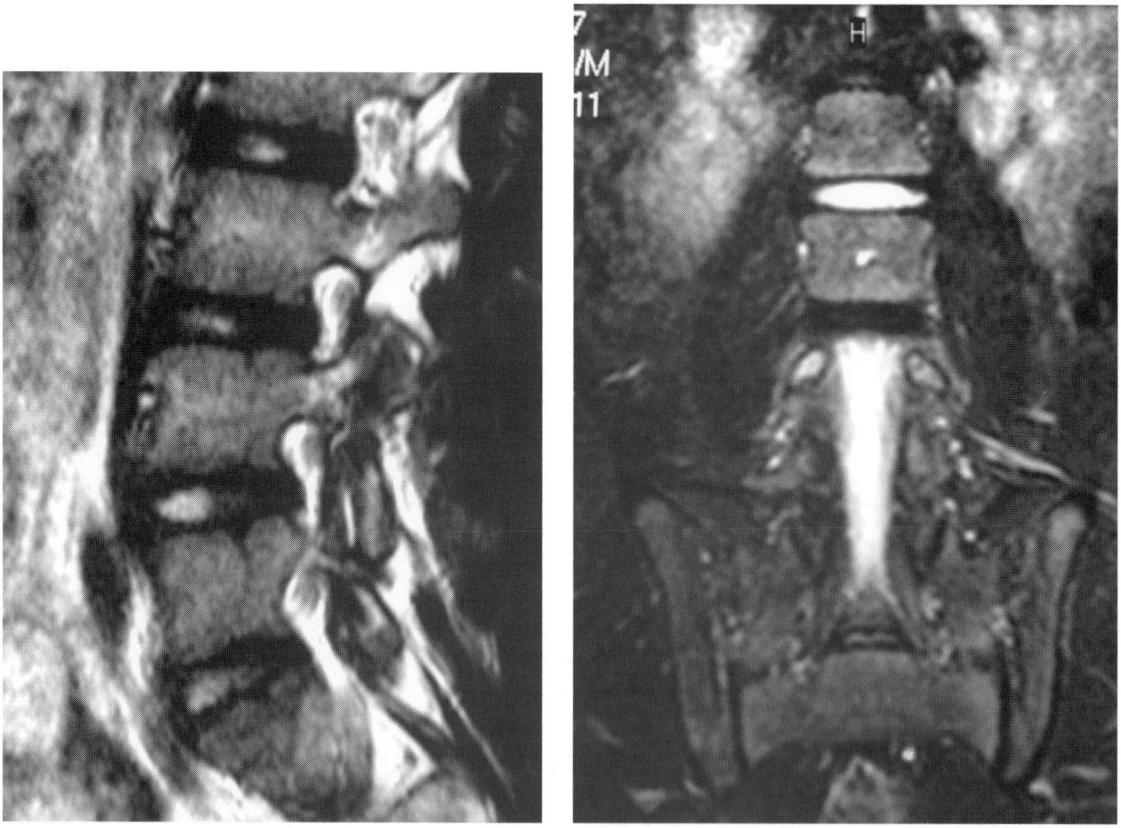

(a) (b)



**Fig. 11.19** (**a**) Sagittal $T_2$-weighted image showing a vertical spondylolysis of L4, (**b**) with bone edema in the right L4 pars on the fat-suppressed image indicating recent fracture.

## History and clinical findings

- In affected individuals, up to 75% of patients remain asymptomatic.
- Almost 25% of patients develop chronic back pain, usually secondary to complicating facet disease, nerve entrapment or spondylolisthesis.
- Spondylolisthesis is the term used to describe a forward slip of an upper vertebral body on a lower vertebral body (in contrast to backward slippage described as retrolisthesis).
- The degree of slippage is graded 1–4:
  - grade 1 represents a slip of 0–25%
  - grade 2 represents a slip of 25–50%
  - grade 3 represents a slip of 50–75%
  - grade 4 represents a slip of more than 75%.
- Although spondylolisthesis is most commonly secondary to spondylolysis, it is also commonly identified in the elderly secondary to facet joint disease and rarely secondary to a structural deficiency in the vertebral body.
- Although unexplained, only 50% of patients with spondylolysis develop spondylolisthesis, of whom only half become symptomatic.

- Pathria has previously demonstrated that almost 70% of patients over 40 years old have evidence of significant facet joint osteoarthritis at CT.
- According to Pathria, facet disease is graded 0–3:
  - grade 1 is mild osteoarthritis
  - grade 2 is moderate osteoarthritis
  - grade 3 is severe osteoarthritis.
- In contrast to spondylolysis, spondylolisthesis complicating facet disease is most commonly identified at the L4–5 level.
- Adolescents presenting with back pain usually have it more marked to the affected side. Episodes of back pain usually resolve over 7–10 days. There are usually no radicular symptoms.
- Focal discomfort may be produced by deep palpation at the affected level.

## Imaging findings

### Radiography

- Oblique views may show an established spondylolysis.

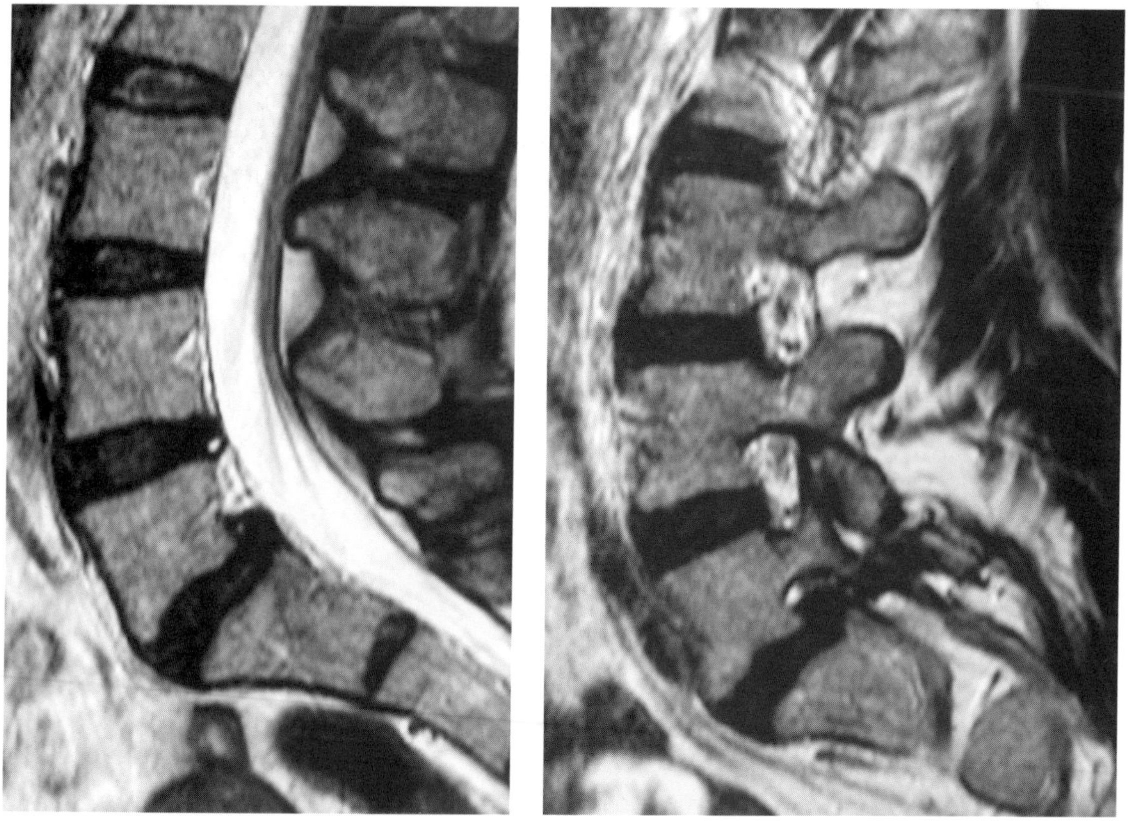

(a) (b)

**Fig. 11.20** (**a**) Sagittal $T_2$-weighted image showing anterior listhesis of L5 on S1 with associated L5–S1 disk disease. (**b**) In the same patient as in (a), a far lateral image showing disk protrusion to the exit foramen with compression of the exiting L5 nerve root, the so-called foraminal encroachment sign.

| | |
|---|---|
| Scintigraphy | • A bone scan will show a concentration of radiotracer at the site of the fracture or lysis. |
| Multislice computerized tomography | • Sagittal reformatted images allow the optimum visualization of the lysis or stress fracture. |
| Magnetic resonance imaging | • Sagittal images show spondylolysis occasionally before becoming radiographically apparent even at CT. Stress-induced marrow changes or bruising may precede the development of lysis (Fig. 11.20). |

## Management

| | |
|---|---|
| Non-surgical | • Weight reduction.<br>• Rest.<br>• Core stability; physiotherapy.<br>• Antiinflammatories.<br>• Targeted steroid bupivacaine hydrochloride to the spondylolysis, injected with fluoroscopic guidance. |
| Surgical | • Undisplaced spondylolysis fails to heal as a result of motion at the lysis margins with lumbar flexion extension. Healing could theoretically occur if affected patients were completely immobilized by body bracing or prolonged bed rest. However, this is somewhat impractical. Undisplaced spondylolysis may be fixed surgically with immobilizing screw fixation localized with C arm guidance. |

# Infection

## Mechanism

- Spinal infection is generally a sequel to hematogenous spread, either arterial or venous, and rarely complicates medical intervention.
- Reflecting vascularity, infection in childhood is frequently confined to the vascular disk. In adulthood, infection is initially to vascular red marrow adjacent to the anterior margin of the end-plate, with disk infection complicating local osteomyelitis.
- Occasionally infection spares the disk and spreads via the anterior subligamentous space, particularly in tuberculous or fungal infections.
- Staphylococcus infection accounts for up to 60% of cases, even in immunocompromised patients.
- In contrast, isolated posterior element infection is invariably secondary to tuberculosis.

## History

- Progressive back pain.
- Fever.
- General debility.
- Radiculopathy (occasionally).
- Psoas spread may lead to groin pain in the femoral nerve distribution.

## Imaging findings

### Radiography

- Shows the disk space narrowing and with erosion.

### Computerized tomography

- CT scan may show a paraspinal collection.



### Scintigraphy

- A bone scan will show a concentration of radiotracer at the level of the infection secondary to induced osteoblastic activity.

### Magnetic resonance imaging

- MRI with contrast is the optimum diagnostic test as it allows the identification of fluid within the disk space and whether or not there is extension of infection to the epidural space or paraspinal soft tissues (Fig. 11.21).

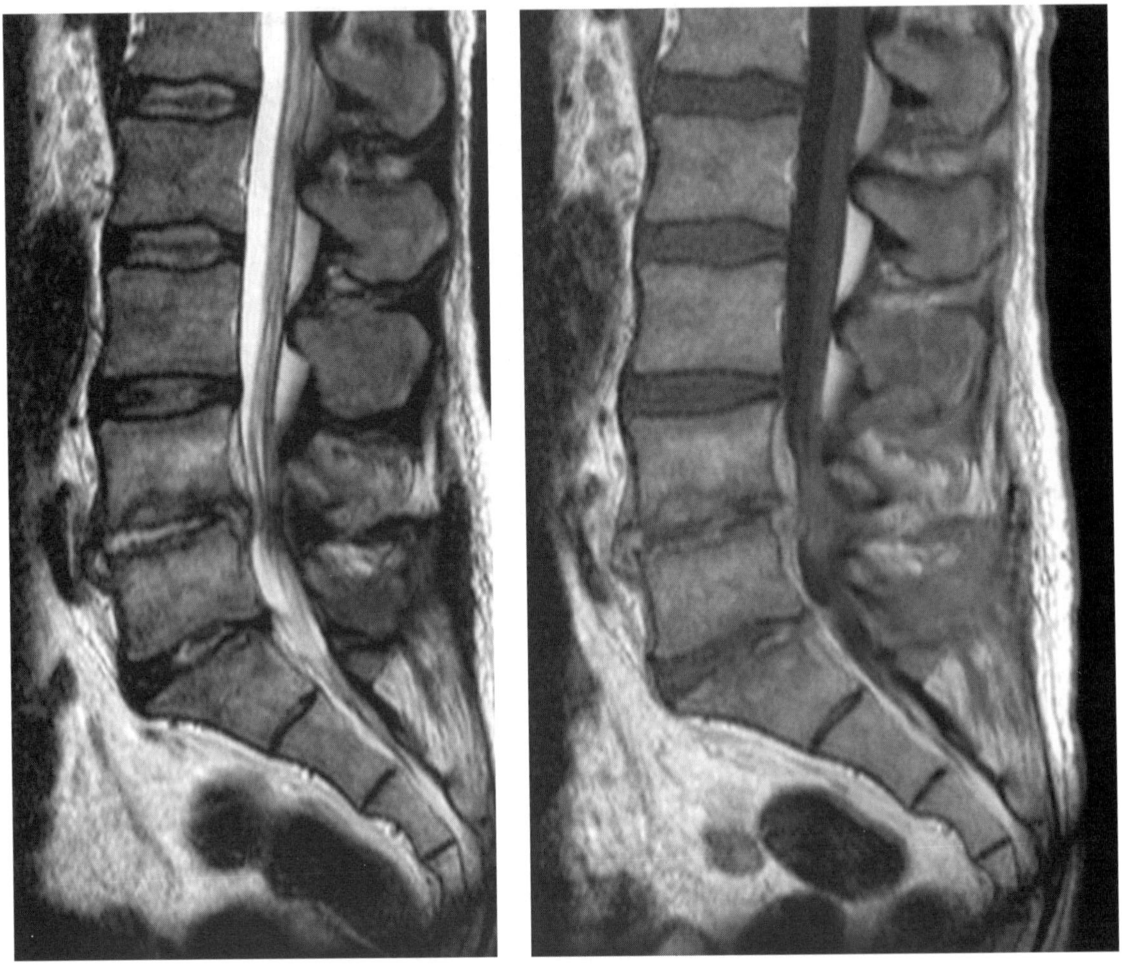

(a) (b)

**Fig. 11.21** (**a**) Sagittal $T_2$-weighted image showing active diskitis at the L4–5 disk space where there is disk space pus and fluid (**b**) with enhancement of inflammatory debris following the administration of Gd.



## Management

### Non-surgical

- Blood cultures.
- Disk space aspiration will allow culture and sensitivity. Disk space aspiration is invariably unproductive once i.v. antibiotic therapy has been commenced.
- Antibiotic therapy.
- Analgesia.
- Paraspinal collections are catheter drained following radiologic placement (Figs 11.22, 11.23).
- Epidural collections, if producing neurologic compromise, require surgical drainage.

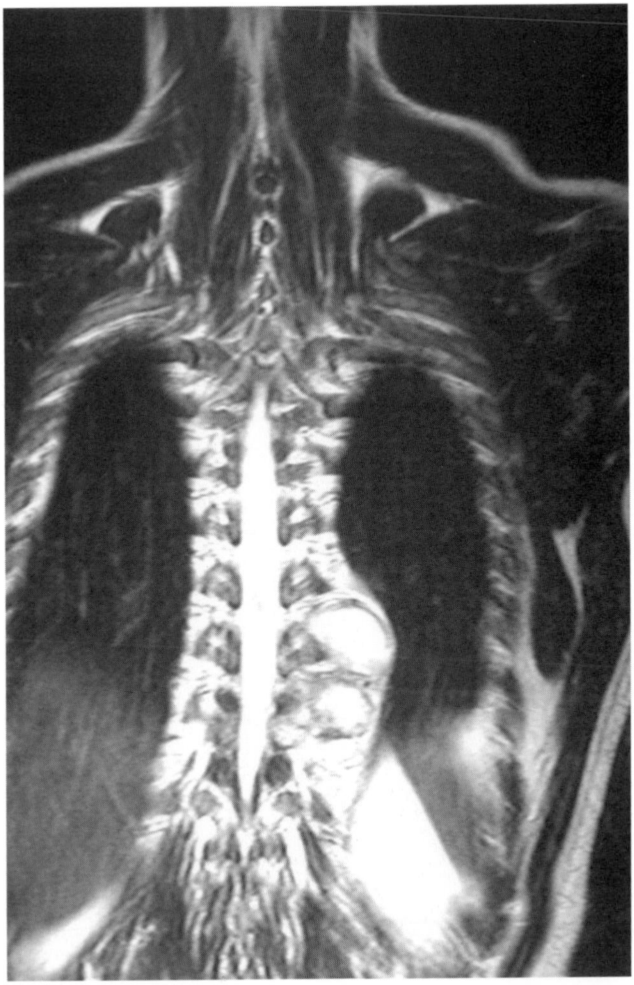

**Fig. 11.22** Coronal $T_2$-weighted image showing loculated paraspinal fluid in a patient with tuberculous infection.

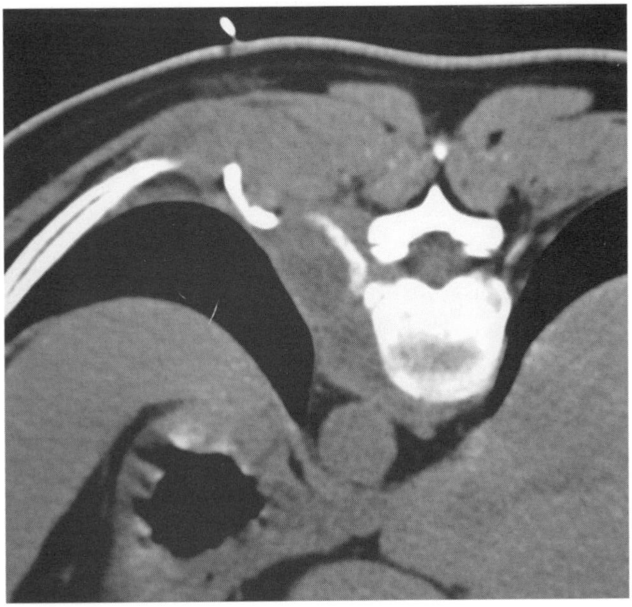

**Fig. 11.23** CT-guided catheter drainage of paraspinal tuberculous abscess.

# Dorsolumbar fracture

## Predisposing factors in thoracolumbar junction fractures

- Approximately 90% of thoracic and lumbar vertebral body fractures occur at the thoracolumbar junction between T11 and L4.
- Fractures occur at this site because:
  - it is the junction of two opposing spinal curvatures: the dorsal kyphosis and the lumbar lordosis
  - of a loss of the stabilizing effect of the bony and soft-tissue thoracic cage
  - at this point there is change in the orientation of the articular facets from the thoracic coronal to the lumbar sagittal planes (Fig. 11.24).
- Injuries involving the vertebral body are considered to be major injuries.

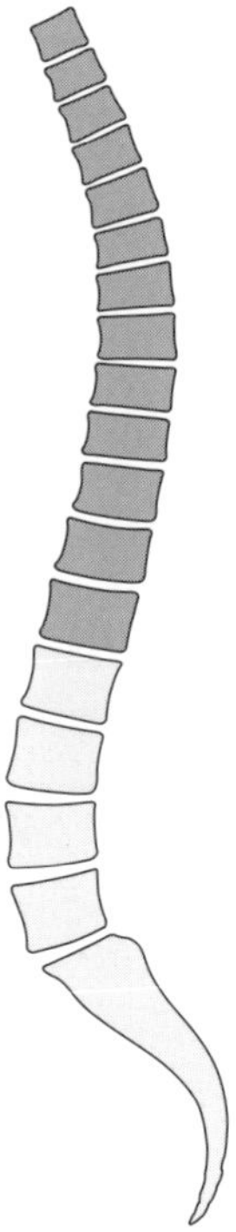

**Fig. 11.24** Diagram of the junction between the fixed dorsal spine and the flexible lumbar spine, which accounts for the high incidence of fractures at this site.

- Injuries involving the posterior elements (the transverse processes, the pars interarticularis and the spinous processes) are considered to be minor injuries. Minor injuries, tend to be stable, not associated with neurologic compromise and do not produce progressive deformity.
- Major injuries of the vertebral body may be secondary to anterior wedging (compression fractures), axial loading (burst fractures) or acute hyperflexion (seat-belt fractures) with or without rotation.
- Denis and Ferguson divide the spine into three columns:
  - the anterior column incorporates the anterior longitudinal ligament, the anterior two-thirds of the vertebral body and the anterior two-thirds of the annulus fibrosis and disk. (It is the site of wedge or compression fractures.) (Fig. 11.25)
  - the middle column incorporates the posterior third of the vertebral body, the posterior third of the annulus fibrosis and disk, and the posterior longitudinal ligament. (Both the anterior and middle columns are involved in burst fractures.) (Fig. 11.26)
  - the posterior column incorporates the posterior bony elements (pedicles, articular processess, and the lamina and spinous processes) and the posterior ligamentous complex (ligamentum flavum and the interspinous and supraspinous ligaments). (The middle and posterior columns are involved in lap seat-belt injuries.) (Fig. 11.27)
- All three columns are disrupted in fracture dislocations where rotation is typically superimposed on hyperflexion and distraction forces (Box 11.2).



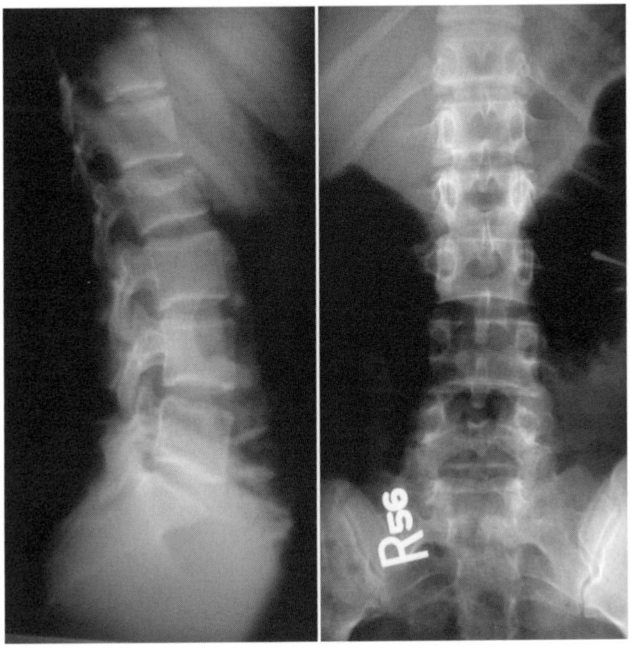


**Fig. 11.25** Lateral radiograph showing superior end-plate wedge compression fracture at L2.

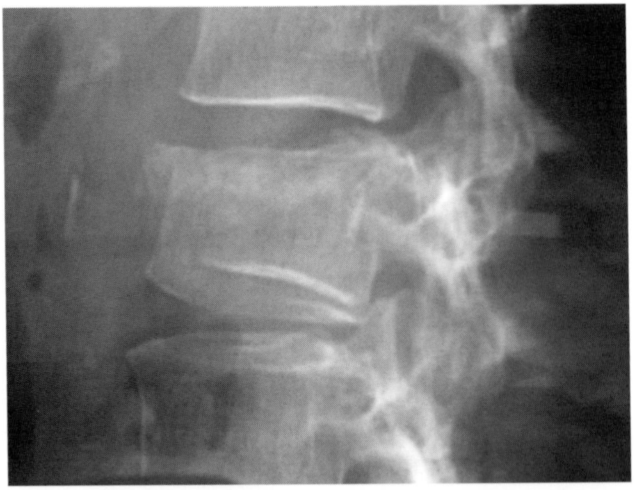

**Fig. 11.26** Burst fracture of L2 with posterior bowing and disruption of the anterior and posterior walls of the vertebral body.

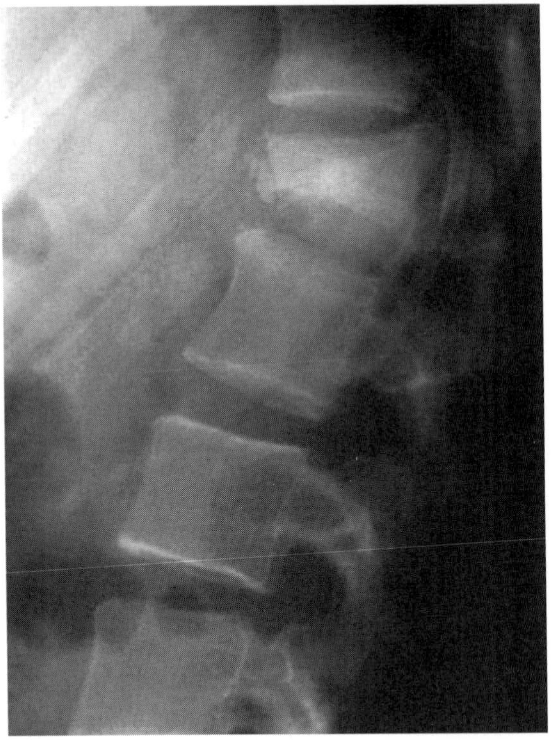

(a)

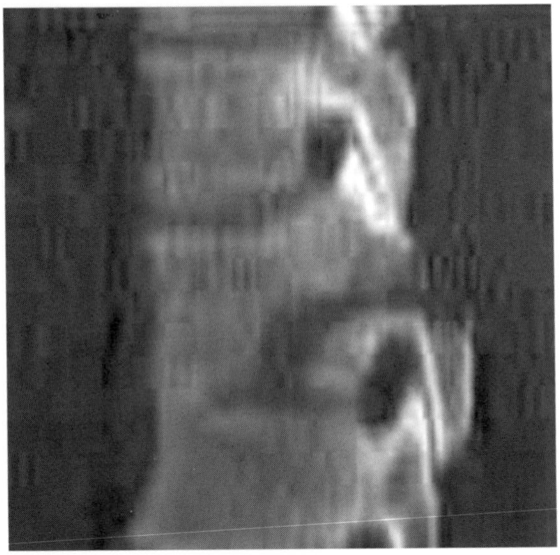

(b)

**Fig. 11.27** Lateral image showing a fracture of L2 extending through the anterior and posterior vertebral walls to the posterior element; this is the so-called seat-belt fracture.



**Box 11.2 Three-column classification of dorsolumbar spine fractures**

- Anterior column: wedge compression fractures
- Anterior and middle columns: burst fractures
- Middle and posterior columns: lap seat-belt fractures
- Three columns: fracture dislocations

# Wedge compression fractures

- Secondary to trauma or more frequently secondary to vertebral body softening in osteoporosis.
- Wedge compression fractures follow acute hyperflexion with impaction, accounting for almost 50% of dorsolumbar fractures.
- Mechanical failure of vertically oriented trabeculae within the cancellous bone of the vertebral body, particularly of the anterior column, results in vertebral body wedging with mechanical compression of the superior end-plate, which may become comminuted in the presence of bony demineralization.
- Being confined to the anterior column, sparing the middle and posterior columns, wedge compression fractures are generally stable. Instability is conferred by the loss of more than 50% of the anterior vertebral body height or compressions at multiple levels.

## History

- There will be history of an acute event or, in the presence of osteoporosis, a history of back pain often without a recognizable event.

## Imaging findings

### Radiograghy

- Allows the clear identification of fractures. Differentiation of wedge and burst fractures requires CT guidance.

### Scinitgraphy

- A bone scan shows concentration of radiotracer at the site of the injury.

### Computerized tomography

- Wedge fractures are poorly visualized in the axial plane at CT as the fracture lines are almost parallel to the imaging plane. This is the 'in-plane' fracture phenomenon. Sagittal reformatted images are valuable in patient assessment.

### Magnetic resonance imaging

- Sagittal images clearly allow the identification of the fracture.

## Management

### Non-surgical

- Management is usually conservative (non-surgical). Persistent weight bearing and activity in an unrecognized acute wedge may result in progressive compression with the development of instability.
- In the presence of severe wedging, MRI may be undertaken in order to differentiate an acute stable wedge fracture from an unstable two-column burst fracture (Fig. 11.28).

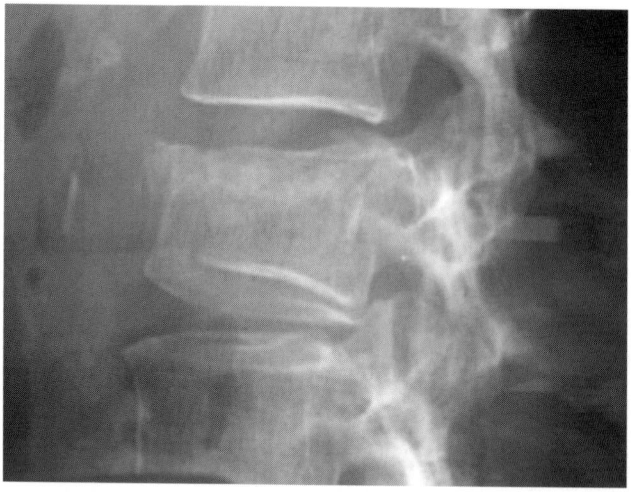

**Fig. 11.28** Radiograph showing an osteoporotic wedge fracture of L4.

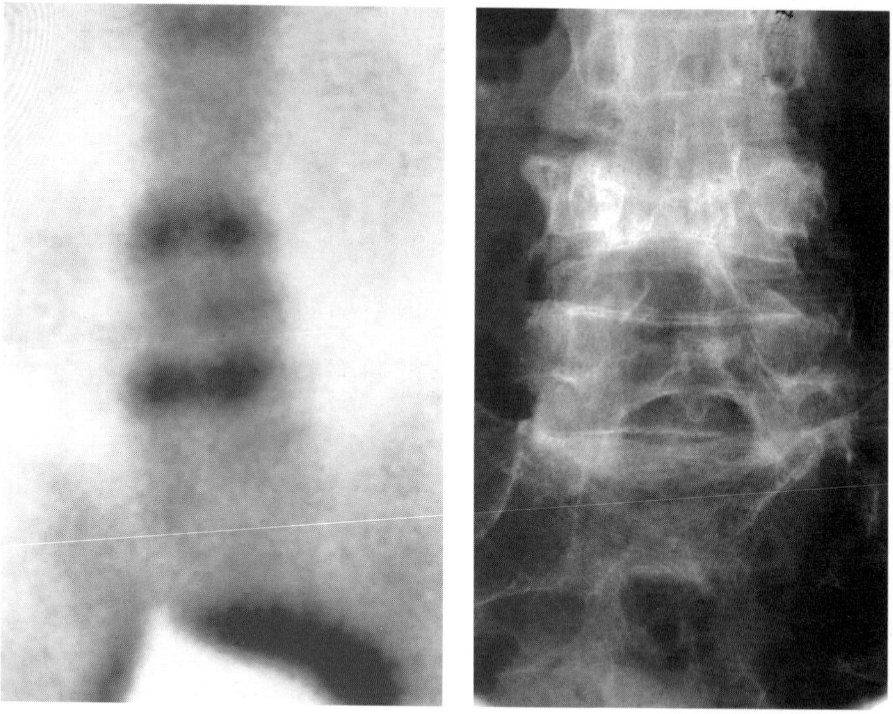

(a) (b)

**Fig. 11.29** Isotope bone scan showing the concentration of radiotracer at (**a**) L2 and (**b**) L4 secondary to active recent osteoporotic compression fractures.



- Vertebroplasty: percutaneous cement injection is undertaken in patients with painful osteoporotic compression fractures. Although not reducing the fracture, cement placement produces marked reduction in symptoms almost immediately following placement (Figs 11.29 and 11.30).

## Surgical

- Surgical stabilization with a pedicle screw and rods is undertaken in unstable fractures.

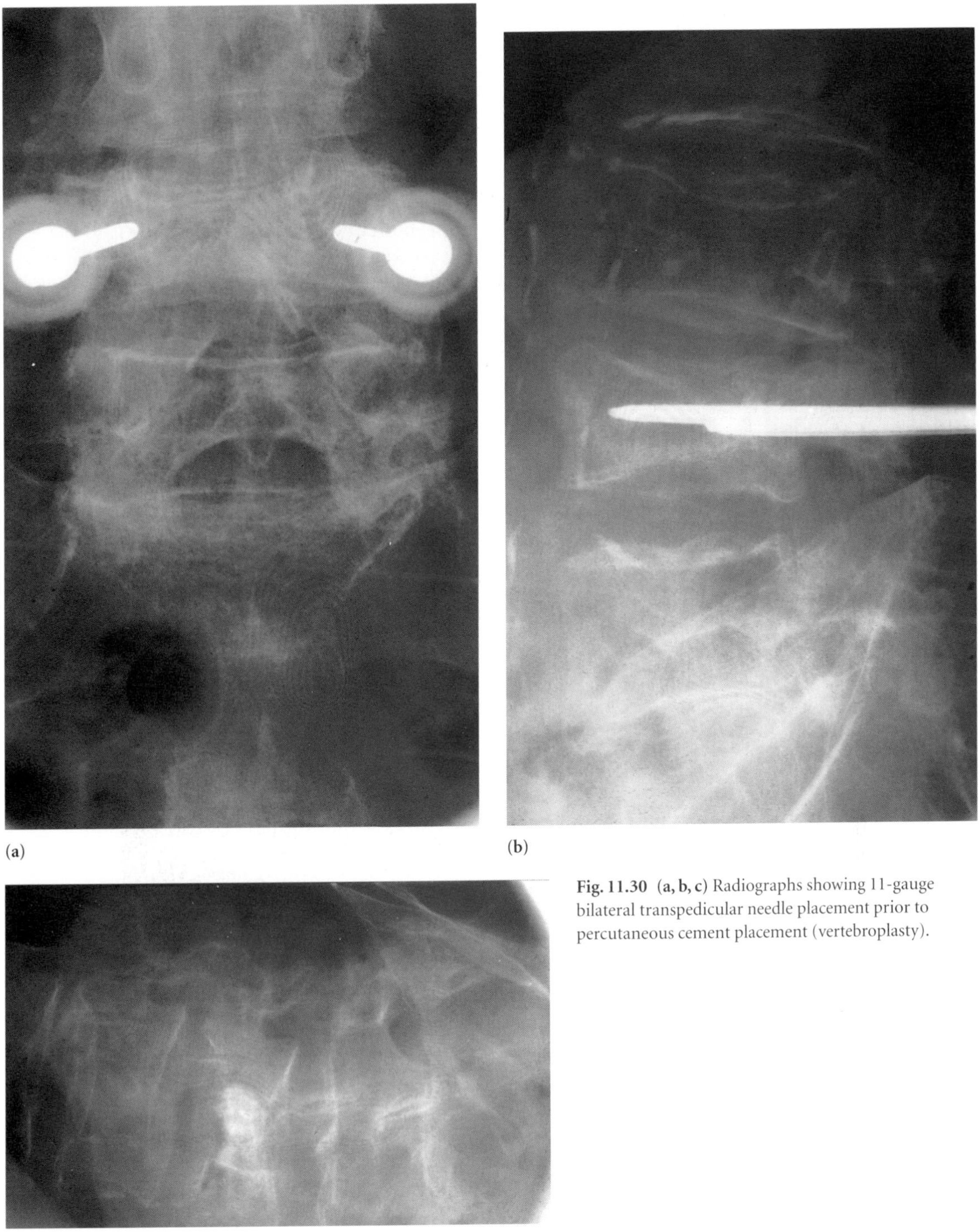

(a) (b) (c)

**Fig. 11.30** (**a, b, c**) Radiographs showing 11-gauge bilateral transpedicular needle placement prior to percutaneous cement placement (vertebroplasty).

# Lumbar burst fracture

- Burst fractures are usually the result of acute axial loading such as occurs following a fall from a height. They account for up to 15% of dorsolumbar fractures and are of importance as they are frequently associated with neurologic injury.
- Burst fractures are comminuted fractures involving the anterior and middle columns, the superior or inferior end-plates, or both, occasionally associated with vertical fractures through the posterior elements.
- Frequently comminution is associated with loss of vertebral body height both anteriorly and posteriorly and with retropulsion of bone fragment to the spinal canal.

## History

- There is frequently a history of a fall from a height.

## Imaging findings

### Radiography

- Allows fracture detection.

### Computerized tomography

- CT is routinely undertaken in this injury as it allows specific evaluation of the degree of vertebral body comminution and localization of retropulsed osseous fragments.

### Magnetic resonance imaging

- MRI in coronal, sagittal and axial planes allow similar fracture assessment.
- MRI allows the improved detection of concomitant disk prolapse and differentiation of acute cord edema and hemorrhage.



## Management

- Burst fractures are generally considered to be unstable fractures requiring operative fixation. Associated vertical fracture of the posterior element, particularly the pedicles, is a marker of definite instability (three-column injury).

## Lap seat-belt fractures: chance fractures

**Mechanism of injury**

- Acute hyperflexion over a seat-belt, preventing forward propulsion following motor vehicle accidents, may lead to a severe fracture and distraction of the middle and particularly of the posterior columns. Such injuries account for 5% of dorsolumbar spine fractures in adults.

**Definition**

- Classic chance fractures represent a horizontal fracture through the posterior arch, pedicle and posterior vertebral body. However, many variations in this injury are now recognized ranging from purely ligamentous disruption through a combination of bone and soft tissue, with disruption of the disk rather than vertebral body with variations often involving more than one vertebral body level.

### Imaging findings

Radiography

- This shows widening of the posterior elements following this injury but may not show extension to the vertebral body or disk.

Computerized tomography

- Similarly to wedge fractures, the plane of this injury often limits its visualization using CT ('in-plane' fracture phenomenon) without sagittal reformatting.

Magnetic resonance imaging

- Using MRI, sagittal images clearly delineate extension of these fractures through either the vertebral body, disk or posterior elements.
- Similar to other injuries, sensitivity to edema facilitates the identification of cord contusion, and associated disk disease.

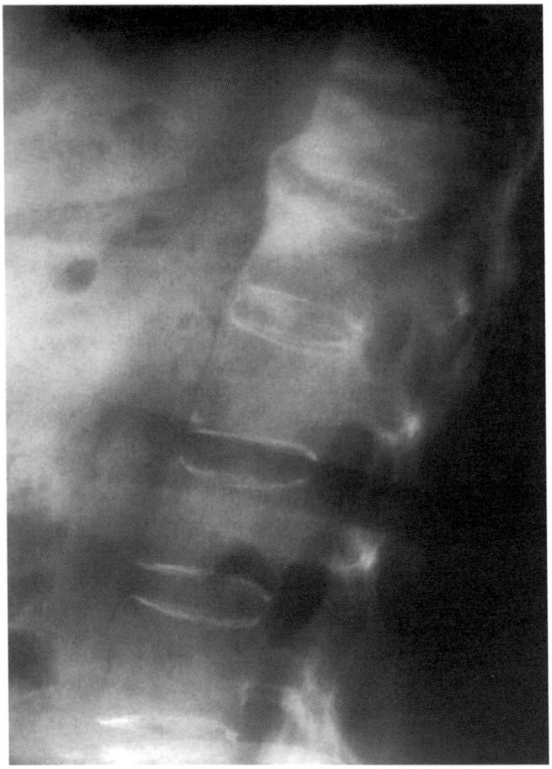

(a)

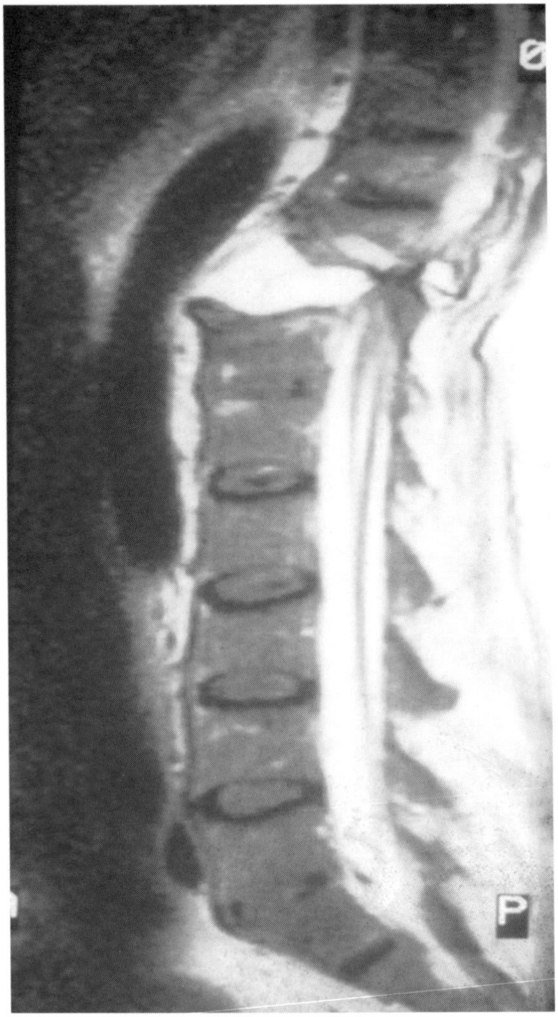



(b)

**Fig. 11.31** (**a, b**) Lateral radiograph showing an Anderson lesion at the dorsolumbar junction in a patient with ankylosing spondylitis, with sagittal $T_2$-weighted image showing complicating catastrophic fracture.



## Management

- Lap seat-belt fractures are generally considered to be stable, stability being conferred by an intact anterior column and anterior longitudinal ligament. These fractures are unstable in flexion.

# Fracture dislocation

- Fracture dislocations of the dorsolumbar spine account for 15% of fractures of the dorsolumbar spine. They are the result of either acute severe hyperflexion (in which dislocation is anterior), acute shear or acute flexion/rotation injury, often following motor vehicle or motorcycle accidents.
- Complete disruption of three columns confers gross instability, which is usually complicated by acute cord compression or transection.

## Imaging findings

### Radiography

- The injury is readily identified on conventional radiographs and the degree of osseous injury usually requires no further evaluation.

### Computerized tomography

- CT is occasionally undertaken to evaluate the position of articular processes and the integrity of the spinal canal, although it has now been replaced for this purpose by MRI.

### Magnetic resonance imaging

- Using MRI in the axial plane, displaced vertebral bodies may be seen in the same plane (the 'double rim' sign) and unpaired articular processes of the facet joints may be identified (the 'naked facet' sign).

# Injuries accompanying fractures of the dorsolumbar spine

- Reflecting severe trauma, fractures of the dorsolumbar spine are commonly associated with concomitant non-contiguous spinal fractures in 5% of cases.
- Fractures are often accompanied by posterior rib fractures (costovertebral dislocation) and injury to the sternum.
- Sternal fractures may be secondary to direct impaction against the steering column, in which case the inferior fragment is displaced posteriorly, or may be secondary to forces applied from above, secondary to acute spinal hyperflexion. Fractures may also be indirect, in which case the superior fragment is displaced posteriorly.
- Isolated dorsal fractures are commonly associated with mediastinal hematoma and hemothorax (mimicking aortic injury).
- Seat-belt fractures are associated with traumatic duodenal hematomas.
- Burst fractures are often associated with compression fractures of the calcaneus.

## Pitfalls and variants

- Physiologic wedging of the anterior margins of the vertebral bodies is commonly identified at the thoracolumbar junction between T8 and T12.
- The ratio of the height of the anterior margin of the vertebral body to the posterior margin is 0.8 in men and 0.87 in women.
- Thinning of the pedicles is commonly identified at the thoracolumbar junction, resulting in apparent widening of the intervertebral foramina.

# Scheuermann's disease

- Scheuermann's disease is a self-limiting osteochondrosis of the vertebral body. It is initially manifest as anterior corner apophysitis, and subsequently as end-plate sclerosis, irregularity and depression. Herniation of the nucleus pulposus through the end-plate infraction results in the formation of a Schmorl's node, a process repeated at multiple contiguous levels. Anterior apophysitis over four contiguous segments produces wedging manifest as an acquired kyphosis. This is a hallmark feature.

## History and clinical findings

- Onset during adolescence.
- Dorsal back pain.
- Limited range of motion.
- Loss of lordosis, exaggerated dorsal kyphosis.

## Imaging findings

### Radiography

- Radiographs show end-plate irregularity and Schmorl's nodes at multiple levels in the dorsal spine. There is also multilevel disk disease in association with a dorsal kyphosis (Fig. 11.32).

### Magnetic resonance imaging

- MRI shows multilevel Schmorl's nodes, disk disease and end-plate irregularity.

## Management



### Non-surgical

- Analgesia/antiinflammatories.
- Rest.
- Mobilizing physiotherapy.

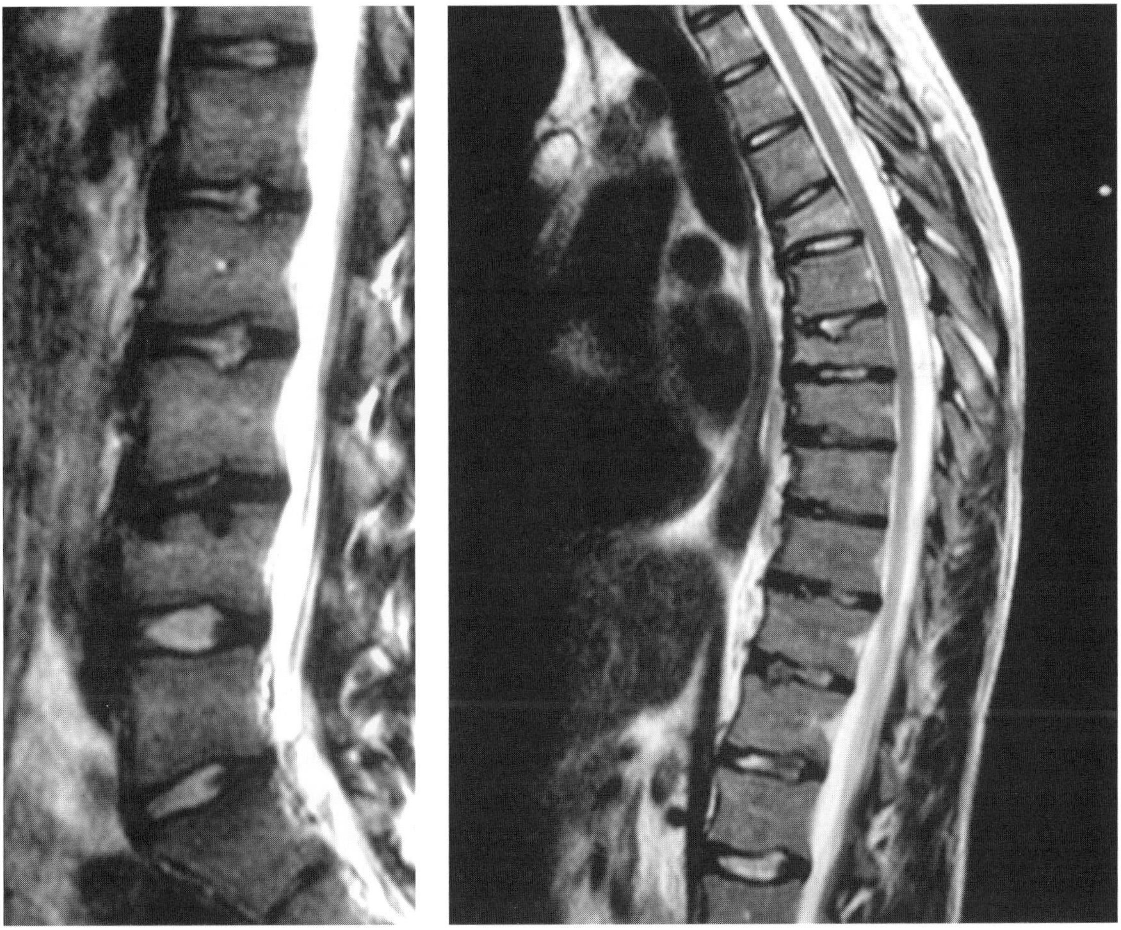

(a) (b)

**Fig. 11.32** (**a**) Sagittal $T_2$-weighted image showing end-plate infractions at multiple levels with herniation of the nucleus pulposus typical of Schmorl's nodes. (**b**) Image of the dorsal spine showing multiple Schmorl's nodes in association with mild vertebral body wedging and kyphosis, features of Scheuermann's disease.



## Complications of spinal injury

- In addition to direct injury to the cord, with either hemorrhage or edema, fracture of the dorsolumbar spine may be complicated by dural tear in up to 15% of cases. If the dura is torn, it is possible for nerve roots to become tangled within fracture fragments. When identified, surgical repair is undertaken from a posterior rather than an anterior approach. Dural tear should be suspected in the presence of a laminar fracture or if a hematocrit level is identified within the dependent portion of the thecal sac.
- Post-traumatic cord atrophy or central spinal cord cysts may produce progressive neurologic signs several years after spinal injury. Spinal cysts are easily identified at MRI and are an indication for surgical decompression.

# Complications of spinal injury: ankylosing spondylitis

- This is a spondylarthropathy characterized by the development of bilateral sacroiliitis and ascending spondylitis progressing to spinal fusion: a 'bamboo spine'. See Figures 11.33 and 11.34(a).

## History and clinical findings

- More common in males at a ratio of 9:1.
- Early morning back pain and stiffness.
- Impaired flexion/extension.
- Impaired side-to-side flexion.
- Impaired chest expansion.

## Complications

- Pulmonary fibrosis: mean onset 15 years in less than 5% of patients.
- Aortic incompetence.
- Bundle branch block.
- Amyloidosis.
- Pseudarthrosis complicating an end-stage bamboo spine occurs at a point of relative instability within an otherwise stable spine, most frequently at the thoracolumbar junction.
- As the disease progresses, the spine becomes progressively fused.
- At the dorsolumbar junction, greater motion prevents complete fusion.
- As the remainder of the spine becomes progressively fixed, motion at this site becomes increasingly more important.
- Progressive motion leads to degeneration of the intervertebral disk with the development of secondary osteoarthritis at this level, with end-plate sclerosis mimicking infection. This is Anderson's lesion.
- Following minor trauma, forced motion is transmitted to the site of the pseudarthrosis, often resulting in catastrophic hyperflexion, and fracture through or just above the disk. Extending through the posterior elements, the injury is usually complicated by acute cord impaction, hemorrhage and edema. See Figures 11.31 and 11.34(b).
- Unlike the primary disease, where enthesopathy generates osteophytes oriented to the long axis of the spine, pseudarthrosis is characterized by degenerative osteophytes with an orientation parallel to the end-plate.

## Management

- Antiinflammatories.
- Physiotherapy.
- Swimming.
- SI joint steroid injections with fluoroscopic guidance.
- Spinal bracing in patients with pseudoarthrosis.

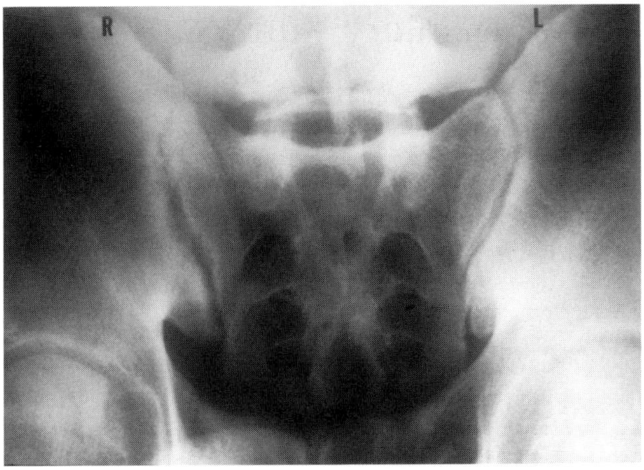


**Fig. 11.33** PA radiograph showing erosions of the articular surfaces of the right sacroiliac joint, secondary to asymmetric sacroiliitis.

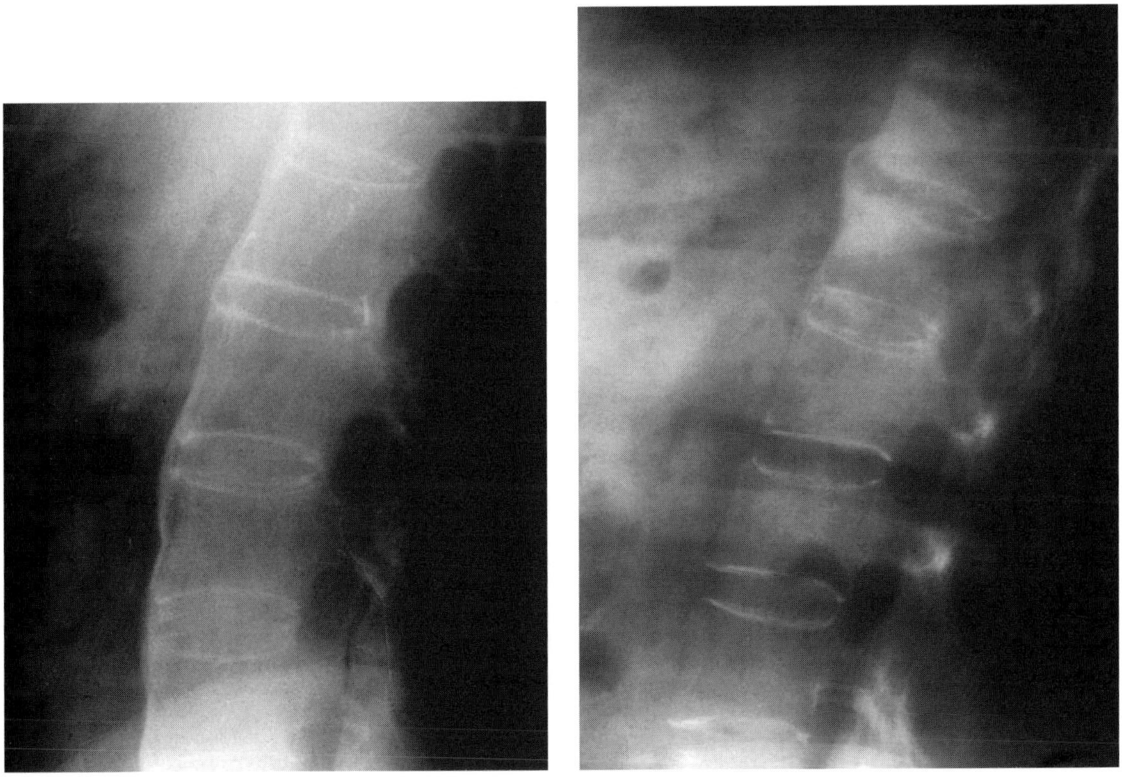

(a) (b)

**Fig. 11.34** (**a**) Lateral radiograph showing ossification of the anterior longitudinal and paraspinal ligaments typical of a bamboo spine. (**b**) Image showing an Anderson's lesion superimposed on a partly fused spine of ankylosing spondylitis

## Complications of spinal injury: Kümmell's disease

- Kümmell's disease is an uncommon cause of vertebral body collapse, usually several weeks (6 weeks) following direct spinal trauma.
- Following insult, serial radiographs or MR scans show progressive vertebral body collapse over 6 weeks, the benign nature of which is suggested by the presence of characteristic intravertebral body gas.
- Although the etiology is unclear, post-traumatic osteonecrosis appears to be the likeliest cause.

## Further reading

Czervionke LF. Lumbar intervetebral disc disease. Neuroimaging Clin N Am 1993; 465–485.

Denis F. The three-column spine and its significance in the classification of acute thoracolumbar spinal injuries. Spine 1983; 8: 817–831.

El-Khoury GY, Whitten CG. Trauma to the upper thoracic spine: anatomy, biomechanics, and unique imaging features. Am J Roentgenol 1993; 160: 95–102.

Hackney DB. Neoplasms and related disorders. Top Magn Res Imaging 1992; 4: 37–61.

Modic MT, Ross JS. Morphology, symptoms, and causality. Radiology 1990; 175: 619–620.

Porter RW, Hibbert CS. Symptoms associated with lysis of the pars interarticularis. Spine 1984; 9: 755–758.

Rauch RA, Jinkins JR. Lumbosacral spondylolisthesis associated with spondylolysis. Neuroimaging Clin N Am 1993; 3: 543–555.

Steel HH. Kümmell's disease. Am J Surg 1951; 81: 161–167.

Wagner M, Sether LA, Yu S et al. Age changes in the lumbar intervertebral disc studied with magnetic resonance and cryomicrotomy. Clin Anat 1988; 1: 93–103.

Watanabe R, Parke WW. Vascular and neural pathology of lumbosacral spinal stenosis. J Neurosurg 1986; 64: 64–70.

Wenger DR, Bobechko WP, Gilday DL. The spectrum of intervertebral disc-space infection in children. J Bone Joint Surg Am 1978; 60: 100–108.

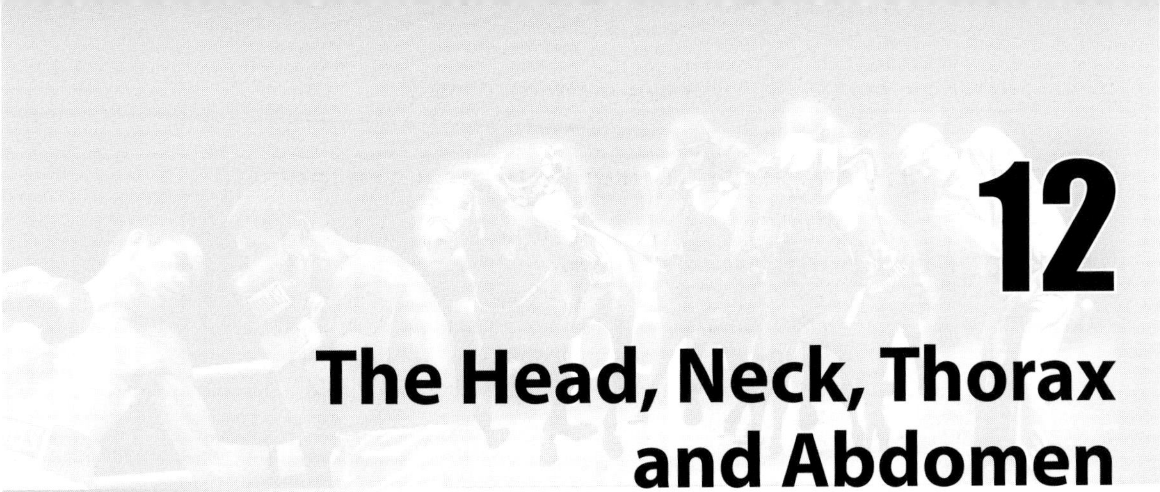

# 12 The Head, Neck, Thorax and Abdomen

## PATHOLOGIES

# Traumatic brain injury

### Anatomy

- The brain is contained within the rigid skull.
- Because of this, only small increases in volume within the intracranial compartment can be tolerated before pressure within the compartment rises dramatically.
- In adults, normal intracranial pressure (ICP) is 0–15 mmHg; the upper limit for ICP in children is lower.
- Severe elevations of ICP are dangerous because, in addition to creating a significant risk for ischemia, uncontrolled ICP may cause herniation of the brain across fixed dural structures, resulting in irreversible and often fatal cerebral injury.

### Mechanism of injury

- Most patients with traumatic brain injury (TBI; 75–80%) have mild head injuries.
- The most common causes include motor vehicle accidents (about 50%), falls, assaults, sports-related injuries and penetrating trauma.
- Traumatic brain injury may be divided into primary and secondary brain injury:
  - primary brain injury is defined as the initial injury to the brain as a direct result of the trauma (i.e. the initial structural injury caused by the impact on the brain) and patients recover poorly
  - secondary brain injury is defined as any subsequent injury to the brain after the initial insult. Secondary brain injury can result, for example, from systemic hypotension, hypoxia and elevated ICP.



### History and clinical examination

- The Glasgow Coma Scale (GCS) is used to describe the general level of consciousness of patients with TBI and to define broad categories of head injury.
- It is divided into three categories: eye opening (E); motor response (M); and verbal response (V).
- There is a maximum score of 15 and a minimum of 3, as shown in Table 12.1.
- In addition to determining the GCS score, the neurologic assessment of patients with TBI should include the following:
  - brainstem examination: pupillary examination; ocular movement examination; corneal reflex; and gag reflex
  - motor examination
  - sensory examination
  - reflex examination.

### Imaging findings

#### Radiography

- Rarely used as the sole method in patients with closed head injury.
- Occasionally used in the evaluation of penetrating head trauma.
- Can help provide a rapid assessment of the degree of foreign body penetration in non-missile penetrating head injuries, e.g. stab wounds.

| Table 12.1 Categories of the Glasgow Coma Scale | |
|---|---|
| **Category** | **Response** |
| Eye opening (E)<br>To verbal command<br>To pain<br>No response | Spontaneously |
| Best motor response (M)<br>Localizes pain<br>Flexion withdrawal<br>Flexion abnormal (decorticate)<br>Extension (decerebrate)<br>No response | Obeys command |
| Best verbal response (V)<br>Disoriented and converses<br>Inappropriate words<br>Incomprehensible sounds<br>No response | Oriented and converses |

## Computerized tomography

- This is the diagnostic study of choice in the evaluation of TBI.
- A non-contrast scan that spans from the base of the occiput to the top of the vertex in 5-mm increments (see Figs 12.1 and 12.2).
- Bone windows settings used for fracture detection.
- Soft-tissue windows settings used to detect the presence of:
  - extra-axial hematomas (e.g. epidural hematomas and subdural hematomas)
  - intraparenchymal hematomas
  - contusions.
- General survey of the brain for any evidence of pneumocephalus, hydrocephalus, cerebral edema, midline shift or compression of the subarachnoid cisterns at the base of the brain.

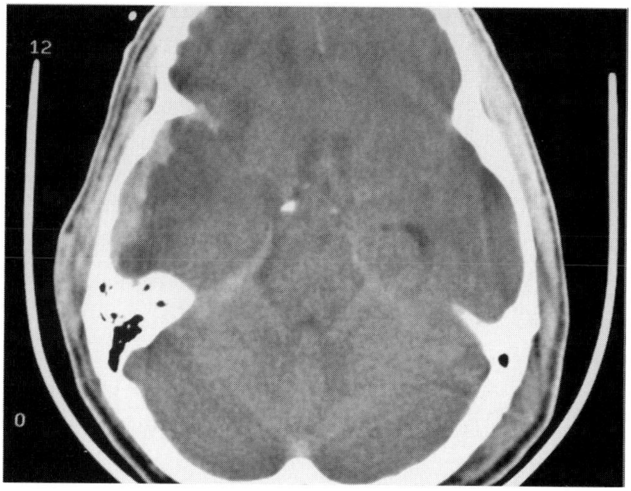


**Fig. 12.1** Axial non-contrast CT showing right-sided extra-axial hyperdense fluid secondary to post-traumatic subdural hematoma.

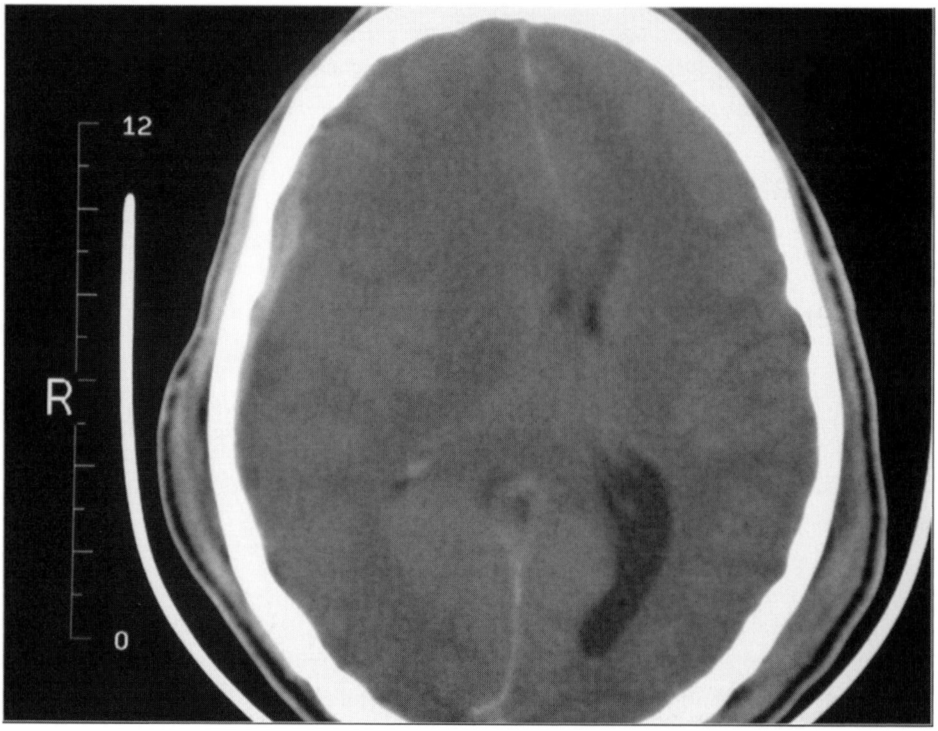


**Fig. 12.2** Axial non-contrast CT scan showing right subdural hematoma with associated cerebral edema producing mass effect, compression of the lateral ventricle and midline shift.

## Skull fractures

- Extra-axial hematomas include epidural and subdural hematomas.
- See also 'Skull fracture', page 452.

## Epidural hematomas

- See 'Extradural hematoma (epidural hematoma)', page 449.

## Subdural hematomas

- Located between the dura and the brain.
- The outer edge is convex while the inner border is usually irregularly concave.
- Not limited by the intracranial suture lines. This is an important feature as it helps with their differentiation from epidural hematomas.
- Usually venous in origin. Classically it is an injury to a bridging vein that travels from the cerebral cortex to the dura.
- Intra-axial hematomas include intraparenchymal hematomas, intraventricular hemorrhages and subarachnoid hemorrhages:
  - subarachnoid hemorrhages that occur because of trauma are typically located over gyri on the convexity of the brain
  - cerebral contusions are post-traumatic lesions in the brain that appear as irregular regions, in which high-density changes (i.e. blood) and low-density changes (i.e. edema) are present
  - contusions are most often caused by the brain gliding over rough surfaces, such as the rough portions of the skull that are present under the inferior frontal and temporal lobes.



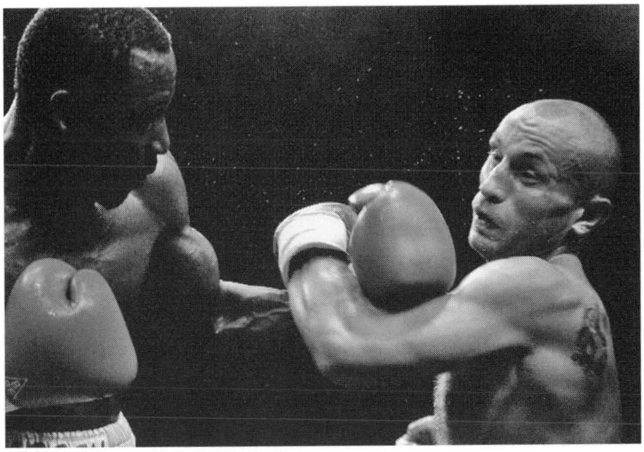

**Fig. 12.3** Sportfile.

## Imaging findings

### Magnetic resonance imaging

- Has a limited role in the evaluation of acute head injury. Although MRI provides excellent detail, it has long acquisition times.
- MRI is superior to CT for helping identify diffuse axonal injury (DAI) and small intraparenchymal contusions.
- DAI is defined as neuronal injury in the subcortical gray matter or the brainstem as a result of severe rotation or deceleration. DAI is often the reason for a severely depressed level of consciousness in patients who lack evidence of significant injury on CT scan images and have an ICP that is within the reference range.
- MRI may also be used in some patients with TBI to assess for arterial injury or venous sinus occlusion.

### Angiography

- Rarely used in the evaluation of acute head injury today, only when a vascular injury may be present. This includes patients with clinical evidence of a potential carotid injury.

## Management

### Non-surgical

- The treatment of head injury is directed at either preventing or minimizing secondary brain injury.
- Most people presenting with mild head injuries will not have any progression of their head injury and may be discharged with an instruction sheet for head injury care.
- Medical attention should be sought if patients develop severe headaches, persistent nausea and vomiting, seizures, confusion or unusual behavior, or watery discharge from either the nose or the ear.
- After a mild head injury, patients displaying persistent emesis, severe headache, anterograde amnesia, loss of consciousness or signs of intoxication by drugs or alcohol are considered to have a moderate-risk head injury. These patients should be evaluated with a head CT scan. Patients with moderate-risk mild head injuries can be discharged if their CT scan findings reveal no pathology, their intoxication is cleared and they have been observed for at least 8 hours.
- sedatives, anticonvulsants and measures to decrease raised ICP (hyperventilation, diuretics, barbiturates, hypothermia) may be required.



### Surgical

- Indications for surgery in patients with head injuries are:
  extra-axial hematoma with midline shift greater than 5 mm, intra-axial hematoma with volume greater than 30 mL
  an open skull fracture or a depressed skull fracture with more than 1 cm of inward displacement
  any temporal or cerebellar hematoma that is over 3 cm in diameter. These high-risk temporal and cerebellar hematomas are usually evacuated immediately.
- Factors that correlated with a poor outcome include:
  - age greater than 60 years
  - initial GCS score of less than 5
  - presence of a fixed dilated pupil
  - prolonged hypotension or hypoxia early after injury
  - presence of a surgical intracranial mass lesion.

# Extradural hematoma (epidural hematoma)

## Anatomy

- Bleeding between the dura mater (the outermost of the meninges) and the inner skull vault results in a hematoma that increases ICP and causes a shift of the brain away from the affected side.

## Mechanism of injury

- Head injury with or without skull fracture that tears the middle meningeal artery.
- Skull fractures are seen in about 90% of adult cases.
- Extradural hematoma is more common in young people because the dura covering the brain is not as firmly attached to the skull as in older people (where venous bleeding is more common).
- Extension of the hematoma is usually limited by suture lines owing to the tight attachment of the dura at these locations.
- Risk increases with contact sports and lack of head protection.

## History and clinical findings

- The following symptoms usually develop within 1 to 96 hours after a head injury:
  - unconsciousness for a short period followed by a headache that steadily worsens
  - drowsiness or unconsciousness
  - nausea or vomiting
  - focal neurologic signs
  - the pupil on the affected side may be dilated (from uncal herniation with compression of the oculomotor nerve) and unresponsive to light stimulation
  - bradycardia and/or hypertension indicative of elevated ICP
  - cerebrospinal fluid (CSF) otorrhea or rhinorrhea resulting from a skull fracture with disruption of the dura.

## Imaging findings

### Radiography

- May show a skull fracture on the affected side (especially at the squamous portion of temporal bone, which overlies the course of the middle meningeal artery).
- Cervical spine radiographs with AP, lateral and odontoid views are useful to identify associated traumatic fractures.

### Computerized tomography

- Has largely replaced plain radiography.
- Visualizes skull fractures but also directly images an epidural hematoma.
- Acute epidural hematoma may appear as a hyperdense lenticular-shaped mass situated between the brain and the skull, though regions of hypodensity may be seen with serum or fresh blood (cf. subdural hematoma, which is crescent shaped).
- Midline shift, ventricular dilatation and compression of the basal cisterns are also readily identifiable (Figs 12.4 and 12.5).

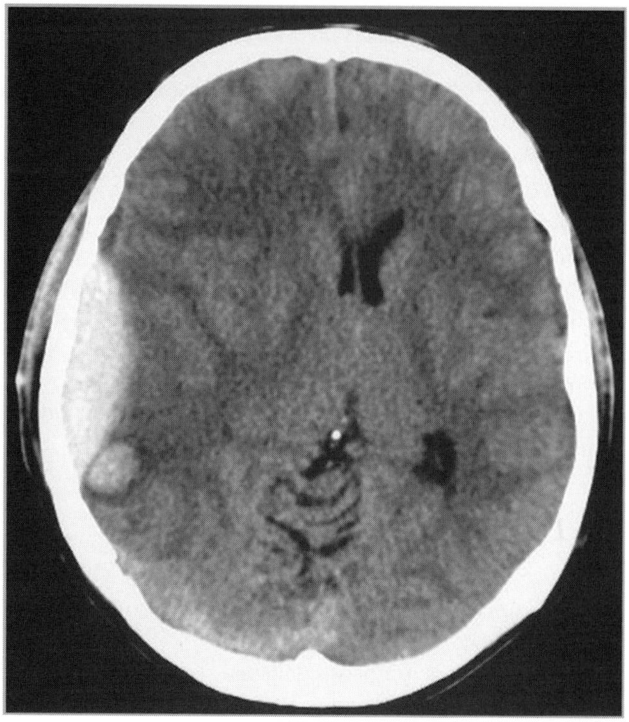

**Fig. 12.4** Axial non-contrast CT showing a biconvex extra-axial hyperdense fluid collection typical of an extradural hematoma with mass effect and midline shift.



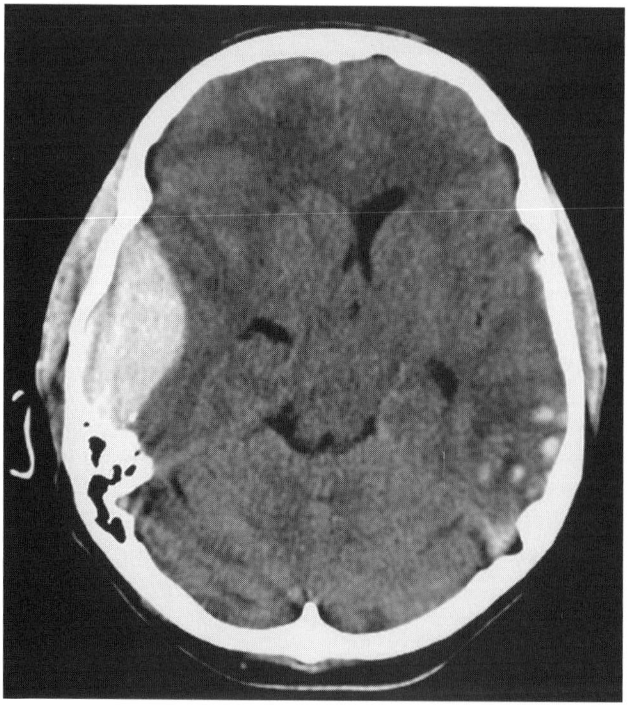

**Fig. 12.5** Axial non-contrast CT showing right extradural hematoma with a contrecoup injury in the left parietal lobe.

## Management

### Non-surgical

- The initial presentation is as for any head injury:
  - if the patient is wearing headgear with a face guard, cut the face guard without removing the headgear or moving the head or neck
  - if the patient vomits, support the head and neck completely and carefully while rotating the entire body to the side to prevent aspiration
  - splint the head and neck and transport the patient to the nearest well-equipped emergency facility
  - watch closely for vomiting, convulsions, changes in consciousness, paralysis or impaired breathing. Be ready to render CPR if needed.

### Surgical

- Emergent surgery (burr hole or craniotomy for large clots) to remove the clot causing pressure on the brain.
- Craniotomy or laminectomy is followed by evacuation of the hematoma, coagulation of bleeding sites and inspection of the dura. The dura is then tented to the bone. Epidural drains may be employed.
- Corticosteroids or osmotic agents, e.g. mannitol, may be used perioperatively to reduce cerebral edema.
- Anticonvulsants may be required postoperatively to control seizures.

## Rehabilitation

- Physical therapy for rehabilitation if there is residual paralysis or disability.
- The degree of residual deficit depends upon general health, age, severity of the injury, rapidity of the treatment and extent of bleeding.
- Avoidance of contact sports.

# Skull fracture

## Anatomy

- Different causative forces are involved in the various fracture patterns.
- The skull is thickened at the glabella, external occipital protuberance, mastoid processes and external angular process, and so is less prone to fracture at these sites.
- The skull vault is composed of cancellous bone (diploë) sandwiched between two layers (laminae). The diploë does not form where the skull is covered with muscles, leaving the vault thin and prone to fracture.
- The skull is prone to fracture at certain anatomic sites including the thin squamous temporal and parietal bones over the temples and the sphenoid sinus, the foramen magnum, the petrous temporal ridge and the inner parts of the sphenoid wings at the skull base.
- The middle cranial fossa is the weakest area with thin bones and multiple foramina.
- Other places prone to fracture include the cribriform plate and the roof of orbits in the anterior cranial fossa, and the areas between the mastoid and dural sinuses in the posterior cranial fossa.

## Mechanism of injury

- Fractures of the skull can be classified as linear or depressed. Linear fractures are either vault fractures or skull base fractures. Vault fractures and depressed fractures can be either closed or open.
- A linear fracture results from low-energy blunt trauma over a wide surface area of the skull. It runs through the entire thickness of the bone and, by itself, is of little significance except when it runs through a vascular channel, venous sinus groove or suture. In these situations, it may cause epidural hematoma, venous sinus thrombosis and occlusion, and sutural diastasis, respectively.
- Linear fractures may be differentiated from sutures by their size (usually >3 mm), straighter course, darker appearance (both sides of the skull vault affected) and characteristic locations, e.g. the temporoparietal region.
- *Basilar skull fracture* – this is a linear fracture at the base of the skull. It is usually associated with a dural tear and is found at specific points on the skull base (temporal bone and occipital condyle).
- Temporal fractures are most commonly longitudinal fractures occurring in the temporoparietal region and involving the squamous portion of the temporal bone, the superior wall of the external auditory canal and the tegmen tympani.
- *Occipital condylar fracture* – this results from high-energy blunt trauma with axial compression, lateral bending or rotational injury to the alar ligament. These fractures are subdivided into stable and unstable fractures, i.e. with and without ligamentous injury.
- *Depressed skull fracture* – this results from a high-energy direct blow to a small surface area of the skull with a blunt object such as a baseball bat.
- Most occur over the frontoparietal region because of the location and thinness of the bone.
- A free piece of bone should be depressed greater than the adjacent inner table of the skull to be of clinical significance and require elevation.
- A depressed fracture may be open or closed.



## History and clinical examination

### Linear skull fracture

- Most patients are asymptomatic and present without loss of consciousness. Swelling may occur at the site of impact.

Basilar skull fracture

- Presenting symptoms depend on the location of the fracture:
  - petrous temporal bone: CSF otorrhea and bruising over the mastoids (Battle's sign)
  - anterior cranial fossa: CSF rhinorrhea and bruising around the eyes ('raccoon eyes').

Longitudinal temporal bone fracture

- Ossicular chain disruption with conductive deafness which lasts longer than 6 weeks. Facial palsy, nystagmus and facial numbness are secondary to involvement of the VII, VI and V cranial nerves, respectively.

Depressed skull fracture

- Approximately 25% of patients with a depressed skull fracture do not report loss of consciousness, and another 25% lose consciousness for less than an hour. The presentation may vary depending on other associated intracranial injuries such as epidural hematoma, dural tears and seizures.

## Imaging findings

Radiography

- Not as sensitive as CT for basilar skull fractures but may be of value in fractures of the vertex.
- May show fluid level in the sphenoid sinus on lateral view in base of skull fracture.

Computerized tomography

- Best for bone detail.
- Shows secondary signs of injury (intracranial hemorrhage, contusion, midline shift).

## Management

Non-surgical

- Patients with simple linear or linear basilar fractures who are neurologically intact do not require any intervention and may even be discharged safely and asked to return if symptomatic.
- Temporal bone fractures are managed conservatively initially as tympanic membrane rupture usually heals on its own.
- Simple depressed fractures in neurologically intact infants are treated expectantly. They usually heal well and smooth out with time, without elevation.
- Open fractures, if contaminated, may require antibiotics in addition to tetanus toxoid.

Surgical

- The role of surgery is limited.
- Infants and children with open depressed fractures require surgical intervention, especially if the depressed segment is more than 5 mm below the inner table of adjacent bone. Indications for immediate elevation are gross contamination, dural tear with pneumocephalus, and an underlying hematoma.
- Delayed surgical intervention is required in ossicular disruption resulting from a longitudinal skull base fracture of the temporal bone, or a persistent CSF leak after a skull base fracture.

# Eye injuries

## Anatomy

- The globe is protected within the bony orbit.

## Mechanism of injury

- Injuries to the orbit itself generally occur from relatively sharp objects (hockey sticks, fingers, squash balls) whereas larger blunt objects tend to result in periorbital soft-tissue damage.
- Significant direct trauma may severely damage internal structures. Anterior chamber and vitreous hemorrhage, retinal hemorrhage or detachment, laceration of the iris, cataract, dislocated lens, glaucoma, orbital floor fractures and rupture of the globe may result.
- Conjunctival and corneal foreign bodies are also very common eye injuries but intraocular foreign bodies occur rarely. Seemingly minor trauma can be serious if ocular penetration is unrecognized or if secondary infection follows a corneal injury.

## History and clinical examination

- Trauma to the eye and adjacent structures requires meticulous examination to determine the extent of injury.
- Vision, range of extraocular motion, depth of anterior chamber, location of lid and conjunctival lacerations and of foreign bodies, and presence of anterior chamber or vitreous hemorrhage or cataract should be determined.

## Imaging findings

- Generally, the role of imaging studies is limited.
- Fluorescein staining with examination of the entire cornea and conjunctiva with a slit lamp is favored for foreign bodies and abrasions.

## Management



### Foreign bodies

- Conjunctival foreign bodies are lifted out with a moist sterile cotton applicator. A corneal foreign body that cannot be dislodged by irrigation may be lifted out carefully on the point of a hypodermic needle under slit-lamp magnification.
- For larger foreign bodies, treatment is as for any corneal abrasion: pupillary dilatation with a short-acting cycloplegic, antibiotic instillation and application of a patch firmly enough to keep the eye closed overnight. Ophthalmic corticosteroids tend to promote the growth of fungi and herpes simplex virus and are contraindicated.
- Intraocular foreign bodies require immediate surgical treatment by an ophthalmologist. The pupil is dilated to allow for examination of the crystalline lens, vitreous and retina. Systemic and topical antimicrobials are given and a protective shield is placed over the eye.

## Lid contusion (black eye)

- In the first 24 hours, treat with ice packs to inhibit swelling. The next day, hot compresses may aid absorption of the hematoma.

## Lid lacerations

- Repair with fine silk sutures for minor lacerations. An ophthalmic surgeon should repair lid-margin lacerations and more significant lacerations, especially those involving the lacrimal canaliculus.

## Trauma to the globe

- Emergency treatment before specialist ophthalmologist care consists of pain relief, keeping the pupil dilated, applying a protective shield and combating possible infection with local and systemic antimicrobials.
- If the globe is lacerated, topical antibiotics should be instilled in the form of drops only. Because fungal contamination of open wounds is dangerous, corticosteroids are contraindicated until after the wounds are closed surgically.

## Anterior chamber hemorrhage (traumatic hyphema)

- This is potentially serious and requires attention by an ophthalmologist. It may be followed by recurrent bleeding, glaucoma and blood staining of the cornea. A shield is needed to protect the eye from further trauma. If intraocular pressure rises, a carbonic anhydrase inhibitor should be given, e.g. acetazolamide.
- Drugs containing oral and topical NSAIDs are contraindicated because they may contribute to re-bleeding. Rarely, recurrent bleeding with secondary glaucoma requires evacuation of the blood by an ophthalmologist.

# Facial fractures

## Mechanism of injury

- Blunt injuries, including sports-related injuries; more common than penetrating trauma.
- Lower impact forces may result in nasal bone or zygoma injury.
- Progressively higher forces required to fracture the angle of the mandible, the glabellar region of the frontal bone and the supraorbital rim.
- Uncommonly seen in accidents in such sports as skiing, snowboarding, hockey and football.

## Types of fracture

- Simple nasal fractures are the most common of all facial fractures. They must be distinguished from the more serious nasoethmoidal fractures, which extend into the nose through the ethmoid bones. Fractures through the ethmoid are prone to CSF leaks from dural tears.
- Zygomatic arch fractures tend to occur in two or three places along the arch. There are often three breaks: one at each end of the arch and a third in the middle, forming a V-shaped fracture. This may impinge on the temporalis muscle below, causing trismus.
- Zygomaticomaxillary (tripod) fractures result from a direct blow to the cheek. Fracture occurs at articulations of the zygoma with the frontal bone maxillae and zygomatic arch and often extends through the orbital floor. Because the infraorbital nerve passes through the orbital floor, hyposthesia often occurs in its sensory distribution.
- Alveolar fractures occur just above the level of the teeth through the alveolar portion of the maxilla. Usually a group of teeth is loose, and blood is noted at the gum line.
- Le Fort or mid-face fractures are classified into three types:
  - Le Fort I – a horizontal maxillary fracture separates the maxillary process (hard palate) from the rest of the maxilla. The fracture extends through the lower third of the septum and involves the maxillary sinus. This is below the level of the infraorbital nerve and thus does not cause hypoesthesia
  - Le Fort II – a pyramidal fracture which starts at the nasal bone, extends through the lacrimal bone and courses downward through the zygomaticomaxillary suture. It travels posteriorly through the maxilla and below the zygoma into the upper pterygoid plates. The inner canthus of the nasal bridge is widened. Because the fracture extends through the zygoma, near the exit of the infraorbital nerve, hypoesthesia is often present. Bilateral subcutaneous hematomas are also often present
  - Le Fort III – craniofacial dysjunction also starts at the nasal bridge. It extends posteriorly through the ethmoid bones and laterally through the orbits below the optic foramen and through the pterygomaxillary suture into the sphenopalatine fossa. This fracture separates facial bones from cranium, causing the face to appear long and flat ('dish face').

## History and clinical findings

- Significant force is required to cause facial bone fractures other than simple nasal bone fractures.
- Important points in history include loss of consciousness, visual or hearing problems, facial numbness or weakness, and inability to close the mouth and bite down.

- Examination includes assessment of facial asymmetry, palpation for bony injury and foreign body, and palpation of the bony supraorbital ridge and frontal bone for step-off fractures.
- Eyes must be examined for injury, abnormality of ocular movements and visual acuity.
- Inspect the nose for widening of the nasal bridge, tenderness and crepitus, and the septum for hematoma and rhinorrhea, which may suggest a CSF leak.
- Palpate the zygoma along its arch as well as its articulations with the frontal bone, temporal bone and maxillae.
- Check facial stability by grasping the teeth and hard palate and gently pushing back and forth, then up and down, feeling for movement or instability of the mid face.
- Inspect the teeth for fracture and bleeding at the gum line (a sign of fracture through the alveolar bone).
- Check the teeth for malocclusion and step-off.
- Palpate the mandible for tenderness, swelling and step-off along its symphysis, body, angle and condyle anterior to the ear canal.
- Evaluate supraorbital, infraorbital, inferior alveolar and mental nerve distributions for hypoesthesia or anesthesia.

## Imaging findings

### Nasal bone fractures

- History and physical examination may be sufficient without the need for X-rays as most nasal fractures do not require reduction.
- Plain nasal films consisting of a lateral view coning down on the nose and a Waters' view can confirm the diagnosis but are of little practical use. If edema has resolved and no deformity is noted, X-rays are unnecessary.
- If deformity persists after resolution of edema, films may be obtained at follow-up to help plan the repair.



### Nasoethmoidal fracture

- If a nasal fracture is suspected and evidence suggests ethmoidal bone involvement (CSF rhinorrhea, widening of the nasal bridge), plain films are of little use.
- A coronal CT scan of the facial bones is the best test to determine the extent of fracture.

### Zygoma fracture

- Underexposed submental view to evaluate the zygomatic arch.
- This fracture may also be seen on a Waters' view of a facial series.

### Tripod fracture

- If a tripod fracture is suspected, plain films should include Waters', Caldwell's and underexposed submental views:
  - Waters' view is best to evaluate the inferior orbital rim, maxillary extension of the zygoma and the maxillary sinus.
  - Caldwell's view evaluates the frontal process of the zygoma and the zygomaticofrontal suture.
  - underexposed submental view evaluates the zygomatic arch.
- A coronal CT scan of the facial bones with a 3D reconstruction used to better evaluate these fractures.

### Le Fort fractures

- A coronal CT scan of facial bones has replaced plain films in the evaluation of Le Fort fractures, especially with 3D reconstruction. If CT is not available, a facial series with lateral, Waters' and Caldwell's views can be used to evaluate the fracture. Almost all Le Fort fractures cause blood to collect in the maxillary sinus.
- *Le Fort I fractures* – imaging demonstrates a fracture extending horizontally across the inferior maxilla, sometimes including a fracture of the lateral sinus wall, extending into the palatine bones and pterygoid plates.
- *Le Fort II fractures* – imaging demonstrates disruption of the inferior orbital rim lateral to the infraorbital canal and a fracture of the medial orbital wall and nasal bone. The fracture extends posteriorly into the pterygoid plates.
- *Le Fort III fractures* – imaging demonstrates fractures at the zygomaticofrontal suture, zygoma, medial orbital wall and nasal bone extending posteriorly through the orbit at the pterygomaxillary suture into the sphenopalatine fossa.

## Management

- Initial management as for any significant head injury: ABC; spinal injury precautions; early ET intubation; and assessment for other injuries.
- Referral to maxillofacial/plastics/ENT/orthopedic surgeons for definitive surgical fixation.
- Adequate analgesia, including opiates.
- If there has been nasal packing for epistaxis, prophylactic antibiotics should be used to prevent infection.
- If the patient has an open wound, tetanus immunization should be administered.

# Neck trauma

## Anatomy

- The neck is protected by the spine posteriorly, the head superiorly and the chest inferiorly.
- The anterior and lateral regions are most exposed to injury. The larynx and trachea are therefore readily exposed to injury.
- The spinal cord lies posteriorly, cushioned by the vertebral bodies, muscles and ligaments.
- The sternocleidomastoid separates the neck into anterior and posterior triangles.
- Important vascular and visceral organs lie within the anterior triangle.
- Musculoskeletal structures at risk include: the cervical spine; the cervical muscles, tendons and ligaments; clavicles; the first and second ribs; and the hyoid bone.
- Neural structures at risk include the spinal cord, phrenic nerve, brachial plexus, recurrent laryngeal nerve and cranial nerves (specifically IX–XII).
- Vascular structures at risk include the carotid (common, internal, external) and vertebral arteries and the vertebral, brachiocephalic and jugular veins.

## Mechanism of injury

- Penetrating or blunt trauma.
- Airway occlusion and catastrophic hemorrhage are the major dangers.
- Penetrating injuries are rarely the result of sports injuries.
- Blunt trauma to the neck typically results from motor vehicle accidents but it can also occur with sports-related injuries, e.g. a rugby tackle.

## History and clinical findings

- Clinical manifestations may vary greatly, and delayed presentation of an arterial injury may occur.
- Events surrounding the traumatic event, the amount of time that elapsed, the amount of blood loss and whether the patient lost consciousness should be obtained.
- Cardiovascular manifestations range from bleeding to symptoms normally associated with a cerebrovascular accident.
- Symptoms relating to the aerodigestive tract include dyspnea, hoarseness, dysphonia and dysphagia.
- CNS problems include paresthesias, weakness, hemiplegia and paresis.

### Physical

- Airway patency, breathing and adequacy of circulation.
- If the platysma is not breached by a penetrating injury, there is less likelihood of a significant underlying injury.
- Consider an arterial injury of the neck in patients manifesting gross bleeding, a hematoma, asymmetry of arterial pulses, a bruit on auscultation, and neurologic deficits, especially lateralizing neurologic findings; or hypotension.
- Signs of spinal cord or brachial plexus injury include:
  - focal arm numbness or weakness; bilateral neurologic findings imply a spinal cord injury until proven otherwise
  - signs of larynx or trachea injury: voice change, hemoptysis, stridor, crepitus
  - signs of tracheal or lung injury: subcutaneous emphysema, cough, respiratory distress, tachypnea
  - signs of carotid artery injury: decreased level of consciousness, contralateral hemiparesis, pulse deficit.
- Specific signs of cranial nerve injuries may be apparent.

## Imaging findings

### Radiography

- Cervical X-rays.
- In general, at least a 3-view series is required.
- Review the cervical radiographs for: subcutaneous emphysema; fractures; displacement of the trachea and foreign bodies.

### Chest X-ray

- Check for hemothorax, pneumothorax, widened mediastinum, mediastinal emphysema, apical pleural hematoma and foreign bodies.

### Computerized tomography

- Most useful when bony or laryngeal damage is a consideration, especially with 3D reformats.

### Magnetic resonance imaging and magnetic resonance angiography

- Evaluation of the patient exhibiting neurologic impairment with minimal or absent abnormalities on plain radiographs of the cervical spine.
- Suitable for stable patients only due to time required for examinations.

### Ultrasound/ Doppler

- Doppler ultrasonography may be used as a screening test in low-risk patients or those thought to have a carotid injury.
- Sensitivity remains variable and its sole use is controversial.

### Contrast study

- Although a normal gastrograffin study occasionally proves useful in the evaluation of the cervical esophagus, it does not rule out a pharyngoesophageal leak.



### Angiography

- To evaluate stable patients sustaining penetrating wounds that pierce the platysma.
- A 4-vessel study is needed.
- Important when there is a question of intrathoracic involvement that may necessitate a thoracotomy, or to confirm adequacy of collateral circulation if carotid artery ligation is contemplated, or when therapeutic embolization or occlusion of the affected vessel is being considered.

## Management

- Initial measures include:
  - securing the airway
  - controlling bleeding
  - providing cervical spine precautions
  - identifying life-threatening conditions.

### Non-surgical

- Most blunt traumatic neck injuries can be managed non-operatively.
- Many patients are discharged with the diagnosis of whiplash injury (neck pain following sudden flexion/extension of the head, e.g. with a rear-end motor vehicle accident). By definition, whiplash injury implies that bony damage or other significant injuries are excluded.

## Surgical

- Surgical assessment of penetrating neck wounds usually requires operative intervention, especially when a cut violates the platysma.
- Virtually all patients with hard signs of an arterial injury require operative repair.

# Blunt chest trauma

## Anatomy

- The thorax is bordered superiorly by the thoracic inlet, through which the major arterial blood supply to and venous drainage from the head and neck pass.
- The thoracic outlets form the superolateral borders of the thorax and transmit branches of the thoracic great vessels, which supply blood to the upper extremities. The nerves that comprise the brachial plexus also access the upper extremities via the thoracic outlet. The veins that drain the arm, most importantly the axillary vein, empty into the subclavian vein, which returns to the chest via the thoracic outlet.
- Inferiorly, the pleural cavities are separated from the peritoneal cavity by the hemidiaphragms. Communication routes between the thorax and abdomen are supplied by the diaphragmatic hiatuses, which allow egress of the aorta, esophagus and vagal nerves into the abdomen and ingress of the vena cava and thoracic duct into the chest.
- The chest wall is composed of layers of muscle, bony ribs, costal cartilages, the sternum, clavicles and scapulae. In addition, important neurovascular bundles course along each rib, containing an intercostal nerve, artery and vein. The inner lining of the chest wall is the parietal pleura. The visceral pleura invests the major thoracic organs. Between the visceral and parietal pleurae is a potential space, which, under normal conditions, contains a small amount of fluid that serves mainly as a lubricant.

## Mechanism of injury

- Blunt injury to the chest can affect any one or all components of the chest wall and thoracic cavity. These include the ribs, clavicles, scapulae, sternum, lungs and pleurae, tracheobronchial tree, esophagus, heart and great vessels of the chest.



### Rib fractures

- Rib fractures are the most common blunt thoracic injuries.
- Ribs 4–10 are most frequently involved.

### Flail chest

- When three or more consecutive ribs are fractured in two or more places, a free-floating, unstable segment of chest wall is produced: this is 'flail chest'.
- A significant amount of force is required to produce a flail segment. Therefore, associated injuries are common, including closed head trauma.

### Clavicular fractures

- Clavicular fractures are one of the most common injuries to the chest wall and shoulder girdle area.
- Common mechanisms include a direct blow to the shaft of the bone, a fall on an outstretched hand or a direct lateral fall against the shoulder.
- Approximately 75–80% of clavicular fractures occur in the middle third of the bone.

### Pneumothorax

- Pneumothoraces are most frequently caused when a fractured rib penetrates the lung parenchyma. This is not absolute.
- Pneumothoraces can result from deceleration or barotrauma to the lung without associated rib fractures.

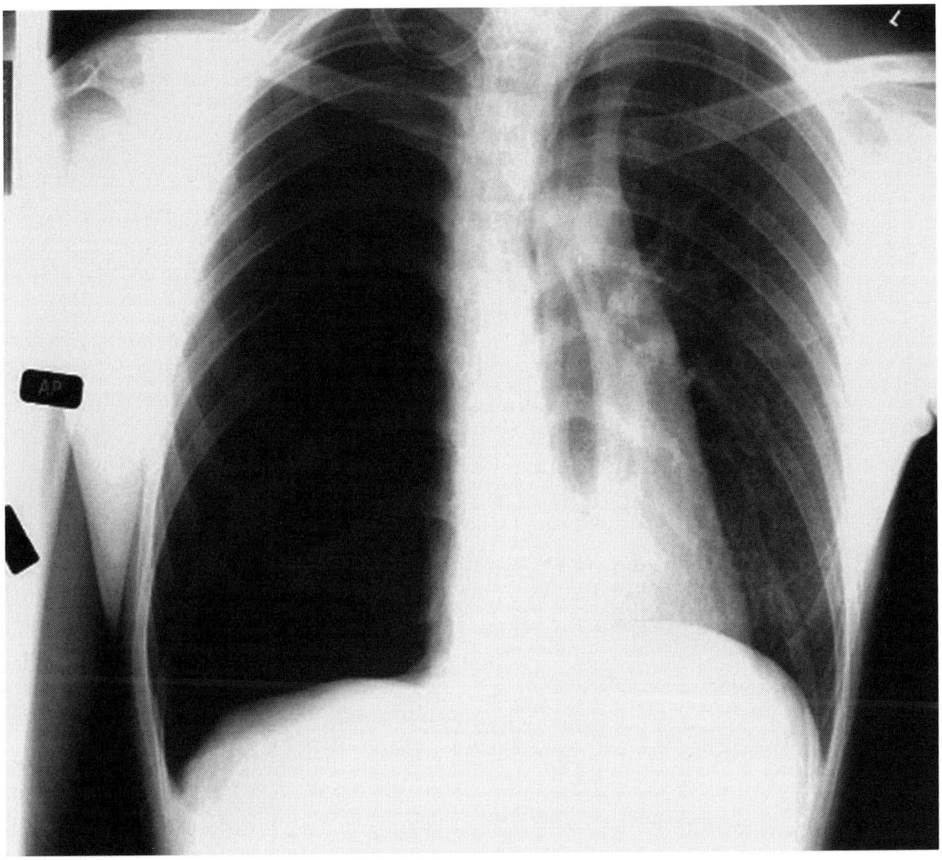


Fig. 12.6 Chest radiograph showing right tension pneumothorax with midline shift following blunt chest trauma.



Tension pneumothorax

- The mechanisms that produce tension pneumothoraces are the same as those that produce simple pneumothoraces. However, with a tension pneumothorax, air continues to leak from an underlying pulmonary parenchymal injury, increasing pressure within the affected hemithorax (Fig. 12.6).

Hemothorax

- The accumulation of blood within the pleural space can be due to bleeding from the chest wall (e.g. lacerations of the intercostal or internal mammary vessels attributable to fractures of chest wall elements) or to hemorrhage from the lung parenchyma or major thoracic vessels (Fig. 12.7).

## Imaging findings

Radiography

- The chest radiograph (CXR) is the initial radiographic study of choice in patients with thoracic blunt trauma.
- A CXR is an important adjunct in the diagnosis of many conditions, including chest wall fractures, pneumothorax, hemothorax and injuries to the heart and great vessels, e.g. enlarged cardiac silhouette or widened mediastinum.

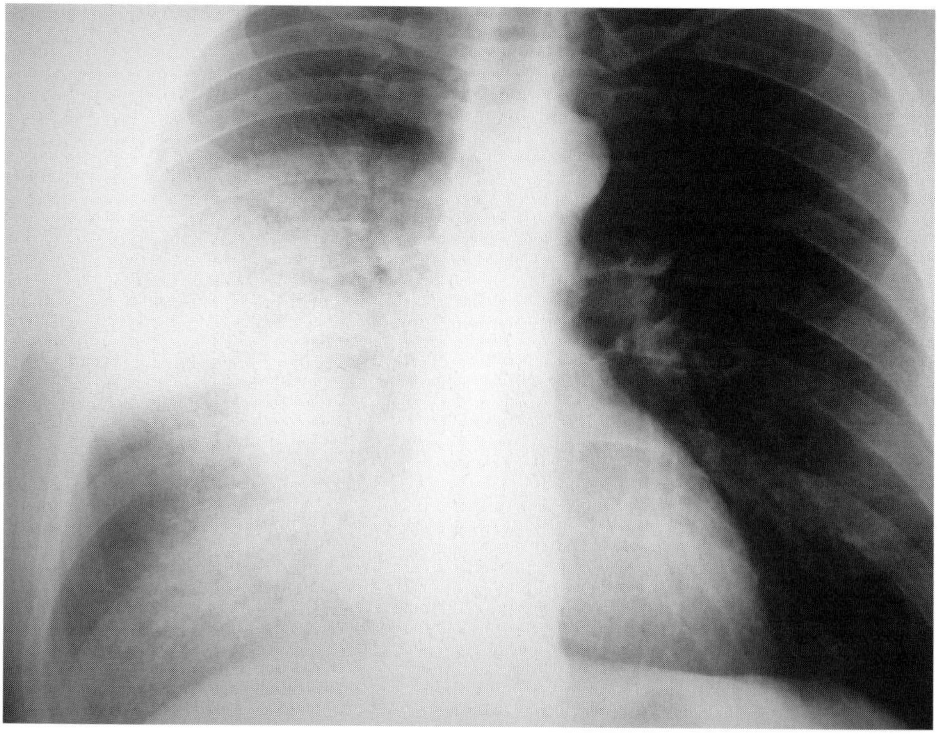

**Fig. 12.7** Chest radiograph showing diffuse right lung opacity and consolidation secondary to parenchymal hemorrhage following lung contusion.



- Certain cases arise in which physicians should not wait for a CXR to confirm clinical suspicion. The classic example is a patient presenting with a tension pneumothorax. This should be immediately decompressed before obtaining a CXR.

## Computerized tomography

- Chest CT scans are more sensitive than CXRs for the detection of injuries such as pneumothoraces and pulmonary contusions. Their use to confirm the diagnosis of pulmonary and chest wall trauma should be restricted to patients in whom an undetected or occult injury is considered (Fig. 12.9).

## Aortogram

- In the setting of severe chest trauma and possible aortic injury, thoracic aortography may provide a more exact delineation of the location and extent of aortic injuries compared to CT scan or transesophageal echocardiography (TOE) images. Aortography is superior at demonstrating injuries of the ascending aorta.

## Thoracic ultrasound

- Ultrasound examinations may show pericardial effusions or tamponade and hemothoraces associated with trauma.
- Other more specialist examinations (including upper GI contrast studies and TOE) are required in more serious cases of trauma.

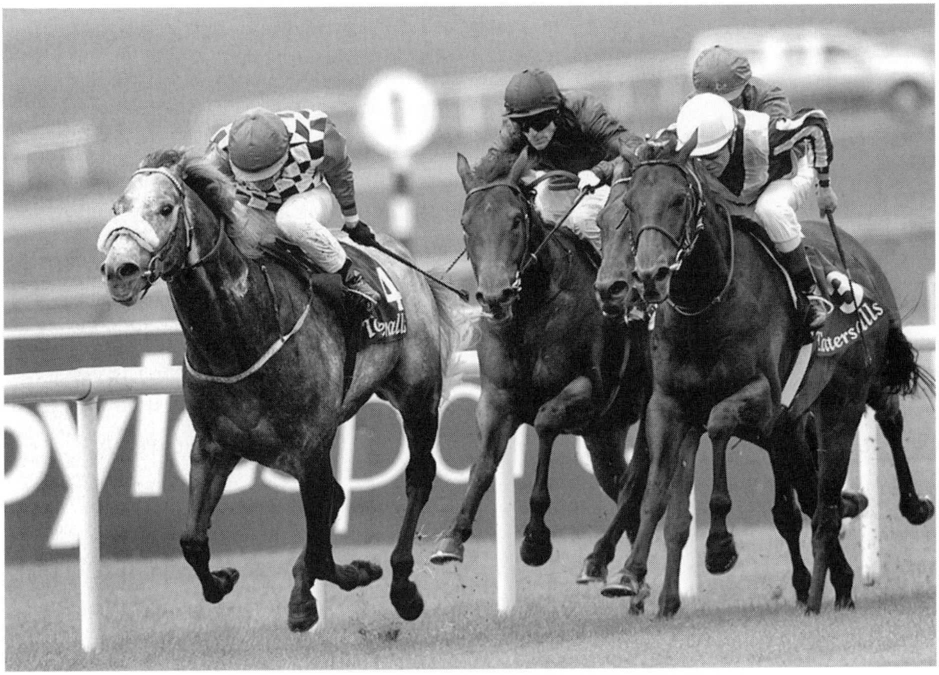


Fig. 12.8 Sportsfile.

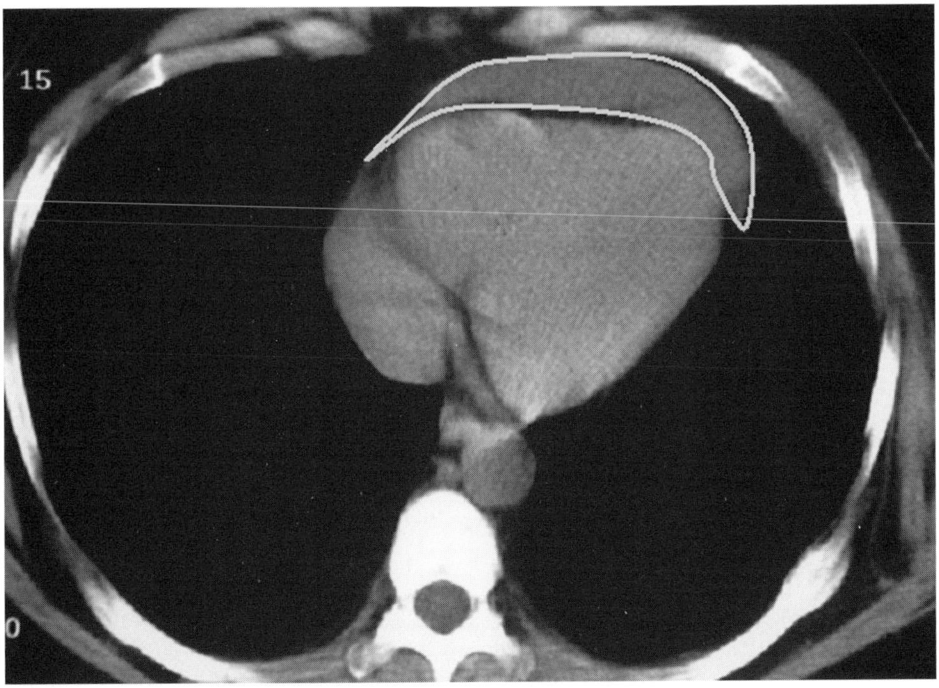


Fig. 12.9 Axial non-contrast CT showing a pericardial effusion following chest trauma.

## Management

### Rib fractures

- Effective analgesia is important.
- Patients with multiple rib fractures, whose pain is difficult to control, can be treated with epidural analgesia.
- Adjunctive measures include early mobilization and aggressive pulmonary toilet.
- Rib fractures do not require surgery.
- Rarely, a fractured rib lacerates an intercostal artery or other vessel; this requires surgical control to achieve hemostasis.

### Clavicular fractures

- Nearly all clavicular fractures can be managed without surgery.
- Primary treatment consists of immobilization with a figure-of-eight dressing, clavicle strap, or similar dressing or sling.
- Surgery is rarely indicated. Surgical intervention is occasionally indicated for the reduction of a badly displaced fracture.

### Pneumothorax

- Pain control and pulmonary toilet.
- All patients with pneumothoraces due to trauma need a tube thoracostomy. The chest tube is connected to a suction system and underwater seal.
- When the lung remains fully expanded, the chest tube may be removed and another CXR obtained to ensure continued complete lung expansion.

### Tension pneumothorax

- Immediate therapy for this life-threatening condition includes decompression of the affected hemithorax by needle thoracostomy.
- A large-bore needle (i.e. 14- to 16-gauge) is inserted through the second intercostal space in the mid clavicular line. A tube thoracostomy is then performed.
- Pain control and pulmonary toilet are instituted.



### Hemothorax

- Hemothoraces are evacuated using tube thoracostomy. Multiple chest tubes may be required.
- Pain control and aggressive pulmonary toilet are provided.
- Large, clotted hemothoraces may require an operation for evacuation to allow full expansion of the lung and to avoid the development of other complications such as fibrothorax and empyema (Fig. 12.10).

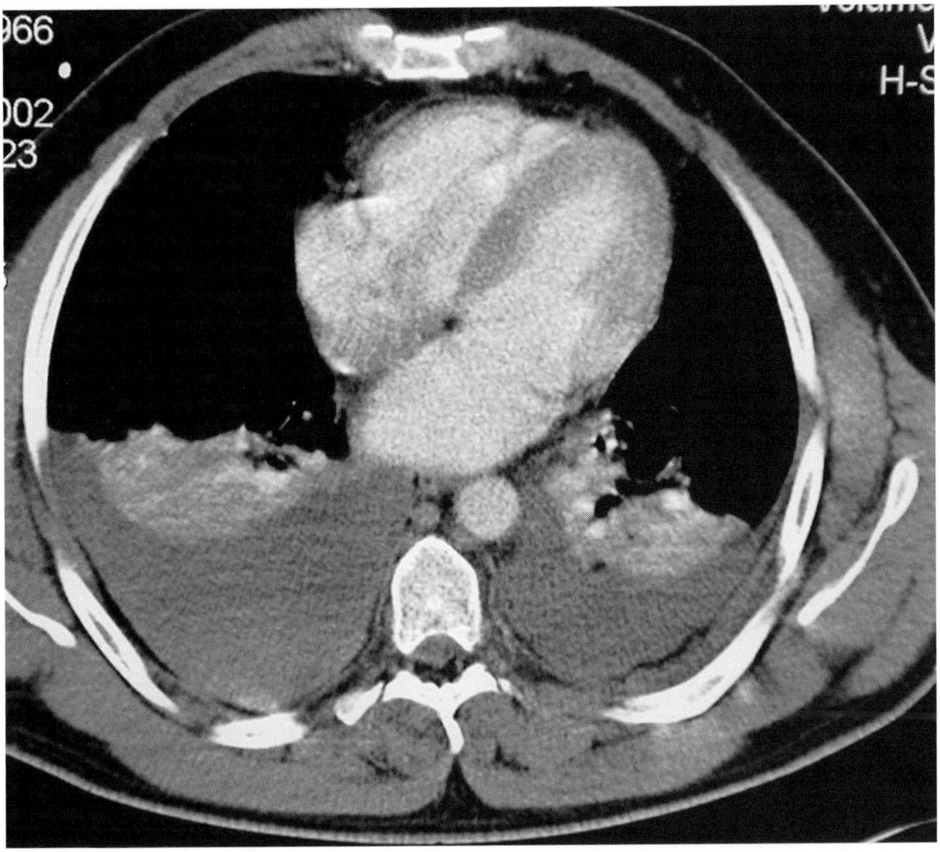


**Fig. 12.10** Axial non-contrast CT showing bi-basal pleural effusions with basal consolidation secondary to parenchymal contusion complicating blunt chest trauma.

# Blunt abdominal trauma

## Anatomy

- See under specific following sections (Fig. 12.11).

## Mechanism of injury

- Injury to intra-abdominal structures can be classified into two primary mechanisms: compression forces and deceleration forces.
- Compression forces result from direct blows or external compression against a fixed object (e.g. a lap belt) and most commonly cause tears and subcapsular hematomas to solid viscera. These forces may also deform hollow organs and transiently increase intraluminal pressure, resulting in rupture. This transient pressure increase is a common mechanism of blunt trauma to the small bowel.
- Deceleration causes stretching and shearing forces between relatively fixed and free objects, which tends to rupture supporting structures at the junction between free and fixed segments, e.g. hepatic tear along the ligamentum teres and intimal injuries to the renal arteries. As bowel loops travel from their mesenteric attachments, thrombosis and mesenteric tears, with resultant splanchnic vessel injuries, can result.
- The liver and spleen seem to be the most frequently injured organs.

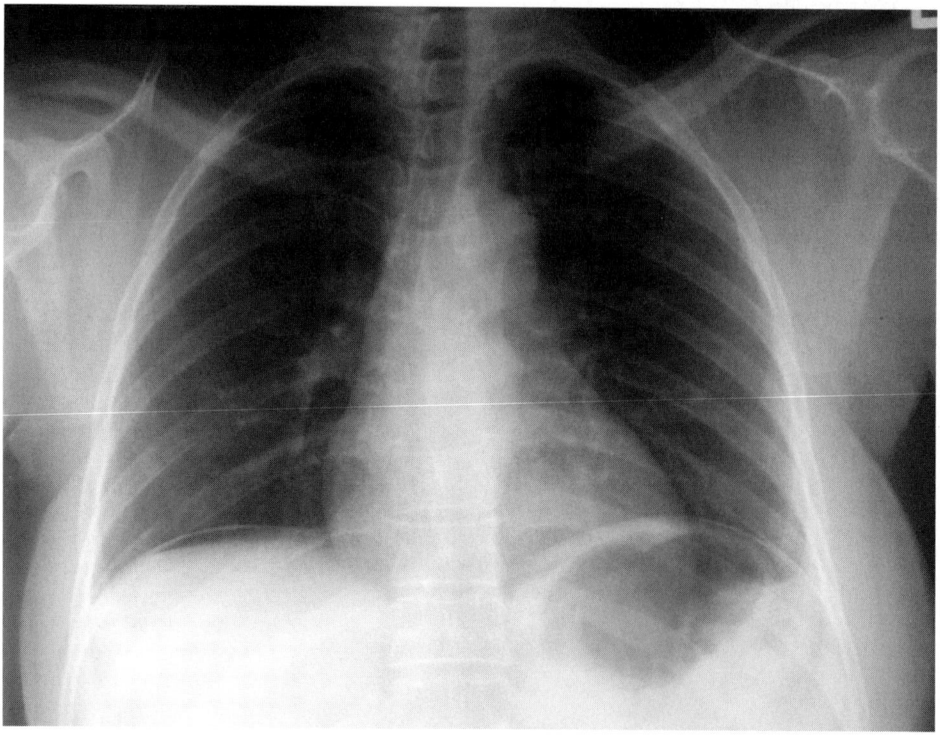

Fig. 12.11 Erect CXR shows subdiaphragmatic air below the right hemidiaphragm following rupture of an intra-abdominal viscus.

## History and clinical findings

- As with any significant trauma, evaluation and resuscitation simultaneously occur.
- The fundamentals of resuscitation (airway, breathing, circulation) take precedence.
- A secondary survey of the abdomen should include:
  - inspection: external signs of injury and any injury patterns, e.g. lap-belt ecchymosis and small bowel injury
  - observation: abdominal distension/discoloration, bradycardia (free intraperitoneal blood?), periumbilical ecchymosis (retroperitoneal hemorrhage?)
  - auscultation (bruit?)
  - palpation: abnormal masses, tenderness and deformities. Lower rib cage crepitus (splenic or hepatic injury?) or pelvic instability (urinary tract injury?). Also rectal and bimanual vaginal pelvic examinations
  - percussion: tenderness on percussion indicates peritonism (Fig. 12.12).

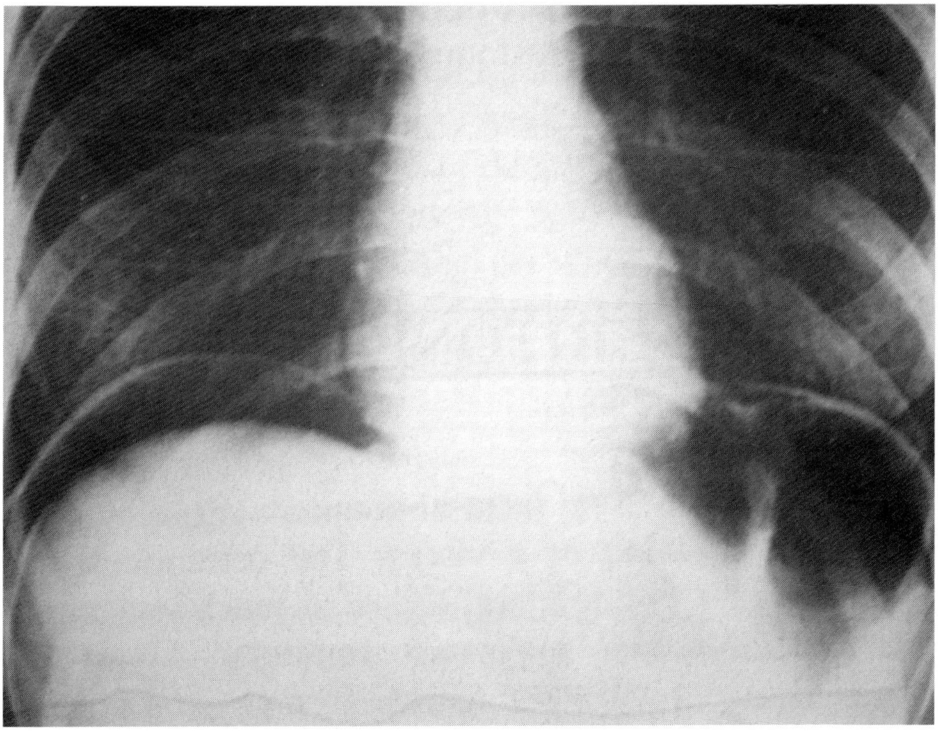

**Fig. 12.12** Radiograph showing extensive subdiaphragmatic free air following bowel rupture.

Diagnostic peritoneal lavage

- Rapidly determines the presence of intraperitoneal blood. Useful if the history and abdominal examination of an unstable patient is unreliable.
- Abdominal exploration is indicated if approximately 10 mL of blood is aspirated upon insertion of the peritoneal catheter (grossly positive) in the unstable patient.
- If findings are negative, 1 L of crystalloid solution is infused into the peritoneum and allowed to drain by gravity, after which analysis is performed.
- Over 100 000 RBC/$mm^3$ or over 500 WBC/$mm^3$ is considered a positive finding.

## Imaging findings

Ultrasound

- Focused abdominal sonogram for trauma (FAST).
- Diagnostic accuracy generally is equal to that of diagnostic peritoneal lavage (DPL).
- Rapid evaluation of hemoperitoneum.
- Studies demonstrate a degree of operator dependence.
- Sensitivity for solid organ-encapsulated injury is moderate at best.
- Hollow viscous injury is rarely identified.
- Complementary measure to CT scan, DPL or exploration.
- FAST evaluation of the abdomen consists of visualization of the pericardium (from a sub-xiphoid view), the splenorenal and hepatorenal spaces (e.g. Morrison's pouch, which is the most sensitive), the paracolic gutters and the pouch of Douglas in the pelvis.
- Free fluid, generally assumed to be blood in the setting of abdominal trauma, appears as an anechoic black stripe.

Computerized tomography



- Examination of choice for hemodynamically stable patients.
- Highly specific and useful for guiding non-operative management of solid organ injuries.
- Additional time required if both oral and i.v. contrast are administered, the use of which is controversial.

## Management

Non-surgical

- Free fluid in a hemodynamically unstable patient indicates exigent laparotomy. However, a CT scan may further evaluate the stable patient with free fluid.
- Resuscitative measures take precedence, including securing the airway, cervical immobilization if necessary, volume resuscitation and venous access.
- Detailed management is beyond the scope of this book and so a specialized text should be consulted (see 'Further reading' below).

# Liver trauma

## Anatomy

- The liver is the largest solid abdominal organ with a relatively fixed position deep to the right lower ribs.
- Due to its great size and proximity to the ribs, the right lobe is injured more often than the left.
- Functional anatomic division is into four sectors and eight segments by vertical and oblique planes defined by the three main hepatic veins and a transverse plane following a line drawn through the right and left portal branches.
- Determining the anatomy of the liver segments allows accurate localization of hepatic masses relative to the hepatic vasculature, which is important for assessment regarding possible hemihepatectomy and segmental and subsegmental resections.

## Mechanism of injury

- The liver is the second most frequently injured organ in abdominal trauma (injured in 15–20% of blunt abdominal injuries) but accounts for the most common cause of death (>50%).
- Children are at greatest risk.
- Usually liver injury is secondary to more significant impact (e.g. motor vehicle accident) but is occasionally secondary to sports.
- The liver's ligamentous attachment to the diaphragm and the posterior abdominal wall can act as sites of shear forces during deceleration injury.
- Increasing numbers of central liver hematomas caused by accidents involving mountain bikes are being encountered.
- Liver trauma may result in:
  - subcapsular hematoma or intrahepatic hematoma
  - laceration
  - contusion
  - hepatic vascular disruption
  - bile duct injury.

## History and clinical findings

- Signs and symptoms of hepatic injury are related to loss of blood, peritoneal irritation, right upper quadrant tenderness and guarding.
- Rebound tenderness is common but non-specific.
- Patients may present with severe peritonism due to bile peritonitis resulting from bile leaks.
- Signs of blood loss (shock, hypotension and a falling hematocrit level) may be present.
- Elevation of serum liver enzyme levels in a patient with blunt abdominal trauma suggests that the liver has been injured.
- Diagnostic peritoneal lavage has been shown to be useful in evaluating patients with blunt abdominal trauma, with reported sensitivities as high as 95%.

## Imaging findings

### Radiography

- Findings are non-specific and may be normal.
- No direct visualization of liver injury.
- May show right lower rib fractures and pneumoperitoneum.

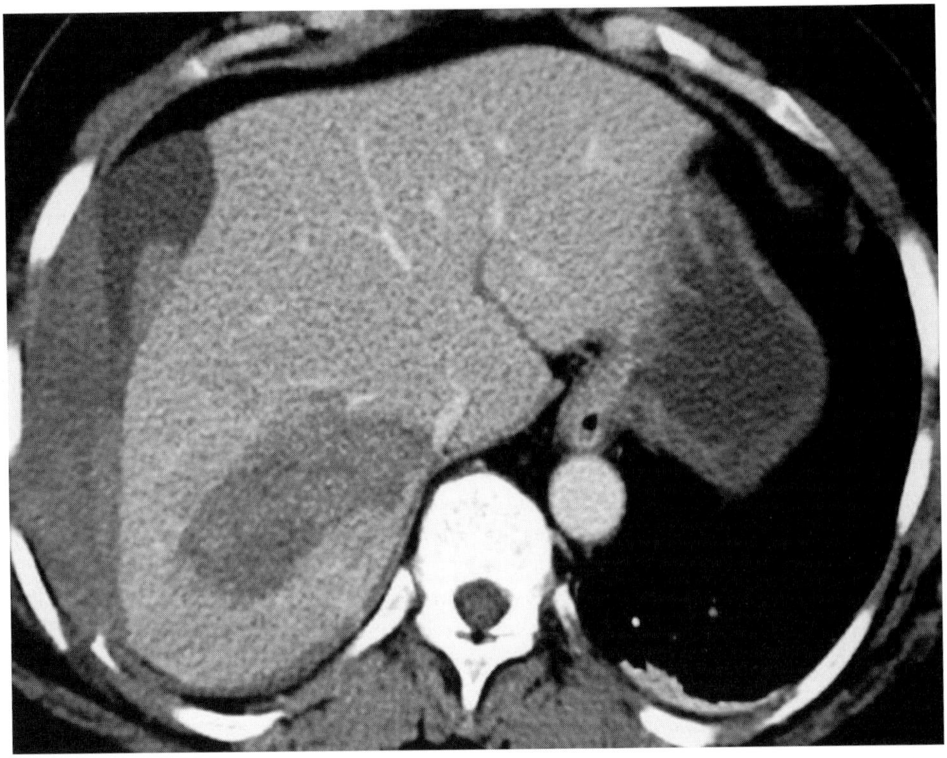

**Fig. 12.13** Axial CT scan, post i.v. contrast, showing laceration of the right lobe where there is subcapsular hematoma and intraparenchymal contusion.



## Computerized tomography

- Contrast-enhanced CT is the examination of choice in patients with blunt abdominal trauma.
- CT has a significant impact on the treatment of patients with liver trauma, resulting in a marked reduction in the number of patients requiring surgery and non-therapeutic operations (80% of adults and >95% of children are treated conservatively) (Fig. 12.13).
- Severity of injury (grades I–VI) based on American Association for the Surgery of Trauma guidelines:
  - grade 1: subcapsular hematoma <1 cm in maximal thickness, capsular avulsion, superficial parenchymal laceration less than 1 cm deep and isolated periportal blood tracking
  - grade 2: parenchymal laceration 1–3 cm deep and parenchymal/subcapsular hematomas 1–3 cm thick
  - grade 3: parenchymal laceration >3 cm deep and parenchymal or subcapsular hematoma >3 cm in diameter
  - grade 4: parenchymal/subcapsular hematoma more than 10 cm in diameter, lobar destruction or devascularization
  - grade 5: global destruction or devascularization of the liver
  - grade 6: hepatic avulsion.

- Acute intrahepatic hemorrhage is seen as irregular areas of contrast agent extravasation.
- On non-enhanced CT scans, the liver appears hyperattenuating compared with a hematoma.
- On enhanced CT scans, a hematoma appears as a low-attenuating lesion relative to the enhancing liver parenchyma.
- Over time, the attenuation of the hematoma is reduced and the hematoma eventually forms a well-defined serous fluid collection.
- Acute lacerations have a sharp or jagged margin but, over time, lacerations may enlarge and the margins may develop rolled edges.

### Ultrasound

- Emergency FAST findings based on the demonstration of free fluid and/or parenchymal injury have overall sensitivities for the detection of blunt abdominal trauma of >70%.
- The sensitivity is higher for injuries of grade 3 or higher.
- However, negative ultrasound findings do not exclude hepatic injury.
- A subcapsular hematoma usually appears as a curvilinear fluid collection with echogenicity varying with age.
- Initially, hematomas are anechoic, becoming progressively more echogenic by 24 hours.
- Over time, echogenicity of the hematoma begins to decrease.
- Septa and internal echoes may develop within the hemorrhagic collection by 1–4 weeks.
- Lacerations appear slightly echogenic, becoming hypoechoic or cystic when scanned days after the injury.
- The most common ultrasound pattern observed with liver parenchymal injuries is a discrete hyperechoic area.
- Bilomas appear as rounded, anechoic and loculated structures in close proximity to the liver and bile ducts.



### Nuclear medicine

- Radionuclide study with technetium-99m IDA is useful for suspected bile leaks.

### Angiography

- May be useful to localize the site of hemorrhage prior to transcatheter embolization of bleeding sites.
- Angiographic images can fail to depict active bleeding if intermittent and/or the flow rates are low.

## Management

### Non-surgical

- A finding of pooled contrast material within the peritoneal cavity on CT indicates active and massive bleeding; patients with this finding may require emergency surgery.
- Intrahepatic pooling of contrast material with an intact liver capsule usually indicates a self-limiting hemorrhage; most patients with this finding can be treated conservatively.
- Mild hepatic injuries, which involve less than 25% of one lobe, resolve within 3 months. Most moderate injuries involving 25–50% of one lobe heal within 6 months whereas severe injuries require 9–15 months to heal.

# Splenic rupture

## Anatomy

- The spleen is invested with peritoneum except for the insertion of the splenic artery and vein.
- The capsule around the spleen, especially the thicker layer in young patients, provides added protection against blunt injury.
- The spleen is primarily fixated to the posterior aspect of the left upper quadrant by gastrosplenic and splenorenal ligaments.
- The major arterial supply to the spleen is through the splenic artery, which branches off the celiac artery and runs superior and posterior to the pancreas.
- The artery commonly bifurcates externally to the spleen, supplying upper and lower poles separately, a finding that may make splenorrhaphy much easier for the operating surgeon.
- The tail of the pancreas is often intimately positioned near the splenic hilum and can be easily damaged during splenectomy if adequate care is not taken to identify and protect the organ.

## Mechanism of injury

- Although protected under the bony ribcage, the spleen is the most commonly affected organ in blunt injury to the abdomen in all age groups.
- Splenic injuries are common in sporting events and accidents involving bicycle handlebars, and in situations of rapid deceleration.
- The spleen is a highly vascular organ that filters 10–15% of total blood volume every minute.
- As much as 25% of the circulating platelets are estimated to be held in reserve in the spleen.
- Because of the immunologic function of the spleen, recent interest has turned to salvage rather than splenectomy.



## History and clinical findings

- Clinical presentation of splenic injury is highly variable.
- In most patients with minor focal injury to the spleen, complaints include left upper quadrant abdominal tenderness. Left shoulder tenderness may also be present as a result of subdiaphragmatic nerve root irritation with referred pain.
- With free intraperitoneal blood, diffuse abdominal pain and rebound are more likely. If the intra-abdominal bleeding exceeds 5–10% of blood volume, clinical signs of early shock may manifest.
- With increasing blood loss into the abdominal cavity, abdominal distension, peritoneal signs and overt shock may be observed.
- Hypotension in a patient with a suspected splenic injury, especially if young and previously healthy, is a grave sign and a surgical emergency. This should prompt immediate evaluation and intervention.
- Diagnostic peritoneal lavage may be a valuable adjunct if time permits and multiple other injuries are present.

## Imaging findings

- Unstable patients suspected of splenic injury and intra-abdominal hemorrhage should undergo exploratory laparotomy and splenic repair or removal.

### Ultrasound

- FAST in experienced hands is helpful in documenting the presence or absence of blood in the peritoneal cavity, which highly suggests the possibility of splenic injury.

- However, FAST is poor for delineating organ-specific anatomy with any reliability in the emergency setting.

### Computerized tomography

- The advent of CT scanning has made conservative management more practical and safer for victims of splenic injury.
- In the stable trauma patient, CT scanning provides the most ideal non-invasive means for evaluating the spleen.
- Intravenous contrast injected at the time of scan improves the clinician's ability to determine the severity of injury.
- A splenic blush noted at CT has a greater propensity to require splenic exploration in most series.
- Splenic injury is graded using the standards published by the Organ Injury Scaling Committee of the AAST. Categories range from grade I (minor) to grade V (major) and correlate to the need for laparotomy. These grades are used in conjunction with non-operative assessment, e.g. CT scanning. Studies comparing CT staging with operative staging indicate that CT overestimates the injury by as much as 10%. However, CT scan findings correlate well with the need for operative intervention.

### Angiography

- Angiography is rarely the first choice for evaluation of the patient with a splenic injury.
- Angiography is usually performed after CT images are obtained. Angiography is less of a diagnostic modality and more of a preparation for therapeutic embolization of active bleeding sites.

## Management

### Non-surgical

- The trend in management of splenic injury continues to favor non-operative or conservative management, especially for patients with stable hemodynamic signs, stable hemoglobin levels over 12–48 hours, minimal transfusion requirements (2 U or less), CT scan injury scale grade of 1 or 2 without a blush and patients younger than 55 years old.

### Surgical

- In the cases of CT scan-documented splenic injury, the decision for operative intervention is determined by the grade of the injury, the patient's current and pre-existing medical conditions and the facilities available at the hospital, including the availability of interventional angiographic services.
- Signs of persistent bleeding or hemodynamic instability are clear indications for surgery.
- Surgical therapy is usually reserved for patients with signs of ongoing bleeding or hemodynamic instability.
- In some institutions, CT scan-assessed grade V splenic injuries with stable vitals may be observed closely without operative intervention but most patients with these injuries undergo an exploratory laparotomy for more precise staging, repair or removal.
- In less emergent situations, splenorrhaphy is the preferred method of surgical care. Multiple techniques are described but they all attempt to tamponade active bleeding either by partial resection and selective vessel ligation or by putting pressure on the spleen via an absorbable mesh bag or sutures.

**Fig. 12.14** Sportsfile.

- Other measures include revaccination with pneumococcal vaccine after 4–5 years one time only.
- Patients should be warned about the increased risk of post-splenectomy sepsis and should consider lifelong antibiotic prophylaxis for invasive medical procedures and dental work.

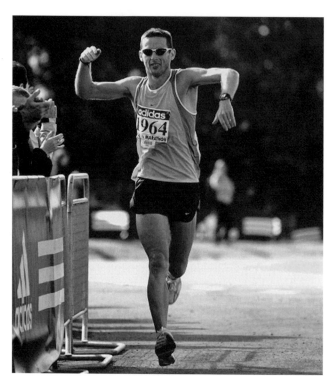

## Renal trauma

### Anatomy

- Paired retroperitoneal structures.
- The superior aspect of the kidneys is somewhat protected by the lower ribs.
- Segmental arterial supply, which is important in the management of renal lacerations.
- Blunt injuries tend to fracture along the planes between the segmental vessels, while penetrating injuries cross the segmental vessels.
- The closed retroperitoneal space around the kidney also promotes tamponade of bleeding renal injuries.

### Mechanism of injury

- Occurs in up to10% of patients who sustain abdominal trauma.
- Most occur secondary to blunt trauma.
- Renal injuries may be divided into renal laceration, renal contusion and renal vascular injury.

### History and clinical findings

- The mechanism of injury is important.
- Particular attention should be paid to flank or abdominal pain.
- Urinalysis should be performed: if gross hematuria is not present, a microscopic examination is advisable.

### Imaging findings

#### Computerized tomography

- CT allows unsurpassed functional and anatomic assessment of the kidneys and urinary tract and provides assessment of any concurrent injuries.
- Full urinary assessment may be provided by performing delayed scans in order to view the bladder and ureters.

#### Ultrasound

- Non-invasive and may be performed in real time in conjunction with resuscitation.
- Bladder injuries may be missed.

#### Intravenous pyelogram

- A 'one-shot' intravenous pyelogram (IVP) is favored over traditional IVP in the urgent evaluation of renal trauma.
- IVP allows the functional and anatomic assessment of both kidneys and ureters.
- IVP is time-consuming and provides high patient dose.
- IVP has largely been superseded by CT.

#### Angiography

- Has the capacity to aid in both the diagnosis and treatment of renal injuries.
- May further define injury in patients with vascular injuries but is relatively invasive.

### Management

#### Non-surgical

- A trend towards non-operative or expectant management has increased, even in the most seriously injured kidneys, replacing the past tendency toward aggressive renorrhaphy.
- Indications for emergent exploration include hemodynamic instability.

- Expanding hematomas or active hemorrhage suggest the possibility of high-grade renal injury.
- Patients with penetrating trauma who are stable and do not require urgent laparotomy for other intra-abdominal injuries may be observed without immediate renal exploration.
- Unrelenting gross hematuria may require urgent exploration. However, the presence of a renal contusion does not typically require specific intervention as most renal contusions resolve, particularly if the lesion is of low grade.
- Interventional radiology has extended the ability to use a non-operative approach, including percutaneous drainage of perinephric fluid collections or urinomas, and ureteric stenting.
- Angiography with selective embolization has been used in the setting of isolated renal trauma.

## Surgical

- In the appropriate clinical setting, operative therapy may include:
  - nephrectomy: shattered kidney, multiple concurrent injuries and uncontrolled hemorrhage
  - partial nephrectomy: avulsed fragments, polar penetrating mechanism and collecting system repair.

# Bladder trauma

## Anatomy

- The bladder is located within the bony pelvis and is a mostly extraperitoneal organ.
- It has four primary surfaces (superior, posterior and two inferolateral).
- The posterior surface (fundus) is anterior to the rectum but remains mostly retroperitoneal.
- The pelvic floor musculature and overlying fatty tissue support the inferolateral margins of the bladder.
- The pubovesicular, medial and paired lateral umbilical ligaments strengthen the association with the anterior body wall.
- There is little preventing motion of the bladder, in that the only rigidly fixed point is the bladder neck.

## Mechanism of injury

- Blunt or penetrating trauma.
- Bladder disruption occurs in 5–10% of patients with pelvic fractures.
- Approximately 65% of ruptures are extraperitoneal (many with associated pelvic fractures), 30% are intraperitoneal, and only 1–10% of disruptions are both (Fig. 12.15).

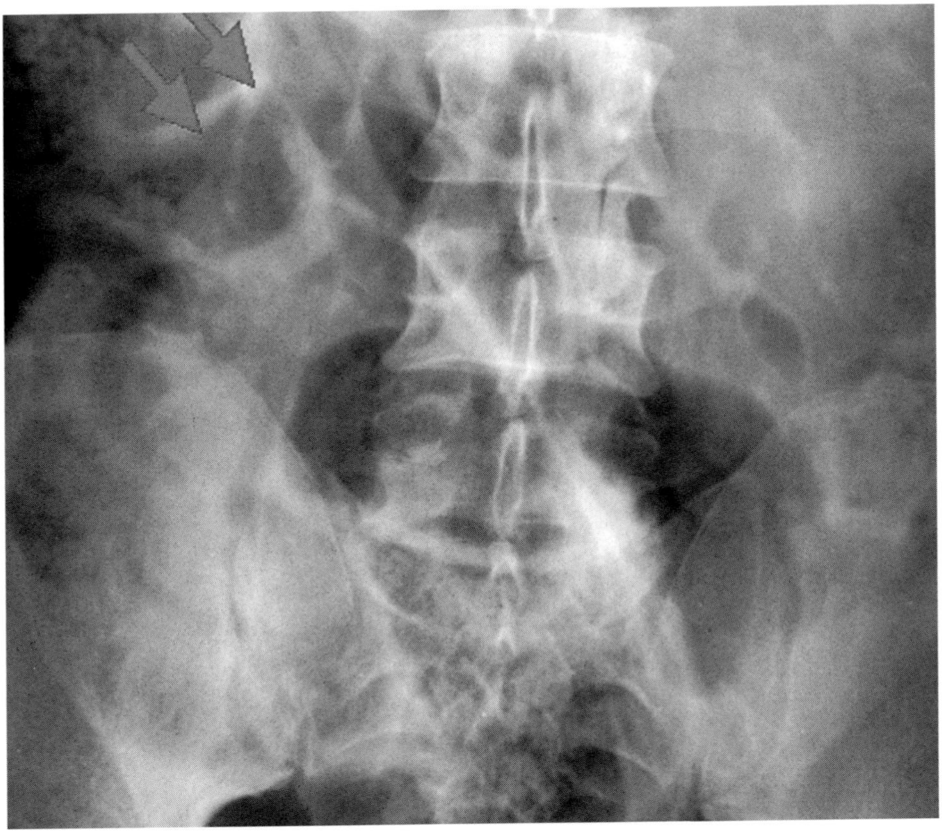

**Fig. 12.15** Radiograph showing intraperitoneal bladder rupture with free contrast within the peritoneum

- Classification of injury – five grades are recognized:
  - type I: partial tears of the mucosa. This is the most common injury pattern of multisystem trauma patients and associated with blunt trauma. This pattern is not a major bladder injury
  - type II: intraperitoneal bladder rupture (10–20% of all major bladder injuries). Most commonly, this is the result of a direct blow to the distended organ. The bladder dome is the weakest point, thus intraperitoneal rupture usually occurs as a result of a tear in the bladder dome. Intraperitoneal fluid is observed in the paracolic gutters and mesenteric folds
  - type III: intramural or partial-thickness laceration of the intact serosa (interstitial pattern). CT cystography is commonly diagnostic and demonstrates intramural contrast within the bladder wall
  - type IV: extraperitoneal bladder injury. It is the most common bladder rupture. In blunt trauma, one theoretic cause for laceration of the lower bladder is from secondary injury from pelvis fragments
  - type V: combined rupture (both intraperitoneal and extraperitoneal urine).

## History and clinical findings

- Trauma to the bladder is associated with significant trauma to the pelvis and intra-abdominal organs.
- Commonly, patients have few symptoms secondary to their bladder injury or even rupture.
- Physical examination findings suggestive of bladder trauma include vague peritoneal signs or abdominal tenderness; more suggestive findings include isolated suprapubic tenderness, pelvic instability or lap-belt ecchymosis.
- Bladder injury is essentially ruled out when no red blood cells are observed in the urine. Gross hematuria is present in 95% of patients; the remaining patients have microscopic hematuria.
- When a pubic rami fracture is present or if pubic symphysis diastasis is present, a high index of suspicion for rupture should be held.
- The ability to urinate does not exclude bladder injury or perforation.



## Imaging findings

### Computerized tomography retrograde cystography

- The same retrograde introduction of contrast agent is generally performed as with retrograde cystography. However, multiple images, including post-voiding and oblique views, are not necessary (as in plain radiography).
- The technique is both sensitive and accurate, provided that adequate bladder distension with at least 300–400 mL of contrast material is achieved.
- CT cystography is commonly diagnostic and demonstrates intramural contrast within the bladder wall in type III injuries, and contrast around loops of bowel and in the paracolic gutters and mesenteric folds in intraperitoneal ruptures.
- In extraperitoneal ruptures, contrast may be seen in the perivesicular space tracking between different fascial planes or even in the thigh or scrotum with disruption of the inferior fascia of the urogenital diaphragm (perineal membrane).

| | |
|---|---|
| Retrograde cystography | • Nearly 100% sensitive for detecting rupture provided adequate distension is accomplished and post-voiding images are obtained.<br>• Time consuming and requires additional radiographic views. |
| Ultrasound | • Ultrasound is not sensitive or specific enough to be useful for evaluation of bladder rupture. |

## Management

- Radiologic examination is of paramount importance and should be performed to identify and classify the injury and to plan surgical repair but it should not hinder patient treatment and stabilization.
- One semi-emergent condition is trauma to the bladder, especially trauma that results in uroperitoneum. Sepsis can develop within 24 hours in these injuries if surgery with repair is not performed.

### Non-surgical

- Most extraperitoneal ruptures can be managed safely with simple catheter drainage (i.e. urethral or suprapubic) for 7–10 days, after which a cystogram should be performed.
- Approximately 85% of the time, the laceration is sealed and the catheter is removed for a voiding trial.
- Virtually all extraperitoneal bladder injuries heal within 3 weeks.

### Surgical

- Intraperitoneal bladder rupture.
- Most, if not all, intraperitoneal bladder ruptures require surgical exploration. These injuries do not heal with prolonged catheterization alone. Urine takes the path of least resistance and continues to leak into the abdominal cavity. This results in urinary ascites, abdominal distension and electrolyte disturbances.

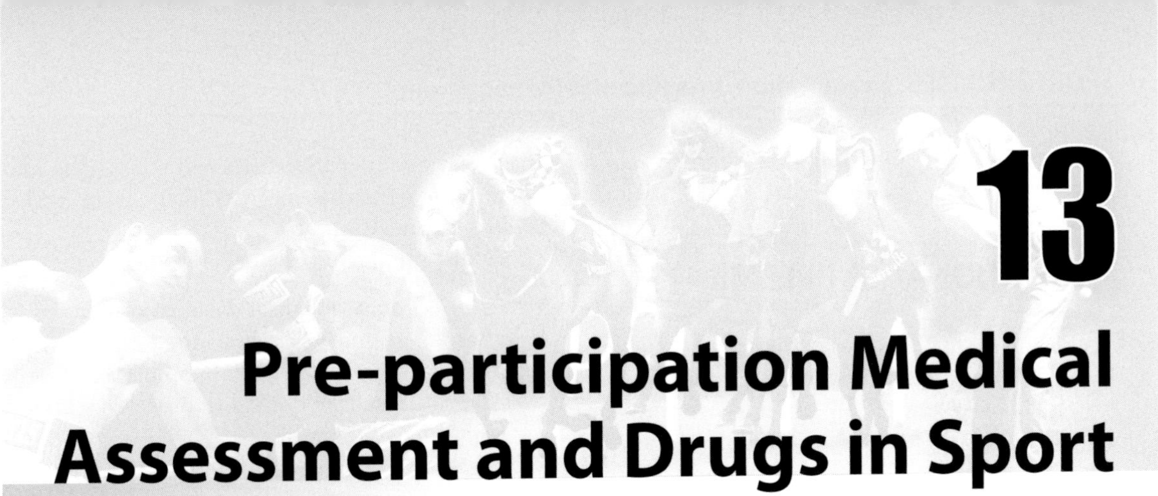

# 13

# Pre-participation Medical Assessment and Drugs in Sport



## DRUGS IN SPORT

In 1968 formal drug testing was adopted for the first time for the Summer and Winter Olympics in an attempt to control the use of drugs being taken by athletes specifically to improve performance. Since this time, formal testing has been adopted by all sporting governing bodies, although there is still a lack of uniformity in agents banned by differing bodies.

### Categories of banned drugs

- Stimulants
- Narcotics
- Anabolic steroids
- Beta-blockers
- Diuretics
- Growth hormone.

### Restricted drugs

- Alcohol
- Local anesthetics
- Corticosteroids
- Beta-agonists.

*The use of any of the above agents by an athlete requires a declaration of medical need by a registered physician and completion of a drugs exemption form. At the time of writing the use of bronchodilators requires a formal diagnosis of asthma on the basis of pulmonary function tests and restricted $FEV_1$ or an asthma stress test although a lack of scientific confirmation that bronchodilators are performance* *enhancing suggests that their restricted use may be short term.*

## NUTRITIONAL SUPPLEMENTS

A nutritional supplement describes any supplement that either improves or is thought to improve one's health (dietary aids) or physical performance (ergogenic aids). These agents fall outside the Food and Drug Administration's (FDA) umbrella and are therefore largely unregulated.

### Creatine (an ergogenic aid: not banned)

Creatine or methylguanide-acetic acid is an amino acid identified in 1835 by Michel-Eugène Chevreul. It is naturally synthesized in the liver, pancreas and kidneys, and is available from normal diets containing meat and fish. In 1993 creatine monohydrate was introduced as an agent to promote muscle strength when taken, 20–30 g daily and combined with resistive exercise. Many athletes naturally increase creatine synthesis endogenously. Equally, levels may be lower in females and vegetarians who hence appear to benefit maximally from added creatine to diet.

Two actions are recognized:

- Creatine intake enhances the bioavailability of phosphocreatine in skeletal muscle cells and therefore allows faster resynthesis of ATP from ADP and results in quicker recovery from brief high-intensity exercise.
- Creatine delays fatigue by buffering intracellular hydrogen ions, which accumulate during exercise. Hydrogen ions are thought to produce muscle fatigue by induced pH changes.

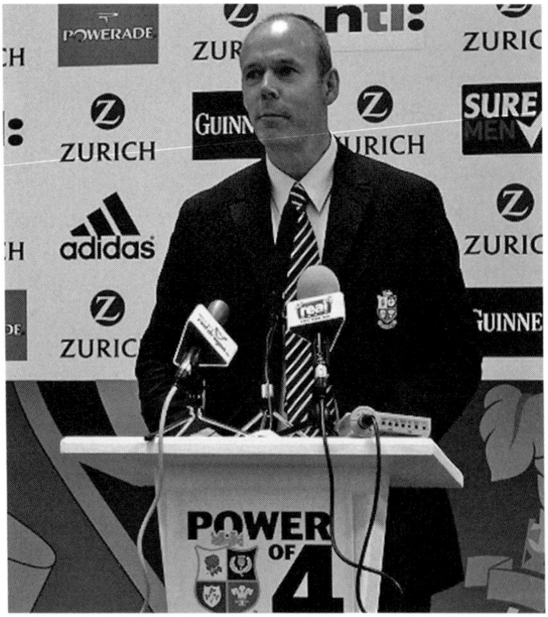


**Fig. 13.1** Sportslife.

### Dehydroepiandrosterone (ergogenic aid: banned substance)

Dehydroepiandrosterone (DHEA) was taken off the market by the FDA because of a potential association with liver damage. However, in 1994, following the passage of the Federal Dietary Supplement Health and Education Act, DHEA was reclassified as a dietary supplement and reintroduced to the consumer. Despite such a classification, DHEA is a banned substance according to the NCAA and the USOC.

DHEA is produced by the adrenal gland and is an endogenous precursor to the production of both androgens and estrogens. In health, endogenous levels of this hormone fall from 20 years onwards, hence the role of supplementation. Data suggest that DHEA increases testosterone levels with associated anabolic impact. In studies of adults over 40 years of age, a dose of 50–100 mg per day DHEA has been shown to significantly increase androgenic steroid plasma levels and produce subjective improvements in physical and psychological well-being. The impact of DHEA on healthy adults between 20 and 40 years has yet to be scientifically evaluated.

Potential adverse effects of this agent include virilization in women, hirsutism and alopecia. Although unproven, it has been suggested that long-term use may increase the risk of prostate and uterine carcinoma because of the prolonged elevation of sex hormones. There is also a concern that long-term use may induce insulin resistance, a fall in HDL levels and induce liver carcinoma.

## Androstenedione

Androstenedione at ingestion levels of 100–300 mg per day over an 8-week period has been shown to significantly increase serum testosterone and estradiol levels with normalization of levels occurring rapidly within 24 hours.

Androstenedione, by virtue of its impact on testosterone, appears to have an effect on muscle strength and bulk. Similar side-effects to DHEA are reported.

## Beta-hydroxy-beta-methyl butyrate (ergogenic aid: not banned)

Beta-hydroxy-beta-methyl butyrate (HMB) is a metabolite of the essential amino acid leucine and is produced endogenously in small amounts. It is found in the normal diet in milk and citrus fruits. Promotors of this supplement suggest that HMB regulates enzymes responsible for protein breakdown therefore slowing muscle degradation and indirectly increasing muscle bulk.

# PRE-PARTICIPATION PHYSICAL EXAMINATION

## Objectives

- Detect any underlying condition that would restrict athletic participation.
- Identification of potential problems and previous injuries.
- Injury prevention evaluation.
- Fulfillment of legal and insurance requirements.
- Establish a database and record-keeping system.

## Timing

It is suggested that the Pre-participation Physical Examination (PPE) should be performed 6–8 weeks before the start of the sporting season. A formal medical should be performed on entry to a sporting program followed by an annual check-up with the examination focused on specific problems or injuries at that time.

## Technique

For PPE technique see review sheets proposed by a consensus group reflecting guidelines of the American Academy of Family Physicians, the American Academy of Pediatrics, the American Medical Society for Sports Medicine, the American Orthopedic Society for Sports Medicine and the American Osteopathic Academy of Sports Medicine, all of which are published by *The Physician and Sports Medicine.*

*The PPE should include a detailed medical history focusing on previous medical illnesses, injuries, surgeries and possible cardiovascular problems* (Fig. 13.2 and Tables 13.1 and 13.2).

## Preparticipation Physical Evalution

### HISTORY

**DATE OF EXAM** ______________________

Name ______________________ Sex ______ Age ________ Date of birth ____________
Grade ____ School ______________ Sport(s) ______________________________
Address __________________________________________ Phone ____________
Personal physician ______________________________________________
*In case of emergency, contact* ______________________________________
Name ______________ Relationship __________ Phone (H) ____________ (W) ____________

**Explain "Yes" answer below.**
**Circle questions you don't know the answer to.**

| | Yes | No |
|---|---|---|
| 1. Have you had a medical illness or injury since your last check up or sports phsysical? | ☐ | ☐ |
| Do you have an ongoing or chronic illness? | ☐ | ☐ |
| 2. Have you ever been hospitalized overnight? | ☐ | ☐ |
| Have you ever had surgery? | ☐ | ☐ |
| 3. Are you currently taking any prescription or nonprescription (over-the-counter) medications or pills or using an inhaler? | ☐ | ☐ |
| Have you ever taken any supplements or vitamin to help you gain or lose weight or improve your performance | ☐ | ☐ |
| 4. Do you have any allergies (for example, to pollen, medicine, food, or stinging insects)? | ☐ | ☐ |
| Have you ever had rash or hives develop during or after exercise? | ☐ | ☐ |
| 5. Have you ever passed out during or after exercrise? | ☐ | ☐ |
| have you ever been dizzy during or after exercise? | ☐ | ☐ |
| Have you ever had chest pain during or after excercise? | ☐ | ☐ |
| Do you get tired more quickly than your friends do during execrise? | ☐ | ☐ |
| Have you ever had racing of your heart or skipped heartbeats? | ☐ | ☐ |
| Have you had high blood pressure or high cholestrol? | ☐ | ☐ |
| Have you ever been told you have a heart murmur? | ☐ | ☐ |
| Has any family member or relative died of heart problems or of sudden death before age 50? | ☐ | ☐ |
| Have you had a severe viral infection (for example myocarditis or mononucleosis) within the last month? | ☐ | ☐ |
| Has a physician ever denied or restricted your participation in sports for any heart problems? | ☐ | ☐ |
| 6. Do you have any current skin problems (for example, itching, rashes, acne, warts, fungus, or blisters)? | ☐ | ☐ |
| 7. Have you ever had a head injury or concussion? | ☐ | ☐ |
| Have you ever been knocked out, become unconscious, or lost your memory? | ☐ | ☐ |
| Have you ever had a seizure? | ☐ | ☐ |
| Do you have frequent or severe headaches? | ☐ | ☐ |
| Have you ever had numbness or tingling in your arms, hands, legs, or feet? | ☐ | ☐ |
| Have you ever had a stinger, burner, or pinched nerve? | ☐ | ☐ |
| 8. Have you ever become ill from exercising in the heat? | ☐ | ☐ |
| 9. Do you cough, wheeze, or have trouble breathing during or after activity? | ☐ | ☐ |
| Do you have asthma? | ☐ | ☐ |
| Do you have seasonal allergies that require medical treatment? | ☐ | ☐ |

| | Yes | No |
|---|---|---|
| 10. Do you use any special protective or corrective equipment or devices that arent' usually used for your sport or position (for example, Knee brace, special neck rool, foot orthotics, retainer on your teeth, hearing aid)? | ☐ | ☐ |
| 11. Have you have any problem with your eyes or vision? | ☐ | ☐ |
| Do you wear galsses, contacts, or protective eyeswear? | ☐ | ☐ |
| 12. Have you ever had a sprain, strain or swelling after injury? | ☐ | ☐ |
| Have you broken or fractured any bones or dislocated any joints? | ☐ | ☐ |
| Have you had any other problems with pain or swelling in muscles, tendons, bone, or joints? | ☐ | ☐ |

*If yes, Check appropriate box and explain below*

| | | |
|---|---|---|
| ☐ Head | ☐ Elbow | ☐ Hip |
| ☐ Neck | ☐ Foream | ☐ Thigh |
| ☐ Back | ☐ Wrist | ☐ Knee |
| ☐ Chest | ☐ Hand | ☐ Shin/calf |
| ☐ Shoulder | ☐ Finger | ☐ Ankle |
| ☐ Upper arm | | ☐ Foot |

| | Yes | No |
|---|---|---|
| 13. Do you want to weigh more or less than you do now? | ☐ | ☐ |
| Do you lose weight regularly to meet weight requirements for your sport? | ☐ | ☐ |
| 14. Do you feel stressed out? | ☐ | ☐ |

15. Record the dates of your most recent immunizations (shots) for:
Tetanus ____________ Measles ____________
Hepatitis B ____________ Chickenpox ____________

**FEMALES ONLY**

16. When was your first menstrual period? ____________
When was your most recent menstrual period? ____________
How much time do you usually have from the start of one period to the start of another? ____________
How many periods have you had in the last year? ____________
What was the longest time between periods in the last year? ____

Explain "Yes" answers here: ______________________________

I hereby state that, to the best of my knowledge, my answers to the above queslions are complete and correct.
Signature of athlete ______________ Signature of parent/gaurdian ______________ Date ________

**Fig. 13.2** (a) Pre-participation Physical Examination. Reproduced with permission from Leawood KS. American Academy of Family Physicians, American Academy of Pediatrics, American Medical Society for Sports Medicine, American Orthopedic Society for Sports Medicine, American Osteopathic Academy of Sports Medicine, 1992, 1996.

## Preparticipation Physical Evaluation

PHYSICAL EXAMINATION

Name ______________________ Date of birth ______________

Height ______ Weight ______ % Body fat (optional) ______ Pulse ______ BP ___ /___ /(___/___, ___/___)

Vision R 20/ ____ L 20/ ____ Corrected: Y N Pupils: Equal ____ Unequal ____

| | NORMAL | ABNORMAL FINDINGS | INITIALS* |
|---|---|---|---|
| **MEDICAL** | | | |
| Appearance | | | |
| Eyes/Ears/Nose/Throat | | | |
| Lymph Nodes | | | |
| Heart | | | |
| Pulses | | | |
| Lungs | | | |
| Abdomen | | | |
| Genitalia (males only) | | | |
| Skin | | | |
| **MUSCULOSKELETAL** | | | |
| Neck | | | |
| Back | | | |
| Shoulder/arm | | | |
| Elbow/forearm | | | |
| Wrist/hand | | | |
| Hip/thigh | | | |
| Knee | | | |
| Leg/ankle | | | |
| Foot | | | |

*Station-based examination only

CLEARANCE

❑ Cleared

❑ Cleared after completing evaluation/ rehabilitation for: ______________________

❑ Not cleared for: ______________ Reason: ______________

Recommendations ______________________

Name of physician (print/type) ______________________ Date ______________

Address ______________________ Phone ______________

Signature of physician ______________________ MD or DO

**Fig. 13.2** (**b**) Pre-participation Physical Examination. Reproduced with permission from Leawood KS. American Academy of Family Physicians, American Academy of Pediatrics, American Medical Society for Sports Medicine, American Orthopedic Society for Sports Medicine, American Osteopathic Academy of Sports Medicine, 1992, 1996.

**Table 13.1** Medical conditions and sports participation*

| Condition | May participate |
|---|---|
| Atlantoaxial instability (instability of the joint between cervical vertebrae 1 and 2) | Qualified yes |
| Explanation: Athlete needs evaluation to assess risk of spinal cord injury during sports participation. | |
| Bleeding disorder | Qualified yes |
| Explanation: Athlete needs evaluation. | |
| Cardiovascular disease | |
| Carditis (inflammation of the heart) | No |
| Explanation: Carditis may result in sudden death with exertion. | |
| Hypertension (high blood pressure) | Qualified yes |
| Explanation: Those with significant essential (unexplained) hypertension should avoid weight and power lifting, body building, and strength training. Those with secondary hypertension (hypertension caused by a previously identified disease) or severe essential hypertension need evaluation. The National High blood Pressure Education Working group [3] defined significant and severe hypertension. | |
| Congenital heart disease (structural heart defects present at birth) | Qualified yes |
| Explanation: Those with mild forms may participate fully; those with moderate or severe forms or who have been undergone surgery need evaluation. The 26th Bethesda Conference [4] defined mild, moderate, and severe disease for common cardiac lesions. | |
| Dysrhythmia (irregular heart rhythm) | Qualified yes |
| Explanation: Those with symptoms (chest pain, syncope, dizziness, shortness of breath, or other symptoms of possible dysrhythmia) need evaluation. All others may participate fully [5]. | |
| Heart murmur | Qualified yes |
| Explanation: If the murmur is innocent (does not indicate heart disease), full participation is permitted. Otherwise, the athlete needs evaluation (see congenital heart disease and mitral valve prolapse) [5]. | |
| Cerebral palsy | Qualified yes |
| Explanation: Athlete needs evaluation. | |
| Diabetes mellitus | Yes |
| Explanation: All sorts can be played with proper attention to diet, blood glucose concentration, hydration, and insulin therapy. Blood glucose concentration should be monitored every 30 minutes during continuous exercise and 15 minutes after completion of exercise. | |
| Diarrhea | Qualified no |
| Explanation: Unless disease is mild, no participation is permitted, because diarrhea may increase the risk of dehydration and heat illness. See fever. | |
| Eating disorders | Qualified yes |
| Anorexia nervosa | |
| Bulimia nevosa | |
| Explanation: Patients with these disorders need medical and psychiatric assessment before participation. | |

*Continued*

**Table 13.1** Medical conditions and sports participation*—*Cont'd*

| Condition | May participate |
|---|---|
| Eyes<br>Functionally one-eyed athlete<br>Loss of an eye<br>Detached retina<br>Previous eye surgery or serious eye injury<br>Explanation: A functionally one-eyed athlete has a best-corrected visual acuity of less than 20/40 in the eye with worse acuity. These athletes would suffer significant disability if the better eye were seriously injured, as would those with loss of an eye. Some atheletes who previously have undergone eye surgery or had a serious eye injury may have an increased risk of injury because of weakened eye tissue. Availability of eye guards approved by the American Society for Testing and Materials and other protective equipment may allow participation in most sports, but this must be judged or an individual basis [6, 7]. | Qualified yes |
| Fever<br>Explanation: Fever can increase cardiopulmonary effort, reduce maximum exercise capacity, make heat illness more likely, and increase orthostatic hypertension during exercise. Fever may rarely accompany myocarditis or other infections that may make exercise dangerous. | No |
| Heat illness, history of<br>Explanation: Because of the increased likelihood of recurrence, the athlete needs individual assessment to determine the presence of predisposing conditions and to arrange a prevention strategy. | Qualified yes |
| Hepatitis<br>Explanation: Because of the apparent minimal risk to others, all sports may be played that the athlete's state of health allows. In all athletes, skin lesions should be covered properly, and athletic personnel should use universal precautions when handling blood or body fluids with visible blood [8]. | Yes |
| Human immunodeficiency virus infection<br>Explanation: Because of the apparent minimal risk to others, all sports may be played that the athlete's state of health allows. In all athletes, skin lesions should be covered properly, and ahtlete personnel should use universal precautions when handling blood or body fluids with visible blood [8]. | Yes |
| Kidneys, absence of one<br>Explanation: Athlete needs individual assessment for contact, collision, and limited-contact sports. | Qualified yes |
| Liver, enlarged<br>Explanation: If the liver is acutely enlarged, participation should be avoided because of risk or rupture. If the liver is chronically enlarged, individual assessment is needed before collision, contact, or limited-contact sports are played. | Qualified yes |

*Continued*

**Table 13.1** Medical conditions and sports participation*—*Cont'd*

| Condition | May participate |
|---|---|
| Malignant neoplasm | Qualified yes |
| Explanation: Athlete needs individual assessment. | |
| Musculoskeletal disorders | |
| Explanation: Athlete needs individual assessment. | Qualified yes |
| Neurologic disorders | |
| History of serious head or spine trauma, severe or repeated concussions, or craniotomy [9, 10]. | Qualified yes |
| Explanation: Athlete needs individual assessment for collision, contact, or limited-contact sports and also for noncontact sports if deficits in judgment or cognition are present. Research supports a conservative approach to management of conclusion [9, 10]. | |
| Seizure disorder, well-controlled | Yes |
| Explanation: Risk of seizure during participation is minimal | |
| Seizure disorder, poorly controlled | Qualified yes |
| Explanation: Athlete needs individual assessment for collision, contact, or limited-contact sports. The following noncontact sports should be avoided: archery, riflery, swimming, weight or power lifting, strength training, or sports involving heights. In these sports, occurrence of a seizure may pose a risk to self or others. | |
| Obesity | Qualified yes |
| Explanation: Because of the risk of heat illness, obese persons need careful acclimatization and hydration. | |
| Organ transplant recipient | Qualified yes |
| Explanation: Athlete needs individual assessment | |
| Ovary, absence of one | Yes |
| Explanation: Risk of severe injury to the remaining ovary is minimal. | |
| Respiratory conditions | |
| Pulmonary compromise, including cystic fibrosis | Qualified yes |
| Explanation: Athlete needs individual assessment, but generally, all sports may be played if oxygenation remains satisfactory during a graded exercise test. Patients with cystic fibrosis need acclimatization and good hydration to reduce the risk of heat illness. | |
| Asthma | Yes |
| Explanation: With proper medication and education, only athletes with the most severe asthma will need to modify their participation. | |
| Acute upper respiratory infection | Qualified yes |
| Explanation: Upper respiratory obstruction may affect pulmonary function. Athlete needs individual assessment for all but mild disease. See fever. | |
| Sickle cell disease | Qualified yes |
| Explanation: Athlete needs individual assessment. In general, if status of the illness pemits, all but high exertion, collision, and contact sports may be played. Overheating, dehydration, and chilling must be avoided. | |

*Continued*

**Table 13.1** Medical conditions and sports participation*—*Cont'd*

| Condition | May participate |
|---|---|
| Sickle cell trait | Yes |
| Explanation: It is unlikely that persons with sickle cell trait have an increased risk of sudden death or other medical problems during athletic participation, except under the most extreme conditions of heat, humidity, and possibly increased altitude [11]. These persons, like all ahtletes, should be carefully conditioned, acclimatized, and hydrated to reduce any possible risk. | |
| Skin disorders (boils, herpes simplex, impetigo, scabies, molluscum contagiosum) | Qualified yes |
| Explanation: While the patient is contagious, participation in gymnastics with mats; martial arts; wrestling; or other collision, contact, or limited-contact sports is not allowed. | |
| Spleen, enlarged | Qualified yes |
| Explanation: A patient with an acutely enlarged spleen should avoid all sports because of risk of rupture. A patient with a chronically enlarged spleen needs individual assessment before playing collision, contact, or limited-contact sports. | |
| Testicle, undescended or absence of one | Yes |
| Explanation: Certain sports may require a protective cup. | |

*This table is designed for use by medical and nonmedical personnel. "Needs evaluation" means that a physician with appropriate knowledge and experience should assess the safety of a given sport for an athlete with the listed medical condition. Unless otherwise noted, this is because of variability of the severity of the disease, the risk of injury for the specific sports listed in Table 1, or both. From Academy of pediatrics Committee on Sports Medicine. Recommendations for participation in competitive sports. Pediatrics 1988;88:737.

**Table 13.2** Classification of sports by strenuousness

| High to moderate intensity | | |
|---|---|---|
| High to moderate dynamic and static demands | High to moderate dynamic and low static demands | High to moderate static and low dynamic demands |
| Boxing* | Badminton | Archery |
| Crew or rowing | Basketball | Auto racing |
| Cross-country skiing | Basketball | Diving |
| Cycling | Field hockey | Horseback riding (jumping) |
| Downhill skiing | Lacrosse | Field events (throwing) |
| Fencing | Orienteering | Gymnastics |
| Football | Race walking | Karate or judo |
| Ice hockey | Racquetball | Motorcyling |
| Rugby | Soccer | Rodeo |
| Running (spring) | Squash | Sailing |
| Speed skating | Swimming | Ski jumping |
| Water polo | Table tennis | Water skiing |
| Wrestling | Tennis | Weight lifting |
| | Volleyball | |
| **Low intensity (low dynamic and low static demands)** | | |
| Bowling | | |
| Cricket | | |
| Curling | | |
| Golf | | |
| Riflery | | |

*Participation not recommended by the American Academy of Pediatrics.

# Index

Note: page numbers in **bold** refer to tables and figures.

# D



# E



# F

# N



# O



# P

# Q



# R



# S

# T



# U



# V



# W